INTRODUCTION TO MICROBIOLOGY FOR THE HEALTH SCIENCES

INTRODUCTION TO MICROBIOLOGY FOR THE HEALTH SCIENCES

Second Edition

MARCUS M. JENSEN
Professor of Microbiology
Brigham Young University

DONALD N. WRIGHT
Professor of Microbiology
Brigham Young University

Clinical Professor of Pathology
University of Utah

PRENTICE HALL, Englewood Cliffs, New Jersey 07632

Library of Congress Cataloging-in-Publication Data

Jensen, Marcus M.
  Introduction to microbiology for the health sciences.

    Rev. ed. of: Introduction to medical microbiology.
    Includes bibliographies and index.
    1. Medical microbiology. I. Wright, Donald N.
II. Jensen, Marcus M. Introduction to medical
microbiology. III. Title.
QR46.J46 1989   616'.01   89-3598
ISBN 0-13-487364-5

Editorial/production supervision:
  Fay Ahuja and Zita de Schauensee
Interior design: Linda Conway
Cover design: Bruce Kenselaar
Manufacturing buyer: Paula Massenaro

Cover illustration: Colonies of *Cryptococcus neoformans*
(dark blue) and *Candida albicans* (light blue) as cultured
on trypan blue medium. (Photo by Glenn S. Bulmer,
University of Oklahoma)

Printed in the United States of America
10 9 8 7 6 5 4 3 2 1

ISBN 0-13-487364-5

Prentice-Hall International (UK) Limited, *London*
Prentice-Hall of Australia Pty. Limited, *Sydney*
Prentice-Hall Canada Inc., *Toronto*
Prentice-Hall Hispanoamericana, S.A., *Mexico*
Prentice-Hall of India Private Limited, *New Delhi*
Prentice-Hall of Japan, Inc., *Tokyo*
Simon & Schuster Asia Pte. Ltd., *Singapore*
Editora Prentice-Hall do Brasil, Ltda., *Rio de Janeiro*

CONTENTS

Clinical Notes

PREFACE

Introduction to Microbiology for the Health Sciences has been designed with the student in mind. The authors have carefully constructed the content to represent the state of the art in medical microbiology. The text was prepared with the idea that beginning microbiology can be provided for the health-science oriented student in a single semester or quarter of study without the necessity of demanding an earlier introduction to the subject or an extensive background in chemistry and mathematics. We believe that students can learn the principles of microbiology necessary for them to perform in allied health professions through a single exposure to the subject presented. We are also aware that some students may wish to add to this course and believe that the text provides the necessary background support for such extended study. The purpose of the text is to provide a useful and thorough introduction to the host-parasite relationship and a thorough understanding of the microbe in its role as a disease-producing agent.

In addressing the specific subjects of medical microbiology, the authors have designed the book principally toward students in nursing and other allied health areas. Because of its somewhat limited scope, the content has been reduced in an effort to provide only that information essential to an appreciation of the role of microorganisms in the disease process. The text is neither an encyclopedic reference of general microbiology nor a detailed analysis of host responses to parasitic microorganisms. The reader will find that the text provides an excellent background of the agents of infectious disease and human disease processes associated with microorganisms.

This second edition has retained the innovative style of the first edition, including a student-oriented presentation which contains the following advantages for student use:

Introductory Sketch Each chapter begins with a brief introductory sketch of the content to be covered in the chapter.

Taxonomic Presentation Microorganisms are presented in a pathogen-oriented sequence that provides an understanding of the microbe in its clinical setting regardless of the site of infection.

Concept Summary Each chapter contains a concept summary with a brief review of the most significant aspects of each subject.

Key Words Words with significant subject or vocabulary meaning are italicized for emphasis and ease of retrieval.

Appendix A brief appendix is included for students interested in extending their study of specific topics.

Glossary The text-end alphabetized glossary is provided for student access to new and significant scientific terms.

In addition to these useful pedagogic aspects of the text, there are a number of features of significant value to student learning which are new to this edition including:

Clinical Notes This edition contains an expanded number of new clinical notes for student interest and awareness as well as subject application. These notes focus on pertinent on-going concerns in infectious disease microbiology.

Study Summary A study summary consisting of questions designed to help the student focus on critical concepts is provided with each chapter.

Running Glossary A running glossary is provided to expand the student's understanding of terms as they are used. This glossary will facilitate both the learning process and reduce the time required to read the text.

Bibliography A current bibliographic reference list is included with each chapter.

Illustrations A section of full color illustrations of microbes and microbial processes is included.

Much of the text itself has been rewritten for this edition. Each chapter has been up-dated and includes numerous new illustrations and tables. There are several completely new chapters including an update on AIDS. The new format includes a judicious use of color to highlight the most significant aspects of subject presentation.

The text is accompanied by a variety of available pedagogic and instructor resources including:

 laboratory manual
 instructor's manual
 student guide
 transparency package

The authors wish to express their appreciation to the following individuals, who reviewed the manuscript and provided timely insight and suggestions for the text.

Louis Giacinti
Milwaukee Area Technical College

Helen B. Hanten
University of Minnesota, Duluth

Joy A. McMillan
Madison Area Technical College

Raymond B. Otero
Eastern Kentucky University

David Saltzman
Sante Fe Community College

Carmen V. Sciortino
Medical University of South Carolina

George F. Wendt
Long Island University

Provo, Utah   Marcus M. Jensen

                                               Donald N. Wright

chapter 1

HISTORICAL DEVELOPMENTS IN MEDICAL MICROBIOLOGY

Infectious disease

a disease, such as tuberculosis or AIDS, caused by a living organism. Some infectious diseases are communicable and can be transmitted from person to person.

Epidemic

the occurrence of a common disease such as influenza in greater than expected numbers; or the occurrence of a rare disease even in small numbers.

P erhaps nowhere has the application of the scientific method been more rewarding than in the medical sciences. This method of systematic study involving the rational organization of information was largely responsible for the development of the science of microbiology. Microbiology as a discipline didn't exist 125 years ago and the men and women who developed the concepts that today are associated with this discipline were largely trained as chemists or physicians. It should not be surprising, therefore, that the development of the science of microbiology was associated primarily with concerns for improving the health of the human population and reducing the ravages of infectious diseases.

Infectious diseases have been the greatest pestilences in human history. Only in the past 75 to 100 years have many of our major infectious diseases been brought under control. In past years, severe outbreaks of infectious diseases periodically swept across nations and through cities ravaging their inhabitants. Classic examples of these **epidemic** scourges include smallpox, typhus, cholera, and plague. Outbreaks of smallpox, which periodically struck cities, would often kill from 10% to 90% of the inhabitants; the great plague pandemic of the Middle Ages killed an estimated one-fourth of the inhabitants of Europe. The disease of tuberculosis, which develops slowly in the body and rarely causes explosive outbreaks, has always been with us. Until the present century approximately 30% of the world's inhabitants who reached adulthood died of tuberculosis before reaching old age. Childhood infectious diseases have always been present as well; before 1900 about one of every two children died before reaching 10 years of age, primarily due to these diseases.

Today the number of persons dying from infectious diseases in developed countries is only a small portion of what it was in earlier times. Developments that led to the control of many devastating human microbial diseases represent some of the great triumphs of modern technology. Yet many infectious diseases are still not effectively controlled. Moreover, as social and physical living conditions change, new patterns of older diseases, as well as entirely new diseases, such as AIDS, develop. These new patterns result from new medical procedures that, while benefiting patients in some ways, render them more susceptible to certain types of infections in other ways. A person working in health care must be aware of conditions that cause these changing patterns of infectious diseases and must then be able to adapt procedures to minimize or control such infections. Serious infectious diseases are still widespread in many underdeveloped countries, particularly those diseases caused by parasites and those transmitted because of unsanitary conditions.

Germ theory
the theory that infection is caused by microorganisms.

The discoveries that led to an increased understanding and control of infectious diseases involved many people over many years. By the latter half of the nineteenth century the contagious nature and mode of transmission of many diseases had been demonstrated. This information, coupled with an increased ability to study microorganisms, led to the formation of the **germ theory** of disease and ushered in the Golden Age of Microbiology. This period of discovery spanned the years from about 1875 to 1900, during which time the foundations of the science of microbiology were established.

Developments that preceded and established the basis for the germ theory of disease came from three independent branches of research: (1) observations on the contagious nature of disease, (2) experiments with vaccination or immunization, and (3) basic research on the nature of microorganisms. Once the central concept of the germ theory of disease had been established, various subdisciplines arose that specialize in the study of different types of microbial agents as well as the methods used to treat and control infectious diseases. Some historical highlights of medical microbiology are outlined in Figure 1-1 and are discussed next.

DEVELOPMENTS PRECEDING THE GERM THEORY

Observations of Contagion

The idea that certain diseases could be passed from person to person by contact existed in many ancient cultures. The most notable examples of awareness of contagion are biblical references to the disposal of human wastes and regulations to avoid contact with lepers. The ancient Greek civilization was more aware of this concept than many later cultures. Aristotle reportedly instructed Alexander the Great to have his armies boil their drinking water

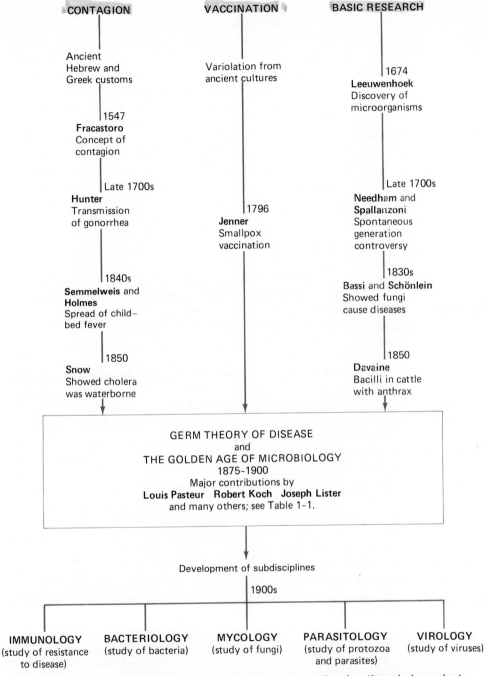

Figure 1-1 Historical highlights in medical microbiology, showing three independent branches of research coming together in the latter part of the nineteenth century to formulate the germ theory of disease and usher in the "Golden Age of Microbiology." In the twentieth century, subdisciplines of medical microbiology developed.

and bury their dung. Yet many later cultures seemed unaware of the contagious nature of diseases. One dominant philosophy common before the nineteenth century held that diseases resulted from contaminations of earthly influences, planetary conjunctions, or supernatural forces. The name *influenza* stems from the Middle Ages when it was thought that certain positions of the stars "influenced" the onset of this disease. Yet despite such philosophies, some scientists correctly observed the contagious nature of infectious diseases. One such interpretation was recorded in a book entitled *De Contagione et Contagiosis Morbis* (Contagion and Contagious Diseases) written in 1547 by an Italian physician, *Girolamo Fracastoro.* Fracastoro theorized that tiny imperceptible particles ("seeds of disease") spread from person to person. He postulated three forms of contagion: (1) by direct contact, (2) by fomites (a term first introduced by Fracastoro in referring to contaminated inanimate objects), and (3) at a distance—that is, by air or water. Unfortunately, his concepts were several hundred years ahead of their time and generally did not become part of the medical philosophy of his day.

Convincing work on the contagious nature of infectious disease was done in the 1700s by *Antonio Micheli, Mathieu Tillet,* and *Isaac Prevost,* who studied the transmission of plant diseases and the prevention of transmission by the use of chemical agents. This work, however, had little impact on those concerned with diseases of humans or animals. In the latter half of the eighteenth century, self-inoculation with the germs of syphilis and gonorrhea by the noted British surgeon *John Hunter* helped emphasize the concept of contagious diseases. Yet Hunter inadvertently, and somewhat tragically, confused the entire concept. In an attempt to prove the contagious nature of gonorrhea, he purposely inoculated the skin of his arm with pus from a person with gonorrhea. His concept was proven when he developed a gonorrheal lesion at the site of inoculation. Unfortunately, the experiment was confused because the patient from whom the pus was taken had syphilis as well. This disease was also successfully transmitted to the unfortunate Dr. Hunter and resulted in his untimely death. Because of this error, for years afterward, many persons believed gonorrhea and syphilis were different manifestations of the same disease.

During the first 30 years of the nineteenth century some chemical antimicrobials, mostly chlorine compounds used primarily for odor control, came into use in some medical facilities. Other antimicrobials were used to treat infected wounds, purify water, and disinfect hands. Notable observations were made between 1830 and 1860 on the mode of spread of childbed or puerperal fever, measles, and cholera. During the 1830s and 1840s independent observations on the transmission of a serious disease called *childbed fever* were made by the noted American physician-poet

Oliver Wendell Holmes and a young Hungarian physician, *Ignas Semmelweis*. They proposed methods for controlling this disease by having physicians wash their hands regularly with chloride solutions. Semmelweis, trained in obstetrical service, secured a position in that service at the general hospital of Vienna, and while there became greatly concerned about the high death rate from childbed fever in women in that hospital. By careful observation (Figure 1-2), he detected certain patterns of this disease. Patients examined shortly after a physician had autopsied a cadaver frequently contracted childbed fever. He theorized that "cadaveric particles" carried by the physician from the cadaver to the patient were responsible for the disease. He then instructed those working under him to wash their hands thoroughly with chlorinated water after having examined a cadaver or a diseased patient. Consequently, the mortality rate from childbed fever on his service was greatly reduced.

Figure 1-2   A table from the research of Semmelweis showing a higher death rate (9.92%) from childbed fever in women giving birth in the clinic attended by physicians (Klinik für Aerzte) compared to a death rate of 3.38% in the clinic attended by midwives (Klinik für Hebammen). Translations: *Geburten* = births; *Todte* = deaths; *Abtheilung* = division.

I. Abtheilung.

Klinik für Aerzte.

1841	Geburten 3036,	Todte 237,	Percent-Antheil		7.80
1842	» 3287,	» 518,	»	»	15.75
1843	» 3060,	» 274,	»	»	8.95
1844	» 3157,	» 260,	»	»	8.83
1845	» 3492,	» 241,	»	»	6.90
1846	» 4010,	» 459,	»	»	11.44
	» 20042,	» 1989,	»	»	9.92

II. Abtheilung.

Klinik für Hebammen.

1841	Geburten 2442,	Todte 86,	Percent-Antheil		3.52
1842	» 2659,	» 202,	»	»	7.59
1843	» 2739,	» 164,	»	»	5.98
1844	» 2956,	» 68,	»	»	2.80
1845	» 3241,	» 66,	»	»	2.03
1846	» 3754,	» 105,	»	»	2.79
	» 27791,	» 691,	»	»	3.38

Unfortunately, the theories of Semmelweis were largely based on an incomplete application of the scientific method. Although Semmelweis was meticulous in his observations, his hypotheses were not brought to experimental study. Thus, his method was largely a matter of making observation from which he then constructed a hypothesis. This was followed by additional observations and further hypotheses. The missing, and critical, step recognized by today's scientists is associated with the development of experiments that can be used to test the validity of each hypothesis. Owing partly to a lack of validation and partly due to the volcanic nature of his personality, Semmelweis was more abused than honored for trying to introduce "radical new concepts of little value."

In 1846 *Peter Panum*, a 26-year-old Danish physician, was sent by his government to investigate an outbreak of measles in the Faroe Islands. After interviewing thousands of patients, he determined that measles was contracted by contact with a person who already had measles and that the disease did not arise spontaneously as some authorities thought. He also determined the incubation time for the disease and clearly observed that those who had had the disease were immune when reexposed. His work presented a clear and accurate picture of the epidemiology of measles.

Communicable
a synonym for *contagious*. A communicable disease can be transmitted from one person to another.

Further important observations were made on the **communicable** nature of cholera through a detailed study by *John Snow*. In 1854 he showed that persons using water from the Broad Street pump in London were much more likely to contract cholera than those obtaining their water from other pumps (Figure 1-3). He further showed evidence of human fecal contamination at the Broad Street pump and correctly deduced that this contamination was responsible for the outbreaks of cholera.

Immunization

Since antiquity people have observed that individuals surviving one attack of certain diseases were often immune to a second attack. Most notable were observations on the disease smallpox (also called *variola*). It was further noted that both a major and a minor form of smallpox occurred and that recovery from one conferred immunity against both forms of the disease. Death rates from the minor form of smallpox were considerably less than the risk of dying from the naturally acquired major form. Therefore in some countries before the nineteenth century, primarily in Asia, Africa, and, to some extent, North America, a procedure called *variolation* was practiced. This procedure entailed purposely exposing persons to the minor form of smallpox. The English physician *Edward Jenner*, who was aware of the practice of variolation, carried the concept a step further. Jenner observed that milkmaids, who often contracted a mild disease called *cowpox*, rarely

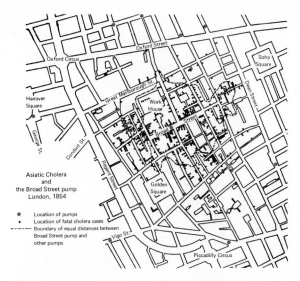

Figure 1-3   A map of the Broad Street London showing the clustering of outbreaks of cholera among persons using water from the Broad Street pump. From the study of John Snow in 1854. (Modified from J. P. Fox, C. E. Hall, L. R. Elveback: *Epidemiology Man and Disease,* Figure 10-10, p. 227. Copyright© 1970 by Macmillan Publishing Company)

came down with smallpox. Therefore in about 1796 he deliberately inoculated persons with materials taken from cowpox lesions (Figure 1-4). This process came to be known as **vaccination,** a term based on the Latin word for cow (*vacca*). In spite of some early opposition, the practice of vaccination against smallpox eventually became widely accepted and started a process that in time led to the complete eradication of this disease.

Discovery of Microorganisms and Early Basic Research

The discovery of microorganisms in 1674 came not from research by scholars or scientists of that day, but from the astute observations of a layman. *Antony van Leeuwenhoek* of Delft, Holland, was not well educated in the classical manner of his day, but he had become very skilled in his hobby of grinding glass lenses and making simple one-lens microscopes (Figure 1-5). These microscopes gave magnifications of up to 300 times and through a special method of illumination, which he kept a secret but which was probably a form of dark-field lighting, he was able to observe the fine structure of many materials. While observing pond water in 1674, he was amazed to see many very small creatures, apparently

Vaccination

a process by which small amounts of infective material, or material similar to that which is infective, is introduced into individuals to increase their resistance to disease. Sometimes used in the general sense to refer to the process of immunization.

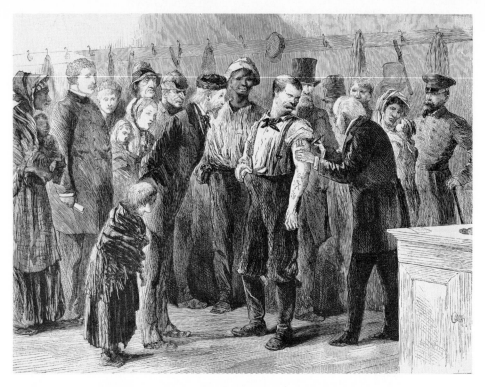

Figure 1-4 Early smallpox vaccination procedure in which cowpox material was introduced into the skin. (The Bettmann Archive)

algae or protozoa. He called these creatures *animalcules*. This discovery greatly intrigued Leeuwenhoek, who spent most of his spare time over the next 50 years making observations of microorganisms that he found in various materials. Encouraged by friends, he communicated his discoveries to the Royal Society of London. Leeuwenhoek wrote his first letter to the Royal Society somewhat apologetically, for it was in his own simple Dutch dialect and not in the scholarly Latin then customary in scientific writing. Yet using this simple language, he was able to accurately describe his important discovery (Figure 1-6). Impressed with Leeuwenhoek's discovery, the Royal Society encouraged him to continue his observations and correspondence. Between 1673 and the time of his death in 1723 Leeuwenhoek sent over 150 letters to the Royal Society. In his simple, colorful way Leeuwenhoek accurately described protozoa, fungi, algae, and bacteria. He was honored by being made an honorary member of the Royal Society, the preeminent society for scientific research of his time. Today he is recognized as the "Father of Microbiology." Neither Leeuwenhoek nor his contemporaries made any connection between these recently discovered "animalcules" and diseases, however.

Studies of microorganisms were limited during the first 150

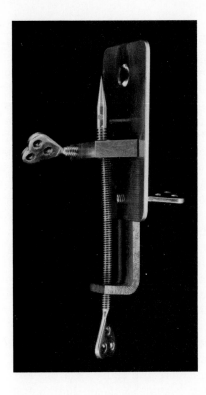

Figure 1-5   A replica of the type of single-lens microscope used by Leeuwenhoek. The object was placed on the pointed tip and brought into focus by turning the screws. (From Thomas D. Brock, *Biology of Microorganisms,* Third Edition, Figure 1.2, p. 3. Copyright © 1979 by Thomas D. Brock. Reprinted by permisssion of Prentice Hall, Inc.)

years after their discovery and were considered little more than biological curiosities. Because of technical difficulties, most biologists of that era found it unprofitable to study microorganisms. The Swedish naturalist *Carl Linnaeus,* in an attempt to include microorganisms in his scientific classification of plants and animals in 1758, referred to them as the class ''chaos.'' This name perhaps best described the contemporary state of knowledge regarding microorganisms in the eighteenth century.

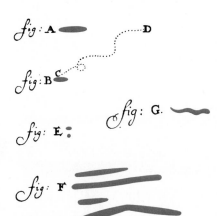

Figure 1-6   Reproductions of microorganisms drawn by Leeuwenhoek in one of his letters to the Royal Society. (From C. Dobell, *Anthony and His Little Animals.* New York: Dover Publications, 1960)

The systematic laboratory investigation of microorganisms accelerated in the latter half of the eighteenth century. During this time microorganisms became the central subject of a controversy concerning the possibility of spontaneous generation (life arising from nonliving matter). Studies by *Francesco Redi* a century earlier had laid to rest notions such that flies arose spontaneously from decomposing meat. In 1784, however, *John Needham*, after conducting a series of experiments in which bacterial growth appeared in broth that had previously been boiled, concluded that only spontaneous generation could explain his results. Today it is clearly understood that Needham's findings were a result of the growth of resistant **bacterial spores** present in the broth and poor aseptic techniques. In any case, Needham's theory received wide support as well as notoriety. *Lazzaro Spallanzani* challenged this theory and conducted an extensive series of experiments to show that microorganisms arose only from other microorganisms of the same type. The controversy between Spallanzani and Needham continued for many years, increasing the scientific interest in microorganisms. A century later the theory of spontaneous generation was finally disproved by *Louis Pasteur* and *John Tyndall*.

Bacterial spore

an environmentally stable and persistent form used by some bacteria as protection against lack of nutrients, heat, or drying.

By the mid-1800s investigators started to recognize the possible role of microorganisms as causative agents of disease. In 1836 *Agostino Bassi* showed that fungi were the cause of a disease in silkworms; and a few years later *Johann Schonlein* demonstrated the association of fungi with a human skin disease called *favus*. *Gerhard Hansen* discovered **bacilli** in cells from leprosy patients as early as 1847. In 1850 *Casimir Davaine* carried out preliminary studies in which he observed large bacilli in the blood of cattle with anthrax, leading him to suggest that these organisms might be the cause of this disease. Then in 1865 *Jean-Antoine Villemin* experimentally transmitted tuberculosis to animals. In spite of their potential significance, the full impact of these early studies was not initially recognized; they were, however, a prelude to the formulation of the germ theory of disease and an introduction to the Golden Age of Microbiology during the latter part of the nineteenth century.

Bacilli

bacteria that are elongated or rod-shaped.

THE GERM THEORY OF DISEASE AND THE GOLDEN AGE OF MICROBIOLOGY

The central figures in establishing microbiology as a science were the French scientist Louis Pasteur and the German physician *Robert Koch*.

Pasteur (Figure 1-7) first gained recognition as a chemist when he successfully separated left- and right-handed crystals of

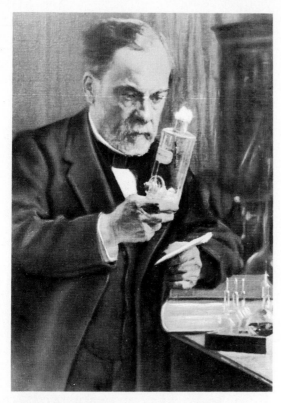

Figure 1-7   A painting of Louis Pasteur by Edelfeld. (The Bettmann Archive)

tartaric acid. Then in the 1850s his studies turned to the process of fermentation and he concluded that microorganisms were responsible for this process. In a short series of studies published in 1860 and 1861, Pasteur helped disprove the lingering theory of the spontaneous generation of microorganisms. Because of his knowledge of fermentation, Pasteur was asked to help solve the problem of the so-called "wine disease." In this study, he scientifically determined that undesirable wine was produced by the presence of undesirable acid-producing microorganisms. To resolve this problem, he applied mild heat to the grape juice in order to destroy the unwanted microorganisms, a process now called *pasteurization* (Figure 1-8). Pasteur was next requested to cure a silkworm disease that was gradually destroying the French silk industry. After many trials and setbacks and five years of effort, Pasteur demonstrated that a protozoan caused this disease and he introduced methods to limit its spread.

By 1876 Pasteur had turned to the study of the contagious diseases of vertebrates. Carrying out extensive experiments with anthrax and chicken cholera, Pasteur helped establish the causative role of specific bacteria in each of these diseases. Among his

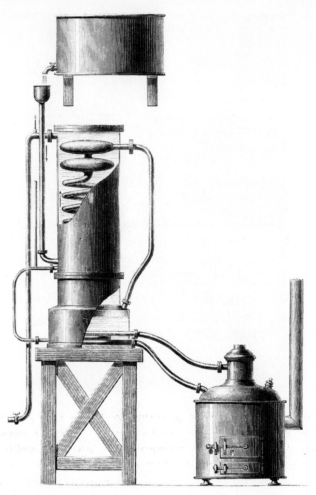

Figure 1-8 An early type of apparatus used for the pasteurization of wine. (Institut Pasteur, Paris)

Vaccine

a preparation of bacteria or products made from bacteria which can be used to immunize against disease.

greatest contributions were the development of **vaccines** for their control. This work laid the foundation for an entire scientific discipline known today as immunology. In the mid-1880s Pasteur developed a successful treatment for persons exposed to rabies. A modification of this treatment continues in use even today. More than any other single individual, Pasteur helped to move medical science from an empirical to an experimental process.

Koch was fascinated with research on microorganisms early in his medical career. Working under makeshift conditions in the 1870s (Figure 1-9), he developed systematic methods for the study of these organisms. His first reports, published in 1876, clearly demonstrated the role of a specific bacterium as the causative agent of anthrax. These efforts enabled him to demonstrate a bacterial cause of disease in large animals and humans. It was while

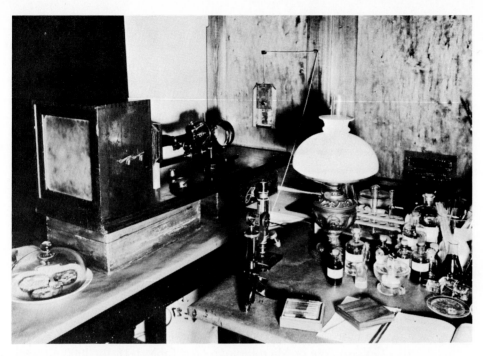

Figure 1-9   A room in Koch's house that was converted into a laboratory and was used during his early studies in microbiology. (The Bettmann Archive)

working with anthrax that he formalized into a set of postulates the ideas of a former colleague, Jacob Henle. Now termed *Koch's postulates*, these maxims (see Chapter 14), are used today as convincing proof of the **etiology** of infectious diseases. By 1880 Koch was receiving increased support for his work and could spend his full efforts in research. He continued to improve the methods used to study microbial diseases, with some of his most important work centering on tuberculosis. By demonstrating the infectious nature of this significant human disease, Koch disproved the then present theory of its genetic basis. Before his death in 1910, Koch became a central force for microbiological research and, with his associates, made many notable contributions to medical microbiology.

Etiology
cause of disease, a study of the cause of disease.

Great research institutes developed around both Pasteur and Koch and became the major centers for microbiological research during the latter part of the nineteenth century. Through the remarkable scientific skill of these two men, the responsibility for control and treatment of contagious disease began to shift from individuals to communities. As long as people had accepted the concepts of spontaneous generation, occurrence of infectious disease was considered as capricious, and control impossible. However, with true understanding of the processes of contagion and with knowledge that organisms were not transmutable, the development and application of vaccines and social control measures became meaningful. The science of medicine became a social endeavor.

While both Pasteur and Koch carried out important work in France and Germany, significant developments were being made in Great Britain by the surgeon *Joseph Lister.* Lister was familiar with the studies of Pasteur on fermentation and putrefaction and in 1865 he reasoned that microorganisms could be causing the putrefaction or pus formation (suppuration) associated with wounds. He further reasoned that dressing the wound with some material capable of killing these germs might help prevent the suppuration. Noting that carbolic acid (phenol) was effective in preventing sewage odors, Lister chose to use this substance as his antiseptic agent. This choice was fortunate and Lister had great success in preventing wound infections. He extended his methods to surgeries by soaking **ligatures** in disinfectants and by performing operations under a spray of phenol (Figure 1-10). Although Lister's methods were not readily accepted, by the end of the nineteenth century aseptic surgery had become a standard procedure.

Numerous discoveries were made by other scientists during this Golden Age of Microbiology (see Table 1-1). By 1900 microbiology was a well-established science and the relationship between microbes and many diseases had been clearly determined. Even more important, methods for treating and controlling some diseases were developed during this time. The secrets of the great human pestilences of history began to yield to the persistent studies of men such as *Emil von Behring, Albert Neisser, Georg Gaffky, Alexandre Yersin,* and *David Bruce.* Together and independently these men unlocked the doors leading to the possibility of human life free from the worry, sorrow and horror of calamitous epidemic disease. In the early 1900s numerous contributions broadened our knowledge of microbiology. Out of this early knowledge came the various subdisciplines of medical microbiology shown in Figure 1-1.

Ligature
suture; material (often silk) used to close an open wound. Commonly referred to as "stitches."

CHEMOTHERAPY

Knowing that living biological agents were responsible for disease in humans led naturally to an investigation of the means by which we could come to control infections. One who engaged in this forward-looking research was a German chemist by the name of *Paul Ehrlich.* Ehrlich had studied the action of aniline dyes on many materials and observed that the various parts of cells could be specifically stained with selected dyes. With this idea in mind,

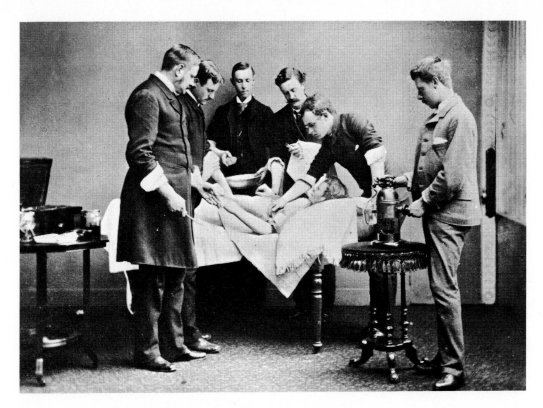

Figure 1-10   An operation in Edinburgh, about 1870, using the carbolic spray method of Lister. Masks, gloves, caps, and gowns were not yet being used. (The Bettmann Archive)

he postulated that it should be possible to find a "magic bullet" that would selectively react with an essential part of a microbial cell and not with the human or host cells. He reasoned that such an interaction could be used to selectively destroy invading microorganisms and restore the patient to health. His prodigious work led him through the trial of hundreds of compounds with but little success. But his hypothesis continued to be tested, leading to the firm establishment of the concept of chemotherapy, the use of chemicals to treat infectious disease.

Later developments in chemotherapy in the 1930s revolutionized our ability to treat bacterial diseases. From England in 1928 *Alexander Fleming* had reported a chance discovery of strong antibacterial properties produced by the secretions of the mold *Penicillium* (Figure 1-11). This substance he called *penicillin*. By 1938 *Howard Florey* and *Ernst Chain* had purified this material and demonstrated its usefulness in treating bacterial infections. Stimulated by the advent of World War II, scientists soon found methods for the mass production of penicillin and the first true antibiotic agent became available to the world. The significance of this single event in terms of the reduction in human suffering and mis-

Table 1-1 Some Important Discoveries Made in Medical Microbiology During the Golden Age of Microbiology, 1875–1900

Year	Discoverer	Discovery
1877	R. Koch	Proved that anthrax is caused by a bacterium
1877	F. Cohn	Demonstrated bacterial spores
1878	J. Lister	First grew bacteria in pure culture
1879	A. Neisser	Discovered the cause of gonorrhea
1880s	L. Pasteur	Developed vaccines and treatment of rabies
1881	A. Ogston	Discovered staphylococci cause wound infection
1882	R. Koch	Discovered the cause of tuberculosis
1883	T. Klebs	Discovered the cause of diphtheria
1884	A. Nicolaier	Discovered the cause of tetanus
1884	R. Koch	Discovered the cause of cholera
1884	G. Gaffky	Discovered the cause of typhoid fever
1884	E. Metchnikoff	First observed phagocytosis by white blood cells
1887	D. Bruce	Discovered the cause of Malta fever
1890	E. von Behring and S. Kitasato	Discovered bacterial toxins and how to develop antitoxins
1892	W. Welch and G. Nuttal	Discovered the cause of gas gangrene
1892	D. Ivanovski	First demonstration of a virus
1894	A. Yersin	Discovered the cause of plague
1897	E. Van Ermengen	Discovered the cause of botulism food poisoning
1898	K. Shiga	Discovered the cause of dysentery
1900	W. Reed	Showed yellow fever was transmitted by mosquitoes and was caused by a virus

ery has been incalculable, and was recognized with the award of the Nobel Prize in medicine to the three principal scientists responsible for developing penicillin.

The development of another important chemotherapeutic agent during this era involved several groups of scientists. In the early 1930s *Gerhard Domagk,* a German pathologist, found that a chemical called *prontosil* had significant antibacterial activity against some bacterial infections. Then in 1935 *Jacques* and *Thérèse Tréfouël,* a husband-and-wife team working in France, discovered that the antibacterial activity of prontosil was due to the sulfanilamide segment of the molecule. This finding rapidly led to the development of numerous ''sulfa'' compounds that continue to be used as effective antimicrobial agents.

Penicillin and sulfa drugs were the first highly effective compounds developed for treating specific bacterial diseases. Over the past 50 years, untold millions of patients have been treated by

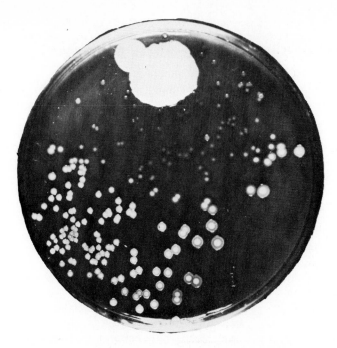

Figure 1-11   A photograph of Alexander Fleming's original plate showing the growth of the mold *Penicillium notatum* and its inhibitory action on bacterial growth. (The Bettmann Archive)

using these two agents. Moreover, these chemicals have been continually improved over the years and since 1940 many additional chemotherapeutic agents have been developed for use against all forms of infectious disease agents.

MOLECULAR BIOLOGY

Many advances in each of the subdisciplines of microbiology have occurred since the 1940s. The most impressive contributions, however, are those that have led to a preliminary understanding of how molecules work together inside a living cell—a field of study now referred to as *molecular biology.* Because of their relative structural simplicity, microorganisms and, in particular, viruses have been extensively used in these studies. Using bacterial cells, *Oswald Avery, Colin MacLeod,* and *Maclyn McCarty,* working in New York, first reported the genetic role of DNA (deoxyribonucleic acid) in 1944. Then in 1953 *James Watson* and *Francis Crick,* working in England, resolved the structure of DNA. These early discover-

Molecular Biology and Immunization

From the days of Edward Jenner it has been clear that the process of immunization is not without risk to the patient. Many potential vaccines have either not been developed or are not generally used because of such risks or because of biological limitations. Now, after nearly 200 years of immunization practice, we recognize many of the characteristics of a good vaccine, as well as many of the undesirable effects of vaccine use. While Jenner was able to use cowpox as a vaccine for smallpox, most infectious disease agents have no closely related, relatively harmless microorganisms that can be used for immunization. This has required scientists to consider numerous alternative approaches in their quest for useful vaccines.

In principle, the development of a microbial vaccine should be relatively simple. It consists of exposing an individual to the causative agent (or part of the agent) of the disease and allowing the individual's body to respond by producing protective antibodies against the disease-causing microbe. As with many concepts, theory is easier than practice. To create a vaccine that is maximally useful, scientists must consider questions like these: Which is the route of vaccine administration; that is, is the best vaccine most effective when given by mouth or must it be injected? Is a single dose of the vaccine adequate or must it be repeatedly administered? Can more than one vaccine be administered at the same time, or will multiple components compete with each other and reduce the immunity to all? How old should an individual be in order to receive the vaccine, and what is the optimal age of administration. How can a toxic (poisonous) vaccine be modified such that it can still be used? These and many more concerns have been addressed by scientists as they have attempted to increase our resistance to serious infectious disease.

With the advent of recombinant DNA technology, a way has been opened to resolve many of the problems associated with the development and use of vaccines. Scientists have been able to identify the specific chemical molecules, known as *epitopes,* of an infecting microorganism that are used by individuals to develop immunity to the microorganism. With this information, they have been able to select the microbial gene that is responsible for producing the epitope. The scientists can then engineer the gene into non-disease-producing microorganisms so that it will produce large quantities of the desired epitope. When the specific purified chemical molecules that stimulate immunity to the disease-producing microbe are available in large quantities (without the rest of the organism) it is relatively easy to find answers to the questions raised in the previous paragraph.

There are presently only a few genetically engineered vaccines available, but it can be expected that within very few years these techniques will be used to develop vaccines against viral diseases such as AIDS for which no vaccines are now available. It is also likely that presently available vaccines will be discontinued in favor of vaccines made by these new scientific methodologies. Such vaccines can be expected to be effective even if multiple epitopes are included in the vaccine. They will facilitate immunization of younger children and will reduce the toxic properties that limit the present usefulness of many vaccines.

**Table 1-2   Some Possible Products and Potential Applications
of Genetic Engineering**

Products	Applications
Enzymes that metabolize petroleum	Clean up oil spills
Insulin	Treatment of diabetics
Human-growth hormones	Treatment of growth disorders
Animal-growth hormones	Stimulate growth for increased meat production
Interferons	Treatment of viral infections and possibly cancer
Pheremones (insect hormones)	Insect control
Endorphins	Pain killers
Antigens	Preparation of vaccines not easily produced by regular methods
Antibiotics	Improved or less expensive antibiotics
Methane or alcohol	More efficient formation of these products from cellulose waste
Nitrogen fixation	Increased soil fertility

ies preceded a rapid advance in understanding as various scientists demonstrated how DNA functions as the genetic storehouse of information and how that information is used to direct the various cellular activities.

Most recently, a subdiscipline of molecular biology referred to as *genetic engineering* has become the central focus of research into the understanding of infectious disease. As recently as 1973, the first report of the successful cloning of a gene was received by the scientific community. This breakthrough was shortly followed by genetically engineered production of proteins, development of animal vaccines, and the availability of other pharmaceutical compounds such as human insulin made from cloned genes, Table 1-2. The use of microbial genetic engineering processes has extended far beyond medicine and concern for health. Industrial processes relating to petroleum degradation, nitrogen fixation, cellulose digestion, production of organic chemicals and the uses of single-cell protein have each been significantly improved through the techniques of molecular biology.

It can be expected that the application of the scientific method to the problems of human welfare will result in an almost unending series of scientific breakthroughs. Whereas in the past, advances in science seemed to await the rare genius of a Pasteur or a Lister, today the broad application of the scientific method by numerous careful investigators appears to ensure a steadily increasing understanding of the natural world.

CONCEPT SUMMARY

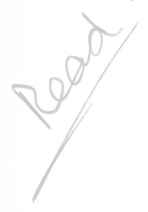

1. Microbiology is a rather recent scientific discipline that has grown rapidly during the past 100 years. Historically the primary concern and interest regarding the microorganism centered around its ability to produce serious, often fatal, disease. Later microorganisms proved a great tool in the study of life and much that we know regarding genetics, biochemistry, cellular physiology, and molecular biology was derived through careful study of these life forms.

2. Microbiology took a great leap forward with general acceptance of the germ theory of disease. This awakening, guided by men such as Pasteur and Koch, led to a period known as the Golden Age of Microbiology during which most infectious disease agents now known were discovered.

3. A parallel science based on a study of resistance to infection developed concurrently with the discovery of infectious agents. This discipline, immunology, ranks today as one of the most challenging and exciting fields of scientific discovery. In time, the development of antimicrobial therapy, centered in the antibiotics, brought a new success to the world of the microbiologist and hope to the whole human family.

4. The recent development and advances in the procedures of molecular biology have rekindled the thinking of scientists throughout the world. With these new technologies, powerful scientific tools have become available by which the secrets of nature are being discovered at an ever-increasing rate.

5. Use of the scientific method evolved slowly into the patterns of research. Application of this process virtually ensures a continuing flow of new understanding about our world.

STUDY SUMMARY

1. What role did the development of the germ theory of disease play in making microbiology a separate scientific discipline?

2. How has the knowledge that some diseases are communicable led to the methods for control of infections?

3. What could Semmelweis have done to ensure acceptance of ideas regarding the transmission of childbed fever?

4. Review the work of Edward Jenner in terms of the scientific method. Write a probable hypothesis, outline the experiment

used to test his hypothesis, and list the results of that experiment.

5. What impact has antimicrobial chemotherapy had on the American lifestyle?

REFERENCES FOR FURTHER STUDY

1. *Milestones in Microbiology,* T. Brock, 1961. Prentice-Hall.
2. *The History of Bacteriology,* W. Bulloch, 1960. Oxford.
3. *Three Centuries of Microbiology,* H. Lechevalier, 1965, McGraw-Hill.
4. *The Microbial World,* 5th ed, R. Stanier, 1986. Prentice-Hall.

METHODS USED TO STUDY MICROORGANISMS

T he progress and development of the science of microbiology had to await the availability of tools, techniques, and procedures that could be applied to the study of very small life forms. This chapter describes some of the methodologies and tools that facilitated the growth of microbiology as a laboratory science. The first section deals with a most valuable tool, the microscope, which has enabled direct visualization of many microbes and indirect observation of others. The second section describes commonly used methods of counting microorganisms.

MICROSCOPY

In order to describe microorganisms it is necessary to use units of measurement which are unfamiliar to most students. As with all scientific measurements, these units are part of the metric system and are shown in Table 2-1.

Because of the inability of the unaided human eye to perceive objects smaller than 0.1 mm (Figure 2-1), a microscope is essential to see microbial cells and to determine their morphological characteristics. Two general types of microscopes are available: the *light microscope* and the *electron microscope.* Light microscopes use visible light waves as the source of illumination and are able to produce meaningful magnifications to about 1000 times (1000×). The electron microscope uses an electron beam as the source of illumination and is able to magnify well in excess of 100,000×. Electron microscopes, on the other hand, are large, expensive, complex instruments that are restricted to specialized laboratories with highly trained personnel.

Table 2-1   The Units of Measurement Used in Microbiology

Unit of Measurement	Abbreviation	Equivalent
Meter	m	39.37 inches
Centimeter	cm	1/100th of a meter (10^{-2} m)
Millimeter	mm	1/1000th of a meter (10^{-3} m)
Micrometer[a]	μm	1/1000th of a millimeter (10^{-6} m)
Nanometer[b]	nm	1/1000th of a micrometer (10^{-9} m)
Angstrom	Å	1/10th of a nanometer (10^{-10} m)

[a]*Formerly called a micron.*
[b]*Formerly called a millimicron.*

Figure 2-1   Relative size of microscopic objects. Visible objects are shown in millimeters (mm); sub-visible are shown in micrometers (μm); and sub-microscopic are shown in nanometers (nm).

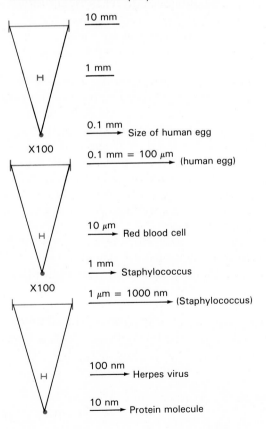

Light Microscopes

The earliest microscopes were little more than sophisticated magnifying glasses. Through these lenses a careful observer, such as Leeuwenhoek (see Chapter 1), could view objects at a magnification of about 400×. A more powerful system of magnification was developed in Denmark by Zachariah Jansens. His system was an imaginative application of optical principles that resulted in the development of the compound microscope. Today virtually all microscopes used in microbiology are compound light microscopes; in other words, they use a series of lenses to magnify the object. The magnifying lenses are called (1) the *objective* lens, and (2) the *ocular* or eyepiece lens. The objective lens is the primary magnifying lens and is positioned close to the material or object to be viewed. The ocular lens is positioned close to the eye of the observer and produces a secondary magnification of the image produced by the objective lens. Light is focused on the object by *condenser* lenses that are not part of the magnification system. The magnifications of the objective and ocular lenses provide the total magnification of the compound microscope. The maximum magnification that can be obtained, under most conditions, from a single glass lens is about 100×; and most compound microscopes have objective lenses that give magnifications of 10×, 40×, or 100×. These lenses are mounted on a rotating base called a *nose piece* so that each lens can be easily moved into position as needed. Most ocular lenses give magnifications of 10×, although lenses of 1.5× to 20× are available. Thus by using the 10× ocular lens with the various objective lenses, total magnifications of 100× (10 × 10), 400× (40 × 10), or 1000× (100 × 10) are obtainable. The lower magnifications are used to observe large areas of the object or relatively large objects and higher magnifications for more detailed observations of selected areas of the object. Magnifications of at least 400× are needed for the observation of most microbial cells and 1000× is customarily used. An outline of an optical microscope is shown in Figure 2-2.

It might be asked, Why not use such lens combinations as a 100× objective and a 50× or 100× ocular lens to obtain magnifications of 5000× or 10,000× and so on? Theoretically it can be done; however, no added value is achieved because this greater magnification shows no added detail. It is called "empty" magnification. The reason is that the *resolving power* (the ability to distinguish between two adjacent objects) is primarily a function of the wavelength of the type of illumination used. This relationship is defined according to the following formula:

$$\text{Resolving power} = \frac{0.5 \times \text{wavelength of light}}{\text{NA}}$$

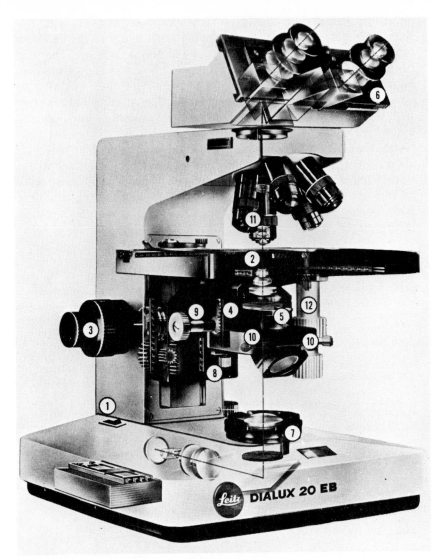

Figure 2-2   A cutaway diagram of a modern light microscope. The light path is shown and the essential parts of the system are indicated: (1) light switch; (2) mechanical stage where the object to be viewed is placed; (3) focus adjustment; (4) substage light condenser; (5) light diaphragm control for condenser; (6) ocular or eye piece; (7) light-focusing lens; (8) condenser adjustment; (9) condenser focus adjustment; (10) condenser light filter; (11) objective lens—this microscope has 5 objectives attached to a rotating turret housing; (12) substage adjustment control. (Courtesy E. Leitz, Inc.)

where NA is the numerical aperture of the lens. The greater the resolving power, the greater is the useful magnification that can be obtained; and obviously the shorter the wavelength of light used and the larger the NA of the lenses (up to about 1.4), the greater is the resolving power of the microscope. The mid-wavelength of visible light used in optical microscopes is 0.5 μm. The maximum resolving power obtainable with usual lenses is about one-half the length of the light waves or about 0.25 μm. The relationship between wavelength and resolving power is shown in Figure 2-3.

The lenses in an expensive microscope must always be corrected for two natural artifacts: *chromatic aberration* and *spherical aberration*. Chromatic aberration is a multicolored fringe that surrounds an object viewed through a single lens, while spherical aberration results from the curvature of the lens itself, and makes part of the microscopic field appear to be out of focus. These aberrations can be corrected by adding additional lenses into the light path, each with an aberration that cancels the apparent aberration of the other.

Figure 2-3   The effects of wavelength of radiation source on resolving power of a microscope. (a) Visible light does not detect objects smaller than 0.25 μm, and in this example does not show the fimbriae, the virus, or the space between the two bacteria. (b) The electron beams do detect the fimbriae, the virus, and the space between the bacteria.

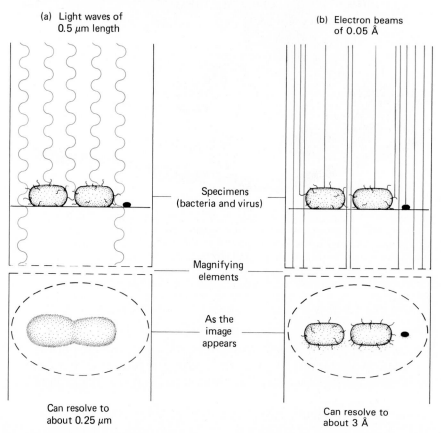

(a) Light waves of 0.5 μm length

(b) Electron beams of 0.05 Å

Specimens (bacteria and virus)

Magnifying elements

As the image appears

Can resolve to about 0.25 μm

Can resolve to about 3 Å

Types of Optical Microscopy

Bright-field microscopy   In the most common form of microscopy, the light is focused directly on the object and the resulting image is magnified and observed (Figure 2-4). Thus the image appears as a shaded object in a bright field (background). Most small objects, such as microorganisms, have only slight optical contrast (refractive index) from their surroundings and are very difficult to see. To enhance this visual contrast, bacteria are stained with various **dyes** (Figure 2-5).

Dark-field microscopy   In the dark-field microscope, light is directed onto the object at an angle so that only the light reflected from the object is magnified and observed (Figure 2-6). The image appears bright in a dark background. This form of microscopy is

Dye
a colored compound from which a stain can be made.

Figure 2-4   Photomicrograph of unstained parasite, *Giardia lamblia* (top) and same parasite stained with iodine stain (bottom). (Courtesy Centers for Disease Control, Atlanta)

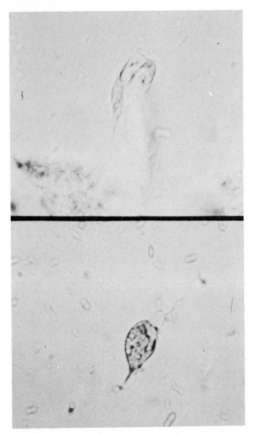

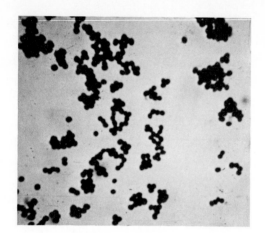

Figure 2-5
Photomicrograph of stained
bacteria.

particularly useful for observing the movement of microorganisms, because no staining is needed (Figure 2-7) and living objects can be observed. This procedure is also used to examine organisms that do not stain with simple staining procedures such as the spirochete causing syphilis.

Phase-contrast microscopy Phase-contrast microscopy uses a special optical system that renders the details of unstained cells much more visible. It is particularly useful in observing living cells. Different components of a cell have slight differences in their

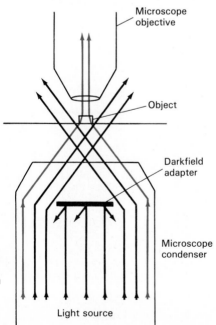

Figure 2-6   Schematic of darkfield
microscopy. The only light visible in
the microscope is that which is
reflected by the object into the
eyepiece.

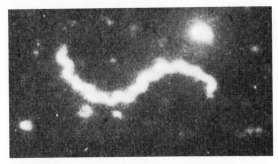

Figure 2-7 Photomicrograph of *Treponema pallidum* taken by darkfield microscopy. (Courtesy Centers for Disease Control, Atlanta)

refractive indices. These differences cause light rays to be bent or refracted as they pass from one portion of the cell to another. The refracted light is intensified by the optical system of a phase-contrast microscope and forms an image in which much of the fine detail of the cellular components can be seen. Staining is not needed and movement of cellular components can be observed (Figure 2-8).

Fluorescence microscopy Fluorescence microscopy allows us to observe materials that fluoresce—that is, materials that give off light of one color when subjected to light of another color. Most fluorescence microscopes use ultraviolet light as the primary light source; light given off by the fluorescent material is orange, yellow, or green, depending on the type of fluorescing material. To

Refractive index
a numerical value used to indicate the ability of a substance to transmit light. The refractive index is a property of the chemical composition of the substance. Light rays are bent (change direction) as they pass from a substance of one refractive index to that of a different refractive index.

Figure 2-8 Phase contrast micrograph of sheep erythrocytes surrounding mouse peritoneal cells. (Courtesy I. R. Tizard, Bacteriol. Rev 35:365)

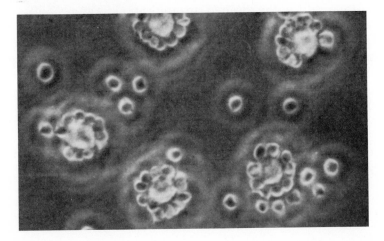

Antibody

a serum protein made by an individual in response to an antigenic stimulus. Antibodies are able to combine with the same kind of antigens that were responsible for signaling their production.

prevent injury, the ultraviolet light must be filtered out before its rays reach the eyes of the observer. Some microorganisms contain naturally fluorescent materials, but in most applications of fluorescence microscopy the microorganisms to be observed must be stained with special fluorescent dyes. The dyes rhodamine, auramine, and fluorescein are most commonly used. They are used directly or attached to specific antibodies (see Chapter 13), thus allowing attachment to selected microbial cells or only to specific subcomponents of these cells. This procedure has made fluorescence microscopy a useful tool in diagnostic laboratories. Rapid detection and identification of an unknown microbe are possible by adding a known fluorescent-tagged **antibody** to a clinical specimen and then watching for the presence of fluorescence. This procedure not only allows a specific identification of microbes but also increases the accuracy and speed of their detection.

Electron Microscopes

Electron microscopes can provide much greater magnifications than optical microscopes because they use an electron beam as the source of illumination. The electron beam has a wavelength of only 0.05 Å; this produces great resolving power. Due to technical problems, however, electron microscopes cannot actually resolve to 0.05 Å. Although several special microscopes can resolve to 3 Å, most have a resolving power of about 0.001 mm. This latter figure allows useful magnifications of well over 100,000×. Two general types of electron microscopes exist: *transmission* and *scanning* (Figure 2-9).

Transmission electron microscopes (TEMs) The transmission electron microscope sends a high-voltage electron beam through the center of a vacuum column. The beam strikes the object to be viewed, which then casts a shadow of the object. As the beam continues down the column, electrons are deflected by a magnetic field to produce the desired magnification (Figure 2-10). The greater the deflection, the greater is the magnification. Ultimately the electron beam strikes a fluorescent screen at the bottom of the column, where an outline of the shadow of the object becomes visible. A photographic film is located under the fluorescent screen and a photograph of the object can be made by moving the screen and allowing the electrons to expose the film. The transmission electron microscope has made it possible to see particles as small as viruses and much of the internal structure of cells (see Figures 2-11, 5-5, 27-3, 28-13, and 42-3). This information has been a tremendous aid in increasing our understanding of how biological systems function.

Various methods can be used to coat or stain an object with electron-dense materials. These metals or salts increase the ability

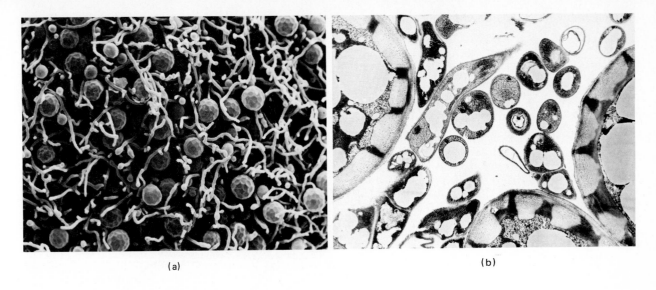

(a)

(b)

Figure 2-9 Electron micrographs of fungal spores of *Tilletia controversa:*
(a) taken with scanning electron microscope; (b) taken with transmission
electron microscope. (Courtesy W. M. Hess, Brigham Young University)

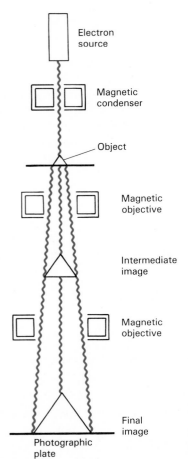

Electron source

Magnetic condenser

Object

Magnetic objective

Intermediate image

Magnetic objective

Final image

Photographic plate

Figure 2-10 Operational schematic of electron microscope. Magnetic fields are used both to focus and enlarge the electron image of the object.

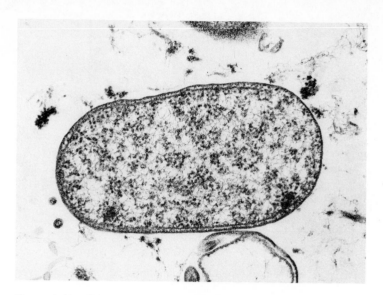

Figure 2-11   Electron photomicrograph of bacterial cell (x 49,000). (Courtesy W. M. Hess, Brigham Young University)

of the electron microscope to show contrast and details of minute structures (Figure 2-11). Certain limitations are inherent in the transmission electron microscope, however. Because the specimen must be observed in a vacuum, it requires dehydration, a factor that along with the treatment with electron-dense staining materials frequently causes distortions of the original structure. Moreover, the electrons cannot readily penetrate very dense or thick materials; consequently, the specimen must be spread in a thin film or cut into very thin sections in order to allow observation of internal components.

Scanning electron microscopes (SEM)   The scanning electron microscope also uses an electron beam. The beam, however, is not magnetically amplified within the column as with the TEM but is focused into a narrow beam that rapidly scans back and forth over the specimen. The electrons reflected from each scan of the beam are picked up by an electron collector in the same orientation as they are reflected. These electrons produce an electrical current that is sent from the collector to amplifiers where each scan is amplified and the image is reconstructed line by line on a CRT (television) screen. The scanning electron microscope is able to produce magnifications up to $100,000\times$. Nevertheless, much of the work with these microscopes is done at lower magnifications. Important advantages of the scanning electron microscope include its capability to create images in a three-dimensional reproduction with only slight distortion of the specimen (because the specimen need not be cut into thin sections or stained). As a result, materials can be viewed in their natural orientation (see Figures 7-4, 15-1, 17-1, 18-1, 19-1, 24-6, and 27-1).

Today innovations in electron microscopes are appearing rapidly. Instruments are now available that have the capabilities of both the transmission and the scanning microscopes. For example, some scanning electron microscopes are equipped with x-ray analysis equipment that permits areas of the specimen to be analyzed for the types of chemical elements it possesses.

Preparation of Microorganisms in Microscopy

In order for an object to be seen, it must contrast with its background. Often, however, objects that we wish to view through a microscope are very similar to the medium in which they are suspended. In order to provide the needed contrast when observing with the bright-field microscope the microorganisms are **stained.** An aqueous or broth suspension of the microorganism is spread in a thin film over an area of a microscope slide and allowed to dry. The slide is then passed two or three times through a flame, which fixes the cells to the surface, and the cells are stained. *Simple, negative,* or *differential* staining procedures may be used. Simple staining involves adding a stain to the cells for a time, followed by rinsing of the slide to remove excess stains. The most commonly used simple stains are *methylene blue, crystal violet,* and a red dye called *safranin.* Negative staining is a procedure that stains the background but not the cells. For this procedure, either a black dye, called *nigrosin,* or India ink is mixed with the bacteria and is spread in a thin film on a microscopic slide. The stain will form a dark film over the background but will leave the cells as clear structures. Negative staining is generally used to show the presence of bacterial surface structures such as capsules. Differential staining procedures use more than one stain and are able to define bacteria or bacterial components, based on their staining characteristics. The most widely used differential staining procedure is the *Gram stain.* This process divides bacteria into two major groups: *Gram-positive* and *Gram-negative.* The steps leading to the reactions of the Gram stain are shown in Table 2-2. The *acid-fast* stain is a differential stain that helps identify the bacteria that cause tuberculosis or leprosy (Figure 2-12). The process is discussed in Chapter 22. Other special staining procedures help to visualize specific cellular structures, such as bacterial endospores.

Stain
a solution of dye that can be used to color objects to improve their visibility. Stains can be prepared that are very selective and will attach only to specific kinds of cells or parts of cells.

COUNTING MICROORGANISMS

It is often necessary to determine the number of microorganisms present in a culture or other material for research or industrial purposes. These determinations help to provide an assessment of

Clinical Microscopy

The word *microbiologist* often evokes a mental image of a scientist looking through a microscope for endless hours. Like many other impressions, however, this one is generally false. Considering the great uniformity of shape and staining properties among bacteria, it is not likely that such intense attention to the microscope would be very productive. There are, however, several circumstances where the microscope is an invaluable tool to the clinical microbiologist. When specimens from infected patients are received by the laboratory, there are generally two questions that need to be answered: Are there any bacteria in the specimen? If there are, what kind are they? The microscope can provide good answers to the first question, and can give considerable help in answering the second.

Specimens from sick patients come either from areas of the body that are normally sterile (e.g., blood, urine, or cerebral spinal fluid), or from areas that are the normal habitat of diverse bacteria (e.g., feces, throat, or skin). Proper use of the microscope can help evaluate both kinds of specimens. The microscopic observation of bacteria in a normally sterile body fluid is a strong indicator that these organisms are the cause of a patient's illness. Therefore, with a little practice, a microscopist can provide in a few minutes important diagnostic information that otherwise might take 24–48 hours to obtain. There are limitations to such procedures, however. If, for example, you were to place 10 bacteria into 1 ml of water and then try to detect these bacteria by microscopy, you would probably never be successful. In fact, the concentration of bacteria necessary to see even 1 bacterium per high-power microscope field is on the order of 100,000 organisms per milliliter. Therefore, in order to improve the probability that smaller numbers of bacteria will not escape observation, specimens are usually concentrated by centrifugation before they are placed on a microscope slide. When procedures like this are used, bacteria can be detected in nearly 80% of the specimens from patients with meningitis, and in over 90% of urine specimens from patients with cystitis.

When specimens are collected from areas of the body where there is a normal bacterial flora, the microscopic examination is almost invariably positive for bacteria. The problem is to determine the meaning of such bacteria from a sick patient. Under these conditions, the microscopist looks for other clues to disease such as the presence of white blood cells (pus) in addition to the bacteria. If such cells are present, then it is a reasonable conclusion that the specimen was obtained from the true site of infection in the patient. With this information, the microscopist then begins the careful examination of the bacterial cells in order to interpret the meaning of their presence: do they represent normal bacteria or are they responsible for the infection?

Other useful information can be obtained by microscopic examination of clinical specimens. It is usually possible to distinguish bacterial from fungal infections, to identify animal parasites such as protozoa, and to give clinical management support to physicians who submit tissue biopsies or material from an abscess for examination. In some instances it is even possible to make definite diagnosis, for example, of gonorrhea in males or of primary syphilis in any patient. Use of special stains makes up to 70% of the diagnoses of tuberculosis and Legionnaires' disease possible by microscopy. The use of special stains and fluorescent antibody procedures continues to increase the number of disease agents that can be rapidly detected and identified by microscopic techniques.

Table 2-2 Steps in the Gram Stain

		Results	
Step	**Procedure**	**Gram +**	**Gram −**
Initial stain	Crystal violet for 30 seconds	Stains purple	Stains purple
Mordant	Iodine for 30 seconds	Remains purple	Remains purple
Decolorization	95% ethanol for 10–20 seconds	Remains purple	Becomes colorless
Counterstain	Safranin for 20–30 seconds	Remains purple	Stains pink

the quality of food products or the general sanitary state of a given environment. The more common direct and indirect methods of counting microorganisms are discussed here.

Direct Microscopic Counts

Direct microscopic counting is a quick and relatively easy method of determining approximate numbers of microorganisms. Special counting chambers, such as the Petroff-Hausser chamber (Figure 2-13), have measured grids marked on the surface and a cover slip that is held at a precise distance over the chamber. The space between the **slide** and the cover slip is filled with a fluid containing microbial cells; the number of cells in a specified number of squares of the grid is counted. Because the volume of fluid over

Slide
a thin, rectangular piece of glass used to support material for microscopic examination.

Figure 2-12 *Mycobacterium tuberculosis* stained with the acid fast technique.

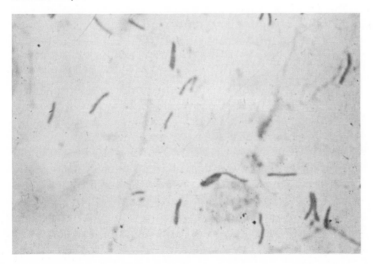

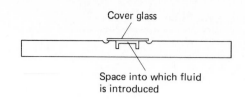

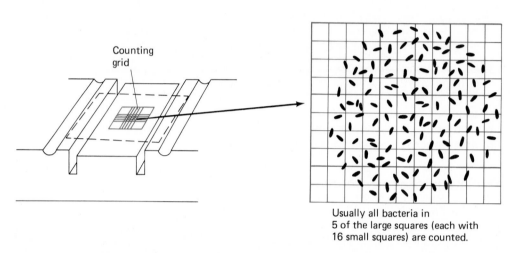

Usually all bacteria in
5 of the large squares (each with
16 small squares) are counted.

Figure 2-13   A Petroll-Hauser cell counter for making direct microscopic counts of the number of bacteria in a fluid.

each square is known, the number of microorganisms per unit volume can be determined. Suspended microbial cells are best seen with a phase-contrast microscope.

Another method of direct microscopic counting is to spread a small known volume of fluid uniformly over a 1 cm^2 area of a slide. The fluid is dried and stained and the number of cells counted with the high-power (40×) lens of a bright-field microscope. This procedure is often used in counting the number of bacteria in milk.

These direct counting methods have certain disadvantages that may lead to inaccuracies: counting both living and dead cells, difficulty of seeing small cells, and inability to count cells in low concentrations.

J. A. Coulter invented an electronic system known as the *Coulter counter* (Figure 2-14), which can be used to directly enumerate bacteria. This counter uses changes in electrical impedance created as the bacteria are drawn through a small opening in an electric field to count the bacteria. Although relatively accurate, the instrument is expensive and requires that the bacterial suspending fluid be absolutely clean and free of all dust or particles

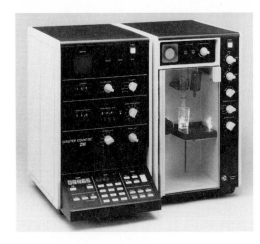

Figure 2-14   Coulter counter model ZM. Used to count human or bacterial cells. (Courtesy Coulter Elecronics, Hialeah)

which, like bacteria, would be counted as they pass through the electric field.

Plate counts   Among the most frequently used methods of counting bacteria are the plate-counting procedures. Such processes are quite accurate in determining the number of living bacteria in a fluid and can measure low concentrations of cells. One method of obtaining plate counts is the *spread-plate method*. For this procedure the fluid to be examined is spread evenly over the surface of a bacterial growth medium. After incubation for 24 to 48 hours, colonies develop where each **viable** bacterium was deposited. The number of colonies is then multiplied by a dilution factor to give the original concentration of cells per milliliter. Another process is the *pour-plate method* in which a measured volume, usually 0.1 or 1.0 ml, of test fluid is mixed with a melted **agar** medium that has been cooled to 48° C. The agar is then poured into a **petri plate,** where it solidifies. The bacteria are trapped in the agar and each viable organism develops into a colony after incubation for 1 or 2 days.

The number of bacteria is so great in many samples that if undiluted samples were plated directly, the many colonies would fuse to form a solid layer of bacteria and the number could not be determined. It is necessary in most cases to dilute the sample before plating. The dilution technique is illustrated in Figure 2-15. The original sample is diluted through a series of tubes; using separate agar plates, 0.1 to 1.0 ml is added to an agar plate from each tube. The colonies are counted on those plates that produce between 30 and 300 colonies. These numbers have been shown to give the most reliable indication as to the correct number of cells. The number of cells in the original undiluted sample can be determined by making the proper multiplication of the number of colonies counted in a known volume at the known dilution.

Viable
living or capable of being alive.

Agar
an extract of seaweed, which is semisolid at room temperature and is used as a growth support medium in the cultivation of microorganisms. A variety of nutrients can be added to the agar to grow specific organisms.

Petri plate
a small circular dish with a close-fitting lid used to cultivate microorganisms.

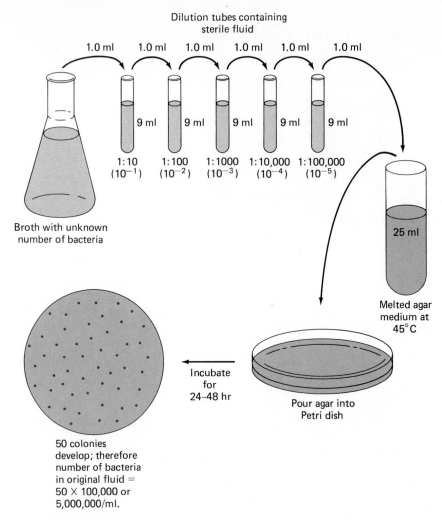

Figure 2-15 Determining the number of bacteria in a broth sample by serial tenfold dilutions and pour plates.

Indirect Counting Methods

When repeated microbial counts must be made from the same type of liquid, as is often the case in research projects or industrial processes, an indirect method of determining the approximate number of cells can be used. The most frequently used indirect measurement is to determine the degree of *turbidity* produced in the broth by bacterial growth. The amount of turbidity is directly proportional to the mass of cells present and hence indirectly proportional to the number of cells. The amount of turbidity can be accurately measured by placing a tube of the microbial culture in an instrument called a *spectrophotometer,* which electronically measures the amount of light that is able to pass through the fluid. A turbidity reading can be correlated with a reference number obtained by doing spread-plate counts at different intervals during the growth at the same time that the turbidity is determined (Figure 2-16). Once this curve is obtained, estimates of the number of cells from similar cultures can be quickly made with the spectrophotometer.

Environmental Sampling

In many areas, such as a hospital environment, it may be important to know how many bacteria are present in the air, on a surface, or in a fluid. It is necessary to maintain environments with

Figure 2-16 Estimation of the number of bacterial cells based on the amount of turbidity as measured with a spectrophotometer. Sample A is clear broth and shows 100% light transmittance. Sample B has moderate cell concentration and sample C has a heavy cell concentration; they allow decreased amounts of light transmittance proportional to the number of cells.

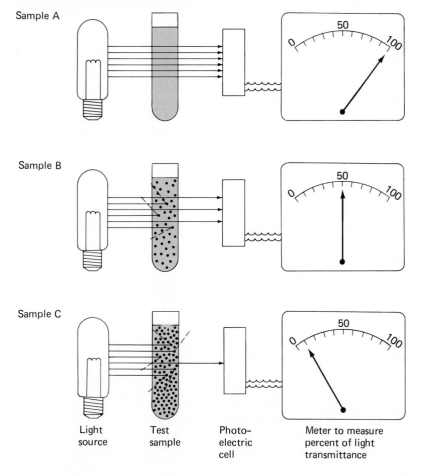

Sample A

Sample B

Sample C

Light source   Test sample   Photo-electric cell   Meter to measure percent of light transmittance

very low numbers of microorganisms in such hospital areas as operating rooms, nurseries, intensive care units and protective isolation rooms. Various procedures are used to control microbial contamination in these areas, and several air and surface microbial sampling techniques have been developed in order to monitor the effectiveness of these procedures.

Air sampling   One of the simplest methods to detect airborne microorganisms is to expose open petri plates containing nutrient agar to the air for a specified length of time. This is called the *settling plate method*. A certain percentage of the microbes in the air settles onto the surface, and after incubation colonies form that can be readily counted. Settling plates give only approximations of the actual number of bacteria present. More precise results are obtained with *impaction air samplers*. Impaction samplers draw a given volume of air through a series of limiting openings so that the velocity of air is increased to a point where airborne particles are impacted onto nutrient agar surfaces (Figure 2-17). The number of colonies developing on the agar surface gives a fairly reliable count of the number of airborne microorganisms in the sampled air.

Surface sampling   The two most common surface sampling methods are *swabbing* and *contact plates*. Swabbing procedures are used for uneven surfaces, corners, or crevices. The swab is prepared by firmly twisting a material like nonabsorbent cotton over one end of a wood applicator stick and then sterilizing it. In order to take a sample, the tip of the swab is rubbed slowly and thoroughly over a measured surface area three times. The swab is returned to a known volume of solution and vigorously rinsed. Next, a measured sample of the solution is assayed by the spread- or pour-plate method. About 50% of the bacteria on a surface is picked up via the swabbing method.

Another process that is also about 50% efficient involves the RODAC-type plate (*RODAC* is an acronym for *r*eplicate *o*rganism *d*etection *a*nd *c*ounting) and is the most widely used method of contact sampling (Figure 2-18). Sampling with these plates, however, is primarily limited to flat surfaces. RODAC-type contact plates are disposable plastic plates that are filled with an agar medium to form a 25-cm (2-in.) -square convex surface above its sides. A contact sample is taken by pressing the surface of the contact plate on the surface to be sampled for several seconds. The contact plates are then covered and incubated. The number of bacterial colonies that develop can be directly counted on the surface of the plate. When sampling surfaces have been treated with chemical disinfectants, which would inhibit bacterial growth, neutralizers, such as lecithin or Tween 80, must be added to neutralize any chemical that might be transferred to the agar surface.

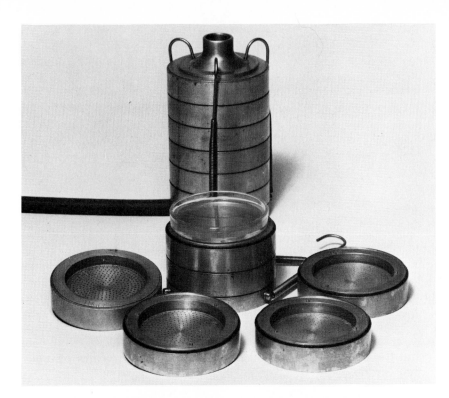

Figure 2-17 The Andersen cascade impaction air sampler. This sampler consists of six metal stages (assembled in background and partially disassembled in foreground) each pierced with 400 holes. The holes in the top stage are larger (far left) and become progressively smaller through to the bottom stage. A petri dish containing nutrient agar is placed under each stage and air is drawn through the unit at the rate of 28 liters per minute. Airborne bacteria are impacted onto the agar surfaces, and as the velocity of air increases as it flows through the progressively smaller holes in the descending stages, the larger particles are impacted onto the upper plate and the progressively smaller particles onto the sequential lower plates. This sampler resembles the respiratory tract, where larger particles are impacted in the upper regions and smaller particles are impacted in the lower region.

RODAC plates are commonly used to directly monitor the bacterial contamination of burn wounds. Used as described, they are less destructive of the injured tissue than swabbing procedures.

Sampling of fluids When fluids may contain moderate to large numbers of microorganisms, counts can be made by the spread- or pour-plate methods, using appropriate dilutions. If very small concentrations of bacteria are present, as is often the case with drinking water, the bacteria may be concentrated by passing a measured volume through a membrane filter that will retain the bacteria. This filter is then placed on the surface of an agar plate

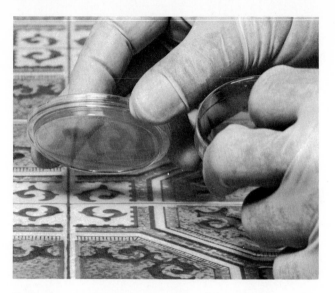

Figure 2-18   A rodac-type contact plate being used to collect a surface sample off a floor.

and the bacteria trapped on the filter will grow to form colonies that can be counted.

CONCEPT SUMMARY

1. A number of laboratory procedures and tools have proven invaluable in the development and understanding of microbiology. There is a variety of microscopic systems which use either visible light or electrons as sources of illumination. Microscopy has provided understanding of cell structure and has also been used to define cell composition and function.

2. A variety of procedures are available to enumerate microorganisms. Direct counting methods usually depend on growth of the organism; indirect systems rely on the detection of any of several cell components by use of scientific instruments.

STUDY SUMMARY

1. Why isn't it possible to increase the useful magnification of a light microscope by any desired amount such as 5,000× or 10,000×?

2. List four possible advantages of the light microscope as compared to the electron microscope.

3. List two possible advantages of the electron microscope as compared to a light microscope.

4. Contrast the uses of a simple stain with the uses of a differential stain for light microscopy.

5. A researcher counted the number of bacteria in a suspension by direct microscopic methods and by plate counting. It was determined that there were 6.7×10^8 bacteria per milliliter by direct counting but only 5.3×10^6 bacteria per milliliter by plate count. Explain the possible basis of difference in these two results.

6. The principle of counting bacteria by indirect methods is based upon what premise?

REFERENCES FOR FURTHER STUDY

1. *The Use of the Microscope,* P. Gray, 1967. McGraw-Hill.

2. *Microbiology for the Allied Health Professions,* A. Delaat, 1973. Lea and Febiger.

3. *Theory and Practice in Experimental Bacteriology,* G. Meynell, 1970. Cambridge University Press.

THE SCOPE OF MICROBIOLOGY

The cell is the basic unit of all living systems and each cell contains the unique components of life. Life forms exist either as multicellular forms or as single cells. The multicellular forms such as familiar plant and animals consist of millions of cells of diverse types that function together and depend on each other. In contrast, microorganisms are single-cell life forms; each cell is an individual and is able to carry out the biological functions necessary to perpetuate itself. Because most single-celled life forms can be seen only with the aid of a microscope, they are called *microorganisms* and are the primary subjects of microbiology. The total number of individual microorganisms is staggering and far exceeds the number of all other forms of life combined. Microorganisms have adapted such that they are able to grow in diverse environmental niches (Table 3-1). For example, within the digestive tract of humans or other animals, as many as 10^{10} microorganisms may be present in 1 gram of fecal material, and 1 g of fertile topsoil may contain more than 10^9 microorganisms. Yet other environments may be relatively free of microorganisms; for example, outside air may contain less than one microorganism per liter or a clean surface exposed to sunlight may contain no viable microorganisms.

The environments to which microorganisms have adapted are diverse and, in some cases, extreme. Certain microorganisms grow in hot springs at temperatures above the boiling point, whereas others are able to grow on snow banks and have been found in environments as hostile as those of Antarctica. Microorganisms often have a profound effect on their surroundings and are responsible for many essential biological phenomena that ensure the maintenance of balanced life systems on the earth. By and large, the overall effect of microorganisms on other life forms is beneficial. Without microorganisms other life on this planet would probably be unable to survive. Although this textbook deals

Table 3-1 Common Habitats Where Bacteria Are Present

Habitat	Approximate Number of Bacteria
Garden soil (surface)	9.7×10^6/g
Garden soil (30 cm deep)	5.7×10^5/g
Lake water (shallow)	10^4/ml
Lake water (deep)	10^2/ml
Seawater	1.1×10^3/ml
Human skin	10^6/sq cm
Human mouth	10^7/ml
Human intestine	4×10^{10}/g
Milk	10^3 to 10^6/ml
Cheese	10^8/g
Sunlit surface	Few
Air	Few

primarily with microorganisms that cause diseases in humans, it is also important for readers to be aware of the ecological role of microorganisms in general. This chapter briefly introduces the various groups of microorganisms and nonmedical microbiology.

BASIC CELL TYPES

Life forms are composed of one of two basic cell types: *eucaryotic* or *procaryotic*. Generally, eucaryotic cells are larger and more complex than the procaryotic cells and possess a membrane-enclosed nucleus; *eucaryotic* means "true nucleus" (*eu* = true; *karyon* = nucleus). All plants, animals, fungi, protozoa, and algae are composed of eucaryotic cells. Only the microorganisms classed as bacteria and cyanobacteria are procaryotic cells. Procaryotic cells have no nuclear membrane and therefore lack a true nucleus. The Latin prefix *pro* means "early" and in this instance suggests the somewhat primitive nuclear structure found in bacterial cells.

Eucaryotic organisms are sometimes simply referred to as *eucaryotes* and the procaryotic microbes as *procaryotes* (Figure 3-1). The morphology of these cell types is discussed in greater detail in Chapter 4. The differences between eucaryotic and procaryotic cells are of more than academic interest to the medical microbiologist. Much of the rationale in the treatment of many microbial infections capitalizes on these differences, a concept that will be expanded in subsequent chapters.

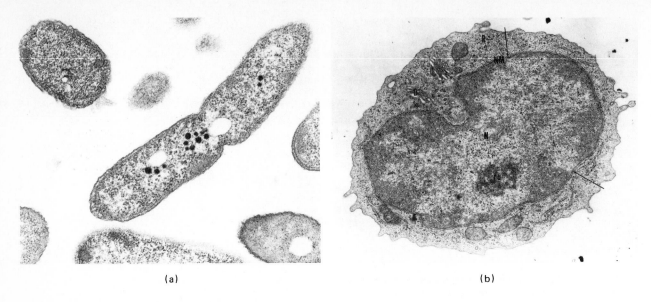

(a)   (b)

Figure 3-1 Electron micrographs of (a) procaryotic cells, and (b) eucaryotic cells (× 19,000). Note absence of nucleus in procaryotic cells.

CLASSIFICATION OF MICROORGANISMS

Classification of microorganisms, and all other forms of life, is an endeavor to arrange the various life forms into related groups. *Taxonomy* is the term used when referring to the science of classification. All biological classification schemes start out with major divisions (kingdoms) and move down through a series of progressively smaller and less inclusive categories. The smallest category (species) is one in which all members are alike in all or most major characteristics. The various taxonomic categories used by biologists are defined in Table 3-2. While these taxonomic categories have been very useful in helping the biologist organize the myriads of life forms, the system is somewhat idealized as applied to bacteria.

The most useful system of classification is one that makes use of known or implied genetic relationships and places every known living organism into a "family tree." Such a system is

Table 3-2   The Taxonomic Categories of Living Organisms

Kingdom (major division)
  Phylum (groups of related classes)
    Class (groups of related orders)
      Order (groups of related families)
        Family (groups of related genera)
          Genus (groups of related species)
            Species (living organisms that are alike)

called a *phylogenetic* classification (Figure 3-2) and shows evolutionary relatedness. Because of the extremely poor bacterial fossil record, however, the classification of these organisms is largely based on apparent relatedness as demonstrated by similarities of function and appearance. This is known as a **phenetic** or *phenotypic* classification. Unfortunately, a phenetic system is not perfect and the classification of microorganisms has been extremely unstable. With the discovery of new microorganisms or new phenotypic properties of an old species, the phenotypic classification of the entire microbial world is subject to change. This problem was evidenced when, in 1980, the International Committee on Systematic Bacteriology agreed to reduce the accepted number of named species of bacteria from more than 30,000 to about 2500 species.

Phenetic
based on the visible features of organisms and their apparent ability to modify their environment.

Figure 3-2   A "family tree" showing phylogenetic relationships among some plants and animals. The basis of the relationships is the amino acid composition of a protein common to each of the organisms.

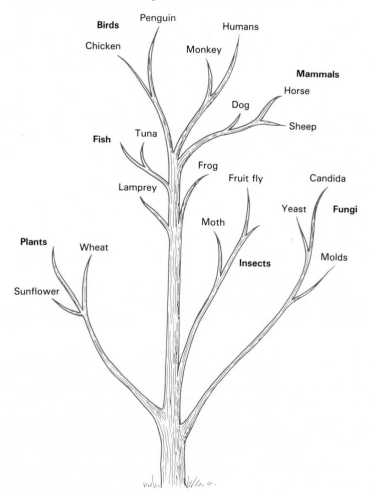

Attempts at a more realistic (genetic) classification of bacteria have recently been more successful than in previous decades. Rather than depending on gene expression (phenotype) to characterize bacteria, present-day microbial taxonomists can use the tools of the molecular biologist to assist in this difficult problem. Specifically, three genetic techniques have been used to show relationships among the bacteria. The first of these examines the deoxyribonucleic acid (DNA) of each organism to compare the concentration of the nucleotide bases guanine (G) plus cytosine (C) (referred to as the G + C content) found in the chromosome of one organism to the G + C content of other bacteria. Two organisms would be considered closely related if their G + C contents were similar. A second molecular genetic technique depends on the complementary pairing of DNA molecules from two organisms (DNA homology). It is possible to bring together the DNA from two separate microorganisms in such a way that they "stick" or anneal together. The tightness of the bond between the DNA from the two organisms is directly proportional to the closeness of their taxonomic relationship. Thus, by doing DNA homology comparisons among many bacteria, it has been possible to construct a useful family tree for these microorganisms. A third technique, and in some a ways a more useful analysis of species relatedness, involves a comparison of the ribonucleic acid (RNA) found in the **ribosomes** of each organism. This technique has allowed the determination of relationships even among very distantly related species.

Ribosome
a ribonucleic acid–protein complex used by cells for the synthesis of new protein.

Nomenclature

Following the recommendations of the great biologist Carl Linnaeus, a system of *binomial nomenclature* is used in which a dual scientific name is given to each biological species and includes both the *genus* and the *species* name of the organism. These names are given in Latin, or are Latinized forms, and are usually descriptive or honorary. The species *Pasteurella multocida*, for example, has a genus name to honor Louis Pasteur, who discovered this bacterium, and the species name *multocida* because it is able to infect the cells of many different animal hosts. Likewise, the species *Neisseria gonorrhoeae* has a genus name that honors Albert Neisser, who discovered this bacterium, and a species name that indicates it is the causative agent of gonorrhea. When a species is mentioned repeatedly in the same report, the genus name is written out in full the first time but thereafter is abbreviated to its first letter (e.g., *P. multicida, N. gonorrhoeae*). By agreement, the genus name is always capitalized and the species name is in lower case, and because of their Latin origins both names are either underlined or italicized. Often a common name may be used in general

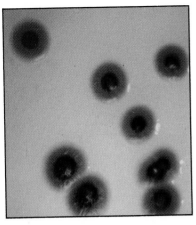

10. Colonies of *Salmonella* (see Chap. 24) growing on Hektoen agar. (Courtesy *Laboratory Medicine*,vol.16, no. 8)

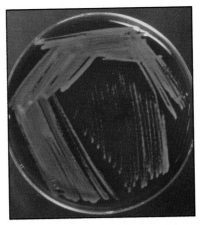

11. Culture of Campylobacter (see Chap. 26) on blood agar plate.

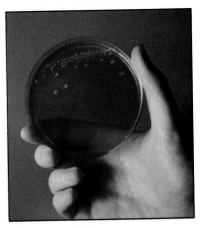

12. *Escherichia coli* growing on Mac-Conkey agar (see Chap. 24).

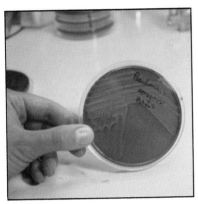

13. *Pseudomonas aeruginosa* (see Chap. 25) growing on blood agar.

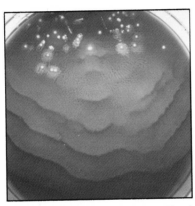

14. *Proteus vulgaris* swarming on blood agar.

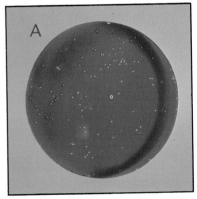

15. *Bordatella pertussis* growing on Bordet-Gengou agar (see Chap. 23).

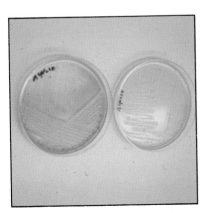

16. *Vibrio cholerae* (see Chap. 26) growing on TCBS (left) and MacConkey (right) agar.

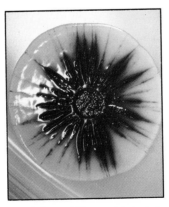

17. Colony of *Chromobacterium violaceum* on nutrient agar. (Courtesy J. A. Shapiro)

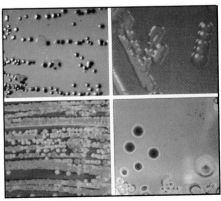

18. Growth of Enterobacteriaceae (see Chap. 24) growing on four different selective enteric agars. (Courtesy *Laboratory Medicine*, vol. 15 no. 4)

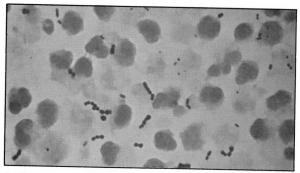

1. Gram stain of specimen from patient with streptococcal pharyngitis (see Chap. 16).

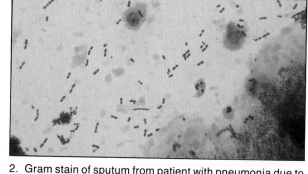

2. Gram stain of sputum from patient with pneumonia due to *Streptococcus pneumonia* (see Chap. 17).

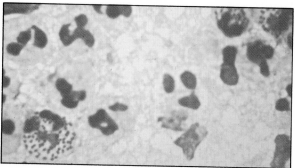

3. Gram stain of pus from urethra of patient with gonorrhoea (see Chap. 18).

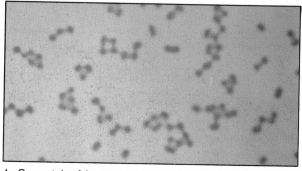

4. Gram stain of the coccobacillus *Acinetobacter calcoaceticus* (see Chap. 25).

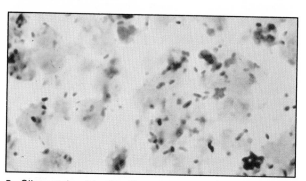

5. Silver stain of *Legionella pneumophila* (see Chap. 27).

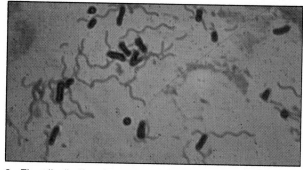

6. Flagella (Leifson's) stain of *Salmonella* (see Chap. 24).

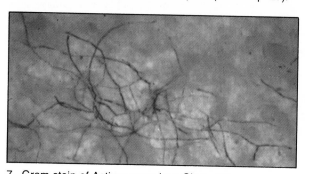

7. Gram stain of Actinomyces (see Chap. 22).

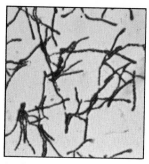

8. Gram stain of *Corynebacterium* (see Chap. 21).

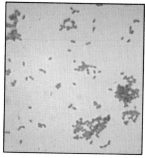

9. Gram stain of *Bacteroides melaninogenicus* (see Chap. 20).

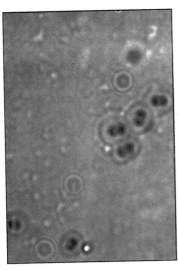

28. Positive quellung reaction (see Chap. 17).

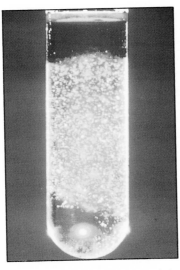

29. Growth of anaerobic bacteria in broth medium.

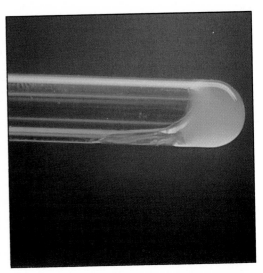

30. Positive staphylococcal (see Chap. 15) tube coagulase test.

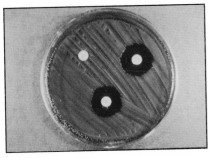

31. Inhibition of bacterial growth by anti-biotics which diffuse into medium from paper disks (see Chap. 9).

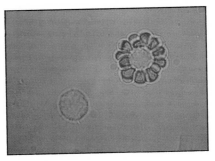

32. Rosette of red blood cells surrounding T-cell lymphocyte (see Chap. 12).

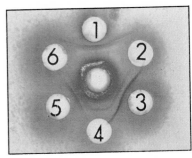

33. Positive (1, 3, 5) and negative (2, 4, 6) immunodiffusion tests (see Chap. 13).

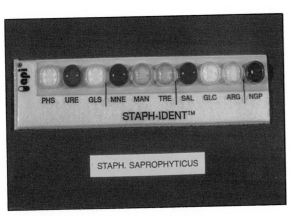

STAPH-IDENT™

PHS URE GLS MNE MAN TRE SAL GLC ARG NGP

STAPH. SAPROPHYTICUS

34. Rapid staphylococcal identification procedure based on interaction of bacterial enzymes with chromogenic substrate (see Chap. 4).

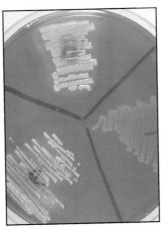

35. Positive (pink) and negative tests for DNAse production by bacteria.

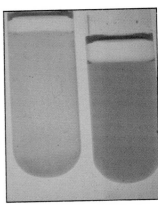

36. Positive (left) and negative (right) sugar fermentation tests.

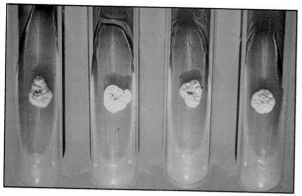

19. *Nocardia* (see Chap. 22) species growing on nutrient agar slants.

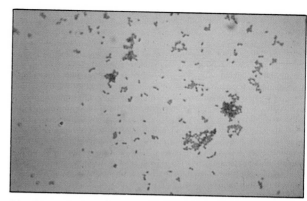

20. Gram stain of *Bacteroides fragilis.*

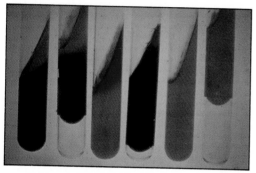

21. Biochemical reactions occurring on triple sugar iron agar (see Chap. 24).

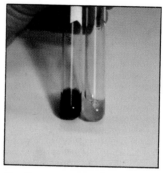

22. Positive (left) and negative (right) phenylalanine deaminase test (see Chap. 24).

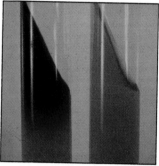

23. Positive (left) and negative (right) bile-esculin reaction (see Chap. 16).

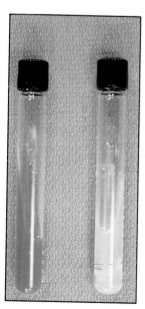

24. Positive (left) and negative (right) urease reaction (see Chap. 24).

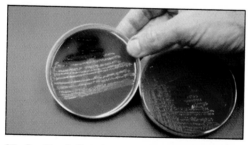

25. Positive (left) and negative (right) oxidase reaction (see Chap. 18).

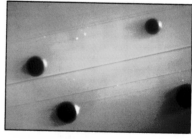

26. Colonies of *Bacteroides melaninogenicus.*

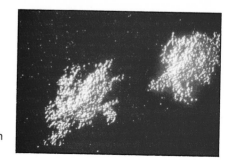

27. Colonies of *Clostridium tetani* on blood agar.

references to a given bacterium. For example, *N. gonorrhoeae* may be called the gonococcus.

In order to achieve uniform naming of microorganisms, an International Code of Nomenclature of Bacteria has been adopted by microbiologists in all parts of the world. Even so, occasional changes in nomenclature are proposed that are not accepted by all of them. In order to assure some degree of uniformity, all names must be published in the *International Journal of Systematic Bacteriology* to be properly recognized. A periodically updated publication called, *Bergey's Manual of Systematic Bacteriology* serves as the standard reference source for the classification and naming of bacteria.

Early classification schemes divided all forms of life into either the plant or the animal kingdom. As early as 1866 Ernst Haeckel, a German biologist, recognized that microorganisms could not readily be classified into either the traditional plant or animal kingdom because they shared properties of both kingdoms. He proposed the addition of a third kingdom to be called Protista ("first life"), which would contain all single-celled microorganisms. Subsequent studies demonstrated that the bacteria were remarkably different from other protists and a separation of the procaryotes (bacteria) from the protists (Table 3-3) is now generally accepted. The following list represents a current general agreement regarding microbial classification. Proposals have been made to divide microorganisms into the following three kingdoms:

1. *Kingdom Procaryotae* (also called Monera in one scheme), which contains the procaryotes—that is, the cyanobacteria, which are photosynthetic microbes (formerly classified as blue-green algae)—and the bacteria (including the rickettsiae and chlamydiae)

2. *Kingdom Protista,* which consists of the protozoa and the microscopic algae.

3. *Kingdom Fungi,* which consists of the molds and yeasts.

Table 3-3 Taxonomic Kingdoms

Kingdom	Members
Animalia	Multicellular animals
Plantae	Multicellular plants
Fungi	Molds, yeast, and mushrooms
Protista	Protozoa and microscopic algae
Procaryotae	All procaryotic microbes

Viruses, subcellular microbiological agents, do not fit well into this classification scheme, but are often listed separately close to the bacteria for convenience.

MAJOR GROUPS OF MICROORGANISMS

The purpose of this section is to give a brief overview of the characteristics of the major groups of microorganisms, with an emphasis on nonmedical areas. The medical aspects will be covered in later chapters.

Fungi

The fungi (singular *fungus*) are a large group of nonphotosynthetic, plantlike eucaryotes, including such diverse organisms as yeasts, molds, and mushrooms (Figure 3-3). Yeasts are globular-shaped cells about 10–30 μm in diameter that multiply by budding. They are best known for their use as a leavening agent for bakery goods and for their ability to produce alcohol.

Molds are organisms that consist of masses of branchlike filaments called *hyphae* and are most frequently recognized by their fuzzy growth on various foods and other organic matter. Reproduction in fungi usually results from the formation of large numbers of seedlike structures called *spores*. These spores, which are usually asexual structures, enable the organism to withstand det-

Figure 3-3   Three different types of fungi. The mushroom is close to natural size. The bread mold and yeast are greatly enlarged.

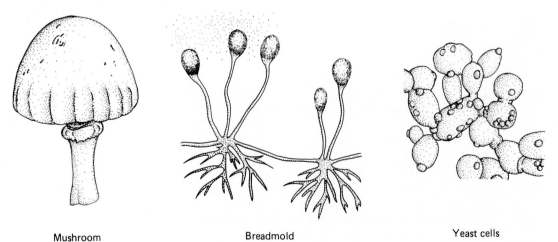

Mushroom   Breadmold   Yeast cells

rimental environmental conditions, thus ensuring species survival. Interestingly, even though sexual reproduction is used as the basis of fungal classification, the sexual stages are often difficult to find. Mushrooms, although not microscopic in size, are actually complex arrangements of single, independently functioning cells that have the appearance of multicellular structures. Fungi are widely distributed in nature and because they are not **photosynthetic** they readily grow in dark, damp places where organic matter is found. Only a relatively small number of molds and yeast is able to cause disease in humans (see Chapter 30). A large variety of fungal species can cause diseases in plants and lower animals, however, and have a significant impact on reducing the world's food supply.

The most notable function of fungi is their ability to decompose **organic** matter. They secrete powerful enzymes that dissolve such food sources. When moisture is present and other environmental factors are not extreme, fungi grow on a wide variety of organic substances. Organic matter in contact with the soil is rapidly decomposed by fungi as part of the natural, essential recycling process in nature. Such products as foods, paper, lumber, fabrics, paint, and rubber can all be decomposed by fungi. This decomposition process may be either beneficial or detrimental depending on the circumstances; for example, the decomposition of dead plants in the soil is beneficial whereas the decomposition of lumber stored for building is detrimental. Human societies spend a great deal of time and effort to treat and store materials so that they will not be damaged by fungal growth; even so, large quantities of foods and other materials are lost each year due to fungi. On the other hand, some by-products of fungal growth have commercial value and large-scale industrial fermentation processes produce such fungal products as antibiotics, alcohols, cheeses, and solvents.

Photosynthetic
capable of using light to provide one's requirement for energy.

Organic
composed of carbon and hydrogen. Organic molecules are characteristic of living organisms and often include a variety of elements such as oxygen and nitrogen.

Algae

Algae (singular *alga*) are a large morphologically and physiologically diverse group of eucaryotic micro- and macroscopic organisms (Figure 3-4). All contain chlorophyll, which allows them to carry out photosynthesis. This process results in the production of both energy-containing compounds and gaseous oxygen. Many algae occur as single cells, ranging in size from less than 1 μm to upward of 60 μm in diameter. They may be shaped as spheres, rods, or spindles. Others occur in multicellular colonies that are often visible to the naked eye and take on a wide variety of shapes. Some, such as seaweeds, grow to great sizes and appear much like multicellular plants.

The presence of chlorophyll gives diverse pigmentations to the algal cells and this characteristic is used in their classification.

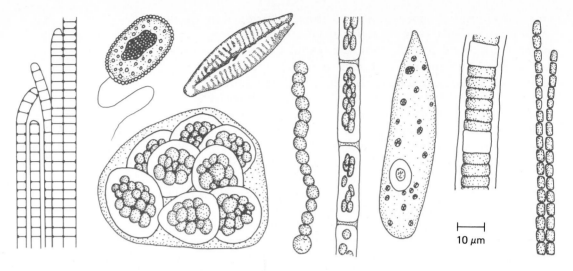

Figure 3-4   Different species of algae and cyanobacteria reproduced to scale (see 10 μm bar).

Toxin

a poisonous substance produced
by a living organism. Microbial
toxins are among the most
poisonous substances known.
Toxins are frequently responsible
for the characteristic symptoms
associated with infectious
diseases.

Along with their scientific names, they are also referred to as
yellow-green, green, red, or brown algae. One major group, the
blue-greens, have recently been discovered to be true procaryotes
and as such are now classed as bacteria with the name *cyanobacteria*. Thousands of different species of algae exist and are found
in most moist environments. Many algae are free-living in waters;
others grow in soils or on the surfaces of plants and rocks. The
wide diversity of algae is reflected by the fact that some grow on
ice or snow whereas others are able to grow in hot springs. The
only human health problem commonly associated with algae is
the result of their ability to produce **toxins** that may be consumed
by aquatic animals, such as shellfish. When algae levels are high,
during the summer months, enough toxins may be retained in the
shellfish that they cause illness when eaten by humans.

Because algae are involved in many biological cycles and are
important contributors to the overall balance in nature, they play
important roles in the well-being of humans and most other forms
of life. They are a primary source of atmospheric oxygen, they aid
in soil fertility by adding organic matter, and some species are able
to fix atmospheric nitrogen. Some algae are harvested from the
sea and used directly as human or animal food. *Agar*, a solidifying
agent used in microbial culture media or as a thickening agent in
various foods, is extracted from seaweeds. Currently a great deal
of interest is being shown in the mass culture of algae as a direct
source of food. Large numbers of algae are found in oceans, seas,
lakes, ponds, and streams. Small free-floating algae make up a
part of the life forms referred to as *phytoplankton*. Plankton (Figure
3-5) are at the beginning of the food chain in aquatic environments
and are often consumed by small aquatic animals (zooplankton),

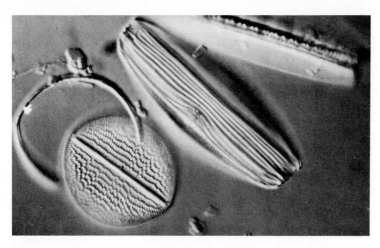

Figure 3-5 Fresh water phytoplankton. Photo is by phase contrast microscopy. (Courtesy Dr. S. Rushforth, Brigham Young University)

which, in turn, are eaten by small fish, which are eaten by larger fish, and so on. Some larger aquatic animals, such as the blue whale, eat plankton directly. Essentially all sea and freshwater animals depend on the presence of algae for food. Algae are found in most bodies of water and in depths up to 180 meters. The amount of organic matter resulting from the photosynthesis occurring in algae in aquatic environments exceeds the amount of similar materials produced from all plants on terrestrial surfaces combined.

Protozoa

The protozoa (singular *protozoan*) are a group of microorganisms that are animallike in their structure and function. They are eucaryotic cells and possess many intracellular components that are characteristic of higher forms of life (Figure 3-6). It is suspected that the protozoa may have evolved from the algae through the loss of chlorophyll-containing structures which has resulted in unicellular, nonphotosynthetic protists. Protozoa vary considerably in their size and shape and have some form of active locomotion. The mechanisms by which they move (flagella, cilia, ameboid) are major factors in the classification of these organisms.

The smallest protozoa are only a few micrometers in diameter whereas others may be seen with the unaided eye. Protozoa are able to ingest food particles by folding their outer membrane around the food and then pinching off the membrane to form an intracellular vacuole, a process known as *phagocytosis*. Protozoa thrive in moist environments. They inhabit most bodies of water, are found in soil, and live in the digestive tract of many higher forms of life. Because of their relatively large size and motility,

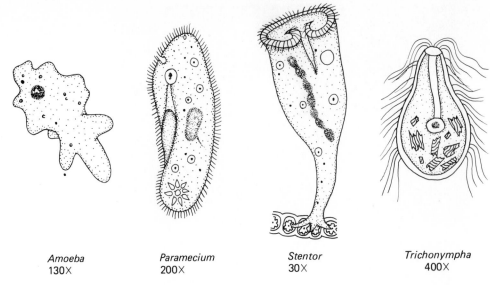

Amoeba	Paramecium	Stentor	Trichonympha
130×	200×	30×	400×

Figure 3-6   Four different types of protozoa with degrees of enlargement indicated.

protozoa are easily seen by the microscopic examination of water from such sources as stagnant ponds. Protozoa have a moderate influence on water quality and on the various biological cycles in nature. While the majority of the protozoa do not cause diseases in higher forms of life, those that do are responsible for two of the most common and serious illnesses: malaria and African sleeping sickness.

Procaryotes

There are three major groups of procaryotes: *archaebacteria* (meaning "primitive" bacteria), *cyanobacteria*, and *eubacteria* ("true bacteria"). The archaebacteria are not true procaryotes, but are more closely related to this group than they are to eucaryotic cells. They include three groups of bacteria: the extreme *halophiles* (salt-loving bacteria), the *thermoacidophiles* (acid-loving bacteria, which grow at high temperatures), and *methanogens* (bacteria that produce methane gas). These organisms share both physiologic and morphologic properties that distinguish them from procaryotes. The unique chemical structures associated with the archaebacteria have led scientists to speculate that eucaryotic cells evolved from this group of organisms. None of the archaebacteria are currently associated with human disease.

The cyanobacteria are photosynthetic bacteria formerly referred to as the *blue-green algae*. These organisms are distinguished from other photosynthetic procaryotes by their ability to produce gaseous oxygen as a product of photosynthesis. They differ from algae in that their chlorophyll is associated with a stack of membranes located just inside the cell membrane, and not in specialized organelles (chloroplasts). Procaryotes that are neither archaebacteria nor cyanobacteria are all classified with the eubacteria.

Eubacteria are procaryotes and are both smaller and less complex than eucaryotic cells. Normally, bacteria have rigid cell walls and are shaped as spheres, rods, or helices (Figure 3-7). Bacteria are found in virtually every environmental habitat and some types have adapted to grow on minimal nutrients or under extreme environmental conditions. Some, for example, are able to grow on simple inorganic compounds, others in hot springs, in cold storage food, or on the bottom of the ocean under extreme pressure; still others grow in areas completely devoid of oxygen. Most bacteria multiply through a process known as *binary fission* whereby a cell simply divides into two daughter cells. Under proper conditions, growth may be very rapid with cell division occurring as often as every 12 to 15 minutes. This rapid growth may lead to profound changes in the surrounding environment. Although many important infectious diseases of humans are caused by bacteria, most bacteria are not able to cause disease and many bacteria produce beneficial environmental changes, such as the decomposition of waste products, aiding in soil fertility, or the production of useful chemicals.

Two groups of small (0.3 to 0.5 μm in diameter) bacteria, called *rickettsiae* and *chlamydiae*, are able to multiply only inside living eucaryotic cells. Because of their small size and dependency on living host cells (characteristics that are also shared by viruses), the rickettsiae and chlamydiae have in the past been grouped next to or with the viruses. It is now well established that the rickettsiae and chlamydiae have definite cellular structures and are best considered small obligately parasitic bacteria. Because of their dependency on living host cells, they have no direct influence on

Figure 3-7 Bacterial cells showing representatives of the three basic cell shapes.

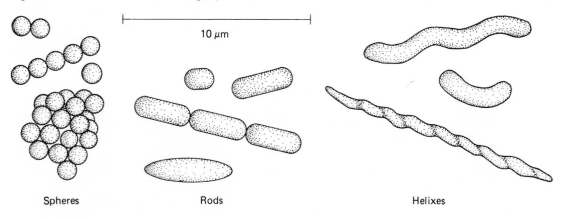

10 μm

Spheres   Rods   Helixes

the outside environment. Nevertheless, these microbes can cause some important human diseases.

Viruses

Viruses are a unique type of biological agent. The organisms described previously are complete cells with the capability of carrying out **metabolic** activities and other functions of life. Viruses, however, are not cells and have no independent metabolic activity. Viruses might best be described as independent genes encased in a protein coat. Each virus has a single molecule of nucleic acid, either DNA or RNA; this molecule contains the genetic information necessary for the manufacture of additional virus particles (see Chapter 6). The virus is covered with a coat called a *capsid* that consists of a geometric arrangement of protein molecules. When a virus enters a living cell, the viral genes are released and the information contained in them may be expressed in the host cell. The information on the viral genes may redirect the cell to make virus particles and eventually the cell may be destroyed or altered. The only effects produced by viruses are on the host cells; when found outside host cells, viruses are simply a collection of molecules with no apparent life functions. Viruses range in size from about 25 to 300 nm in diameter. Most viruses have definite geometric forms, the most common being spherical; some of the others are rod-, brick-, bullet-, or tadpole-shaped (Figure 3-8). Every form of life, including bacteria, has specific viruses that are able to infect its cells. Their effect on living cells can be destructive and many common diseases of both plants and animals are caused by viruses.

There are two subcellular structures, *viroids* and *prions*, that behave in a manner similar to viruses but these structures lack protein capsids. Viroids are relatively small RNA molecules that have the capacity to produce disease in plants. The exact mecha-

Metabolic
related to the chemical processes occurring within a cell. Often associated with energy-producing processes.

Figure 3-8   The shapes and relative sizes of various types of viruses that infect animals.

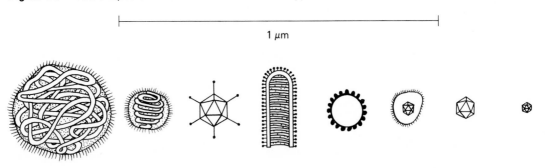

1 μm

Paramyxovirus   Myxovirus   Adenovirus   Rhabdovirus   Coronavirus   Togavirus   Papovavirus   Picornavirus

Clinical Microbiological Specimens

Material sent to the microbiology laboratory for examination is referred to as a *clinical specimen.* Such specimens are obtained from persons who are ill, and come from body materials (secretions, fluids, tissues, exudates, etc.) that are most likely to contain microorganisms of the type responsible for illness in the patient. The responsibility of the microbiology laboratory is to discover disease-causing microorganisms that may be present in the clinical specimen. This task is approached by using both microscopic and cultural techniques to isolate and identify the bacteria or viruses that are in the specimen.

Laboratory processing of clinical specimens can be straightforward and relatively simple. This is particularly true when the specimen is from a body site where there are no normal bacteria. Under these circumstances, any organism that is observed through the microscope or that grows when cultured, likely represents an organism that is associated with the disease. The situation is far more complex when the specimen is from a body site such as the mouth, intestinal tract, skin, or reproductive tract where there is a normal microbial population in healthy persons. Under these conditions, a disease-causing organism may be hidden among the many microbial species that are normally present. To make an appropriate judgment as to the significance of each kind of organism in such a specimen takes much skill and understanding of microbial processes.

There is an additional problem relating to interpreting the significance of microbes that are present in clinical specimens. This problem is created when the individual collecting the specimen for examination is not careful, and contaminating microbes are accidentally collected along with the specimen. Under these conditions, it is almost impossible for a microbiologist to determine whether isolated organisms represent the cause of infection or simply contamination. For example, if a culture of cerebral spinal fluid (which is normally sterile) grows a staphylococcus, the assumption is made that the staphylococcus must play a significant role in the patient's illness. However, if the staphylococcus is a contaminant from the skin, its presence in the specimen would only lead to a misleading diagnosis.

Health care personnel need to be aware of the problem of determining the significance of microbes in specimens sent to the laboratory and ensure that they will aid in the diagnosis rather than confuse the laboratory results. While any specimen may be contaminated, those obtained through puncture of the skin or from a body site near a mucosal surface are most likely to be contaminated. Strict procedures must be followed by individuals collecting specimens if useful laboratory data are to be obtained.

nism by which they carry out this function is unknown. Prions are protein molecules that have been studied as the possible cause of a disease in sheep known as *scrapie.* Little is known about these particles but prions may be responsible for human neurologic diseases such as kuru and Creutzfeldt-Jakob disease.

NONMEDICAL ASPECTS OF MICROBIOLOGY

Most of the material in this textbook will deal with medical microbiology; yet microorganisms are used or play an important role in various other areas. This section briefly discusses several nonmedical aspects of microbiology.

Soil Microbes

Most microbes occur in the upper 0.5 meter of soil, and 1 g of fertile farm soil may contain as many as 4 to 5 billion microorganisms. These microorganisms are actively involved in the decomposition of organic matter, a vital phase in the natural recycling of the elements needed for living systems. The incorporation of nitrogen, sulfur, and carbon into organic matter by plants would quickly deplete the soil of these essential nutrients if they were not recycled by microorganisms. Environmental nitrogen and sulfur cycles have been studied extensively. Microbes have been discovered to play a major role in both of these essential cycles. The photosynthetic algae add organic matter to the soil by their growth and death. Some bacteria and algae are able to convert (fix) atmospheric nitrogen into a form that can be used by plants. Acids produced by microbes aid in dissolving rocks, an important step in the formation of soil. Both the development and the maintenance of fertile soils is to a large extent the product of microbial activities.

Aquatic Microbes

Microorganisms are found in all bodies of fresh- and saltwater. The numbers and types vary greatly, just as the conditions of the water vary. Some microbes are natural inhabitants of water whereas others are transient, having entered from sewage, land runoff, or other external sources. As in soil, microorganisms are vital links in the recycling of nutrients in the aquatic food chain. Much of the world's food supply is made possible by the activities of these aquatic microbes. Maintaining the proper biological balance of these aquatic systems is one of the great challenges of present-day technology and is essential for the continued survival of most life forms on this planet. The important role of algae in the aquatic food chain was mentioned earlier. An overabundance of algal growth, however, may be detrimental to a body of water; this situation may occur when concentrations of nutrients are high and the water is warm. Such massive growth of algae is called a *bloom* (Figure 3-9). Algal blooms rapidly deplete the available oxygen in the water, resulting in the death of fish and making the water unsuitable for recreational activities. All lakes are slowly fill-

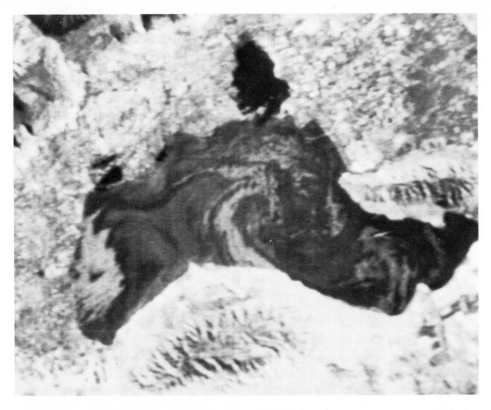

Figure 3-9 A shallow freshwater lake, about 35 kilometers in length and surrounded by mountains, photographed from a space satellite during the summer. The swirls and areas of contrast show massive blooms of algae. (NASA)

ing with sediments and microbial debris which contribute significantly to this process of **eutrophication.** Excess nutrients such as phospate in the water may accelerate the rate of filling, mainly by the increased growth of algae.

In its natural state, water is found either as surface water (lakes, rivers, etc.) or as groundwater, which must be obtained from wells or from natural springs. Groundwater is the most common source of water used for household purposes and is always contaminated by microorganisms. In order to make such water potable (safe for drinking), it must be treated. Treatment generally consists of two processes: *filtration* and *chlorination*. Most water is first treated by sand filtration to remove debris and most microorganisms. Water that has been adequately filtered is then rendered completely safe for human use by the addition of only 0.5 part per million of free chlorine. Chlorine kills those organisms that might have passed through the filtration process and inactivates any that might somehow enter the water system following treatment. Because water can serve as an important vehicle for the

Eutrophication

the process by which a body of water becomes so rich in dissolved nutrients that the resultant algal growth depletes the water of oxygen supplies needed by other organisms.

transmission of disease-causing microorganisms, proper water treatment is an essential aspect of public health.

A second important aspect of proper municipal water management is associated with adequate treatment of waste water. This water is normally collected into extensive sewage collection systems and then carefully processed at a wastewater treatment facility. In these treatment facilities harmful microorganisms are again filtered from the water, solid waste materials and undesirable molecules are removed, and oxygen may be added back to the water by aeration. Water that has been properly treated is not dangerous for the environment and may be returned to the surface water system. Microorganisms are used to decompose organic matter, one of the significant steps in wastewater treatment. Water may serve as an important vehicle for the transmission of disease-producing microorganisms. The proper treatment of water for human consumption and the treatment of sewage are of vital importance in maintaining a healthy environment.

Microorganisms in Dairy Products

Microbial contamination
the addition, usually unintended, of viable bacteria to a previously microbial-free environment, or the addition of unwanted organisms to an environment that contains known or desirable microorganisms.

Milk provides an excellent medium for the rapid growth of many types of microorganisms and great care is needed during the collection and processing of milk to minimize **microbial contamination.** In general, the quality of milk is directly related to the numbers and types of microorganisms it contains; thus the dairy industry spends considerable time and money on controlling microorganisms.

Bacterial contamination of milk comes from two major sources: *external,* the contamination of milk after it has been collected, and *internal,* the contamination of milk directly from an infected cow. Either source of contamination may lead to serious human infection and requires the careful handling of fresh milk and proper animal husbandry for dairy cattle. It is almost impossible to prevent some microbial contamination of milk at the time that it is collected. If left unrefrigerated, bacteria quickly multiply and the milk sours. The number of bacteria present in fresh milk is greatly reduced by the process of *pasteurization.* This procedure, first applied by Louis Pasteur to the manufacture of wine (see Chapter 1), raises the temperature of the milk to 71.5°C for 15 seconds or 90°C for 0.5 second. These temperatures are sufficient to destroy all disease-producing organisms commonly found in fresh milk and render it safe for human use. However, these procedures do not destroy all bacteria that may be present in milk, and even pasteurized milk will quickly spoil if not kept under proper refrigeration. When pasteurization is combined with storage at low temperatures, the storage time of milk is greatly increased.

Testing for adequate pasteurization is accomplished by

means of a *phosphatase test*. Phosphatase is an enzyme, found in milk, that is destroyed through the process of pasteurization. Thus by testing for this enzyme it is possible to determine whether milk has been properly treated to make it safe for human use.

Certain microorganisms, under controlled conditions, induce desirable changes in milk (Figure 3-10). Dairy items such as yogurt, sour cream, and buttermilk result from the fermentation of milk products through the addition of selected acid-producing bacteria. Cheeses are produced by the controlled growth of selected microorganisms on curdled milk, a process called *ripening*. Different cheeses are produced by the action of different microorganisms.

Microorganisms in Food

Like dairy products, most foods provide excellent media for the growth of many types of microorganisms. Generally, microbial growth in food is undesirable and produces changes in texture and flavor commonly called *spoilage*. Because of their relatively high natural bacterial contamination, certain foods such as fish, poultry, and ground meats spoil easily. Spoilage is not the only concern associated with microbial contamination. Some microorganisms such as *Salmonella* and the virus that causes infectious hepatitis are easily transmitted to humans from some foods. Other bacteria such as *Staphylococcus* and *Clostridium botulinum* produce toxic waste materials when grown in foods. These toxic sub-

Figure 3-10   Some of the dairy products that are produced by the action of microorganisms on milk components.

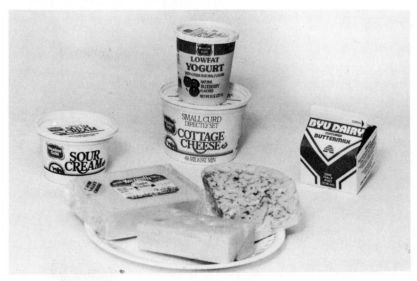

stances can lead to severe illness or even death if they are ingested by an unsuspecting consumer.

Because of such risks, food industries make great efforts to prevent detrimental changes to food by microorganisms. Much of what is done in food processing is directed toward the control of both microbial spoilage and pathogen transmission. Processes such as drying, smoking, salting, freezing, refrigerating, heat processing (canning), and the use of chemical preservatives like sodium benzoate or calcium propionate, are the major methods in preventing or slowing the spoilage of foods. Because of the ever-increasing costs of foods and the limited supplies of certain foods in many countries, reducing waste due to spoilage is increasingly important and offers a challenge to food microbiologists. Some estimates indicate that as much as 25% of the world's food supply is lost to spoilage by microorganisms or by infestation by insects or rodents.

To a limited extent, microbes may be used directly as a food source, such as yeast as a food supplement. The potential for using microorganisms as a food source is great and active research projects are currently underway to develop methods of using the rapid-growth capabilities of microorganisms as a means of producing food substances. When compared to other forms of life, microorganisms are much more efficient producers of proteins. A rapidly growing culture of microorganisms under controlled conditions, for instance, is able to produce as much protein in one day as a meat-producing animal can produce in several weeks. Furthermore, microbes do this in a small space, and often by using waste products or inexpensive organic materials as their food source. This area of research offers a possible means of providing a more adequate food supply for the world's increasing population. Currently the appeal of microorganisms as a basic food for humans is limited. The term *single-cell protein* is used when referring to this type of product to make it sound more appealing. Although most humans are not yet ready to trade their roast beef for "bacterial-protein patties," single-cell protein may become an important food supplement for meat-producing animals that are, in turn, processed for human consumption.

Industrial Uses of Microbial By-products

Many by-products of microbial growth are extremely useful. The field of industrial microbiology uses the action of microorganisms to mass-produce many of these products. In some cases, the useful product can be produced only by microorganisms; in others, the microbial process is the most economical means of production. To be economically feasible, the raw material should be relatively inexpensive and readily available while the end product must be of greater value. These conditions are fulfilled in many processes that have become the basis of large commercial industries. Among the products produced by microorganisms are solvents, organic acids, alcohols (including alcoholic beverages), enzymes, and antibiotics.

The increasing costs and scarcity of petroleum and natural gas have renewed interest in microbial fermentations that can convert plant materials into methane gas and alcohols. These products can then be used for heating or in internal combustion engines. Because plant materials are renewable, these processes could greatly reduce our dependence on nonreplenishable petroleum reserves.

Microorganisms as Biological Tools

Microorganisms are widely used as biological models for scientists who wish to study fundamental principles of living systems. When working with bacteria, it is possible to start with a single cell, which will then replicate so rapidly that within a day trillions of nearly identical cells can be produced. This population of identical cells is much easier to study than is a population of mixed cells that might be obtained from animal or plant tissues. Much of what we know about the biological activities of all cells has evolved through studies of bacteria. Some of these basic biological properties of microorganisms are presented in Chapters 4-7.

It has now become possible to pass some genes from other forms of life into bacteria and from one type of bacterium to another (see Chapter 6). This process, referred to as *genetic engineering* or *recombinant DNA* technology, allows microorganisms to be used in unique ways. One of the first practical developments of genetic engineering was to place the human insulin gene into a bacterium. As this bacterium divided, the insulin gene divided and was passed into each daughter cell. Within a short time trillions of bacteria, each producing human insulin, were available. Consequently, inexpensive human insulin can be produced for the treatment of diabetics. Many other applications of this new technology now being developed will allow common microbial cells to provide new and beneficial products for humankind (Table 1-2).

CONCEPT SUMMARY

1. Microorganisms hold an important place in the world of living things. Although unique in many attributes, these single cells exemplify all the characteristics normally associated with biological systems.

2. The microworld of biology can be divided into several logical major groups. These groups are classified and named according to the systems used for larger life forms. The smallest and simplest forms of these biological structures are the viruses. More complex and larger are the procaryotic bacteria and three groups of eucaryotic microorganisms (fungi, protozoa, and algae) that are often included within the designation *microorganism*.

3. Microorganisms are ubiquitous in their habitat. They are found throughout the world, in, on, and around every conceivable environment. They play a major role in maintaining ecological balance and are often used in procedures that are beneficial to human beings.

STUDY SUMMARY

1. What limitations are associated with a biological classification system that is entirely phenetic?

2. How would you justify a taxonomic proposal that includes both a kingdom Procaryotae and a kingdom Protista?

3. What characteristics of fungi are associated with their ubiquitous presence?

4. Since microscopic algae are rarely involved in human disease, what aspect of these organisms makes them so important?

5. What concerns must be addressed if surface water is to be used for drinking?

6. If all of the bacteria present in milk are not killed during pasteurization, of what value is this process?

REFERENCES FOR FURTHER STUDY

1. *The Microbial World*, 5th ed., R. Stanier, 1986. Prentice Hall.

2. *Microbes, Man and Animals*, A. Linton, 1982. J. Wiley.

3. *Biology: The Unity and Diversity of Life*, 4th ed., C. Starr, 1987. Wadsworth.

4. *Bergey's Manual of Systematic Bacteriology*, 9th ed., N. Krieg, 1984. Williams and Wilkins.

5. Molecular Systematics of Prokaryotes. *Annual Reviews of Microbiology* 37:143. 1983.

chapter 4

CELLULAR ANATOMY

ll cells share some fundamental characteristics in their structural components and biochemical functions. These similarities permit scientists to extrapolate information obtained from the study of one type of cell to other cells, and much of what we know about the biochemical reactions in complex eucaryotic animal cells was first discovered through studies of the simpler procaryotic cells. Still, there are many differences between cell types, particularly between procaryotic and eucaryotic cells. A knowledge of these differences is essential in understanding why chemical agents can be selectively used to treat particular diseases. Chemicals, like penicillin, that specifically interfere with the function of components that are found in procaryotic cells but not in eucaryotic cells have proven to be effective chemotherapeutic agents in treating diseases caused by procaryotic cells. The following discussion deals with the major cellular components of both procaryotic and eucaryotic cells.

PROCARYOTIC CELLS

Because most procaryotic cells of importance in medical microbiology are *bacteria*, this section is limited to a discussion of bacterial anatomy.

Sizes and Shapes

Bacteria are the smallest independently living cells, with most ranging from 0.25 to 3.0 μm in diameter and 1 to 20 μm in length. Some are slightly larger. The thousands of different species occur in one of only three general shapes: (1) spherical, (2) rod-shaped (cylindrical), and (3) curved (helical) (Figure 4-1).

Spherical bacteria are called *cocci* (singular *coccus*) and each species exhibits one of the characteristic arrangements of cells

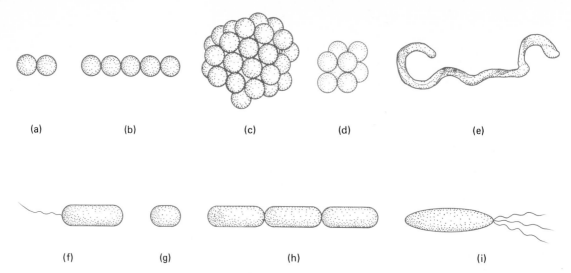

Figure 4-1   Some of the general shapes and arrangements of bacteria: (a) diplococci, (b) streptococci, (c) staphylococci, (d) sarcinae, (e) spirillum, (f) bacillus with monotrichous flagellum, (g) coccobacillus, (h) streptobacillus, and (i) bacillus with lophotrichous flagella.

shown in Figure 4-1. The cylindrical-shaped bacteria are called *bacilli* (singular *bacillus*) or rods; most occur as single cells and not in arrangements like the cocci. However, under some growth conditions, some bacilli also occur in pairs or short chains; some characteristically lie side by side in palisadelike arrangements and others may occur in Y or branching-shaped arrangements. Some bacilli are short, stubby rods between 0.5 and 1 μm in length with a diameter only slightly less than the length. Such cells, especially if they have rounded corners, have an elliptical shape and appear to be as much coccal-shaped as rod-shaped; the term *coccobacillary* is sometimes used to describe this shape. Many bacilli have definite rod shapes with some species being significantly larger than others.

Helical bacteria may be called *spirilla* (singular *spirillum*) whereas others are grouped into the *spirochetes* and usually occur as individual cells. Chains of these organisms rarely occur, however. Many variations exist between species as to length and number and amplitude of spirals.

Components of Procaryotic Cells

Figure 4-2 is a drawing of a composite bacterium showing many of the components found in procaryotic cells.

Cell envelope   Each procaryotic cell is bounded by three or more structures collectively referred to as the *cell envelope*. This envelope differs in both complexity and composition between Gram-

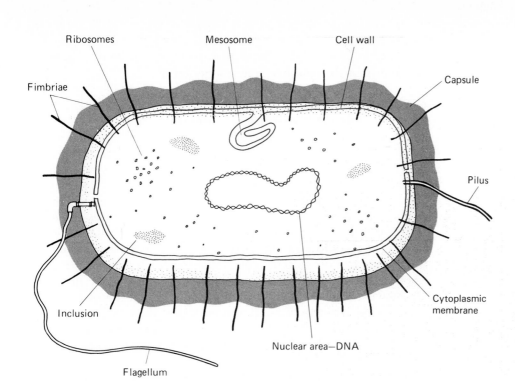

Figure 4-2 A schematic diagram of a composite procaryotic bacterial cell.

positive and Gram-negative bacteria. The Gram-negative envelope is a complex structure including an inner membrane (cytoplasmic, plasma, or cell membrane), a relatively thin **peptidoglycan** layer, and a complex outer membrane composed of
protein, lipid and **polysaccharide.** External to these structures
Gram-negative bacteria frequently have a capsular layer composed of a complex polysaccharide. The space between the outer
and inner membranes is referred to as the *periplasmic space*. The
periplasmic space contains peptidoglycan and a number of enzymes that assist the cell in digesting large, nontransportable molecules into smaller, absorbable molecules. Some of the proteins
found in the periplasmic space assist the cell by binding directly
to molecules used by bacteria as food. Some antibiotics, such as
the penicillins, are also bonded by proteins found in this region
of the cell. The somewhat simpler Gram-positive envelope consists of the inner cytoplasmic membrane, a thick peptidoglycan
cell wall layer, and a **capsule.**

Two types of cell walls are found among the different species
of bacteria and divide bacteria into one of two staining types called
either *Gram-positive* or *Gram-negative*. The *Gram stain*, a cell-stain-
ing procedure developed by Dr. Christian Gram, is used to differentiate the two types of cell walls. Briefly, when subjected to the
Gram stain, the Gram-positive cell walls retain a crystal violet-

Peptidoglycan

a large, complex molecule
primarily made up of acetylated
sugars. This compound is found
only in bacteria and forms the rigid
structural portion of their cell wall.

Polysaccharide

a very large sugar molecule.
Polysaccharides may be composed
of any number of smaller sugars
called *monosaccharides.*
Polysaccharides are often used as
structural building material by the
cell.

Capsule

an amorphous material produced
by bacteria and collected around
the outside of the cell. Most
capsules are polysaccharide
complexes, some are protein.
Capsules are usually hydrated
(contain water) and are protective.

iodine complex whereas the Gram-negative cell walls do not. The use of Gram stain is discussed in more detail in the clinical notes at the end of this chapter and in Chapter 5.

Cell wall   The bacterial cell wall is a unique and important structure. No comparable structure is found in any animal cell, and the cell walls found in higher plants have a different chemical structure. The bacterial cell wall is rigid and gives shape to the cell. Because bacterial cells are directly exposed to the external environment, the cell wall provides a necessary protection for the cell. Bacteria often live in fluids that contain relatively low concentrations of ions (atoms with positive or negative charges) whereas the inside of the cell (cytoplasm) contains high concentrations of ions. Water is drawn to the area of high ionic concentration and thus tends to flow into the cell. This situation creates an osmotic pressure inside the cell of up to 20 times atmospheric pressure. Because the internal osmotic pressure of bacterial cells is relatively high, these cells would swell and burst if it were not for the support of the rigid cell wall. The cell wall is also necessary for cell division. Cell walls are porous and allow the free passage of fluids and small molecules.

   A structure common and unique to both Gram-positive and Gram-negative bacterial cell walls is a large, insoluble chemical structure called *peptidoglycan* (sometimes called *murine* or *mucopeptide*). Peptidoglycan forms a coarse, layered, rigid meshwork that surrounds the cytoplasm and maintains the shape of the cell. A layer of peptidoglycan consists of two types of alternately joined molecules called *N-acetylglucosamine* and *N-acetylmuramic acid* that form long chains. A cell wall may have many such layers. The layers are joined together by short chains of four amino acids (tetrapeptides) that connect above and below with N-acetylmuramic acid and also connect with other short side chains of amino acids that cross-connect the long chains of the peptidoglycan structure (Figure 4-3).

   A number of biologic activities are associated with the cell wall. Each bacterium organizes its cell wall structure in a unique way making its wall different from those of other bacteria. This difference is used by bacterial viruses (bacteriophages; see Chapter 32) as selective attachment sites leading to infection of the bacterial cell. These chemical structures also are antigenically distinct (refer to Chapter 12), making it possible for the host's immune system to distinguish one bacterium from another. The response to these **antigens** often provides the host with the means of resisting repeated infection by the same bacterial species. The type of cell wall possessed by a bacterium may influence the types of clinical signs and symptoms seen in an infection caused by that bacterium; for example, the lipopolysaccharide components of Gram-negative cell walls have toxic effects on infected animal hosts and

Antigen
a chemical that can stimulate antibody production in an animal. Antigens may vary in size but are usually large molecules, and they have unique structure, such that antibodies formed against an antigen will recognize and bind specifically only with that antigen. Proteins and polysaccharides are usually antigenic.

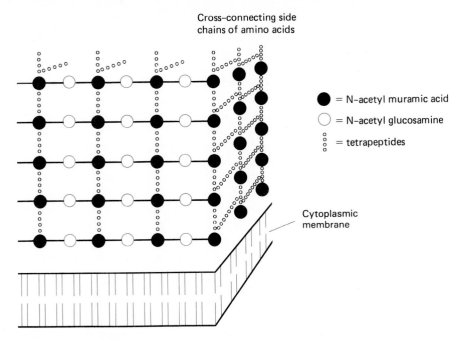

Cross-connecting side
chains of amino acids

● = N-acetyl muramic acid

○ = N-acetyl glucosamine

tetrapeptides

Cytoplasmic
membrane

Figure 4-3   Schematic diagram of Gram-positive cell wall with multiple layers of peptidoglycan.

cause such signs of disease as fever, diarrhea, and shock. These lipopolysaccharides are called *endotoxins* (Chapter 14) and play an important role in the disease-producing capabilities of Gram-negative bacteria.

The cell walls of Gram-positive bacteria may consist of up to 40 layers of peptidoglycan that may form as much as 50% of the cell wall material. Gram-positive cell walls may also contain polysaccharides (complex sugars) and teichoic acids. Teichoic acids appear to be made up of a variety of different type sugar, lipid, and amino acid molecules and are major surface antigens for some Gram-positive bacteria. Like the *N*-acetylmuramic acid and *N*-acetylglucosamine in peptidoglycan, the chemical units of the teichoic acids frequently repeat, forming long chains of interconnected molecules. Some bacteria have teichoic acids primarily connected with the cell wall, and in all Gram-positive bacteria some form of lipoteichoic acid is chemically attached to the cytoplasmic membrane.

The Gram-negative cell wall is more complex than the Gram-positive wall. It contains a thin, rigid inner peptidoglycan component, not more than two layers thick, that constitutes only 5% to 20% of the total cell wall materials. Outside this peptidoglycan layer is an *outer membrane* composed of lipoproteins (large molecules of lipid and protein complexes) and lipopolysaccharides (large molecules of lipid and sugar complexes) associated with a typical double-layer, phospholipid-type membrane (see cytoplasmic membrane, below). The arrangement of these various components in the Gram-negative cell wall is shown in Figure 4-4. The outer membrane forms the major part of the Gram-negative cell wall.

Much scientific research has been centered on the structure of the Gram-negative cell wall. The outer membrane is a lipoprotein bilayer very similar to that of the cytoplasmic membrane. The outer membrane is held in place by abundant lipoprotein molecules and contains a variety of important *outer membrane proteins* (OMPs). The OMPs have a variety of functions including bacteriophage attachment, participation in bacterial conjugation (see Chapter 6), and transport of selected molecules into the cell through porin-type OMPs.

A major difference between Gram-positive and Gram-negative cell walls is the presence of *lipopolysaccharide* (LPS) in the latter. LPS is a relatively complex molecule (Figure 4-5) consisting of three parts. All LPS molecules consist of a lipid-polysaccharide structure known as *lipid A*. The **lipid** portion of this molecule is an integral part of the outer membrane, although the exact arrangement of atoms in this molecule varies from one bacterial species to another. Attached to the outer portion of lipid A is a "core" polysaccharide. This portion of LPS includes a number of unusual

Lipid

synonym for *fat*. Lipids are important structural molecules and are abundant in biological membranes.

Figure 4-4   Schematic diagram of Gram-negative cell wall.

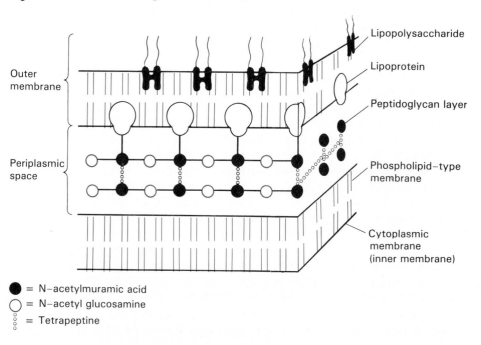

Outer membrane

Periplasmic space

Lipopolysaccharide

Lipoprotein

Peptidoglycan layer

Phospholipid–type membrane

Cytoplasmic membrane (inner membrane)

● = N–acetylmuramic acid
○ = N–acetyl glucosamine
⦙ = Tetrapeptine

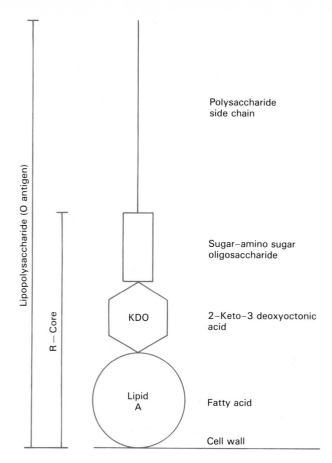

Figure 4-5 Schematic diagram of lipopolysaccharide of Gram-negative bacteria. Antigenic specificity is associated with the terminal polysaccharide. Endotoxicity depends on the lipid A end of the molecule.

chemical structures such as ketodeoxyoctulonate and is in turn attached to a number of repeating sugar molecules such as rhamnose and galactose.

Whether the wall is Gram-positive or Gram-negative may also determine the response of bacteria to certain antibiotics. The classic example is penicillin, which selectively interferes with the formation of the amino acid cross-linkages of the peptidoglycan meshwork when new cells are being formed during cell division. Without the cross-linkages, the cell wall is weak and ruptures; this condition results in the death of the bacterium in most environments. Because the major component of Gram-positive cell walls is peptidoglycan, most Gram-positive bacteria are highly susceptible to penicillin. On the other hand, the peptidoglycan layer forms only a small portion of the Gram-negative cell wall and is covered with the thick outer membrane. The outer membrane hinders penicillin from reaching the peptidoglycan; even with some damage to the peptidoglycan layer, the other components may hold the cell wall together. Therefore penicillin is not effective in treating infections caused by many Gram-negative bacteria. Because animal cells have no peptidoglycan, they are unaffected by penicillin.

As noted earlier, the high internal pressure of bacterial cells requires the support of the cell wall in order to prevent cell rupture. However, if the cell is placed in a solution with a high **osmotic pressure** (e.g., a sucrose solution) it is possible to remove the cell wall without subsequent rupture of the inner membrane. Such living, wall-free structures are referred to as *protoplasts, spheroplasts* or *L-forms* (Figure 4-6). These wall-free cells can be produced by preventing peptidoglycan synthesis with the antibiotic penicillin, or by removal of existing wall material by treating the cells with an enzyme know as *lysozyme* (see Chapter 11). If a small amount of cell wall remains, as with spheroplasts, the bacteria can build new walls when the inhibitor is removed. Cells with no remaining peptidoglycan are not able to construct new cell walls, even in the absence of inhibitor. It is believed that the cell wall material acts as a self-primer, and that new cell wall construction depends on a preexisting structural pattern.

Capsule   Some bacteria produce a slimy or gel-type material that adheres to the outside of the cell wall. It forms a layer around the cell that is called a *capsule* (Figure 4-7). Most, but not all, capsular

Osmotic pressure

pressure on a semipermeable membrane created by unequal concentrations of molecules on the two sides of the membrane

Figure 4-6   Phase contrast photomicrograph of *Mucor racemosus* spheroplast. Note the absence of a cell wall. (Courtesy F. Genthner *et al.*, *J. Bacteriol.* 134:349)

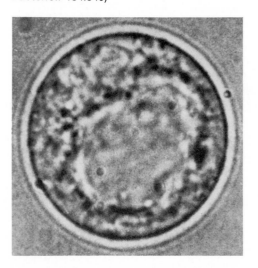

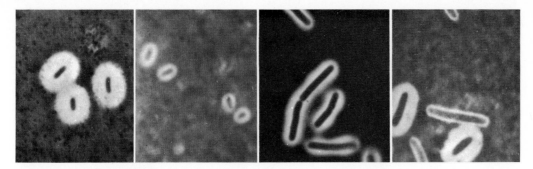

Figure 4-7 Various sized capsules present on different species of the genus *Bacteroides*; magnified 1000 to 1200 x. (J. L. Babb and C. S. Cummins, *Inf. Imm.* 19:1088-1091, Figure 1, with permission from ASM)

materials are polysaccharides (Table 4-1), which are synthesized by enzymes located at the surface of the cells. The capsule often slows the rate at which white blood cells are able to ingest (phagocytize) the bacteria that have invaded the tissues of an animal. The capsule gives the bacteria a greater opportunity for survival and thus a better chance to cause disease. The disease-producing capabilities of some bacteria are directly related to the presence of a capsule. In large amounts this material is termed a *glycocalix* (Figure 4-8) and is important in providing a natural growth environment for some cells. The glycocalix gives some bacterial cells the ability to adhere to a variety of surfaces such as tooth enamel.

Flagella Flagella (singular *flagellum*) are long, hairlike appendages, composed of the protein *flagellin,* that extend out from some bacterial species (Figure 4-9). They are present in many species of bacilli, on some spirilla, but on very few species of cocci. Flagella are attached to the cytoplasmic membrane by a small hook at the end of the structure and are able to rotate rapidly. Flagellin is organized into small aggregate structures that in turn are organized into hollow cylindrical structures (Figure 4-10). Flagella use energy derived from an ion concentration gradient in order to move, and therefore intact flagella that have been removed from the bacterial cell are still capable of rotation.

Table 4-1   Composition of Bacterial Capsules

Type of Capsule	Composition	Organism
Polysaccharide	Glucose-glucuronic acid	*Streptococcus*
Dextran	Glucose	*Leuconostoc*
Colanic acid	Various sugars	*Enterobacteriaceae*
Cellulose	Glucose	*Acetobacter*
Polypeptide	Glutamic acid	*Bacillus*

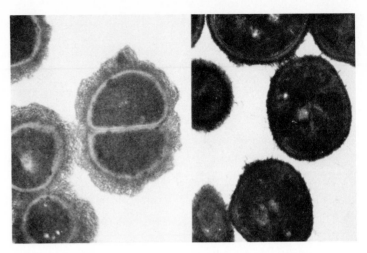

Figure 4-8 Staphylococcus with large glycocaylix (left) and without glycocaylix (right). (Courtesy G. Christensen. *Infect. Immunity* 37:318)

The rotation of some flagella has been measured at over 2000 rpm. This movement propels the bacterium through fluids. Some bacteria are able to move 30 times the length of their cell in one second; such directional movement of bacteria requires a large amount of available energy. The complexity of the flagella attachment mechanism, as well as the structure itself requires a major genetic commitment on the part of a bacterium. Often, upwards of 35 genes are necessary for the formation and operation of these structures.

The term *trichous*, which means "hairlike," is used when referring to the arrangements of flagella on bacterial cells (Figure 4-1). Certain bacteria have only a single flagellum and are called *monotrichous*; some have tufts of flagella and are called *lophotrichous*; still others have flagella protruding from all areas of the cell and are called *peritrichous*.

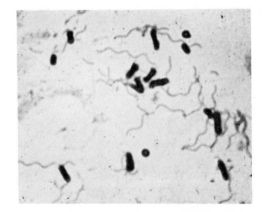

Figure 4-9 Bacteria stained with a flagellan stain. Flagella appear as wavy, threadlike structures.

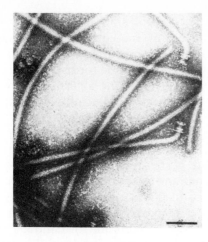

Figure 4-10 Electron micrograph of negatively stained flagella removed from *Salmonella typhimurium.* Bar represents 100 nm. (Courtesy T. Suzuki et al. *J. Bacteriol* 133:904)

Fimbriae and pili The structure of the fimbriae (Latin for "fingers") and pili (Latin for "hairs") is similar in some ways to flagella, but these structures are not associated with motility. Fimbriae and pili are short, hairlike structures that project out from the cell wall. They are present on some bacterial species but not on others. Fimbriae are quite numerous over the entire surface of a bacterium and function as attachment sites between the bacterium and other surfaces. (Figure 4-11). The ability of some bacteria, such as some streptococci and *Neisseria gonorrhoeae,* which causes gonorrhea, to attach to and infect certain tissues is partly a function of their fimbriae. Pili are generally longer than fimbriae and often one or a few may be present on the surface of a bacterium. Certain viruses that infect bacteria (bacteriophages) specifically attach to pili and inject their nucleic acid into the bacterial cell through these hollow structures. Some pili are involved in a bacterial mating process (conjugation) in which they form a tube between two bacterial cells through which DNA may pass. The terms *fimbriae* and *pili* were used interchangeably in the past; however, the preceding definitions are now recommended to distinguish between the two functional types of short, hairlike appendages.

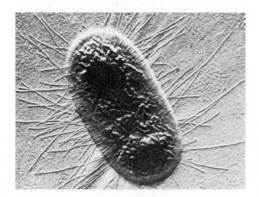

Figure 4-11 Electron micrograph of fimbriae associated with *Escherichia coli.* (Courtesy S. Knutton et al. *Infect. Immunity* 44:514)

Cytoplasmic membrane The cytoplasmic membrane, (*cell membrane* or *plasma membrane*) is a thin, fragile membrane located just inside the cell wall; it completely surrounds the internal cellular components (Figure 4-12). This membrane forms a functional barrier between the inside of the cell and the external environment. Numerous essential biological functions including the synthesis of cell wall materials, the excretion of enzymes (exoenzymes) essential to the nutrition of the cell, and the determination of selective permeability and transport of nutrient and waste products into and out of the cell are carried out by the activities of these membranes. The cell membrane is the physical site of essential energy-producing chemical reactions such as electron transport (Chapter 5), and is the site of enzymes necessary for DNA replication, cell wall synthesis, and new membrane formation. The structure of the cytoplasmic membrane is similar in both procaryotic and eucaryotic cells. The functional integrity of this membrane is essential for the survival of the cell and any process or chemical that disrupts its structure or function causes the death of the cell. Several chemicals that function as disinfectants (Chapter 8) have an effect on this membrane.

The cytoplasmic membrane is only 7 to 10 nm in thickness and consists primarily of phospholipids and proteins. The phospholipid molecules have one end that is soluble in water, or **hydrophylic** (Greek *hydro* = water; *philus* = loving), and another end that is insoluble, or **hydrophobic,** (*phobia* = fear); this situation causes these molecules to form a typical double-layer unit mem-

Hydrophilic

capable of dissolving in water. Table sugar is an example of a hydrophilic compound.

Hydrophobic

incapable of dissolving in water. Oil is an example of a hydrophobic substance.

Figure 4-12 Electron micrograph of a plant cell showing numerous membrane enclosed structures, Golgi, nuclear membrane and cell membrane (× 40,000). (Courtesy W. M. Hess, Brigham Young University)

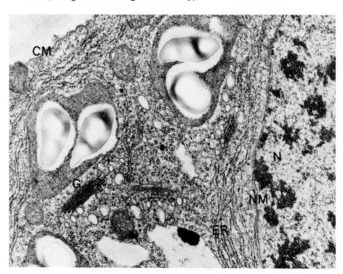

brane with the hydrophilic ends pointing out and the hydrophobic ends pointing inward (Figure 4-13). Protein islands are embedded throughout the phospholipid matrix (Figure 4-14). These proteins are essential for transport of *solute* (dissolved materials) across the membrane and into the cell. Two types of transport are possible: *passive*, which does not require the use of energy to obtain the solute (e.g., water transport), and *active*, which requires that the cell use energy to obtain the solute (e.g., transport of sugar). Protein-enzyme systems called *permeases*, located in the membrane, are involved in both types of transport. Thus a cell that does not have a permease for a specific nutrient is not able to bring that substance across the membrane and into the cell.

Several essential metabolic reactions occur at the bacterial cell membrane (which acts as the functional equivalent of the **mitochondria** found in eucaryotic cells). Therefore, the cell membrane is an essential component of the energy-producing system for bacteria and is an essential part of the process by which **adenosine triphosphate (ATP)** is made available to the cell (see Chapter 5).

Many bacteria contain an invaginated and highly convoluted section of cytoplasmic membrane called *mesosome* (Figure 4-15). Certain mesosomes are thought to be involved with the formation of new cross walls that form when the cell divides, and are often considered to be the site of chromosome (DNA) attachment. Replication of DNA, discussed in Chapter 6, may be initiated by growth-related changes in the membrane.

Cytoplasm All components inside the cytoplasmic membrane are collectively referred to as *cytoplasm*. In all procaryotic and eucaryotic cells, much of the cytoplasm is made up of proteins, nucleic acids, carbohydrates, and lesser amounts of other substances suspended in fluid. Certain anatomically distinct structures called *organelles* are found in the cytoplasm and will be briefly described.

Mitochondria
eucaryotic organelles in which most of the energy-producing chemical reactions take place.

Adenosine triphosphate (ATP)
a molecule containing two high-energy chemical bonds. When either of these chemical bonds are broken, energy is released for use by the cell. These bonds are formed from energy made available from food. ATP acts as "energy currency."

Figure 4-13 The macromolecular phospholipid subunits which are part of bio-membranes. (b) Arrangement of phospholipid molecules in membrane.

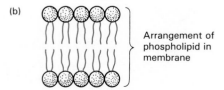

(a) Hydrophilic (phosphate) end

Hydrophobic (fatty acid) end

(b) Arrangement of phospholipid in membrane

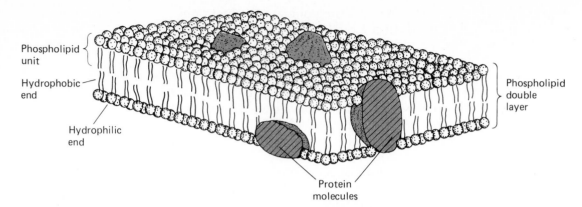

Figure 4-14 Cross section of a cytoplasmic membrane composed of two layers of phospholipid units with their hydrophilic ends pointing to the outside and their hydrophobic ends pointing to the center of the membrane. Protein molecules are "floating" in the "fluidlike" phospholipid membrane.

Ribonucleic acid (RNA)

one of the two kinds of nucleic acid. This molecule differs in structure from DNA but is complementary to DNA in function. In some viruses, RNA (not DNA) is the chromosome.

RIBOSOMES Ribosomes consist of protein and **ribonucleic acid (RNA)** with up to 10,000 ribosomes present in each cell; they are involved in the important function of protein synthesis. Ribosomes are about 20 nm in diameter and are made up of two unequal-sized lobular subunits, a 30-S and a 50-S component (Figure 4-16; the S refers to *Svedberg units,* also known as the *sedimentation constant,* which is determined by the rate that particles can be sedimented in a centrifuge). The two subunits are separated when not involved with protein synthesis. The smaller of the two subunits

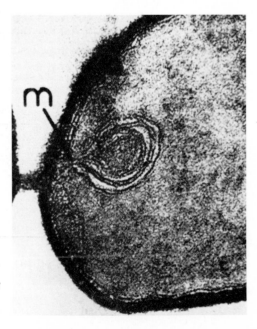

Figure 4-15 Bacterial mesosome (m) as seen with electron microscopy. (Courtesy A. Ryter and O. Landman. *J. Bacteriol* 88:457)

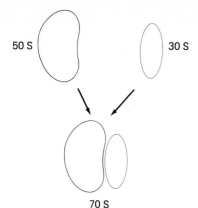

50 S

30 S

70 S

Figure 4-16 The two components of ribosomes that combine to form a 70 S unit when attached to *m*RNA during protein synthesis.

is composed of an RNA molecule and several protein molecules and has a "platform" to which a messenger RNA (mRNA) molecule binds immediately prior to protein synthesis (Chapter 6). With the mRNA in place, the larger subunit attaches and forms the ribosome complex. When directly involved in protein synthesis, ribosomes are arranged in aggregates called *polyribosomes* (Figure 4-17; see also Chapter 6). It is possible to separate such particulate cytoplasmic components such as ribosomes from other organelles by the technique of **ultracentrifugation.** Under high gravitational forces exerted by this procedure, particles separate

Ultracentrifugation

centrifugation at very high speeds. At such speeds, even relatively small molecules can be separated from solution. Because organelles are precipitated as a function of their density, it is possible to separate these structures by using different speeds in the centrifuge.

Figure 4-17 Active genes of a rapidly growing bacterium (*E. coli*). As soon as an *m*RNA molecule begins to be transcribed from DNA (presumed initiation site at arrow), ribosomes begin to attach. As the length of the *m*RNA increases, more ribosomes attach forming longer polyribosomes. In procaryotic cells, where the DNA is not separated from the robosomes by a nuclear membrane, translation may begin before the complete *m*RNA is formed and while it is still attached to the DNA. (Bar = 0.5 μm.) (From Hamkalo and Miller, "Electronmicroscopy of Genetic Material," Figure 6a, p. 379. Reproduced, with permission, from *Annual Review of Biochemistry,* Volume 42. © 1973 by Annual Reviews, Inc.)

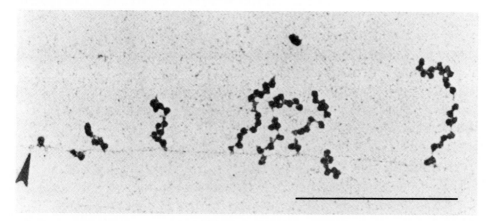

into layers based on their density. The bacterial ribosomes have a density value of 70 S. The 70-S size of the procaryotic ribosome is slightly smaller than the 80-S size of ribosomes of eucaryotic cells, a basic difference that is associated with the ability of the antibiotic streptomycin to selectively combine with the procaryotic ribosome. Consequently, streptomycin can be used as an antibiotic that will interfere with procaryotic cells, but not with eucaryotic ribosome activity.

NUCLEAR REGION The nuclear region is that part of the cytoplasm where the DNA molecule is located (Figure 4-18). Each bacterium possesses a large circular DNA molecule with a molecular weight of about 3×10^9 that contains the genetic information needed by the bacterium. This "chromosome" appears to be attached at one point to the bacterial cell membrane. The absence of a membrane surrounding the nucleus is one of the main characteristics used to distinguish procaryotic cells from eucaryotic cells.

CYTOPLASMIC INCLUSIONS Granules or globules are observed in many bacteria and are collectively referred to as *inclusions*. Many inclusions are aggregates of lipid, sulfur, carbohydrates, or a form of phosphate called *volutin* that can be stored by the cells as reserve food and energy supplies. The volume of the cell that they occupy depends on the growth rate and nutritional state of the cell. Inclusions are not surrounded by membranes but are often made visible by special stains. A form of inclusion called *metachromatic granule* is characteristic of *Corynebacterium diphtheriae* (Figure 4-19; see also Chapter 21).

Endospores Three genera of Gram-positive bacilli, *Bacillus, Clostridium* (Chapter 20), and *Sporosarcina*, are able to form a unique structure called an *endospore* or simply a *spore* (Figure 4-20). These spores are formed inside the bacterial cell, hence the prefix *endo*. The term *vegetative* is used to refer to the actively growing, nonspore stage of a bacterium. Under optimal conditions of growth

Figure 4-18 Electron micrograph of Bacillus species showing nuclear region of cell. Note the absence of a nuclear membrane and the somewhat amorphous nature of the nuclear region. (Courtesy H. Kobayashi et al. *J. Bacteriol* 132:262)

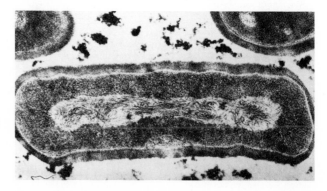

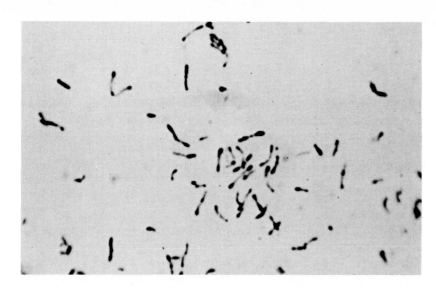

Figure 4-19   Gram stain of bacteria with metochromatic granules. These granules give the cells a rough or irregular staining appearance. (Courtesy Centers for Disease Control, Atlanta)

the vegetative bacteria multiply with or without the formation of spores; that is, the spore is not a necessary step in replication. When growth conditions become unfavorable, such as when nitrogen or an energy source is limited, the formation of endospores is stimulated. One spore develops per cell and forms a dormant, resistant stage for the cell. Bacterial spores are the most stable form of life; consequently, special efforts must be made to destroy them in order to achieve sterile conditions. These structures pose special concerns for medical and industrial microbiologists.

The great environmental stability of the bacterial endospore appears to be related to two major factors, the dehydrated state of the spore and the presence of a unique chemical known as *dipicolinic acid*. Dipicolinic acid is not found in any other living organism. The mature spore is highly resistant to destruction by heat or chemicals and may remain dormant for long periods. Some spores

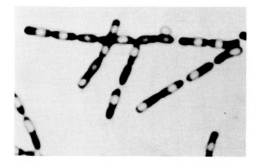

Figure 4-20
Photomicrograph of *Bacillus anthracis* showing endospores (unstained) both within vegetative bacterial cells and free from parental cell. (Courtesy Abbott Laboratories, Chicago)

Germination
the process whereby a bacterial endospore forms a vegetative bacterium.

have germinated—that is, developed back into the vegetative stage—after lying dormant for many years. **Germination** of bacterial spores requires an activation step and an outgrowth process. Activation is accomplished by external damage to the spore coat by heat or mechanical means; outgrowth then occurs if the cell is in a nutritionally favorable environment. The endospore is formed by a sequence of changes called *sporulation*. This process is very complex and involves the activities of a large number of proteins and enzymes. Following initiation, a chromosome near the terminal end of the cell is surrounded by infolding of the cell membrane. In addition to DNA, this membrane-bounded structure includes ribosomes and enzymes that will be needed when the spore germinates to a vegetative cell again (Figure 4-21). This spore "core" is then surrounded successively by a spore wall that contains peptidoglycan (which upon germination will be the nidus of a new cell wall), a relatively thick cortex, and a relatively impermeable proteinaceous layer known as a *spore coat*. Finally, water is removed to dehydrate and mature the spore.

EUCARYOTIC CELLS

Eucaryotic cells are larger and much more complex than procaryotic cells (Table 4-2) Many diverse eucaryotic cells exist, ranging from yeast cells (protists with some similarities to the procaryotic bacteria) to highly specialized cells found in multicellular animals. The major organelles found in eucaryotic cells of animals are shown in Figure 4-22.

Figure 4-21   Major components of a bacterial endospore.

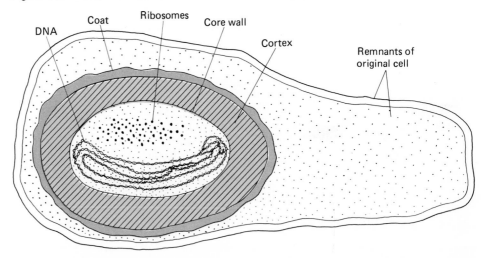

Table 4-2   Comparison of Procaryotic and Eucaryotic cells

Characteristic	Procaryotic Cells	Eucaryotic Cells
Nucleus	Not membrane bound	Membrane bound
Flagella	Submicroscopic	Complex microscopic
Ribosomes	Small (70 S)	Large (80 S)
Cell wall	Complex peptidoglycan	Simple polysaccharide
Mitotic structures	Absent	Present
Chromosomes	Singular-circular, no histone	Multiple with histones
Membrane structures	Mesosome	Endoplasmic reticulum
Endospores	Present	Absent
Membranes	Lack steroids	Contain steroids
Internal membrane-bound organelles	Absent	Numerous; e.g., Golgi, mitochondria, chloroplasts, lysosomes

Components of Eucaryotic Cells

Cell walls Of the eucaryotic cells, only fungi, algae, and plant cells have cell walls. These walls are much simpler than the cell walls of bacteria. Most eucaryotic cell walls are composed of cellu-

Figure 4-22   (a) General eucaryotic cell diagram showing the major cellular components;

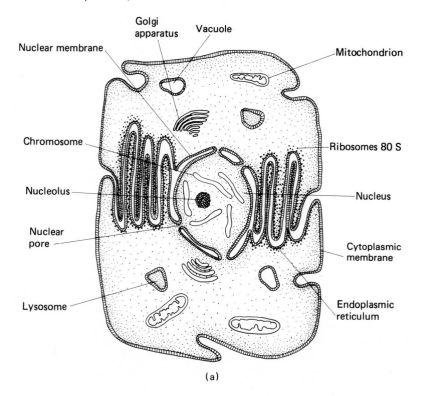

(a)

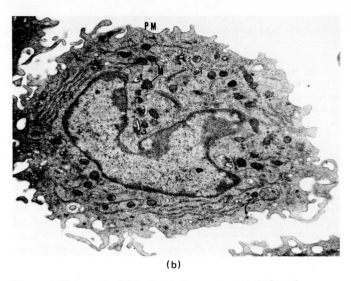

(b)

Figure 4-22 *(cont.)*   (b) (activated mouse macrophage) eucaryotic cell showing nucleus, cell membrane (PM), endoplasmic reticulum, mitochondria and numerous cytoplasmic inclusions (× 14,000).

lose or other carbohydrates. The functions of eucaryotic cell walls are similar to those performed by procaryotic cell walls. Animal cells, lacking cell walls, have a much more irregular shape and are more resilient to external pressures than are cells enclosed within a wall.

Flagella and cilia   Some eucaryotes have flagella or cilia as organs of locomotion. The eucaryotic flagella are more complex than those present on procaryotic cells but perform much the same functions. Flagella, as well as cilia, are composed of microtubules arranged in such a way that as they contract or relax the flagella will bend with a whiplike action. Cilia are structurally similar to the flagella except that they are much shorter and large numbers are usually arranged over the entire surface of the cell (see Figure 17-3). Cilia are found only on some protozoa and some specialized animal cells, such as the ciliated epithelial cells of the respiratory tract.

Cytoplasmic membrane   The cytoplasmic membrane is structurally similar in both procaryotic and eucaryotic cells. Steroid-type lipids are present in eucaryotic cell membranes but not in most procaryotic membranes. The cytoplasmic membrane is the outer limiting membrane of most protozoa (and all animal cells) and it invaginates and convolutes extensively through the interior of the cell to form a structure known as the *endoplasmic reticulum*. The membrane forming the endoplasmic reticulum appears to be continuous with the nuclear membrane. Various membrane-bound vacuoles and organelles (mitochondria, chloroplasts, Golgi apparatus) are located throughout the interior of eucaryotic cells (Figure 4-23).

Vacuoles Vacuoles are membrane-bound areas within the cytoplasm of some cells. They are associated with food storage, digestion, osmotic regulation, and excretion of waste products. Their number and size may change with the physiological state of the cell.

Lysosomes Lysosomes are membrane-bound bodies that contain digestive enzymes and are found in such cells as the white blood cells that ingest (phagocytize) foreign particles. The lysosomes fuse with other vacuoles containing foreign particles to produce a vacuole called a *phagolysosome* in which digestion occurs (see Chapter 11).

Ribosomes The function of the eucaryotic ribosomes is the same as the procaryotic ribosomes. Eucaryotic ribosomes are located along the endoplasmic reticulum and are the sites of protein syn-

Figure 4-23   Electron micrograph of a fungal spore. This freeze-etch replica clearly shows the nuclear pores in the nuclear membrane, cell wall, cell membrane, and cytoplasmic inclusions (× 25,000). (Courtesy W. M. Hess, Brigham Young University)

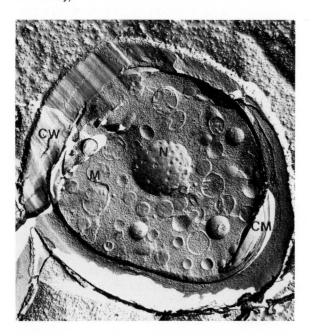

Clinical Application of the Gram Stain

The Gram stain is an extremely useful tool for bacterial identification. In spite of the facts (1) that there are only two reactions (positive and negative), and (2) that all bacteria have only one of three basic shapes (cocci, bacilli, and spirals), these few features can be used to categorize bacteria into fairly specific groups. Under some circumstances, based only on the Gram morphology of a bacterial cell, it is possible to designate the genus if not the species of the bacterium under question. Thus, if a specimen contains paired Gram-negative cocci the identification can quickly be narrowed to only two genera of clinically relevant bacteria. Likewise, if the specimen has relatively large Gram-positive bacilli that have blunt ends, only two genera are possible. By knowing the Gram morphology of a bacterium it is often possible for the microbiologist to provide rapid and very useful data to the physician.

Even if this were the only use of the Gram stain, it would be very valuable, but there is another, perhaps even more significant, contribution that is made by this procedure. The Gram stain can be used as a guide in providing appropriate, early antibiotic therapy for a patient. Bacteria of similar Gram morphologies tend to have similar susceptibility to specific antibiotics. For example, if a patient is reported to have a Gram-negative bacillus as a possible cause of a urinary tract infection, the physician can make a likely choice of antibiotic for treatment even before the identity and antibiotic susceptibility of the organism is known. By this means, application of the Gram stain to clinical specimens can have significant impact on therapy. This situation is particularly true for patients suffering from life-threatening diseases, such as meningitis, where the effects of early therapy are especially beneficial.

thesis (Figure 4-12). These ribosomes have a size of 80 S, which is larger than the procaryotic ribosomes.

Nucleus The nucleus of eucaryotic cells is a prominent membrane-bound structure that contains the genetic material of the cell. A smaller structure inside the nucleus, the *nucleolus*, is the structure involved in the synthesis of ribonucleic acid. Two membranes enclose the nucleus (Figure 4-23). The outer membrane is continuous, at least in part, with the endoplasmic reticulum. Round pores or holes pass through both membranes and allow the passage of large molecules between the nucleus and the cytoplasm.

Other organelles Other major structures found in eucaryotic cells are *mitochondria*, *Golgi bodies*, and *chloroplasts*. Mitochondria are rod-shaped structures about 1×3 μm in size and are associated with energy storage and transfer. Golgi bodies are aggregates of membranes and seem to be associated with the transport of enzymes out of the cell. Chloroplasts are prominent chlorophyll-containing structures found in eucaryotic cells that carry out photosynthesis. The sizes and shapes of chloroplasts vary among the different types of cells.

CONCEPT SUMMARY

1. Bacteria are procaryotic cells with limited variation in shape and unique cell wall structures. The composition of the cell wall is a determinant in the staining characteristics of the bacteria, dividing them into Gram-positive and Gram-negative species.

2. Bacteria possess a number of organelles related to cellular function. Among them, flagella, fimbriae, capsules, and endospores are the most noticeable. Other organelles are similar in shape and function to those observed in eucaryotic cells. An organelle of singular importance in eucaryotic cells, the mitochondria, is not found in procaryotic forms, although a compensating mesosomal structure can often be observed.

STUDY SUMMARY

1. Draw and label a cross section diagram of both a Gram-positive and a Gram-negative bacterial cell.

2. In what ways can the presence of a bacterial capsule increase the likelihood of bacterial survival in a competitive environment?

3. What are the functional differences between bacterial flagella and pili?

4. A major function of bacterial cytoplasmic membrane is selective transport of materials into or out of the cell. What mechanisms are available to the membrane to carry out this function?

5. List the primary function of each of the following: (a) fimbria, (b) ribosome, (c) DNA, (d) endospore, and (e) cytoplasm.

REFERENCES FOR FURTHER STUDY

1. *The Microbial World,* 5th ed., R. Stanier, 1986. Prentice Hall.

2. Molecular Basis of the Permeability of Bacterial Outer Membrane. *Microbiological Reviews* 49:1, 1985.

3. Structure, Function and Assembly of Cell Walls of Gram-positive Bacteria. *Annual Review of Microbiology* 37:501, 1983.

4. Bacterial Motility and the Bacterial Flagella Motor. *Annual Review of Biophysics and Bioengineering* 13:51, 1984.

5. Gram-negative Bacterial Extracellular and Wall Polysaccharides. *Annual Review of Microbiology* 39:243, 1985.

chapter 5

METABOLIC FUNCTIONS

A ny chemical change or reaction that occurs within a cell
is called *metabolism*. Such reactions are involved with
the breakdown of food materials for the release of
energy to the cell, a process called *catabolism*, and with
the production of new cellular components, a process called *biosynthesis* or *anabolism*, which requires energy. Catabolism and biosynthesis are usually coupled together such that the energy released from catabolic reactions can be directly used for
biosynthesis. The rate of metabolic activity in an actively growing
bacterial cell is phenomenal. Some bacteria are able to go through
several generations, reproducing themselves at each generation
in less than 1 hour. This rapid synthesis of new cellular material
requires the catabolism of relatively large amounts of nutrient
with its associated release of energy, and the biosynthesis of
enough new material to double the cell mass for each generation.
The small size of bacterial cells provides for a large surface area
relative to cell mass in order to facilitate this rapid growth. This,
in turn, allows for a rapid interaction between the intra- and extracellular environments.

This chapter briefly outlines the steps involved in the release
and transfer of energy from foodstuffs as well as the production of
new building blocks needed for cell growth. The structure and
functions of enzymes and other proteins are also discussed. The
intention of this chapter is to present a conceptual, generalized
view of cellular metabolism which will, by necessity, omit many
details of this complex subject.

ENERGY METABOLISM

Figure 5-1 presents a simplified outline of the reactions involved
in energy metabolism and the biosynthesis of cellular materials.
The original source of energy used in a vast majority of biological

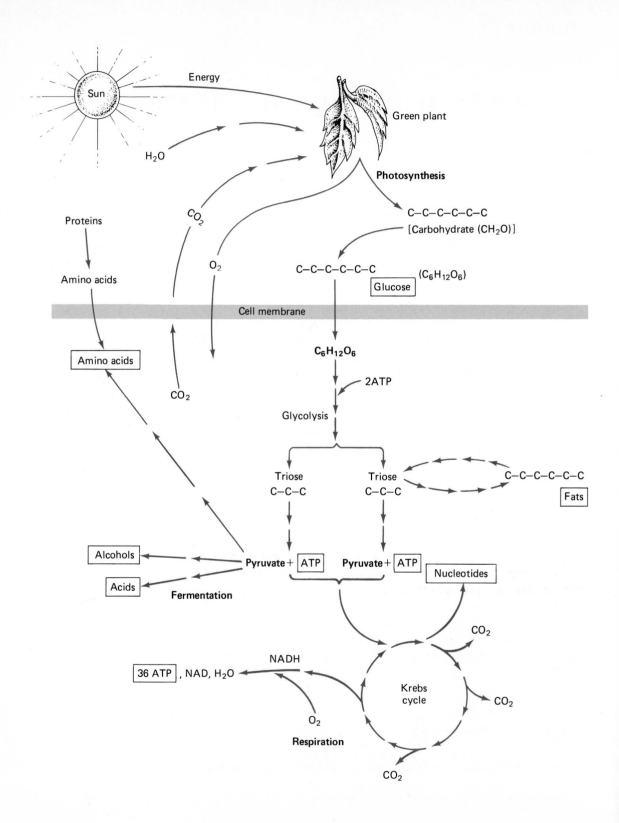

systems is the sun. Autotrophic organisms convert radiant energy from the sun into a form of chemical energy through the process of *photosynthesis*. The available chemical energy can then be used by living organisms that require organic matter as their source of energy (heterotrophs). Green plants growing on land and algae in water are responsible for most of the photosynthetic activity occurring on the earth.

During the process of photosynthesis, radiant energy from the sun is collected by chlorophyll molecules and is used to rearrange the atoms contained in carbon dioxide (CO_2) and water (H_2O) as follows:

$$CO_2 + H_2O \rightarrow CH_2O + O_2$$

Water is broken into its atomic components, hydrogen and oxygen. The oxygen is then released as a molecule and the hydrogen is combined with CO_2 (Figure 5-2). In this **reduced** state, molecules of CH_2O are combined together to form whatever size carbohydrate $(CH_2O)_n$ is required by the cell. Energy is required to form a reduced compound and much of this energy is retained in the compound. In turn, this stored energy can be released for use by a cell at a later time when oxygen is again added to the molecule or when hydrogen atoms are removed, a process called *oxidation* (Figure 5-3).

The above description of photosynthesis is very brief and generalized. In fact, with the exception of the cyanobacteria, bacterial photosynthesis does not include the breakdown of water and proceeds along a somewhat different pathway from photosynthesis in eucaryotic plants. Even so, these organisms are able to convert sufficient solar energy to provide for their own metabolic needs.

Various sizes of carbohydrate molecules are formed by photosynthetic plants and algae. The most common *carbohydrate* molecules are the simple sugars, called *monosaccharides*, usually containing five or six carbon atoms. Two monosaccharides may combine to form a *disaccharide*; many monosaccharides connected together form *polysaccharides*. Starch and cellulose are the major polysaccharides produced by plants and algae (Figure 5-4). These carbohydrates are the major food energy–containing molecules produced by photosynthesis.

Reduced
the condition of a molecule to which electrons have been added. Molecules may exist in either an oxidized or a reduced condition. When electrons are removed from a molecule it is oxidized. Most biochemical reactions add hydrogen (reduction) or remove hydrogen (oxidation) to change the oxidation-reduction condition of the molecule.

Figure 5-1 A simplified schematic diagram illustrating the source of cellular energy and the biosynthesis of cellular materials. The reactions above the cell membrane are representative of photosynthesis (requiring water, carbon dioxide, and light energy for the synthesis of carbohydrate and the release of oxygen). The metabolic reactions occurring in bacterial and animal cells which require chemical energy such as glucose are shown below the cell membrane. These reactions produce the necessary ATP and cellular components for growth while releasing both carbon dioxide and water as end products.

$$\text{Sunlight} + 12\,H_2O + 6\,CO_2 \longrightarrow 6O_2 + C_6H_{12}O_6 + 6H_2O$$

Figure 5-2   Balanced photosynthetic reaction. Water and carbon dioxide are combined to produce oxygen, cabohydrate and water.

Polymer

a relatively large molecule composed of repeating subunit molecules (monomers). Common biopolymers are polysaccharides, polypeptides (proteins), nucleic acids, and lipids.

Energy stored in the chemical bonds of carbohydrates and other molecules, such as proteins and lipids, is made available to the cell through a complex series of metabolic reactions. The main source of energy for most cells is a six-carbon sugar called *glucose,* or a **polymer** of glucose such as starch. Before glucose can be used by the cell, it must be separated from the larger polysaccharide molecule. This splitting is accomplished in microbial cells by digestive enzymes that are released from the cells into the extracellular environment. In Gram-negative bacteria these extracellular

Figure 5-3   Oxidation-reduction reactions involve the transfer of electrons. Losing an electron (A$_1$) results in oxidation while adding an electron results in chemical reduction (A$_2$). In metabolism, hydrogen is often transferred with the electron, thus losing hydrogen (B$_1$, C$_1$) results in oxidized molecules while gaining hydrogen produces reduced molecules (B$_2$, C$_2$).

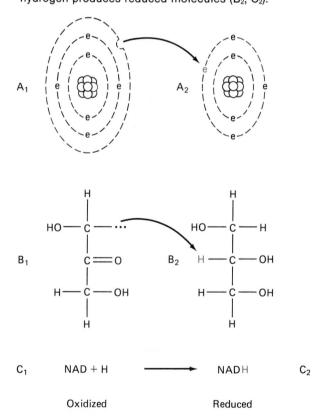

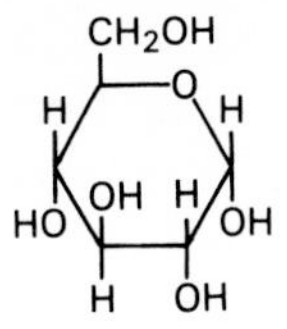

CH$_2$OH

H O H

HO OH H OH

H OH

Glucose
(monosaccharide)

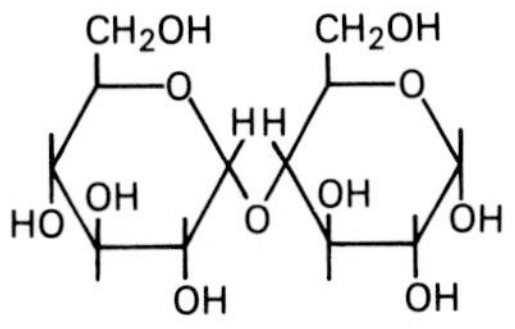

CH$_2$OH CH$_2$OH

O H H O

HO OH O OH OH

OH OH

Disaccharide

CH$_2$OH CH$_2$OH CH$_2$OH CH$_2$OH CH$_2$OH

O O O O O

HO OH O OH O OH O OH O OH OH

OH OH OH OH OH

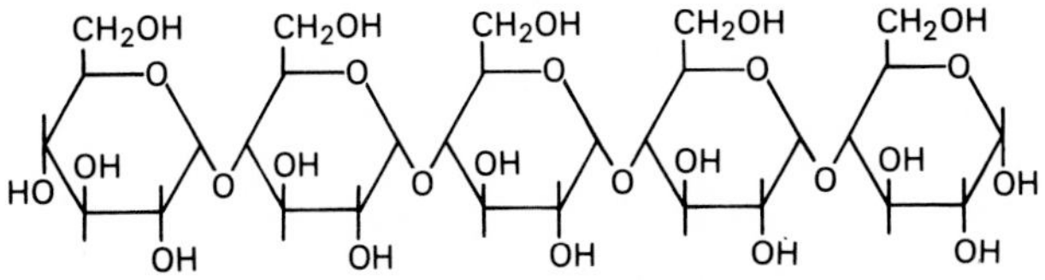

A polysaccharide
such as glycogen

Figure 5-4 A carbohydrate monomer (glucose) used to make a large polymer of glucose molecules—a polysaccharide.

digestive enzymes are often concentrated in the space between the peptidoglycan layer and the outer membrane of the cell wall (periplasmic space) where the larger molecules can be broken down more efficiently (Figure 5-5). The glucose molecules contained in starch are relatively easily split from the larger molecule, whereas the sugars that make up cellulose are more difficult to digest. Some microbes, however, are endowed with a wide array of enzymes that enable them to break down even the most complex and resistant carbohydrates, such as cellulose. Most digestion of the cellulose that is formed by plants is done by microorganisms. Thus, carnivorous animals are unable to digest plant cellulose carbohydrates, whereas herbivorous animals, such as cattle

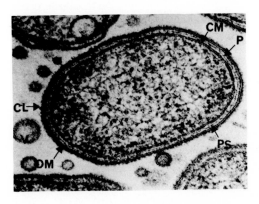

Figure 5-5 Electron photomicrograph of a bacillus. Note the periplasmic space at the end of the cell. (Courtesy T. J. MacAlister, *J. Bacteriol.* 169:3945)

and sheep, are able to feed on plants and digest cellulose because of the kinds of microorganisms that live in their alimentary tract. These microorganisms (bacteria, protozoa, and fungi) are semipermanent residents of the digestive tract of these animals, and break down the large polysaccharide molecules into smaller disaccharides and monosaccharides that can then be absorbed from the intestine of the animal.

Metabolic Energy

Glucose provides a cell with a source of readily available energy. However, it is not convenient for a cell to have glucose involved in every chemical reaction that requires energy *(endergonic* reactions). To make needed energy available for individual reactions, the cell makes use of one of a number of high-energy compounds, the most common of which is *adenosine triphosphate* (ATP)(Figure 5-6). Energy obtained by metabolic processes is briefly stored in ATP molecules. ATP contains three phosphate groups, two of which are connected by high-energy bonds that are readily available for various cellular functions. When energy is released, the ATP molecule loses a phosphate group and is changed to an adenosine diphosphate (ADP) molecule. The ADP molecule can be changed back into an ATP molecule when energy becomes available from the oxidation of other compounds (Figure 5-7).

Glycolysis

Glucose molecules readily pass across the bacterial cytoplasmic membrane; once inside the cell, they enter into a series of reactions that slowly extract the energy stored in these molecules. The

Figure 5-6   Adenosine tri (a), di (b), and mono (c) phosphate showing the position of the high energy (⌣) phosphate bonds.

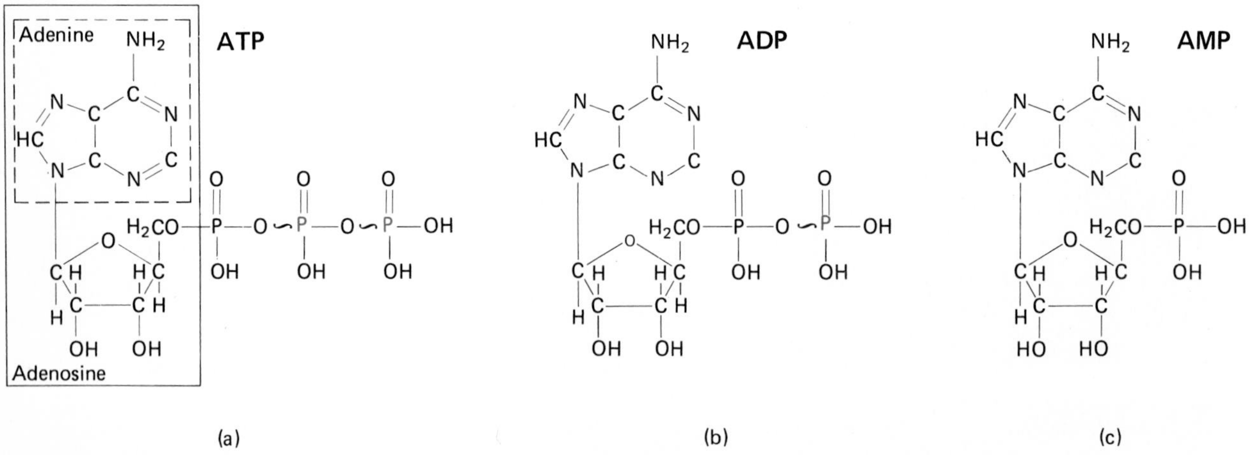

(a)   (b)   (c)

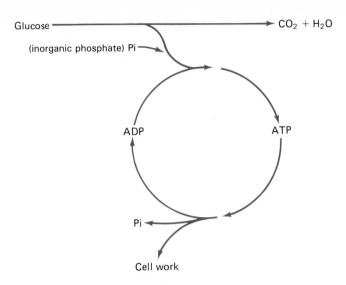

Figure 5-7 The ATP-ADP cycle. Energy obtained through the oxidation of glucose is used to form ATP. This energy is then released by ATP to carry out energy-requiring cellular processes. The resultant ADP is then available to be used in the formation of a new ATP molecule.

first series of reactions in the process of glucose catabolism, called *glycolysis,* begins with several changes occurring in the structure of the glucose molecule. As with most chemical reactions, even those that yield a supply of energy *(exergonic* reactions), it is necessary to initiate the catabolism of glucose by adding energy to the molecule (Figure 5-8). This energy is frequently obtained from the energy available in ATP. In carrying out this reaction, the phosphorus atom that is removed from ATP is attached to the number six carbon of the glucose, producing glucose-6-phosphate; the reaction is as follows:

$$\text{Glucose} + \text{ATP} \rightarrow \text{glucose-6-phosphate} + \text{ADP}$$

In this reaction, the energy from the ATP is transferred to the glucose-6-phosphate molecule, and this molecule becomes less stable and more subject to chemical change than is glucose. **Phosphorylation** of glucose can occur either directly as the glucose crosses the cell membrane, or after it is in the cytoplasm of the cell. After the glucose molecule is phosphorylated it is converted to another six-carbon sugar known as *fructose,* which is again phosphorylated giving a compound known as fructose-1,6-diphosphate. Thus it requires two units of ATP energy (14.6 k cal) in order to prepare glucose for its final oxidation (Figure 5-8). Further glycolysis results in the splitting of these six-carbon sugars into two molecules containing three carbon atoms each. These three-carbon com-

Phosphorylation
the addition of phosphorus to a molecule. This process is usually accompanied by a transfer of a relatively large amount of energy.

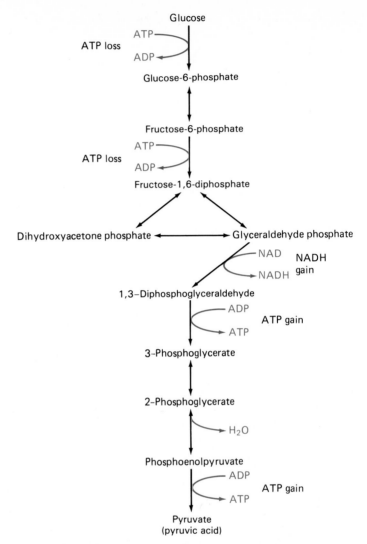

Figure 5-8   Simplified schematic of the glycolytic pathway. Note that two ATP molecules are required to activate this pathway, while ATP is produced in converting glyceraldehyde phosphate to pyruvate. This process results in a net increase of two ATP molecules because the six carbon glucose molecules are converted into two three-carbon glyceraldehyde phosphate molecules.

pounds are further altered to form a compound called *pyruvic acid.* Thus in the reactions that change glucose to pyruvic acid, two ATP molecules are used to prime the reaction; then two ATP units are generated for each of the two pyruvic acid molecules formed. Thus the net gain in energy available to the cell at this point is two ATP molecules because four were generated and two were used to prime the reaction.

A second significant energy-associated reaction occurs during glycolysis. For each molecule of glucose converted to pyruvate, two hydrogen atoms are removed and attached to a carrier molecule known as *nicotinamide adenine dinucleotide* or simply NAD. This molecule, now reduced to NADH, is used later by the cell to obtain additional energy (Figure 5-8). In addition to glycolysis (known as the *Embden-Myerhof pathway*), bacteria have other pathways—for example, the *Entner-Doudoroff pathway* and the *pentose phosphate pathway*—by which important energy-containing sugars can be metabolized. In fact, some bacteria have the ability to choose more than one of these pathways as needed.

After pyruvic acid has been produced from glucose, the cell must make a major metabolic decision. Actually, the decision is made for the cell by the availability of oxygen. The reactions of glycolysis do not use oxygen and if oxygen is not available *(anaerobic* metabolism), pyruvic acid may subsequently be converted into such products as alcohol and organic acids, a process known as *fermentation* (Figure 5-1). To carry out this process, the NADH that was obtained during glycolysis is used to reduce pyruvate either directly to lactic acid (a process that occurs in human muscle cells) or indirectly to ethyl alcohol (a process that occurs with baker's yeast). The reaction leading to lactic acid

$$2 \text{ pyruvic acid } + 2 \text{ NADH} \rightarrow 2 \text{ lactic acid } + 2 \text{ NAD}$$

ensures the cell of a continued supply of NAD for use in glycolysis (Figure 5-8). A net gain of two ATP molecules is produced in the conversion of one molecule of glucose to alcohol. Under these circumstances, most of the energy is still contained in the alcohol molecules. Only certain types of microorganisms are able to produce alcohols or some other products of fermentation. Many such compounds have commercial value and controlled fermentation is carried out on a mass scale in many industrial processes. Because most of the energy originally present in glucose is still found in the alcohol molecules, and because it is easily released by combustion with oxygen, much effort has been directed toward increasing production of alcohol to use as a supplemental fuel for combustion engines.

If oxygen is available and the microorganisms can use oxygen *(aerobic* metabolism) pyruvic acid can be oxidized completely to CO_2 and H_2O with the transfer of the released energy to ADP molecules, which then become ATP. When reactions use oxygen or other appropriate acceptors the process is called *respiration*. This process proceeds when pyruvic acid enters into a series of reactions called the *tricarboxylic acid* (TCA) *cycle* or *Krebs cycle* (Figure 5-9). In the Krebs cycle the carbohydrates are further oxidized and hydrogen is transferred to an appropriate carrier molecule, such as NAD.

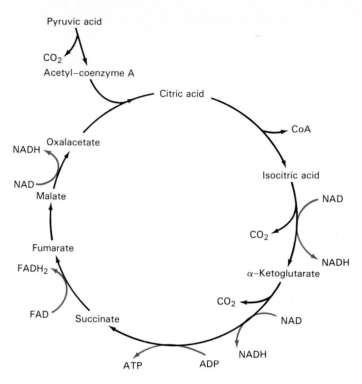

Figure 5-9 Schematic of the chemical reactions occurring within the Krebs cycle. Reactions which yield large amounts of energy are shown in color.

Nucleotide

a compound that contains one of several possible organic nitrogen atoms. The most common nucleotide molecules include adenine, thymine, cytosine, guanine, and uridine. These nucleotides are found in DNA and RNA as well as in a variety of coenzymes and ATP.

Pyruvic acid doesn't directly enter the TCA cycle, but is first modified by the removal of one carbon atom, which is released as CO_2. With each round of the TCA cycle, two additional CO_2 molecules are produced. Thus by the time the TCA cycle goes through two complete revolutions, each of the carbon atoms, originally present in glucose, have been oxidized to CO_2. The organic compounds (e.g., oxaloacetate) that make up the TCA cycle are also important intermediates for the biosynthesis of many necessary cell building blocks such as amino acids (Table 5-1). Therefore, this cycle is also operational in many anaerobic microorganisms as well as all aerobes. Significant energy-associated end products of the TCA cycle include NADH and $FADH_2$. These reduced **nucleotides** enter into an electron transport system where they are oxidized when a hydrogen atom is transferred to an oxygen atom. These reactions release a great deal of energy as ATP (Figure 5-10). Thus the chemical energy contained in pyruvic acid is slowly released through a stepwise series of reactions (TCA cycle and electron transport) involving the passage of electrons from the carbohydrate to oxygen with the resulting formation of water and the release of CO_2. In all, for every glucose molecule metabolized by the cell, 38 ATP molecules are generated by this

Table 5-1   Naturally Occurring Amino Acids

Alanine	Glutamic acid	Leucine	Serine
Arginine	Glutamine	Lysine	Threonine
Asparagine	Glycine	Methionine	Tryptophane
Aspartic acid	Histidine	Phenylalanine	Tyrosine
Cysteine	Isoleucine	Proline	Valine

process (Table 5-2). Because the cell used 2 ATP molecules to initiate the glycolytic reaction, a net total of 36 available ATP molecules are generated by the oxidation of 1 mole of glucose. Respiration is a highly efficient energy-releasing system, returning more than 35% of the available energy to the cell.

The energy demands of human cells are such that their needs cannot be met by fermentation for any length of time. This explains our continuing demand for oxygen to serve as a terminal **electron acceptor.** Anaerobic respiration, which uses compounds such as sulfate or nitrate instead of oxygen as electron acceptors, is known to occur in some bacteria. These reactions make energy available to the bacteria in the absence of oxygen but do not occur in higher life forms. The CO_2 that is formed as a by-product of respiration is released from the cell into the atmosphere where it is again able to enter into the reactions of photosynthesis for conversion back into an energy-containing carbohydrate. On the other hand, the oxygen given off as a by-product of photosynthesis is used in the respiration reactions of the cell, thus forming one

Electron acceptor
an atom or molecule (such as oxygen) that is relatively easily reduced by accepting a hydrogen atom.

Figure 5-10   A schematic diagram representing the transfer of hydrogen from the oxidation of carbohydrate to NAD and from NADH to the electron transport system which ultimately uses two hydrogen atoms to reduce an atom of oxygen to a molecule of water. These reactions result in a concurrent production of ATP (see Appendix A for details).

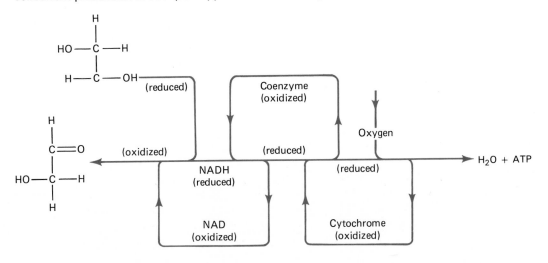

Table 5-2   Sources of ATP from Metabolism of 1 Mole of Glucose

Pathway	Products	ATP Produced
Glycolysis	NADH, pyruvic acid	4
Krebs cycle	NADH, FADH, CO_2	2
Electron transport	H_2O	32

of the important chemical cycles involved in the balance of living systems (Figure 5-1).

Many of the energy-producing reactions occurring within bacterial cells take place at or near the cell membrane (Chapter 4). The membranes serve as physical supports for the enzyme involved. In the electron transport system, the various cytochromes that are used to carry the electrons have a fixed orientation in the cytoplasmic membrane. A number of years ago, this observation provided the basis for the present chemiosmotic theory of active transport in bacteria (Figure 5-11). In this process, electrons are passed from a reduced compound to an oxidized compound by means of the membrane carrier molecules. By means of the orientation of the cytochrome molecules, hydrogen molecules are transported to the outside of the membrane, while electrons are transported to the inside; this results in an unequal concentration of protons on the two sides of the membrane. Such unequal distribution of charges produces a force, or pressure, on the membrane in order to equalize the charge distribution. The cell uses an enzyme, ATPase, to reestablish proton equilibrium by returning protons into the cell, and in the process uses this proton motive force to generate ATP. Other forms of work such as flagellar movement and some permease functions can also be performed with the proton motive force.

Figure 5-11   The use of electron transport to generate ATP. A proton (H) gradient is established as electron carriers (cytochromes) move electrons down an electrochemical gradient. ATP is generated as the proton returns to the inside of the membrane.

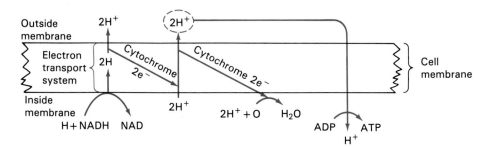

BIOSYNTHESIS

In addition to providing energy through the catabolic reactions just discussed, the metabolic activities of the cell are also engaged in producing building blocks needed for the formation of new cellular components. This process is called *biosynthesis* or *anabolism* and requires energy obtained from the ATP molecules. All living cells consist of a large number of complex organic molecules called *polymers*. Polymers are so called because they are produced by connecting large numbers of smaller subunit molecules called *monomers*. Only about 150 different types of precursor monomers are needed to form the thousands of different polymers found in a living cell. Many monomers are produced through the various metabolic pathways within the cell whereas others come directly from nutrients that are carried into the cell through the cytoplasmic membrane (Figure 5-1). Most biological polymers (also referred to as *macromolecules)* are of the following four general types: (1) *polysaccharides,* (2) *proteins,* (3) *nucleic acids,* and (4) *complex lipids.* Polysaccharides are polymers of simple sugars, and were discussed earlier in this chapter. Proteins are polymers that consist of monomers called *amino acids.* The myriads of protein macromolecules found in any living cell are formed from just 20 different types of amino acids (Table 5-3). The structure and functions of proteins are discussed below. Nucleic acids are polymers composed of chains of subunits called *nucleotide bases.* Their structure and functions are more completely discussed in Chapter 6. The lipid complexes vary in composition, with fatty acids, alcohols, sugars, and amino acids as precursor monomers. Some monomer-polymer relationships are shown in Table 5-1.

STRUCTURE AND FUNCTIONS OF PROTEINS

Proteins serve both as important structural components of the cell and as functional molecules, such as enzymes, that regulate the chemical reactions of cells. Controlling the types of proteins pro-

Table 5-3   The Major Categories of Monomers and the Polymer Formed from Them

Monomers	Polymers
Amino acids	Proteins (polypeptides)
Simple sugars	Carbohydrates (polysaccharides)
Fatty acids, monoglyceride	Lipids
Nucleotide bases	Nucleic acids

duced enables all other characteristics of the cell to be controlled. To help understand this relationship, some knowledge of the structure and enzymatic functions of proteins is needed.

Molecular Structure

The 20 amino acid monomers that constitute the polymeric protein molecules are analogous to letters of the alphabet, whereas the protein molecules are analogous to words of the printed language. The amino acids are connected end to end, forming long chains, and each protein molecule, in order to be formed properly, must contain a specific sequence and number of amino acids, just as correctly spelled words must have a proper sequence and number of letters (Figure 5-12). Yet a protein molecule contains many more amino acids, usually several hundred, than the number of letters in a word.

Amino acids are so called because they contain an amine group (NH_2) at one end and a carboxylic acid group (COOH) at the other end of the molecule. The arrangement of atoms in between the amine and the carboxylic acid groups is different for each amino acid. The structures of two amino acid molecules (alanine and glycine) are shown in Figure 5-12. When the amino acids are brought together under specific conditions, a reaction occurs between the amine group of one amino acid and the carboxyl group of the other. In this reaction a water molecule is removed. The bond that forms between amino acids is called a *peptide bond* and a macromolecule containing many amino acids is called a *polypeptide.*

A complete protein molecule may consist of one or several polypeptides. The sequence of amino acids in the protein is called the *primary structure* of the polypeptide. As the polypeptide forms, it coils into the *secondary structure,* a spiral or helical arrangement called an alpha-helix. The secondary structure of the protein is held together by rather weak chemical bonds known as *hydrogen bonds.* Hydrogen bonding interactions occur because of the unequal distribution of positive and negative electrical charges along the molecule. Each complete helical turn in the alpha-helix requires 3.6 amino acid residues. Next, the helix folds on itself and forms chemical bonds between different segments of the molecule. The result of this folding of the alpha-helix is called the *tertiary structure* and gives the protein molecule a specific three-dimensional shape (Figure 5-12). The tertiary structure is largely maintained by strong chemical bonds that form between individual amino acids.

It is apparent then that the primary structure of the polypeptide determines the secondary, which in turn determines the tertiary configuration. In addition, some protein molecules are formed by connecting several different polypeptides. Such an ar-

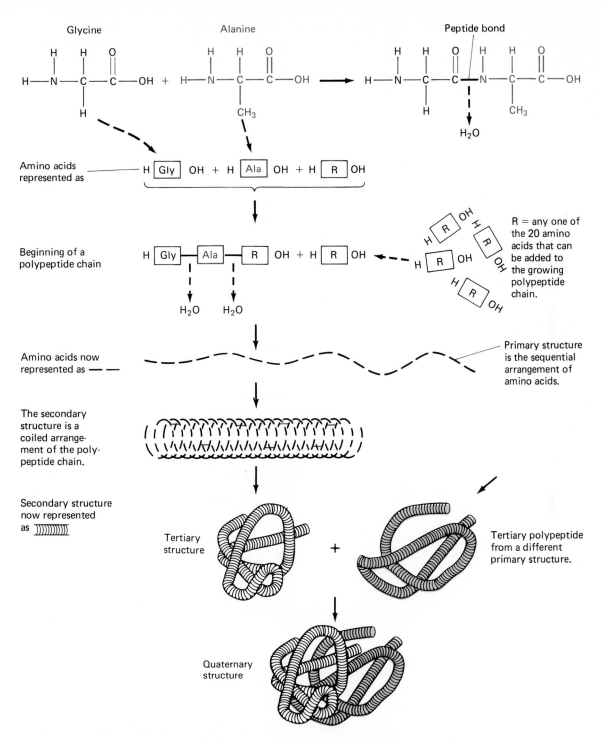

Figure 5-12 Formation of protein molecules from amino acid monomers. Formation and structure of primary, secondary, tertiary, and quaternary structure are shown.

rangement is called a *quaternary structure.* Any amino acid can be connected to any other amino acid; moreover, because of the large numbers of amino acids in a protein, an almost unlimited number of different types of protein molecules can be formed from the 20 amino acids.

Enzymes and Enzymatic Functions

An important function of some proteins is to serve as enzymes. All enzymes are proteins; however, not all proteins are enzymes. Enzymes are the *catalysts* of chemical reactions occurring in living systems. A catalyst is a substance that reduces the energy needed to start a chemical reaction and may increase the rate of the reaction, but the catalyst is not used up in the reaction itself (Figure 5-13). Most chemical reactions that occur in living systems will not proceed without the proper enzymatic catalyst. So without enzymes, life functions, as we know them, would stop. Enzymes are very specific and almost every one of the thousands of chemical reactions that occur in a cell requires a distinct and specific enzyme. Thus, a simple bacterial cell must be able to synthesize hundreds of different types of protein molecules just to supply the needed enzymes. The specificity of an enzyme is a result of the three-dimensional configuration (tertiary structure) of the protein molecule. This shape allows the enzyme to react temporarily with, and properly orient, the compounds involved in chemical reaction so that the energy required to start the reaction is reduced (Figure

Figure 5-13 How a catalyst works. Catalysts such as an enzyme reduce the energy of activation, B, needed to initiate a chemical reaction. The energy available in the substrate is represented by A. The amount of energy conserved by the catalyst is represented by C.

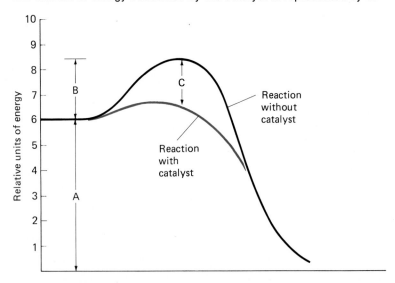

5-14). After the reaction occurs, the enzyme disassociates from the products and is free to repeat the process. Most enzymes are able to catalyze thousands of reactions per second.

Some enzymes direct the synthesis of complex molecules from simpler precursor subcomponents; others may change the arrangement of the atoms within a molecule; still others may break down complex compounds into simpler molecules. The chemical that is acted on by an enzyme is called a *substrate,* and the molecules resulting from the reaction are called *products.* Enzymes are usually named by adding the suffix *-ase* to the name of the substrate or reaction catalyzed. An enzyme that breaks down proteins would be called a prot*ase,* for instance, one that catalyzes the reaction to form a DNA macromolecule would be called a DNA-polymer*ase.* A list of some enzymes and their functions is given in Table 5-4.

What a cell can and cannot do depends on the type of enzymes it possesses. The great diversity of activities of various mi-

Figure 5-14   A catalyst enters a chemical reaction, facilitates the reaction by increasing the interaction between substrate molecules, then leaves the reaction unchanged. (a) This can be exemplified by a bricklayer, who uses brick and mortar (substrates) and combines them into a finished product. (b) An enzyme is a biological catalyst. It facilitates a chemical reaction, makes it go, and is left unchanged by the reaction.

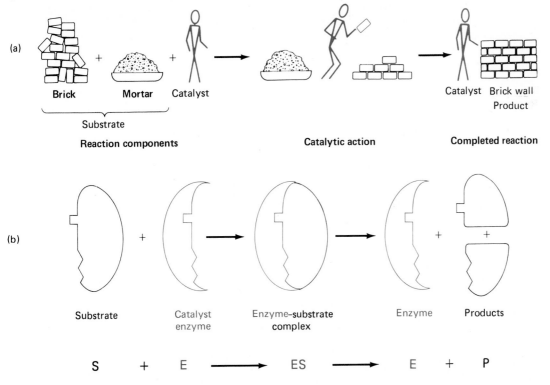

Bacterial Identification

Although procedures are now available that use bacterial genes, antigens, and growth rates for species identification, the most important technique available to microbiologists of the past relied on the metabolic functions of the organisms to identify and classify bacteria. For example, it seemed self-evident to scientists of earlier years that a bacterium that could metabolize a sugar such as lactose was different from one that could not. Therefore, test after test was made first with one sugar (or with one protein, etc.), and then with a second, and a third, and so forth until the metabolic reactions of bacteria were almost completely catalogued. These metabolic fingerprints are well known for most bacteria that cause human disease and are still the most commonly used identification procedures in the diagnostic laboratory.

As clinical laboratorians have made considerable use of information regarding bacterial metabolism, they have devised numerous identification schemas to make their task as simple as possible. Because biochemical processes that are common to all species are not useful in discriminating among them, nearly all such schemas begin with a Gram stain, which divides the bacteria into at least two groups. When that information is obtained, the next step is to determine the microbial response to a second biochemical test that will again separate the organism in question into one of two groups, that is, will provide a positive or a negative response. This procedure is repeated until there is only one species of bacteria that possesses the correct response to each of the tests and the identification is thus secured. For example, if a Gram stain reveals that the organism to be iden-

tified is a Gram-positive coccus, the microbiologist can conclude that it is either a streptococcus or a staphylococcus. To separate these genera, the microbiologist might test the isolate for the presence of an enzyme known as *catalase.* If this test is negative, it would be necessary to pursue the identification of a streptococcus; if it is positive, the bacterial isolate is one of the staphylococci. The next test for a catalase-positive, Gram-positive coccus would be for the presence of an enzyme known as *coagulase.* If this test is positive, the organism is *Staphylococcus aureus;* if it is negative, the organism is one of the other staphylococcal species and additional tests would be used to make a final identification. Using this approach it is possible to obtain a species identification for each microorganism brought into the clinical laboratory. Because there is great need for rapid identification of bacteria that may be causing disease, many of the tests are performed simultaneously.

Knowledge of bacterial metabolism is essential to an understanding of the bacterial identification process. Tests commonly used are able to determine the presence or absence of enzymes, the ability to metabolize various sugars and alcohols, to produce various metabolic end products, to produce various acids during metabolism, to grow on selected energy sources, to grow in the presence of selected growth inhibitors, and the permeability of the cell to a variety of nutritional compounds. Learning how bacteria respond to this broad variety of metabolic opportunities enables the microbiologist to make accurate decisions leading to bacterial identification.

Table 5-4   Enzymes and Enzymatic Functions

Enzyme Class	Examples	Functions
Hydrolase	Amidase, esterase, phosphatase	Breaking of chemical bonds by the addition of water
Isomerase	Mutase, epimerase	Molecular rearrangement producing one isomer from another
Ligase	DNA synthetase	Linking of simple molecules into complex polyers
Lyase	Deaminase, decarboxylase	Nonhydrolytic cleavage of chemical bonds
Oxidoreductase	Dehydrogenase, peroxidase	Catalysis of oxidation and reduction reactions
Transferase	Transaminase, transmethylase	Transfer of atoms or molecules from one compound to another

croorganisms is a function of the types of enzymes they possess. If all the necessary enzymes are formed, the cell will function properly. If an essential enzyme is not properly formed, the cell may die. If an enzyme that catalyzes a minor reaction is missing, the cell may survive but take on different characteristics. Similarly, if a cell acquires the ability to produce a new enzyme, the cell may acquire a new characteristic. Therefore, controlling the synthesis of protein molecules means that all other reactions of the cell are controlled. Fundamentally, the genetic control of a cell or an organism is a function of the control of protein synthesis. The discovery of how a cell can store and transfer to its offspring the information necessary to line up the amino acids into the proper sequences in order to form the proper enzymes has been one of the great scientific achievements of the past 30 years. This topic will be discussed in the next chapter.

CONCEPT SUMMARY

1. Energy for life is primarily a product of the sun. This energy is organized into chemical systems by means of photosynthesis, which occurs in autotrophic life forms. Heterotrophic organisms obtain their needed energy by using autotrophs or the metabolic products of autotrophs for food.

2. Heterotrophic bacteria primarily use carbohydrate as an energy source. The carbohydrate is gradually oxidized through a stepwise rearrangement of the molecule. This energy, obtained in a systemic fashion, is captured in ATP, which is

then used by the cell to perform energy-requiring operations, such as cell synthesis.

3. Cellular metabolism is regulated by the availability of enzymes. These proteins ensure the proper, systematic interaction of those molecules necessary to build new cell material. Other enzymes provide orderly catabolic processes that result in a continuous supply of energy to carry out cell processes.

STUDY SUMMARY

1. Describe the relationship between autotrophs and heterotrophs.
2. How are the processes of photosynthesis and cellular metabolism connected at the molecular level?
3. Why is it important that enzymes have only one or a very limited number of substrates?
4. Draw a diagram showing how the products of glycolysis become the substrates for the Krebs cycle.
5. Explain why it is possible to get a much greater yield of cells when they are grown aerobically rather than anaerobically.
6. How is it possible for single amino acid substitution in a polypeptide to modify the tertiary structure of the protein?

REFERENCES FOR FURTHER STUDY

1. *An Introduction to the Chemiosmotic Theory*, D. Nicholls, 1983. Academic Press.
2. *The Bacteria*, vol. 2, I. Gunsalus, 1961. Academic Press.
3. *The Microbial World*, 5th ed., R. Stanier, 1986. Prentice-Hall.
4. *Biology: The Unity and Diversity of Life*, 4th ed., C. Starr, 1987. Wadsworth.
5. The Respiratory Chains of *Escherichia coli*. *Microbiological Reviews* 48:222, 1984.

chapter 6

THE SYNTHESIS
OF MACROMOLECULES

As was noted in Chapter 5, four classes of macromolecules are essential to normal cell function: (1) polysaccharides, (2) proteins, (3) nucleic acids, and (4) complex lipids. These molecules are unique to biological systems and efforts to understand how they interact together and how they carry out their specific activity is central to the discipline known as *molecular biology*. Most of the recent investigative effort in molecular biology has centered around two of these macromolecular groups: proteins and nucleic acids.

The discovery that protein molecules were intimately associated with cell function, acting both as catalytic molecules (enzymes) and structural molecules, gave great impetus to the study of this important group of compounds. Implied in most of these early studies was the question as to the chemical nature of the genetic information.

Cell genes are information-carrying molecules that contain all the information needed to direct the proper functions of the cell. When a cell divides, a full complement of the genetic information must be passed to each daughter cell. Because the individual chemical reactions of the cell are each catalyzed by a specific enzyme, the information-carrying molecules of the genes must be able to precisely direct the synthesis of such specific proteins.

Although it is now well established that the chemical *deoxyribonucleic acid* (DNA) is the information-carrying molecule of the gene, the discovery of this fact was one of the greatest achievements in science. We will follow the chronology of this discovery as we discuss the nature of the structure of DNA, how equal complements of DNA are passed to each daughter cell, the means of information storage in the gene, and how this information directs the formation of protein molecules.

DNA AS THE GENETIC MOLECULE

By the 1930s it was recognized that the information-carrying molecules of the cell were in the nucleus. Chemical analysis of the nucleus, however, showed that large amounts of both protein and DNA were present. DNA appeared to be a rather unexciting compound composed of only four monomers known as *nucleotide bases*. These bases varied in concentration among different biologic species, but little was known regarding their function within the cell. On the other hand, proteins, which were better known than DNA, were highly variable molecules comprised of an almost limitless arrangement of 20 unique monomers, the amino acids. So scientists of the 1930s had a choice for the genetic information molecule between the limited 4-letter "alphabet" of DNA, and the 20-letter "alphabet" of proteins. It seemed only logical that protein molecules would somehow contain the genetic information so essential to the function of the cell. However, a series of important experiments conducted in the 1930s and 1940s by Oswald Avery, Colin MacLeod, and Maclyn McCarty demonstrated that DNA was in fact the generic material.

These investigators extended the work of Frederick Griffith who had studied two forms of the same bacterium, *Streptococcus pneumoniae.* One of the forms was *virulent* (possessing properties that lead to disease) such that when injected into a mouse it resulted in the death of the mouse. The other form of *S. pneumoniae* was *avirulent* (lacking properties that cause disease) and could be injected into a mouse without causing any ill effect. When Griffith injected a mouse with a living avirulent *S. pneumoniae* and a killed virulent form at the same time, to his surprise, the mouse died. Further investigation revealed that a living virulent bacterium could be isolated from the dead mouse. The only plausible explanation for these results was that some factor relating to virulence must have been transferred from the virulent, but dead, bacterium to the living avirulent form, resulting in a transformation of the avirulent to virulent *S. pneumoniae.* On closer examination just such a factor was discovered in the form of DNA. Using *S. pneumoniae* Oswald, Avery and McCarty performed experiments that demonstrated that the property responsible for virulence in this organism could be passed from one cell to another with pure extracts of DNA (Figure 6-1). Thus, these investigators properly concluded that DNA must be able to carry genetic information that in turn controls cellular function.

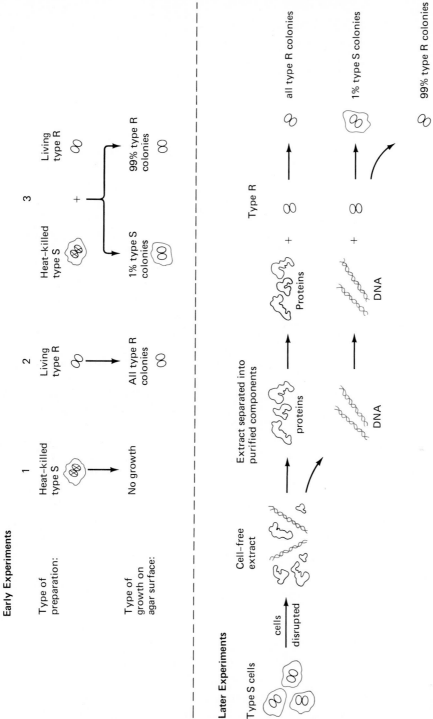

Figure 6-1 The transforming experiments of Avery and coworkers. Two strains of pneumococci were used. One was a strain with a capsule that produced smooth colonies (type S); the other strain had no capsule and produced rough colonies (type R). The early experiments showed that when killed type S cells were mixed with live type R cells about 1% of the living R cells acquired genetic material from the type S cells and were transformed into type S cells. The later experiments demonstrated that the transformation was produced by purified preparations of DNA extracted from type S cells.

Structure of DNA

As is often true with scientific discovery, answers to questions simply lead to new questions. If DNA is the genetic molecule, how could a substance containing only four monomeric nucleotide bases contain the massive amount of information needed to control the myriad of cellular functions. Answers to this question as well as an understanding of the functional properties of DNA became more apparent in 1953 when James Watson and Francis Crick, working in England, were able to construct a model of the DNA molecule showing how the four nucleotide bases fit together. Each nucleotide was known to contain a phosphate group connected to a five-carbon sugar, deoxyribose, which, in turn, is connected to a purine or pyrimidine base. Two pyrimidines, called *cytosine* and *thymine,* and two purines called *adenine* and *guanine,* are associated together in DNA such that the amount of adenine is exactly the same as the amount of thymine, and the concentrations of guanine and cytosine are also equal to each other (Figure 6-2). This creates a configuration known as **complementary pairing.**

The Watson-Crick model showed that the DNA molecule was constructed of two long chains of nucleotides intertwined in a double helix (spiral). The deoxyribose sugar and the phosphate form the backbone of the molecule, and the purine and pyrimidine bases point toward the center and are connected in a specific pairing arrangement to hold the two chains together (Figure 6-3). The DNA molecule is in fact a linear sequence of base pairs. It is the order of base pairs in this sequence that maintains the genetic information and contains the code for all the information necessary to carry out each specific cell function. Complementary pairing is one of the essential features of the model and allows a DNA molecule to replicate into two identical molecules prior to each cell division. This enables each new cell formed by division to receive

Complementary pairing

a structural relationship between nucleotide bases that allows adenine to bond with thymine and guanine to bond to cytosine. These physical configurations ensure that a replicated DNA molecule will have the same structure and base pairs as the original molecule.

Figure 6-2   The structures of the two single-ring pyrimidine bases called cytosine and thymine, and the two double-ring purine bases called adenine and guanine.

Cytosine   Guanine   Adenine   Thymine

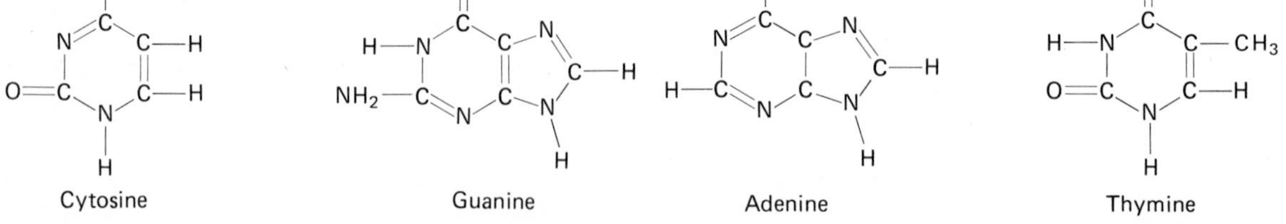

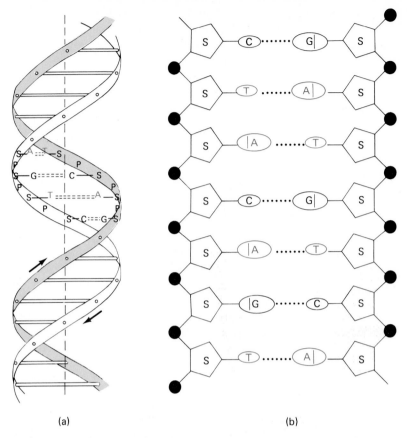

(a)   (b)

Figure 6-3   Structure of DNA molecule. (a) The molecule is made up of two polynucleotide chains. The backbone of the chains is composed of alternate sugars (S) and phosphate (P) units. The two chains are coiled in a double helix and connected by chemical bonds between the complementary bases (A:T, G:C). (b) A diagram of a section of DNA molecule uncoiled showing the alternate sugar (S) phosphate (●) backbones and the cross-connecting purine and pyrimidine bases.

an exact copy of the DNA molecule present in the parental cell. The Watson-Crick model provided a mechanism to show how the DNA molecule could divide and produce exact copies of itself for each new cell.

Replication

The ability of a cell to provide an exact copy of the genetic information for each daughter cell was essential to the genetic model. Each new cell must be able to perform all of the tasks previously performed by the parent cell, and also provide its own daughter cells with this capacity. In addition to providing structural information regarding DNA, the Watson-Crick model provided a

Replication

the process by which a cell produces an exact replica of its chromosome. This process is essential prior to cell division so that each cell will have a full copy of genetic instruction.

mechanism to show how the DNA molecule could replicate—that is, divide and produce exact copies of itself for each new cell.

In order to understand **replication,** it is necessary to know five specific features of this process: (1) base pairing is always complementary—in the DNA molecule adenine always pairs with thymine, and guanine always pairs with cytosine; (2) the two DNA strands in the helix are antiparallel—the base sequence of the two strands is the same, but reads in opposite directions (Figure 6-4); (3) replication of DNA requires a template (pattern) upon which any new DNA is synthesized; (4) it is necessary to have a nucleic acid polymer (a primer) to which the newly synthesized, growing DNA molecule can be attached, and (5) this entire reaction is under the careful guidance of a group of enzymes known as *DNA polymerases.*

When the cell is preparing to divide, or a new copy of the DNA molecule is required, it is first necessary that a single-stranded portion of the DNA molecule be made available as a template. To obtain this single-stranded structure, enzymes carefully unwind a portion of the DNA helix, and the hydrogen bonds between the complementary bases are broken. This produces two single-strand DNA templates that contain the same, but opposite, sequences of bases (Figure 6-4). Synthesis of new double-stranded DNA begins at a point on the DNA template known as the *origin,*

Figure 6-4   The mode of replication of a DNA molecule showing how identical sequences of nucleotide bases are maintained in each replicated molecule.

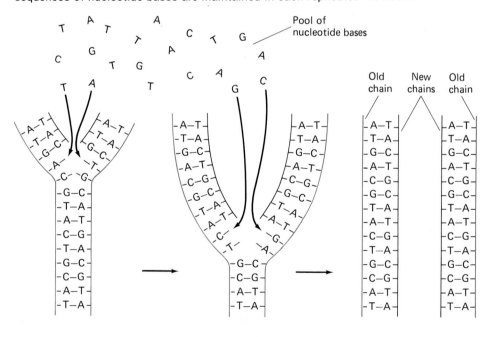

and can proceed along each of the available single strands. As replication proceeds, new nucleotides are positioned at their complementary site on each strand of the DNA molecule. The DNA polymerase enzymes bind each of the bases into proper position and the addition of new nucleotide bases continues along the entire molecule, with the resultant formation of two identical molecules (Figure 6-4). Each new DNA molecule contains one DNA strand from the old molecule and one newly synthesized strand. Although this model requires that the complementary nucleotide pairing between the two strands of the double helix remain rigidly specific, the linear arrangement of the nucleotides along the chains could be variable.

It is apparent that if the replication process makes a mistake by changing any of the bases from the proper linear sequence by addition, deletion, or substitution of the correct base, the nature of the genetic message could be altered. In order to prevent this, one of the polymerase enzymes, known as *polymerase III*, has the interesting task of "proofreading" the newly synthesized DNA strand. If mistakes are noted, appropriate correction is initiated to maintain the integrity of the cell.

RNA SYNTHESIS

The two kinds of nucleic acid, DNA and *ribonucleic acid* (RNA), are very closely related both in terms of structure and function. RNA is a single strand of bases attached to a sugar (ribose)-phosphate back bone and contains the bases guanine, cytosine, adenine, and uracil. This section will include a brief synopsis of the synthesis of RNA molecules. In the cell, there are three kinds of RNA known as **messenger RNA** (mRNA), *ribosomal RNA* (rRNA), and *transfer RNA* (tRNA). Each of these forms of RNA has a unique function related to the synthesis of protein.

The synthesis of each of the forms of RNA is similar. The four nucleotide bases in RNA—adenine, uracil, guanine, and cytosine—share the same complementary relationships as do the bases in DNA. Furthermore, DNA can, and does, act as a template for the synthesis of RNA. In this instance, the cell does not need a primer nucleic acid, but uses an RNA polymerase enzyme to assist the cell in separation of the DNA strands such that the DNA can serve as a template for RNA synthesis. The template ensures the proper sequence of bases in the RNA molecule. The process of RNA synthesis is known as *transcription* because the information encoded on the DNA molecule is transcribed onto an RNA molecule (Figure 6-5). Each base triplet in the DNA molecule is matched by a complementary RNA triplet called a **codon.**

Messenger RNA

a form of RNA that is formed by complementary base pairing with part of a DNA molecule. The messenger has the same base sequence but complementry base from the DNA. Messenger RNA takes the genetic message to the ribosome for protein synthesis.

Codon

three sequential mRNA bases that match a three-base sequence in the DNA code designating the position of a specific amino acid in a protein.

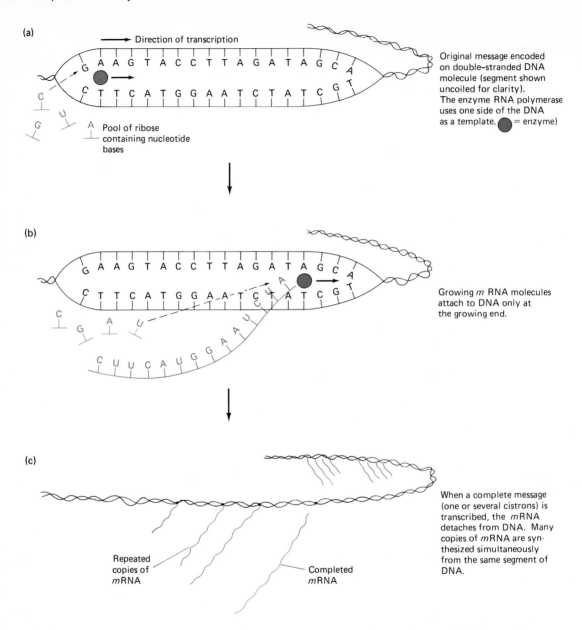

(a)

Direction of transcription →

Original message encoded on double-stranded DNA molecule (segment shown uncoiled for clarity). The enzyme RNA polymerase uses one side of the DNA as a template. ● = enzyme)

Pool of ribose containing nucleotide bases

(b)

Growing *m* RNA molecules attach to DNA only at the growing end.

(c)

When a complete message (one or several cistrons) is transcribed, the *m*RNA detaches from DNA. Many copies of *m*RNA are synthesized simultaneously from the same segment of DNA.

Repeated copies of *m*RNA

Completed *m*RNA

Figure 6-5   Transcription—the passage of genetic information from DNA to messenger RNA.

Transcription

Transcription involves the passage of genetic information from the DNA molecule into an RNA molecule. The process of transcription begins at one of several places in the DNA known as a *promoter site*. At this position, a momentary separation of the strands of the DNA molecule occurs and an RNA nucleotide is brought into the appropriate complementary position on one chain of the DNA molecule. Thus if the base on the DNA molecule is thymine, a ribose-containing adenine nucleotide will attach to it. When the enzyme moves to the next position on the DNA molecule, another RNA nucleotide is brought into a complementary position and is then connected to the adjacent RNA nucleotide through a ribose sugar-phosphate linkage. As the enzyme passes each nucleotide along the DNA molecule, the complementary RNA nucleotide is brought into place and connected to the growing mRNA chain. When the enzyme has passed over the last DNA nucleotide in the message, the end of transcription is signalled by a specific sequence of DNA bases called a *terminator*. The RNA is then separated from the DNA and the complementary DNA nucleotides rejoin to form the double helical orientation of the original DNA molecule. Thus the original message of the DNA molecule is both duplicated in the RNA and preserved in the DNA. The process of transcription is shown in Figure 6-5.

Protein Synthesis

Following the work of Watson and Crick, the challenge was to determine how the genetic information was encoded in the molecule. Obviously the information had to be encoded in the linear sequence of nucleotides along the chains of the DNA. It was therefore necessary to determine how a linear sequence of four nucleotide bases could direct the synthesis of such complex molecules as proteins. That is, how could a 4-letter nucleotide alphabet be used to correspond to a 20-letter amino acid alphabet? Obviously, a one-to-one nucleotide-to-amino acid relationship would not be sufficient to correspond to the 20 amino acids found in protein. The next alternative was to consider two neighboring nucleotides as a code for one amino acid, but this makes only 16 (4×4) possible combinations. The next alternative was to use a sequence of three nucleotides to code for each amino acid, which would give a total of 64 ($4 \times 4 \times 4$) possible combinations of nucleotide bases. This base arrangement has become known as a *triplet code*. Toward the end of the 1950s, sufficient experimental information had accumulated to show that the triplet code was the one used by DNA. Each sequence of three nucleotide bases in the DNA forms a letter of the genetic code. The determination of the genetic code—that is, discovering which triplet corresponded to which amino acid—took an additional 10 years and was completed in the late 1960s. Because there are 64 possible triplets and only 20 amino acids, some triplets were found to correspond to more than one amino acid. Three triplets, however, did not correspond to any amino acid and were shown to function as punctuation marks in the ge-

Termination sequence

a sequence of three bases that does not code for an amino acid, but terminates the length of the mRNA molecule as it is formed on the DNA template.

netic alphabet. These punctuation marks, or **termination sequences,** determine when the messages for specific polypeptides start and end (Table 6-1). The segment of bases in the DNA molecule that codes for one polypeptide is called a *cistron*. The DNA of a bacterial cell is a single molecule (about 1 mm in length) that contains approximately 10 million pairs of nucleotides, more than enough to code for the several thousand different proteins produced by the bacterial cell. That is, three nucleotide bases form one code triplet that corresponds to one amino acid; assuming that an average protein contains 300 amino acids, then 900 nucleotides would be needed in a single cistron to code for that protein.

During the late 1950s important research under the direction of Andre Lwoff, Francois Jacob, and Jacques Monod in France demonstrated how the genetic information of DNA is able to direct the synthesis of proteins. The process of protein synthesis frequently seems complex to most beginning students. However, it is more easily understood if it is remembered what the cell is trying to do. Each chemical reaction carried out by the cell requires the presence of a specific catalyst (enzyme) to make the reaction occur. Thus, if the cell needs to change glucose to glucose-1-phosphate, it can only do so in the presence of the appropriate enzyme (see Chapter 5). All enzymes are protein, and therefore proteins control the activities in the cell. However, the information

Table 6-1   Genetic code

First Letter	Second Letter				Third Letter
	U	C	A	G	
U	PHE	SER	TYR	CYS	U
	PHE	SER	TYR	CYS	C
	LEU	SER	–STOP–	–STOP–	A
	LEU	SER	–STOP–	TRY	G
C	LEU	PRO	HIS	ARG	U
	LEU	PRO	HIS	ARG	C
	LEU	PRO	GLN	ARG	A
	LEU	PRO	GLN	ARG	G
A	ILE	THR	ASN	SER	U
	ILE	THR	ASN	SER	C
	ILE	THR	LYS	ARG	A
	MET	THR	LYS	ARG	G
G	VAL	ALA	ASP	GLY	U
	VAL	ALA	ASP	GLY	C
	VAL	ALA	GLU	GLY	A
	VAL	ALA	GLU	GLY	G

Combining the letters of the codon into triplets composed of 1st, 2nd, and 3rd letters translates directly to a specific amino acid. Thus UUU translates to phenylalanine, AAA to lysine etc.

needed by the cell in order to know which enzyme to synthesize and when to produce it is contained in the DNA chromosome. It should be obvious then, that protein synthesis is under genetic control of the DNA of the cell, and in turn, cell function is under the control of protein molecules. In order to get the genetic information contained in the linear sequence of nucleotides along the DNA molecule into a linear sequence of amino acids in a protein molecule requires two phases: transcription and translation. Transcription has already been discussed; the translation phase of protein synthesis is described next.

Translation

The formation of protein from the mRNA message is called *translation* because it changes the genetic information from the nucleotide "alphabet" into the amino acid "alphabet" of proteins. Translation requires the involvement of each form of RNA: ribosomal RNA, transfer RNA, and messenger RNA. In eucaryotic cells the mRNA passes from the nucleus in the cytoplasm, where translation (Figure 6-6) occurs. In procaryotic cells translation can begin as soon as the mRNA begins to form, for no nuclear membrane separates the DNA from the protein-synthesizing components.

As noted in Chapter 4, each procaryotic ribosome is composed of two subunits, a large 50-S subunit and a smaller 30-S subunit. Both subunits are composed of rRNA and a variety of small proteins ranging in size from 10,000 to 40,000 MW. The two ribosomal subunits are not joined together into the 70-S ribosome complex unless they are involved in the actual synthesis of a polypeptide. The synthesis of protein is initiated when a messenger RNA molecule attaches to the rRNA present in the 30-S ribosome subunit. After this **initiation complex** is formed, the 50-S ribosome attaches to the mRNA completing the ribosome complex necessary for protein synthesis (Figure 6-7). The third form of RNA, transfer RNA, is named by its function. Thus, tRNA transfers amino acids from the cell cytoplasm to the ribosome complex such that the correct amino acid can be added in the growing polypeptide chain. Transfer RNAs are relatively short chains of nucleotides that contain a specific triplet of three nucleotides at one section of the molecule called an *anticodon*. A site exists on an end of the tRNA molecule apart from the anticodon that will combine with only one kind of the 20 different amino acids. After tRNA is synthesized in the nucleus, it is activated by one of a group of enzymes known as aminoacyl-tRNA synthetases. There are 20 of these enzymes, and each is specific for one of the 20 amino acids that may occur in proteins. Because of the **degenerate code** (Table 6-1), some of the enzymes will react with more than one tRNA molecule. The activation reaction requires an expendi-

Initiation complex

an arrangement of the 30-S ribosome and mRNA in a configuration such that the 50-S ribosome can attach, making the synthesis of protein possible.

Degenerate code

the property of the genetic code that allows an amino acid to be represented by more than one codon.

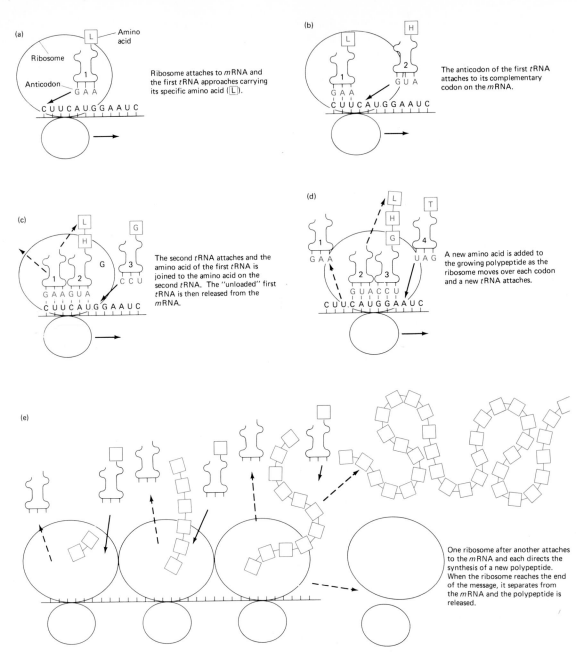

Figure 6-6   Translation of genetic information from a nucleotide sequence to an amino acid sequence.

ture of energy by the cell and the resulting tRNA–amino acid complex is now ready to interact with the ribosome complex (Figure 6-8).

The 70-S ribosome has two reaction sites—an ''A'' site for positioning the activated tRNA, which makes possible attachment

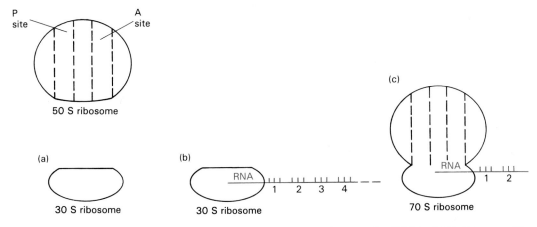

Figure 6-7   Formation of 70 S ribosome complex. (a) Attachment of mRNA to 30 S ribosome (b) initiates the formation of a 70 S ribosomal structure (c) from the 30 S and 50 S ribosome precursor particles. mRNA is shown as a sequence of RNA codons (1, 2, etc.).

of the growing peptide chain, and a ''P'' site where the peptide chain is held until the next amino acid is ready for attachment. This part of protein synthesis depends on three RNA functions: (1) recognition of the codon by the tRNA, (2) transfer of the polypeptide chain from tRNA at the P site to the amino acid at the A site, and (3) **translocation,** movement of the tRNA with its new polypeptide chain from the A site to the P site, thus making the A site available for the next activated tRNA.

    Recognition of the mRNA codon at the A site by an activated tRNA molecule requires that the three identifying bases of the tRNA (the anticodon) be complementary to the three bases in the available codon. Several proteins, called *elongation factors,* assist in the recognition process. During the transfer reaction a peptide bond (see Chapter 5) is formed between the terminal amino acid of the peptide chain and the amino acid held in position at the A site (Figure 6-8). During translocation, the free tRNA at the P site is released and the ribosome complex moves one codon down the mRNA. This puts the tRNA holding the peptide chain into the vacated P position. This process, although it appears to be complex, is repeated by the cell as frequently as 20,000 times per second and makes possible protein synthesis that is both accurate and rapid.

    Each ribosome attaches to one end of the newly formed mRNA and then moves along this molecule. Other ribosomes follow in sequence along the mRNA like beads on a string (Figure 6-9). Usually five or six ribosomes will be strung along a mRNA molecule; this complex of ribosomes is called a *polyribosome.* As ribosomes move along the same mRNA, one after the other, each forms an identical polypeptide. Consequently, thousands of pro-

Translocation
movement of a ribosome along the mRNA such that the tRNA attached to the newly formed peptide chain is moved one codon away from its anticodon.

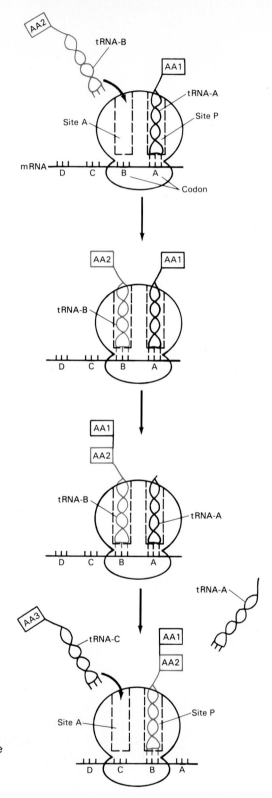

Figure 6-8 Interaction of ribosome with messenger and transfer RNAs for the synthesis of a polypeptide.

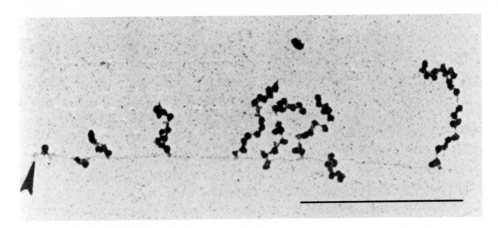

Figure 6·9   Active genes of a rapidly growing bacterium (*E. coli*). As soon as an *m*RNA molecule begins to be transcribed from DNA (presumed initiation site at arrow), ribosomes begin to attach. As the length of the *m*RNA increases, more ribosomes attach forming longer polyribosomes. In procaryotic cells, where the DNA is not separated from the ribosomes by a nuclear membrane, translation may begin before the complete *m*RNA is formed and while it is still attached to the DNA. (Bar = 0.5 μm.) (From Hamkalo and Miller, "Electronmicroscopy of Genetic Material," Figure 6a, p. 379. Reproduced, with permission, from *Annual Review of Biochemistry*, Volume 42. © 1973 by Annual Reviews, Inc.)

teins can be rapidly formed from a single mRNA molecule. The mRNA molecule functions for only a limited period and is then broken down by the cell's enzymes. New copies of the mRNA, however, are transcribed from the DNA as needed. The same genetic code is used by all living systems, with the flow of genetic information going from double-stranded DNA to single-stranded mRNA to polypeptide. The only exceptions are with some viruses, which use the same code but use nucleic acid molecules other than double-stranded DNA for the storage of their genetic information (see Chapter 32).

ALTERATIONS IN GENETIC INFORMATION OF THE CELL

The properties expressed by a microorganism in a given environment are a result of the genetic information contained in the DNA and are modified by environmental conditions. The genetic information—that is, the sequences of nucleotide bases in DNA—in a cell is referred to as the **genotype** of the cell. Nevertheless, when one observes cellular properties or functions, it is not the genotype (DNA) that is seen but the expression of the genes. This observable property of the cell is called its *phenotype*. The phenotype is always influenced by environmental conditions. When the environment changes, the cell responds by using a new portion of

Genotype
the total genetic information in the cell. Normally only selected parts of the genotype are used at any one time. Thus cells may have much greater genetic capability than is observable at any given time.

the genome (i.e., of the complete set of genes) and a different phenotype is expressed. If changes occur in the genotype of a cell, new messages are formed and a new phenotype may be produced.

The genotype of a microbial cell can be altered in three general ways. First, the sequence of nucleotide bases in the existing DNA molecule can be altered; second, the genotype of a cell may be altered by the addition of new DNA, and third, a new genotype results if portions of the DNA are deleted from the cell.

Mutation

Mutation

any change in the DNA base sequence that results in a permanent functional change in the cell.

Any change in the DNA base sequence is referred to as a **mutation,** and may be the result of either base-pair substitution or the insertion or deletion of a nucleotide. The most common mutational event occurs when a mistake in the replication process results in a substitution of one purine for the other (e.g., of adenine for guanine) or one pyrimidine for the other (e.g., of cytosine for thymine). Such substitutions produce a change (e.g., G-C replaced by A-T pairs) in subsequent DNA replications. These *point mutations* (Figure 6-10), if uncorrected by the DNA polymerase proofreading function, cause a change in a codon and may result in the incorporation of one different amino acid into the corresponding protein; this may or may not cause a change in the phenotypic expression of the cell. Purine to pyrimidine and vice versa changes are also known to occur, but are much less frequent than those noted bove.

A mutational event of more concern occurs when one or two base pairs are inadvertently added to or deleted from the DNA code sequence. These changes result in a change (shift) in the translation of all of the genetic message following the addition or deletions. For example, if the correct message was a sequence reading ACC/TAG/CTA/TCG/ . . . a deletion of the second adenine would change the message to read ACC/TGC/TAT/CG. . . . Changes of this type are called *frame-shift mutations* (Figure 6-11). Frame-shift mutations probably occur as a result of a break (nick) in one of the DNA strands, with the resulting addition or deletion of bases. Frame-shift mutation results in an entirely new sequence of amino acids in the corresponding protein; this protein is often nonfunctional, which may cause a pronounced phenotypic change in the cell.

As already noted, the results of a mutation may range from no observable phenotypic change to death of the cell. The question could be asked as to why all mutations are not expressed by a change in phenotype. In some instances the mutational event may be so small, such as with a point mutation, that only one resultant amino acid is different in a protein containing hundreds of amino acids. If the change is not in an amino acid that is critical

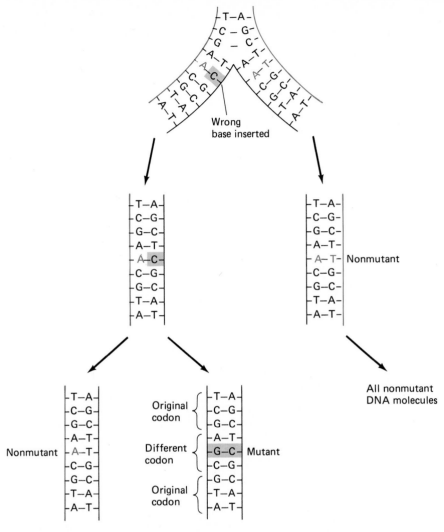

Figure 6-10   A point mutation produced by the wrong insertion of the base cystosine in the place of a thymine base. This results in one different codon in the mutant DNA molecule and one different amino acid in the resulting polypeptide.

to the protein structure, it is unlikely to have an adverse effect on cellular function. If, however, such a change results in the substitution to a **nonsense codon** (e.g., a termination sequence such as UAG, UAA, or UGA), synthesis of the polypeptide will be terminated at that point with a resulting functional loss to the cell. Other changes, such as frame-shift mutations, may result in synthesis of nonfunctional proteins. However, these mutational changes may be reversed if a second frame-shift mutation occurs downstream from the first change. These second mutations may

Nonsense codon

codons that do not correlate with any amino acid. A nonsense codon occurs whenever a termination sequence occurs in the DNA code. A nonsense codon terminates the process of translation whenever it occurs in the mRNA.

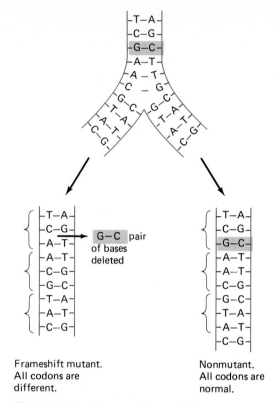

Figure 6-11   A frameshift mutation in which a pair of bases were deleted. This results in a new sequence of codons starting at the position of the deletion.

restore the frame-reading sequence to its proper order, and if the altered sequence of amino acids is not critical to cell function, a normal functioning cell will result.

In cells where there is a mutational loss of a functional protein (enzyme), such a loss will not affect the previously formed protein and the cell will continue to carry out normal activity. However, as the cell continues to divide, each generation will have only half the amount of the preexisting enzyme that was present in the parent cell. Thus, any observable phenotypic change will be delayed until the enzyme level is diluted out by cell division. This delay in phenotypic change is known as *phenotypic lag*. Conversely, mutations leading to the production of a new cellular enzyme (gain mutations) can be detected immediately.

Because most procaryotic cells have multiple copies of the chromosome, a mutation in one copy may not result in a change in cell function. However, as noted above, gain mutations are expressed, even by a single cell, while loss mutations require the segregation of the cells in order for its presence to be demonstrated (Figure 6-12).

Normally mutations occur during cell replication at a frequency of between 1:100,000 and 1:10 billion replications for any given phenotypic characteristic. Certain physical or chemical agents, called **mutagens,** may increase the rate at which mutations occur. A rather lengthy list of mutagens can be compiled and includes such agents as x rays, ultraviolet light, nitrous acid, acridine dyes, alkylating agents, and nucleotide-type bases that are

Mutagen
any environmental influence that increases the rate of mutation.

Figure 6-12   Bacteria grown on medium containing indicator for gene function. (a) Mutation of indicator negative cells gives immediately positive indicator cells (gain mutation). Mutation of indicator positive cells (loss mutation); cells give reduced positive indicator reaction until level of gene product is decreased below indicator threshold.

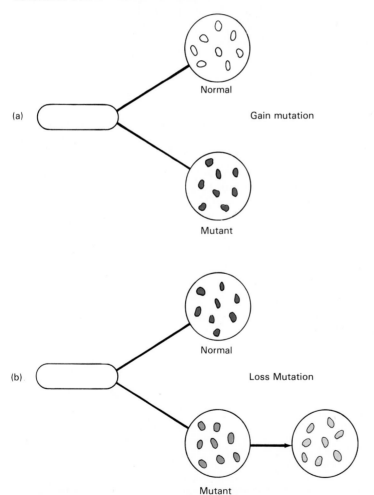

slightly different from the normal nucleotides in DNA (Table 6-2). The agents that increase the mutation rate of bacterial cells are also known to increase the occurrence of cancer in humans and animals. This data would suggest that an increase in gene instability may be an important antecedent to the development of human tumors.

Genetic Exchange

As with higher life forms, bacteria are capable of transferring genetic information (DNA) from one cell to another. However, these small single-celled organisms have evolved not one, but three methods by which they can transfer genes between two cells: *transformation, transduction,* and *conjugation.*

Transformation   The process of transformation is the transfer of cell-free fragments of DNA from one genome to another. This process was referred to earlier in the discussion of the Avery, MacLeod, and McCarty experiments with pneumococci that demonstrated the genetic role of DNA. Transformation of chromosomal DNA depends on a sequence of three distinct events: (1) binding of foreign DNA to a competent cell, (2) uptake of the DNA into the cell and, (3) integration of the foreign (donor) DNA into the chromosome of the recipient cell. These three steps are effectively completed only when the donor and recipient are closely related bacterial species. This process has been demonstrated to occur naturally in only a few species (Table 6-3). In some bacteria, binding of the donor DNA is to a specific DNA-binding protein found on the surface of the recipient cell. After attachment, the DNA fragment enters the recipient cell by passing through the cell wall and plasma membrane. This process is carried out only with relatively small DNA fragments. Enzymes at the cell surface nick (cut) the donor DNA so that the double-stranded DNA breaks upon entering the recipient, and one of the two donor strands is

Table 6-2   Substances That Increase the Frequency of Gene Mutation (Mutagens)

Mutagen	Action on Cell
2-Aminopurine	Base analog; causes transition mutations
Hydroxylamine	Causes G–C to A–T transitions
Nitrous acid	A–T to G–C and G–C to A–T transitions
X-ray irradiation	Breaks chromosome
Ultraviolet light	Breaks one strand of DNA molecule, leading to inaccurate repair
Nitrosoguanine	Alkylating agent; causes transitions and frameshift mutations

Table 6-3   Medically Significant Bacterial Species That Undergo Natural Transformation

Acinetobacter calcoaceticus	*Neisseria gonorrhoeae*
Bacillus subtilus	*Pseudomonas stutzeri*
Bacillus cereus	*Pseudomonas alkaligines*
Haemophilus influenzae	*Streptococcus pneumoniae*
Haemophilus parainfluenzae	*Streptococcus sanguis*
Moraxella osloensis	

digested upon entry, leaving a single strand of DNA free to bind with the recipient chromosome. When donor chromosomal DNA enters a cell, it becomes positioned alongside **homologous** genes (i.e., genes having the same base sequence) of the recipient cell. Enzymes cut out (excise) the homologous genes in the DNA of the recipient cell and the donor chromosomal fragment is integrated into the recipient cell's DNA in place of the excised DNA segment (Figure 6-13). This integration of donor DNA into the recipient DNA is called *recombination*. If the integrated DNA contains genetic information not previously possessed by the recipient cell, the transformation process will cause a genotypic change by adding new information and deleting the information on the excised DNA segment. Plasmids need not recombine with the chromosomal DNA and thus may not delete any information from the recipient cell, but they do add new genetic information.

Transduction   Transduction is a process in which a bacterial virus, known as a **bacteriophage** or phage, carries a small piece of bacterial DNA from a donor to a recipient cell. Transduction is a more frequent method of bacterial genetic transfer than is transformation, and occurs over a wide range (perhaps all) of bacterial species. Two forms of transduction occur: *generalized* (Figure 6-14) and *restricted* (Figure 6-15). A phage infects a bacterial cell by injecting its nucleic acid directly through the bacterial wall (Chapter 32). One type of transduction results when a phage infects a bacterial cell and causes the bacterial chromosome to fragment into many pieces. The phage nucleic acid then directs the bacterial cell to synthesize both new phage nucleic acid and protein coats. As new phage particles are assembled, a fragment of bacterial DNA may accidentally become packaged inside the phage protein coat. When several hundred new phages have been assembled, the bacterial cell bursts and releases the phages into the surrounding medium. When the phage containing bacterial chromosomes later infects a new cell, both the phage DNA and the bacterial DNA inside the phage are introduced into the new host. If the bacterial DNA fragment is carried into the new cell and recombines with the DNA of the recipient cell it will then be expressed. If a plasmid

Homologous

matching in structure. The condition of two pieces of DNA that have the same base sequence.

Bacteriophage

bacterial virus. Bacterial viruses are structurally similar to animal viruses. Each bacteriophage has a limited host range and can infect only specific kinds of bacterial.

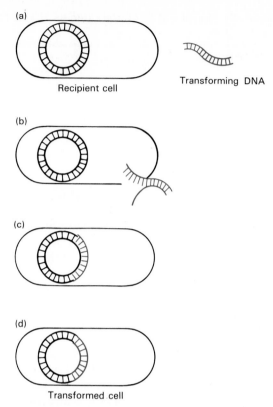

Figure 6-13 Transformation of a bacterial cell by integration of DNA. (a) Competent recipient cell and transforming DNA. (b) Transforming DNA attaches to competent cell and is degraded to single strand by cell nuclease. (c) Single strand DNA pairs with complementary bases of recipient cell chromosome. (d) Integrated transforming DNA is replicated and transformed daughter cells are formed.

Lysogenic
the condition of a bacterial cell that has the DNA of a bacteriophage integrated into its chromosome. Under these conditions the cell does not produce new bacterial viruses, but may carry out function under direction of the virus DNA.

is transported to the recipient cell by the phage, its genetic messages can be expressed without the need to integrate into the DNA of the recipient cell.

In restricted transduction, the bacteriophage does not initially cause the cell to reproduce new phage particles, but the phage integrates into the DNA of the host cell, a condition called *lysogeny*, and replicates along with the bacterial DNA during cell division (Figure 6-15). Periodically **lysogenic** phages are induced to break free from the bacterial chromosome and go through a replicative *lytic cycle*. In some instances, about one in 1 million cells, these phages do not break clean from bacterial DNA, but a

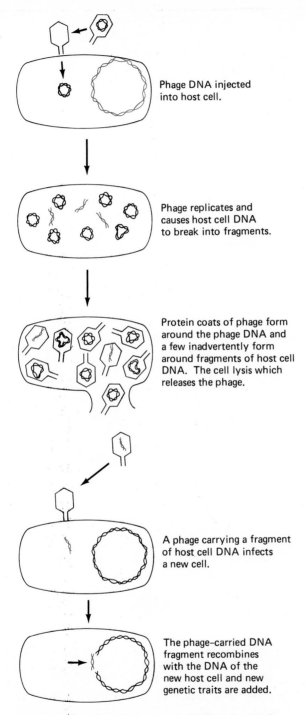

Phage DNA injected
into host cell.

Phage replicates and
causes host cell DNA
to break into fragments.

Protein coats of phage form
around the phage DNA and
a few inadvertently form
around fragments of host cell
DNA. The cell lysis which
releases the phage.

A phage carrying a fragment
of host cell DNA infects
a new cell.

The phage-carried DNA
fragment recombines
with the DNA of the
new host cell and new
genetic traits are added.

Figure 6-14   Generalized transduction in which
bacterial genes are transferred from one cell to
another by a phage.

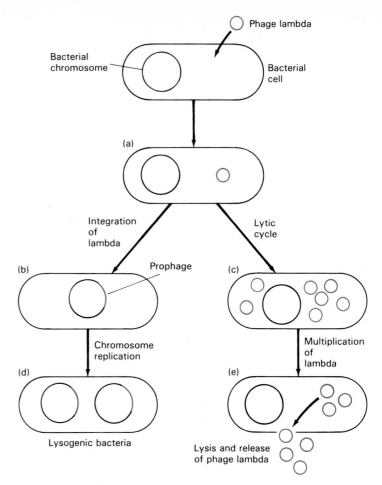

Figure 6-15   Results of bacterial infection by bacteriophage lambda. Following entry to lambda into a host cell (a) the virus DNA either integrates into, and becomes part of, the host chromosome (b), or multiplies independently (c) ultimately leading to bacterial lysis (e). Following integration, the lambda prophage replicates with the host chromosome (d).

Plasmid

circular, extrachromosomal DNA that can be transferred between cells by conjugation. Plasmids replicate independently of cell DNA, and provide genetic information that will be expressed in addition to that of the chromosome.

piece of the host DNA remains attached to the phage chromosome and replicates with it. The host genes are then packaged into the phage coats along with the virus and are transferred with them to new recipients. When these phages infect and integrate their DNA into a new recipient cell, the attached segment of bacterial DNA is also integrated and will induce new genetic traits in the recipient cells.

Conjugation   Bacterial conjugation (Figure 6-16) occurs as a consequence of small extrachromosomal genetic elements called **plasmids.** These small (MW = 10^6–10^8 Daltons) circular pieces of DNA

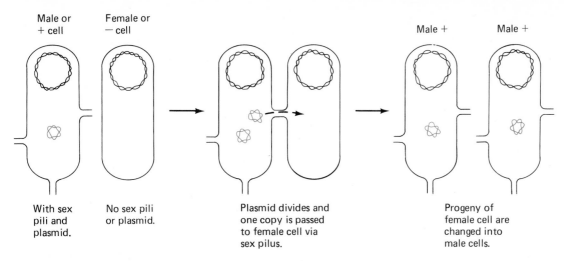

| Male or
+ cell | Female or
− cell | | | Male + | Male + |

Figure 6-16   A mechanism of conjugation in which genetic traits producing the male characteristics are passed with a plasmid to a female cell through a pilus.

frequently contain only a few genes and are similar to bacterial viruses except that they do not have protein coats, nor do they exist in a cell-free phase. As genetic information, plasmids are part of the genome of the bacterial cell.

Bacterial conjugation requires cell-to-cell contact and occurs in a wide variety of both Gram-positive and Gram-negative bacteria. The process of bacterial conjugation is under the direction of plasmids, which facilitate the transfer of both the plasmid and, occasionally, the chromosomal DNA from a donor to a recipient cell. Conjugation is the only known mechanism for the natural transfer of genetic material between different groups of bacteria. Both transformation and transduction appear to be limited to exchanges between closely related bacterial species.

Plasmid replication is under the control of the plasmid and not the bacterial cell. This control enables the plasmid to exist at either a *high copy number* (i.e., the ratio of the number of plasmid copies to the number of chromosome copies is large) or a low copy number (e.g., one). Many plasmids, particularly those associated with Gram-negative bacteria, carry genes necessary to initiate their own transfer between bacterial cells. These plasmid transfer genes code for a variety of proteins, the most notable of which is a long threadlike structure termed a *sex pilus* (see Chapter 4 for a discussion of pili). The end of the sex pilus adheres to any cell with the appropriate receptor site and binds the two cells together. The donor cell (with sex pilus) and recipient cell then join with wall-to-wall contact between the two cells. After the cells join, the plasmid replicates and a single-strand copy of the plasmid DNA is transferred to the recipient (female) cell. A complementary copy of the plasmid DNA is then made in both cells. When the cells break apart, both contain a complete copy of the plasmid and are potential donor (male) cells.

In most cases of conjugation none of the chromosomal DNA is passed. However, a unique plasmid known as F occurs in *E. coli* which may (in about 1 in 100,000 cells) integrate into the host cell DNA chromosome in a manner analogous to that for the lambda prophage (Figure 6-15).

Thus three states are possible with relation to F; the presence of F is F$^+$, the absence of F is F$^-$, and the integration of F is Hfr. Cells that are F$^+$ act similarly to cells containing other plasmids, but when replicative transfer occurs with Hfr cells, the entire bacterial chromosome is replicated and a single strand of DNA representing the bacterial chromosome as well as the Hfr is transferred across the **mating bridge** to the recipient F$^-$ cell. Usually before all the donor chromosome can be transferred, the cells separate and the recipient receives only part of the donor DNA. This transferred DNA becomes integrated into the recipient cell DNA and imparts new genetic characteristics to the recipient cell (Figure 6-17).

As new bacterial genes enter the recipient cell they do so in a linear fashion, one after the other until the entire chromosome is transferred, or the cell-to-cell bridge is broken. Because the transfer of DNA from donor to recipient occurs at a constant rate, it is possible to locate the individual genes on a chromosome in terms of the time it takes for transfer. Therefore, it is possible to determine the **gene sequence** on a bacterial chromosome both in terms of each genetic function (e.g., synthesis of a specific amino acid) and in terms of time of conjugal transfer. In some cases, the plasmid that has integrated into the donor cell chromosome can reverse the process and once again become a free plasmid in the cytoplasm. When the plasmids separate, however, they sometimes carry with them small segments of the donor cell chromosome, which then become a permanent part of the plasmid. When these are passed to a recipient cell, this plasmid carries with it the genetic information picked up from the donor cell chromosome (see lambda phage).

The Significance of Mutations and Gene Transfer

Most mutations that occur in microorganisms result in changes that are detrimental to the optimal performance of the mutant. These mutants are usually eliminated, because they are less able to survive or compete in the environment than normal microbes. Occasionally, however, a mutation or gene transfer occurs that gives a microbe an advantage in a given environment. This is illustrated by the advantage given to a cell that mutates to antibiotic resistance when grown in an environment containing the antibiotic. Such a new genotype may then be able to outcompete and

Mating bridge

a bridge formed between the walls of two adjacent bacteria through which a chromosome may be transferred. Formation of the bridge is under genetic control of the F factor.

Gene sequence

the linear arrangement of functional genetic units along the chromosome. Each gene has a linear position in relation to all other genes on the chromosome.

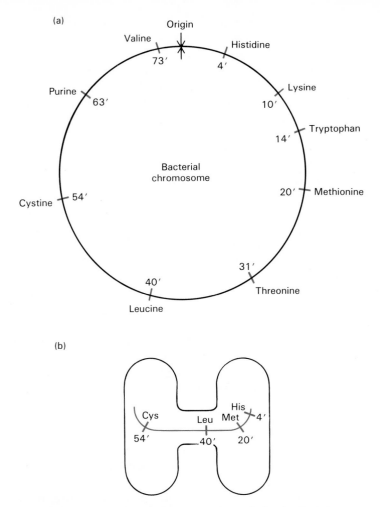

Figure 6-17 Transfer of genetic markers during bacterial conjugation. (a) A partial genetic map of *Pseudomonas aeruginosa* showing the location of various genes as a function of the time needed for transfer during conjugation. (b) A diagrammatic illustration of sequential gene transfer during conjugation.

will replace most normal microbes in that particular environment, or else it may be able to grow in an environment where normal microbes are unable to grow. New genotypes that have an advantage, or have adapted to a new environment, may regularly develop in microbial populations where cell division occurs rapidly.

Mutations may be beneficial or detrimental to human needs. The most troublesome changes associated with medical microbiology are strains of microbes that develop resistance to antimicrobial agents. Antibiotic resistance can be acquired through both mutations and gene transfers. Some genes associated with plasmids, or acquired by transduction, impart disease-producing capabilities

Host range

the kinds of hosts that can be infected by a specific microorganism. Host range is determined by receptors on both the host cells and the microorganism. A parasite with a broad host range can infect many kinds of cells.

(virulence factors) to microorganisms (refer to Table 6-4). Those plasmids with a very broad **host range,** make an immensely large gene pool available to any given bacterial species. Such broad host-range conjugation provides a large genetic reservoir for those bacteria that may be subjected to evolutionary pressures.

Selected mutants and microbes with recombined genes are sometimes of great use. Certain mutants have been selected as highly efficient producers of products of commercial value. For example, when the original *Penicillium* mold (used for the antibiotic) was treated with such mutagens as x rays and ultraviolet light, it was possible to induce a mutant that produced a 1000 times greater yield of penicillin. This mutant allowed penicillin to be produced much more efficiently. Some mutants of disease-producing bacteria that have lost most of their disease-causing capabilities have been effectively used as living vaccines.

The fact that mutagens of bacteria also tend to cause cancer in humans has prompted the testing of many chemicals each year to determine if they are able to increase the mutation rate in bacteria. These tests take only a few days and are relatively inexpensive. Only those chemicals that are mutagenic for bacteria are then further tested by slower and more expensive methods using experimental animals. Thus by using bacteria in the screening tests, the number of chemicals tested in the animal system is greatly reduced and overall many more chemicals can be tested.

GENETIC ENGINEERING

As understanding of DNA function has increased throughout the scientific community, it was natural that studies of laboratory induced changes in gene arrangements would follow. Presently

Table 6-4   Representative Bacterial Virulence Properties That Are Plasmid-Borne

Property	Bacterial Example
Colonization factor	*Neisseria gonorrhoeae*
	Escherichia coli
Invasiveness	*Shigella flexneri*
	Escherichia coli
Enterotoxin (ST, LT)	*Escherichia coli*
Dermal exfoliative toxin	*Staphylococcus aureus*
Antimicrobial resistance	Various; associated with "R factor" plasmids
Neurotoxin	*Clostridium tetani*
Iron sequestration	Various

there is great interest in manipulated gene transfer among microorganisms. This technology, called *genetic engineering* or *recombinant DNA technology*, has the potential of developing microorganisms that are able to produce many useful products that are difficult or impossible to produce by other methods. With this technology it is possible not only to transfer genes from one type of bacterium to another but also to transfer genes from other forms of life into microorganisms. This aspect of science has grown so rapidly and encompasses such a large body of knowledge that it is beyond the scope of this text. Interested students can find additional information by examining the references listed at the end of this chapter.

Perhaps the key discovery associated with genetic engineering was that of enzymes that carry out specific DNA modification functions—for example, *restriction endonucleases* (Table 6-5), which are able to cleave double-stranded DNA molecules, and **DNA ligase** which provides a means of linking DNA molecules together as well as filling in missing bases in the DNA chain. One or more restriction endonucleases occur naturally in most bacterial species and are likely the result of evolutionary selection. These enzymes (more that 200 have been studied) cut DNA molecules at specific base sequences that occur in palindromic order (reading the same in both directions) and protect an organism against the intrusion of unwanted or unneeded DNA from a foreign source. Once cut, foreign DNA is rapidly broken down into nucleotides by nonspe-

DNA ligase
an enzyme that can join two pieces of homologous (complementary) DNA together.

Table 6-5   Representative Restriction Endonuclease Enzymes

Enzyme	Source	Site of Action
Aat II	*Acinetobacter aceti*	GACGTC CTGCAG
Bam HI	*Bacillis amyloliquefaciens*	GGATCC CCTAGG
Bgl II	*Bacillus globigii*	AGATCT TCTAGA
Eco RI	*Escherichia coli*	GAATTC CTTAAG
Hind III	*Haemophilus influenzae*	AAGCTT TTCGAA
Pst I	*Providencia stuarti*	CTGCAG GACGTC
Sma I	*Serratia marcescens*	CCCGGG GGGCCC
Xho I	*Xanthomonas holcicula*	GTCGAG GAGCTC
Xma I	*Xanthomonas malvacaerum*	CCCGGG GGGCCC

cific endonucleases found within the cell. Bacteria are protected against their own restriction endonucleases by a chemical modification of the base sequence at the restriction sites, which are the substrates for restriction endonucleases.

The endonuclease breaks both plasmid and foreign DNA where identical sequences of nucleotides are located. This break is such that a short segment of single-stranded DNA is left at the ends of the broken DNA molecules (Figure 6-18). Using this procedure, the nucleotide sequences at the ends of both DNA molecules become complementary. Such complementary single strands are called "sticky" ends, and they specifically combine with the single-stranded ends of any other DNA molecule that has been treated with the same endonuclease.

Other technical advances that have helped to faciliate genetic engineering are the ability to determine the sequence of bases in DNA molecules (base sequencing), the capacity to synthesize short segments of DNA molecules *(oligomers)* in the laboratory, and the development of ways to use the bacterial enzymes in molecular cloning.

Laboratory manipulation of restriction endonucleases provides a method for carying out molecular cloning as shown in Figure 6-18. To carry out a cloning experiment, a suitable *vector* (plasmid or bacteriophage) is first chosen. This vector must have the ability to infect the desired host bacterium (*E. coli* is most often used) and to multiply within the host. The DNA to be cloned (foreign DNA) is then selected and both the vector and foreign DNA are treated separately with the same kind of restriction endonuclease. When the endonuclease-treated vector and foreign genes are mixed together in the presence of the DNA ligase, their "sticky" ends join together and the foreign gene becomes integrated into the vector. The recombined vector can then be placed back into the host bacterium. The vector now replicates independently of the host, and may produce as many as 2000 copies of both itself and the integrated foreign gene. Procedures are available that will permit the removal of these gene copies, which can then be recut with the restriction endonuclease and purified in large numbers. Alternatively, each progeny bacterium that contains the foreign gene will be able to produce the protein coded by this gene. Because of the rapid growth of microorganisms, large amounts of "foreign" proteins can be produced by such genetically engineered microbes.

Some early applications of genetic engineering included the development of bacteria that could produce human insulin (Figure 6-19) and human-growth hormones. These products have now become available in relatively inexpensive forms for the treatment of diabetics and children with growth defects. Prior to these developments, insulin was obtained from animals and human-growth

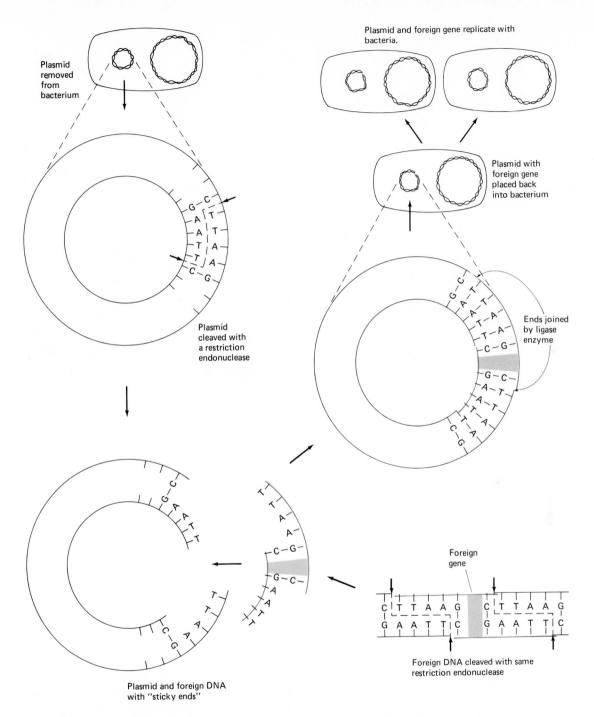

Figure 6-18   A method used to place a foreign gene in a bacterium by genetic engineering.

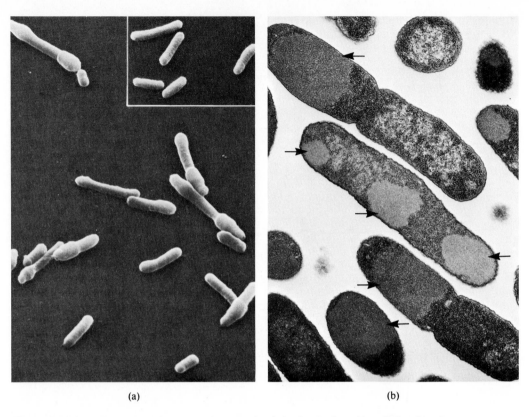

(a)   (b)

Figure 6-19   (a) Scanning electron micrograph of the bacterium *E. coli* that has been genetically engineered to produce components of human insulin. The prominent bulges are caused by the accumulation of insulin inside the bacterial cells; insert shows normal *E. coli* which lack the bulges. (b) Transmission electron micrograph of the insulin producing *E. coli* showing prominent inclusion bodies (arrows) resulting from the accumulation of bacterial-produced human insulin. (Figure 2 and 3 from "Cytoplasmic Inclusion Bodies in *Escherichia coli* Producing Biosynthetic Human Insulin Proteins," D. C. Williams et al., *Science* 215: 687–689. Copyright 1982 by The American Association for the Advancement of Science. Courtesy D. C. Williams, Eli Lilly and Co.)

hormone was obtained from human cadavers and was in very limited supply.

New vaccines, particularly against viral diseases, that could not be produced economically by conventional methods are now being developed through genetic engineering. Large amounts of an antiviral (and possibly anticancer) agent called *interferon* (Chapter 33) are being produced by this new technology; it may soon be possible to treat many diseases that were not previously treatable.

In order to use the rapid growth of microorganisms to increase production and reduce the costs, recombinant DNA technology is being applied in many other areas, such as food and energy production. Genetic engineering is, in fact, creating a technological revolution.

CONCEPT SUMMARY

1. The chemical structure of DNA and its functional operation form the basis for the principles of inheritance and the control of cell activity. Through the process of replication, genetic continuity is maintained while the processes of transcription to RNA and translation to protein account for the maintenance of cell control. Heritable change in the DNA nucleotide sequence is called *mutation* and results in an altered protein synthesis.

2. Bacterial genetic exchange occurs through the processes of conjugation, transduction, and transformation. These processes are analogous to sexual reproduction in higher life forms.

3. Three structural kinds of RNA are found in living cells. These molecules are essential components of genetic translation.

4. Scientific understanding of the functions of DNA and RNA have made possible transfer and redesign of the bacterial chromosomes.

STUDY SUMMARY

1. Describe the concept of complementary pairing and explain how this principle ensures continuity of genetic information from generation to generation.

2. What role does each of the three RNA molecules play in protein synthesis?

3. In principle, why are frame-shift mutations likely to be more damaging to a cell than are point mutations.

4. Why are most mutations harmful rather than beneficial?

5. Construct a table comparing the parameters limiting genetic exchange by (a) conjugation, (b) transformation, and (c) transduction.

6. Why was the discovery of restriction endonuclease such an important step in genetic engineering?

REFERENCES FOR FUTHER STUDY

1. DNA Replication. *Trends in Biochemical Science* 9:122, 1984.
2. *The Microbial World,* 5th ed., R. Stanier, 1986. Prentice-Hall.

3. *The Molecular Biology of the Cell*, B. Alberts, 1983. Garland.

4. *A Dictionary of Genetics*, 3rd ed., Riking, 1985. Oxford.

5. Genetic Transformation. *Annual Review of Biochemistry* 50:41, 1981.

6. The Conjugation System of F-like Plasmids. *Annual Review of Genetics* 14:41, 1980.

7. *Microbiology—1985*, L. Leive, 1985. American Society for Microbiology.

chapter 7

GROWTH AND NUTRITION OF MICROORGANISMS

T he materials and procedures necessary for the laboratory cultivation of microorganisms developed over many years and are still developing. Our understanding of bacterial growth and nutrition is critical to the methods used in isolating and identifying disease agents in the clinical laboratory. This chapter focuses on a working understanding of the growth of bacteria and helps to define processes routinely used in diagnostic microbiology.

NUTRITIONAL REQUIREMENTS OF BACTERIA

Bacteria were first carefully studied in association with infectious diseases. It was early recognized that these microorganisms would not grow on simple substances but required a complex diet, frequently consisting of mammalian body fluids. Such **nutrients** are needed to supply a source of energy and provide the necessary components for cell growth. All disease-producing bacteria—all fungi, protozoa, and animal cells—require organic chemical compounds as a source of carbon and energy; such cells are called *heterotrophs.* The methods used by these cells to obtain energy from organic compounds, primarily glucose, were discussed in Chapter 5.

Certain bacteria, not of direct medical importance, use CO_2 as their source of carbon; such microbes are called **autotrophs.** Some autotrophs obtain their energy from the oxidation of inorganic compounds, such as nitrates, sulfur, and hydrogen, and are called *chemoautotrophs.* Other autotrophs, such as algae and some bacteria, contain chlorophyll and are able to obtain energy from light through the process of photosynthesis; these microbes are called *phototrophs,* or more precisely, *photoautotrophs.*

The most common chemical elements needed by bacterial

Nutrients

ingredients used by a living organism to facilitate growth. This is a general term and applies to energy sources as well as essential vitamins or minerals.

Autotroph

an organism that does not use energy-rich organic compounds for food.

cells are carbon, hydrogen, oxygen, nitrogen, sulfur, phosphorus, potassium, magnesium, calcium, iron, and sodium. In addition, elements like zinc, molybdenum, copper, and manganese are needed in small amounts and are referred to as *trace elements* (Table 7-1). Heterotrophic microbes obtain their carbon from organic compounds, such as sugars, proteins, and lipids. Hydrogen is usually obtained from water, and oxygen is obtained from the atmosphere or from water, where it is found in a dissolved state. Nitrogen, sulfur, and phosphorus can be obtained from either organic or inorganic sources. Most of the other needed elements are obtained from soluble inorganic compounds. Some bacteria, especially several of the disease-producing species, require special growth factors, such as vitamins and amino acids, which explains their need for blood or other animal body fluids.

CULTURE MEDIA

The growth, or *culture*, of a given bacterium requires a culture *medium* (plural *media*) that provides all the essential nutrients, the proper concentration of salts and ions, and the proper pH (relative acidity or alkalinity) for optimum bacterial growth to occur. Moisture is always essential for bacterial growth because the various nutrients must be in a soluble form or in a form that can be solubilized to facilitate diffusion into the cell.

It may be necessary in some studies of bacteria to use a chemically defined medium, called a *synthetic medium,* in which all essential nutrients are supplied as pure chemicals. Such synthetic media are often difficult and expensive to produce for heterotrophic bacteria. Therefore, *complex media* are frequently used in which all necessary ingredients are present but are not precisely defined. Complex media are often mixtures of organic products from plants, animals, or yeasts, along with appropriate salts, and usually contain the nutrients necessary for the growth of a wide range of bacteria. Products like extracts of malted barley, animal tissue, or baker's yeast are frequently used in complex media. Acid or enzyme digests of meats, casein, or soybean protein are also used. These products contain most nutrients, both organic

Table 7-1   Major Elements Essential for Bacterial Growth

Nitrogen	Sulfur	Sodium	Calcium
Oxygen	Phosphorus	Magnesium	Zinc
Carbon	Potassium	Iron	Manganese

and inorganic, that are needed even by the most **fastidious** microorganisms.

Today almost all culture media formulations are produced by commercial companies and supplied to laboratories as dehydrated products (Figure 7-1). To prepare media at the consumer's laboratory, a specified amount of a dehydrated medium is added to a given volume of distilled water. The medium is then sterilized in an autoclave (see Chapter 8) and dispensed in **sterile** test tubes or other appropriate containers (Figure 7-2). Currently, many clinical laboratories purchase their culture media already reconstituted and dispensed in appropriate sterile containers.

Culture media are prepared in both liquid *(broth)* and solid forms. The broth media are made simply by dissolving nutrients in water. Solid media are made by adding a solidifying agent to a broth medium. We are indebted to the laboratory of Robert Koch for the discovery of an appropriate solidifying agent for growth of bacteria. As noted in Chapter 1, many of today's bacteriological techniques were developed in the Koch laboratory. Koch recognized that bacteria would effectively reproduce in broth, but if two or more kinds of bacteria were introduced into a broth medium, the resultant growth was a mixed culture. It was extremely difficult to study the properties of any bacterial species as long as it was mixed with other microorganisms. Earlier studies had shown that when placed on a solid medium, such as bread, solidified egg albumen, or the surface of a freshly cut potato, bacteria would grow into a colony consisting of only one kind of bacterial species.

Fastidious
requiring special nutrient supplementation in order to grow.

Sterile
without life. A microbiologically sterile environment contains no living organisms.

Figure 7-1   Some examples of commercially prepared dehydrated culture media. Components and instructions for preparation and use are given on the labels.

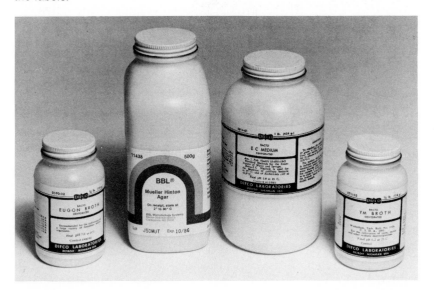

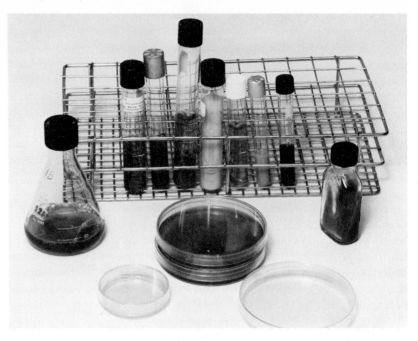

Figure 7-2 Sterilized culture media dispensed into various containers. Petri dishes containing solid agar media are in the foreground. Test tubes and flasks may contain either solid or liquid medium.

The problem for Koch, however, was that such solid surfaces lacked the necessary nutrients to grow disease-producing bacteria, or they produced colonies that could not be easily distinguished from the background surface, or they produced several different kinds of bacterial colonies that were indistinguishable from each other. These problems greatly limited the scientific study of disease-producing microorganisms.

Faced with this problem, Koch tried adding gelatin to clear broth media in order to obtain a solid surface on which to grow microorganisms from infectious processes.

Although this approach enabled Koch to provide the necessary nutritional support for the organisms under study, and growth of various species could be distinguished by their colonial differences, it failed to provide an appropriate solution to the problem because some bacteria digested the gelatin. Further, at optimal bacterial growth temperatures (37° C) gelatin was no longer solid. Therefore, cultures of bacteria in such a system were often equivalent to cultivation in broth.

A solution to the problem came through an observation made by Hesse, one of Koch's assistants. Frau Hesse was aware that in Indonesia a seaweed extract was boiled with fruit juices to provide a jellylike product. Hesse concluded that if such material could be added to the nutrient broths used to grow bacteria, it might be a satisfactory solidifying agent. The seaweed extract, a complex polysaccharide called *agar,* proved to be an ideal product to solidify culture media. Agar is inert for most bacteria and thus does not change the nutritional qualities of the media. It also has the useful property of melting at a temperature just below the boiling point; yet once melted, it will remain in the liquid state until it is cooled to about 44° C. Consequently, the solid medium can be incubated at relatively high temperatures if necessary for the growth of bacteria while the liquid phase can be cooled to a temperature that will not damage heat-sensitive nutrients, chemicals, or live microorganisms that might need to be mixed in the medium before it solidifies. The main advantage of solid media is that they provide a surface on which bacteria can be deposited and grown without mixing with other bacteria. Solid media are widely used for isolating, characterizing, and counting bacteria.

When a bacterial cell is deposited on the solid surface of an agar medium, the cell rapidly divides and its progeny pile up into a mass of identical cells. This mass of cells is called a *colony* (Figure 7-3) and is usually visible to the naked eye by 24 hours. The characteristics of colonies vary among bacterial species and are useful aids in helping to identify a particular species. The colonies may vary in size, texture, contour, margin, and color (Figure 7-4).

Types of Culture Media

Bacteria vary widely in their nutritional requirements, and hundreds of different formulations of culture media have been formulated to provide optimum nutrition for cultivated microorganisms. Some media are formulated to favor the growth of one type of microorganism over others and are called *selective media.* Selective media may contain ingredients that either improve or inhibit the growth of all but a certain group of microorganisms and are used when attempting to isolate these microbes from an environment heavily contaminated with other types of microorganisms. An example of a selective medium is one that contains 7% salt (NaCl). This factor will inhibit or impede the growth of most microorganisms but not the growth of staphylococci; when cultured on this medium, staphylococci will characteristically outgrow other bacteria that may be present. Some types of media contain dyes or other chemicals that specifically react with cellular components or growth products produced by a given bacterium. These reactions produce a specific change in the medium or the microbial colony. Such media are called *differential,* for they help to differentiate one type of bacterium from others that might be growing on the same surface.

Bacterial species vary in the types of carbohydrates they are able to use for energy. Differential media have been made with many of these specific carbohydrates or other organic compounds

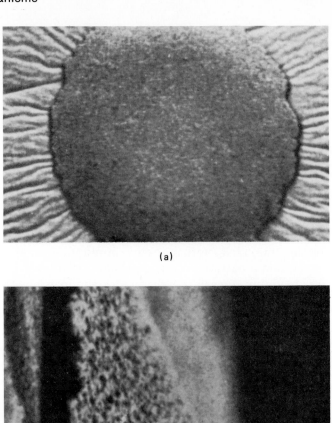

(a)

(b)

Figure 7-3 Scanning electron micrographs of colonies of gonococci shown at increasing magnifications. (a) Viewed from above at 240× magnification, (b) viewed from the side at 1200× magnification and (c) 6000× magnification showing individual cells. (T. Elmros, P. Hörstedt, and B. Winblad, *Inf. Imm. 12*:630–637, Figures 1c, 2c, and 3d, with permission from ASM)

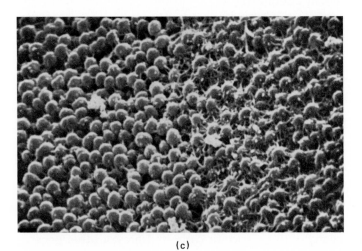

(c)

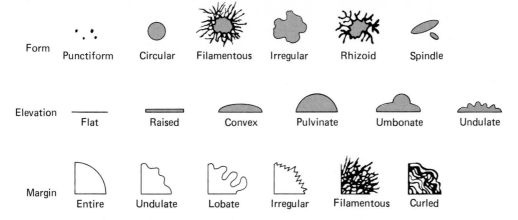

Figure 7-4   Outline drawings of some of the characteristics of various isolated bacterial colonies.

as sources of carbon and energy. These media also contain an indicator dye that will change color when the pH of the medium changes. Thus, when a bacterium is able to use the specific carbohydrate and grows sufficiently in the medium to produce enough acid or alkali to change the color of the indicator dye, the color change can be used to assist in identifying the bacterium. Some microbes also produce gases that can be detected by trapping the gas in small inverted vials *(Durham tubes)* that are placed in tubes of broth (Figure 7-5). The production of gas during metabolism is used as an identifying feature for some bacteria.

Pure Cultures

Microorganisms of various types are found growing together in natural environments. In order to study and characterize a particular microorganism, it must first be separated and grown free of

Figure 7-5   A method used to detect gas production by a bacterium.

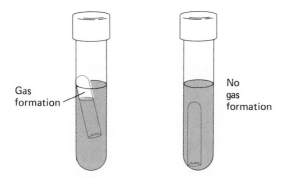

Pure culture

a culture containing only a single species of microorganisms. It is almost impossible to identify microbes unless they can be grown in pure culture.

other microorganisms; this is called a **pure culture.** The development and maintenance of pure cultures are important basic procedures in microbiology and are extensively used in the laboratory diagnosis of infectious diseases.

The most common method of isolating pure cultures is called *streaking* (Figure 7–6). Here a wire loop or cotton swab is first placed in contact with the environmental source to be examined so that the loop or swab picks up a random sample of the microbes present. The loop or swab is then rubbed over one edge of the agar surface contained in a *petri dish*. A petri dish is a small, flat, usually round container with vertical sides and a cover; it permits the liquid agar to harden into a readily available flat surface (Figure 7-2). The loop or swab deposits those bacteria picked up from the source on the surface of the agar. Next, a sterile wire inoculating loop is moved through the deposited bacteria and then streaked over about one-fourth of the untouched agar surface. This step deposits bacteria from the area inoculated by the swab along the lines of the streak. The loop is sterilized and moved through the second streaking, followed by streaking over a fresh one-fourth of the plate. This procedure may be repeated one more time (Figure 7-6). Each streak increasingly dilutes the population of bacteria until single cells are deposited along the streak lines. After incubation for 1 or several days, individual colonies will develop where the single cells were deposited. Bacteria

Figure 7-6 Streak plate showing thinning out of the bacteria with each additional streaking untill well-isolated colonies develop.

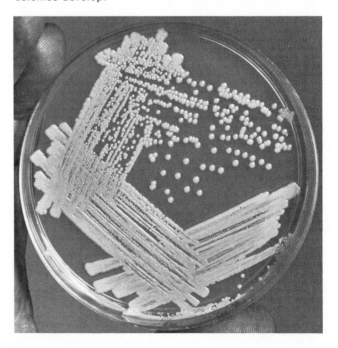

from each colony can then be transferred to a separate sterile medium to produce a pure culture. To ensure that the culture is pure, a second streak plate may be made from a single colony. This procedure may be repeated a number of times until all the colonies appear identical and the culture is assumed to be pure.

IDENTIFICATION OF BACTERIA

Once a pure culture is obtained, a series of tests can lead to identification of the isolated bacterium. To begin with, a trained microbiologist is able to select those colonies from the primary isolation media that are most likely to represent disease-producing bacteria. The morphology and staining characteristics can readily be determined by microscopic examination and a colony from a pure culture is then inoculated into a selected variety of differrential and selective culture media. By comparing the reactions on these media with the known characteristics of different species of bacteria, it is usually possible to determine which disease-producing microbe was isolated from the patient. When organisms produce similar **biochemical reactions,** it is sometimes necessary to use specific antibodies to make a precise identification; this concept will be discussed in Chapter 13.

Biochemical reaction
changes in bacteriologic culture media by the growth of microorganisms.

Besides specifically identifying the microbe that is causing the disease, it is important to know which antibiotics will inhibit its growth and could be used for therapy. Antibiotic susceptibility testing (Chapter 9) is often performed concurrently with the identification tests. Because organism identification and antibiotic susceptibilities are often critical to proper patient care, the time required to obtain these data is an important factor in clinical microbiology. Using traditional procedures, it may require from several hours to several days to complete identification tests on most bacteria; this factor becomes significant in the care of a critically ill patient. Today modern technology is applied in various forms to shorten the time required to obtain the needed information for optimal treatment of the patient.

RECENT LABORATORY INNOVATIONS

Some of the recent laboratory innovations involve miniaturized units that allow rapid **inoculation** of many different types of differential media or enzyme substrates that give rapid identification information (Figure 7-7). Such test kit systems are expensive but they save technician time and reduce the amount of media and space required to run the tests. Instrumentation is now available

Inoculation
a process whereby microorganisms are placed into or on culture media.

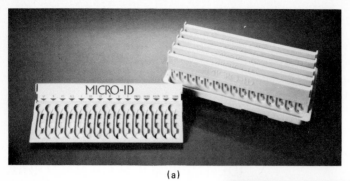

(a)

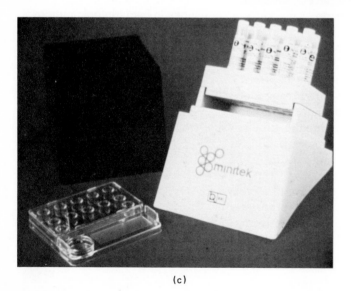

(b)

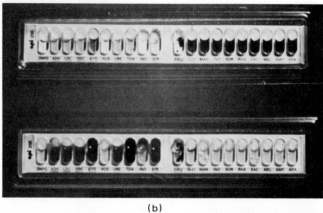

DEXTROSE

LYSINE

ORNITHINE

H$_2$S—INDOLE

LACTOSE

P. A.—DULCITOL

UREA

CITRATE

(c)   (d)

Figure 7-7   A composite of presently available miniaturized, or kit-type, procedures used to identify bacteria in the laboratory. Each of these systems requires isolated organisms in pure culture. The time required for completion of the test varies from 5 to 6 hours for the MICRO-ID (a) and API (b) systems to 24 hours for systems such as Enterotube (d). (a) The MICRO-ID system showing a series of small plastic cuplets which contain identifying chemicals as indicated (courtesy Warner-Lambert Company). (b) The API system showing both a negative (upper set of reactions) and a positive (lower set of reactions) test for the 20 biochemicals used in the identification scheme (Courtesy Analytab Products). (c) Small paper disks containing any of many desired biochemicals are placed into the plastic holder and then inoculated with bacteria; this Minitek system has great versatility. (d) The Enterotube was one of the earliest kit-type approaches to bacterial identification; in this system the inoculating needle (seen in the center of the tube) is drawn through a series of small media chambers and the unit is then incubated.

that can detect the presence of bacteria in normally sterile body fluids, such as blood. Samples of body fluid are introduced into vials of medium containing carbohydrates that have radioactive carbon atoms (Figure 7-8). As the bacteria grow in this medium, radioactive CO_2 is released. This CO_2 can be detected by a sensitive instrument (Figure 7-9), often after as little as 4 to 8 hours of incubation. Other instruments, such as the Autobac (Figure 7-10), can be used to determine antibiotic susceptibility in periods as short as 4 hours.

Continued success of research into molecular genetics has provided a tool for rapid, specific microbial detection and identification directly from clinical specimens, such as tissue or sputum, received by the laboratory. Such specimens can be examined for the presence of individual pathogens by mixing the specimen with a radiolabeled DNA probe. If microorganisms in the specimen have the same DNA base sequence as the DNA probe, the two will bind together. After any excess probe is washed away, remaining radioactivity is directly proportional to the number of microorganisms present in the specimen (Figure 7-11). Thus by using newer technological advances, it is often possible to provide a physician with vital information within a few hours regarding the nature of the microorganism that may be causing the infection in the patient.

Several advances in automation involve the coupling of microgrowth chambers with sensitive electronic detectors of chemical changes. These systems can be interfaced with computers that collect and analyze the data. These instruments, such as the Automicrobic System (Figure 7-12), are able to provide a probable identification of the microbe, as well as information on antimicrobial susceptibility in hours instead of the days required by older traditional methods. New and innovative instruments are being developed each year to aid in the clinical microbiology laboratory, and medical personnel will need continual updating to keep informed of these advances.

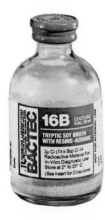

Figure 7-8   Radiolabeled medium used in the BACTEC system for the rapid detection of the presence of pathogens in human body fluids.

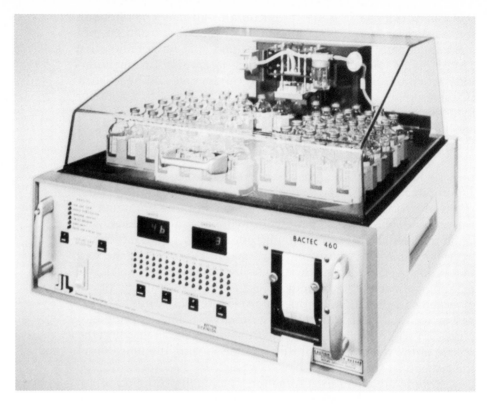

Figure 7-9   The BACTEC instrument used to monitor the development of radiolabeled CO_2 from growing bacteria. This instrument continuously monitors each bottle of medium (see Figure 6-8) and prints a report of all positive cultures.

MICROBIAL GROWTH

Biological growth may be measured by at least two different criteria. The most frequently observed form of growth is the increase in size of an organism. For bacteria, however, such change in size is a poor criterion of growth; rather, increases in the number of organisms are usually used as a measurement. Therefore, when considering microorganisms, scientists usually count the number of living cells *(viable count)* or all cells *(total count)* in order to determine growth. Frequently, some component of cell structure such as protein or DNA is measured as an indirect indication of microbial increase (growth) or decrease (death).

The generation time of a microbial cell is the time required for one complete cell division. Some microbes are able to divide as rapidly as once every 12 to 15 minutes, others require up to several hours, and a few very slow growing bacteria may require more than 24 hours per cell division. When proper nutrients are

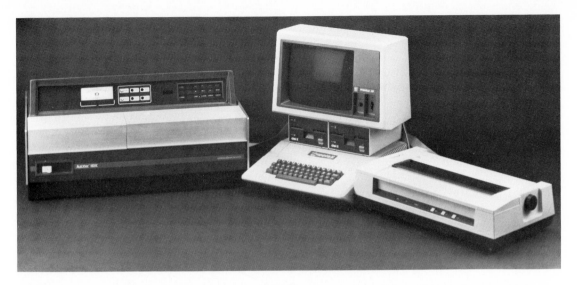

Figure 7-10. The AUTOBAC microbiology system. The unit on the left is a photometer-computer system that can be used to measure the growth of microorganisms. When properly implemented, this system will both identify bacteria isolated from patients and provide the antibiotic susceptibility of such isolates. The units on the right allow instant information retrieval of all cultures processed in the AUTOBAC. (Courtesy Warner-Lambert Company)

available and other conditions are favorable, the growth of microorganisms can be a dynamic event with profound effects on the surrounding environment. If a bacterial cell were to continue to divide once every 30 minutes, for instance, there would be 64 cells in 3 hours, 17 million cells in 17 hours, and 280 trillion cells in 24 hours. If growth could continue for 48 hours at this rate, the mass of cells produced would weigh several thousand times the weight of the earth. Obviously, such rapid growth cannot continue for very long periods. Yet under certain conditions it may occur for a short time.

Growth Curve

When microbial cells are placed in fresh nutrient broth under favorable growth conditions but with limited supply of available nutrient, multiplication follows the typical growth pattern shown in Figure 7-13. This type of growth is referred to as a *batch* or *limited growth* system. When bacteria are first placed in a fresh medium, a period of adjustment follows during which there is an increase in metabolic activity preceding cell division. This interval is called the *lag phase* of growth.

The length of the lag phase is quite variable among different species of bacteria, and is somewhat dependent on the condition of the cells prior to their inoculation into growth medium. Follow-

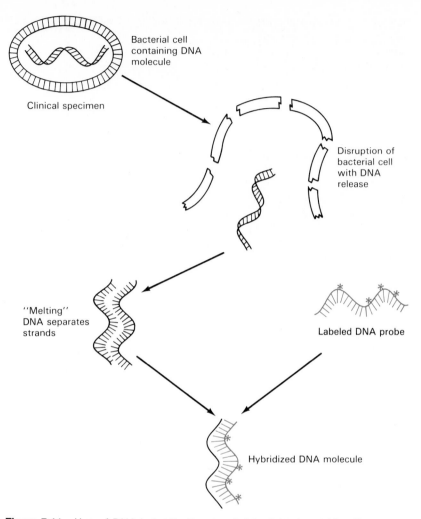

Bacterial cell containing DNA molecule

Clinical specimen

Disruption of bacterial cell with DNA release

"Melting" DNA separates strands

Labeled DNA probe

Hybridized DNA molecule

Figure 7-11 Use of DNA hybridization (*probe*) to detect and identify pathogenic bacteria in a clinical specimen.

Growth rate

the number of generations of a species within a given length of time. *Generation time* is the length of time to go from one generation to the next. For bacteria generation time is usually measured in minutes.

ing adjustment during lag, the cells begin to divide at a constant rate with the number and mass of cells doubling every generation. The number of generations of new cells formed in one hour is known as the **growth rate** of the organism (Figure 7-14). Following the lag phase, the growth rate is maximal and constant during an interval known as the *logarithmic phase* of growth. During this phase, the number of new cells increases exponentially and the cells are in a metabolic condition referred to as *balanced growth*. In balanced growth, all measurable components of the cell such as protein, RNA, DNA or biomass increase at the same rate. Because the ratio of the cell components remains constant during this phase, it is possible to determine changes in the amount of any specific part of the cell simply by measuring changes in a single

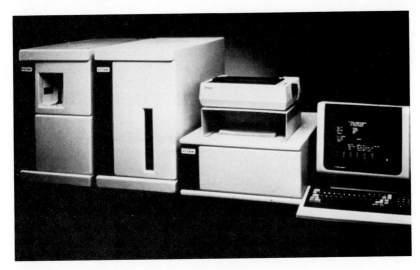

Figure 7-12   The Automicrobic, the only fully automatic bacterial identification and detection system. (Vitek Corporation, Hazelton, Mo.)

component. The exponential growth phase is usually fairly brief, lasting only 4–10 hours for most rapidly growing bacteria.

Logarithmic growth rapidly depletes the available nutrients, and toxic waste products quickly accumulate. As nutrient concentration decreases, or the culture environment becomes more toxic, growth of cells becomes unbalanced and various cellular components are synthesized at different rates. These factors cause a decrease in, and ultimately cessation of, cellular division. The accumulated cells may then remain for a period of time in a static condition—that is, not increasing in the numbers of viable cells.

Figure 7-13   Phases in the growth curve of a pure bacterial culture in a closed system.

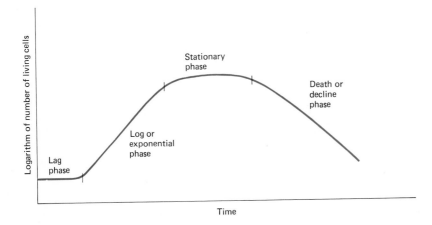

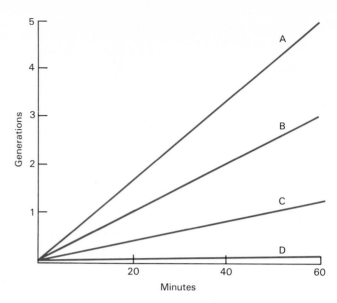

Figure 7-14 Growth rate of *Clostridium perfringens* (a), *E scherichia coli* (b) *Pseudomonas putida* (c) and *Mycobacterium tuberculosis* (d).

Stationary phase

a time during which the number of new cells is equal to the number that die. This is not a static condition and microbes continue to metabolize, multiply, and die during this phase.

This is called the **stationary phase** of the growth curve. Because of unbalanced growth preceding the stationary phase, the cells in this phase are not uniform in composition; they are usually smaller than cells in the logarithmic growth phase and they are most resistant to environmental changes, such as those caused by heat, drying, and radiation.

The stationary phase is followed by a period in which the cells gradually die off—the *decline* or *death phase.* Like growth, the rate at which cells die is a function of both the type of cells and the environment, and under the conditions of batch culture, cellular death is also an exponential function. It should be apparent that measuring the death of microorganisms is somewhat subjective and may be a function of not providing a proper environment for growth rather than an actual loss of viability. Thus we define death as the inability of the organism to multiply when placed into a situation where growth is normally supported and maintained.

Although the characteristic growth curve shown in Figure 7-13 probably only occurs under selected conditions, modifications do happen in nature and in some clinical circumstances. Products like bottled milk, for instance, if not properly refrigerated, could support the growth of microorganisms in the logarithmic phase, thus causing rapid souring, while the change in the number of bacteria follows the normal growth curve. In clinical conditions, such as a wound, where an abscess is forming (Chapter 11), a niche may exist that is filled with dead tissue and body fluids that could support the rapid growth of bacteria for a time. In most abscesses the bacteria have reached the stationary phase of the growth curve; in this condition they do not take in many nutrients or other substances from the surrounding environment. Thus antibiotics given to the patient to cure the infection do not effectively penetrate into the abscess and may not be taken up by the bacteria if they do. Consequently, such therapy may fail to reduce the infection. In order to resolve this problem, it is nearly always necessary to drain abscesses in order to remove the waste products that are inhibiting the growth of the bacteria and preventing penetration of antimicrobial agents. Fresh nutrients then diffuse into the area and the remaining bacteria begin to multiply. If an antibiotic is then given, it will be taken up by the growing bacteria, inhibit their growth, and help cure the infection.

Growth of bacteria in an open environment, such as soil, water, or even the intestine, generally does not follow the curve shown in Figure 7-13. In these circumstances, bacterial growth is most often continuous so that the number of viable microorganisms remains fairly constant over long periods of time.

Laboratory (in vitro) studies of bacteria grown in continuous culture have shown that the organisms grow exponentially in a condition of balanced growth, and that the generation time is determined by the rate at which fresh nutrients are supplied to the culture. Examples of such continuous growth systems in pathogenic microbiology are less common than are batch growth conditions. Humans, however, have "normal" bacteria that inhabit their body surfaces and grow continuously (Chapter 10) and balanced microbial growth may occur to some extent in chronic disease conditions.

Environmental Influences on Microbial Growth

Moisture Microorganisms grow only when adequate moisture is present. Because microbes exist as single cells, they depend on the continual diffusion of nutrients in solution across their plasma membrane. Due to the small size of microbial cells, however, the thin film of moisture often present on many substances is enough to support some microbial growth. Keeping materials free of moisture by dehydration is one of the most common methods of controlling the growth of microorganisms and, in turn, preventing the spoilage or decomposition of food or other materials. Frequently, dehydrated foods such as powdered milk contain large numbers of viable organisms. A lack of moisture, however, maintains the microorganisms in a static state so that multiplication cannot occur.

Temperature The temperatures at which bacteria will grow are primarily determined by the stability of their proteins (Table 7-2).

Table 7-2   Optimal Temperature for Microbial Growth

Classification	Temperature Range	Bacterial Examples
Thermophiles	40°–100°C	*Bacillus stearothermophilus*
		Bacillus coagulans
Mesophiles	20°–40°C	*Escherichia coli*
		Haemophilus influenzae
		Staphylococcus aureus
		Neisseria gonorrhoeae
Psychrophiles	−10°–20°C	*Bacillus globisporus*
		Micrococcus cryophilus

Although most will grow over a range of temperatures, there is an *optimum* temperature at which the growth rate is maximal. Although there is a minimum temperature below which each microorganism will not grow, bacteria are not usually killed at low temperatures, but remain in a stationary state.

Each microorganism has adapted to grow within a specific temperature range (Figure 7-15). Some, able to grow at low temperatures, are called *psychrophiles* (cold-lovers). Even though psychrophiles may grow at temperatures as low as −10°C, most psychrophilic microbes grow best at about 20°C and grow poorly above 30°C. Because of normal body temperatures, psychrophiles are generally unable to cause infections in humans. Still, they may cause spoilage of foods or other products stored at low temperatures.

Many microorganisms grow best at temperatures between 20° and 40°C and are called *mesophiles* (middle-lovers). Most microorganisms that cause infections in warm-blooded animals are mesophiles and usually have optimum growth temperatures of 35° to 37°C.

Certain microbes have very thermostable proteins and are able to grow at temperatures above 45° C. These bacteria are called *thermophiles* (heat-lovers). Generally, thermophiles are unable to

Figure 7-15   Categories of microorganisms based on growth at various temperature ranges. Optimum range indicated.

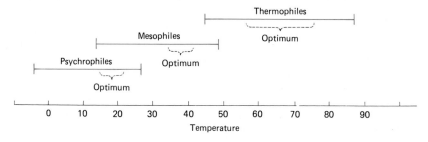

cause infections in humans but are found in such places as natural hot springs. Occasionally thermophilic bacteria cause problems by growing in hot-water systems or in some industrial processes where high temperatures are used. Some thermophiles are able to grow at temperatures as high as 110° C.

Oxygen   Many different microorganisms require free oxygen (O_2) for growth and are called *aerobes.* These organisms utilize oxygen as an electron acceptor in the electron transport pathway (Chapter 5) and will grow only in environments where atmospheric or free oxygen is available. These oxygen-associated reactions are essential to the cell and help to make necessary metabolic energy available. These reactions also produce a highly toxic chemical known as *hydrogen peroxide* (H_2O_2). A second very toxic compound known as *superoxide* (O_2^-) is also frequently produced in small concentrations when cells use oxygen as their electron acceptor. Aerobic bacteria depend on the presence of one or more enzymes such as *catalase* and *superoxide dismutase* to protect them against these toxic metabolic products. At high concentrations, oxygen is toxic to most bacteria, and some aerobes *(microaerophiles)* grow best when only small amounts of oxygen are available.

Certain microorganisms are able to grow in the absence of O_2 and are called *anaerobes.* Several categories of anaerobes exist. Some are able to use O_2 if it is present but can also grow in the absence of O_2; they are termed *facultative* anaerobes. Other bacteria, called *obligate* anaerobes, do not produce protective enzymes such as catalase (Table 7-3) and can grow only in the absence of O_2. Care must be taken to remove O_2 from the media in which these organisms are cultured. An additional group of microorganisms require CO_2 for growth and are called *capnophiles.* Capnophilic bacteria are found among both anaerobes and aerobes. Microorganisms from each of these oxygen-associated categories are able to grow in various habitats of the human body and may cause diseases.

Other factors   Bacteria are able to survive and often grow in water with low concentrations of ions because their rigid cell wall protects against damage due to increased osmotic pressure. This fac-

Table 7-3   Enzymes That Enable Bacteria to Survive in the Presence of Oxygen

Enzyme	Function	Bacterial Example
Catalase	$2H_2O_2 \rightarrow 2H_2O + O_2$	*Escherichia coli*
Peroxidase	$H_2O_2 + XH_2 \rightarrow 2H_2O + X$	*Lactobacillus*
Superoxide dismutase	$2O_2^- + 2H^+ \rightarrow O_2 + H_2O_2$	*Streptococcus faecalis*

Table 7-4   Halophilic Properties of Bacteria

Class	Allowable Salt Concentration (%)	Bacterial Example
Extreme halophile	5–36	*Halococcus morrhuae*
Halophile	2–20	*Vibrio costicolus*
Marine halophile	0.2–5	*Vibrio parahemolyticus*
Nonhalophile	0–4	*Escherichia coli*

Ionic concentration

the concentration of ions in a solution. Compounds with ionic bonds disassociate in solution. The greater the concentration of these compounds the higher will be the ionic strength of a solution.

tor is important, for it allows successful water-borne transmission of many diseases. Bacteria vary in their ability to grow in solutions of high ionic strength (Table 7-4). Those that require high salt concentrations for growth are known as *halophiles* (salt-lovers) and can live even in saturated brine solutions. Nonhalophilic bacteria tolerate only moderate (1% to 20%) salt solution and may be destroyed in highly saline environments.

Most bacteria cannot grow in solutions of very high **ionic concentrations.** This makes possible the preservation of certain foods by the addition of high concentrations of salt or sugar. Sugars are also used to preserve some foods such as jam and jelly. The addition of high concentrations of sugar increases the osmotic pressure of these foods, making it impossible for microorganisms to extract enough moisture for their growth. In fact, bacteria are frequently destroyed under these conditions because water is drawn out from the cell into the surrounding environment. This loss of cell water may result in the collapse of the cell membrane (*plasmolysis*) in Gram-positive bacteria, and collapse of both membrane and wall in Gram-negative cells. The pH of the environment also influences the growth and survival of microorganisms. Most microbes that cause disease in humans grow best at or close to neutrality (pH 7), which is near the pH of most normal body fluids.

CONCEPT SUMMARY

1. Bacterial nutritional needs in the laboratory are met by adding appropriate nutrients to a solidifying material called *agar*. By adding specific substances to the agar, media can be made to enrich, select, or inhibit the growth of desired microorganisms. Use of agar media has simplified the process of obtaining bacteria in pure culture. Such pure cultures are essential for the investigation of organisms and their role in disease processes.

2. Species of bacteria are identified on the basis of their reaction to a variety of ingredients which can be added to an agar or broth medium, and to the conditions for growth imposed on the culture.

3. Culture conditions, such as temperature, atmosphere, moisture, and pH, all impact the growth of microorganisms. Whatever the conditions, cultures of microorganisms follow a reproducible pattern of growth known as a *growth curve*.

STUDY SUMMARY

1. Construct a table which will show a classification of bacteria based on their growth as a function of (a) atmosphere and (b) temperature.

2. What evidence could you suggest to support the statement that most bacteria have a continuous growth pattern in their natural habitat?

3. Use a diagram to show that the change in growth rate from logarithmic to stationary phase is in fact a transition through many growth rate changes.

4. Why was the use of agar as growth medium component such an important step in the history of microbiology?

5. Write a statement that contrasts differential and selective culture media.

6. If you begin at time X with two bacteria that divide regularly, and each of their progeny divides at the same rate as the parent cells, and after 1 hour you have 32 bacteria, what is the generation time of these organisms?

REFERENCES FOR FURTHER STUDY

1. *The Microbial World*, 5th ed., R. Stanier, 1986. Prentice Hall.

2. *Bacterial Nutrition*, H. Lichstein, 1983. Hutchison-Ross.

3. Physiological Responses to Nutrient Limitation. *Annual Review of Microbiology* 37:1, 1983.

4. Growth Control in Microbial Cultures. *Annual Review of Microbiology* 39:299, 1985.

chapter 8

STERILIZATION AND DISINFECTION

Inanimate
not capable of self-movement; usually, but not always, nonliving. Inanimate objects involved in disease transmissions are called *fomites*.

Chemotherapeutic
a compound (chemical) used in treatment of disease. Technically even aspirin is a chemotherapeutic. This term is often reserved for compounds used to treat cancer, but can also be applied to those used to treat infectious disease.

T he control of microorganisms in health care services is extremely important and persons working in these areas should have a fundamental understanding of the principles of sterilization and disinfection. This chapter describes the methods used to control microorganisms on body surfaces and on nonliving materials. The following chapter discusses chemotherapy, the control of microorganisms that infect living tissues. Physical and chemical methods used to destroy microbes on **inanimate** objects are generally nonspecific; that is, they destroy a wide variety of different types of living cells. On the other hand, **chemotherapeutic** agents must be able to destroy selectively only the microorganism and not the host cells.

In certain applications, such as the preparation of bandages or instruments to be used in surgery, successful control requires the complete removal or destruction of all microorganisms. In other applications, such as disinfecting a hospital ward, it is only practical to remove the disease-producing microorganisms or reduce their number to such a low level that the chance of infection is remote.

DEFINITION OF TERMS

Various terms are used to describe the processes involved in the control of microorganisms. Some terms are absolute, others overlap in meaning, and some are relative, having slightly different meanings in different areas of application. The term *sterilization*, which refers to a process that destroys all living organisms, is an absolute term. *Disinfection* refers to a process used to destroy harmful microorganisms but not necessarily including the resistant bacterial spores; a **disinfectant** is an agent that produces this result. *Sepsis* means the presence of microorganisms in blood; thus the term *antiseptic* refers to a substance that opposes or is able to reduce the likelihood of sepsis. Antiseptics are substances that, when applied to microorganisms, render them harmless either by killing them or preventing their growth; such substances are generally applied to living tissues. The suffix *-cide* refers to a killing action—*bactericides* kill bacteria, *fungicides* kill fungi, *germicides* kill a wide range of microorganisms, and so forth. The suffix *-static* refers to agents that stop the growth of microorganisms; for example, a **bacteriostatic** agent prevents the growth of bacteria. Such terms as disinfectant, antiseptic, and bacteriostatic overlap significantly and all might possibly be applied to the same agent. The term *contamination* has different meanings in different settings. In the general clinical environment contamination refers to the presence of disease-producing microorganisms in or on a substance. In more specialized areas, when referring to fluids for intravenous administration or surgical instruments and so on, the presence of any microorganism would be considered contamination. The term *sanitation* is often used in public health regulations and refers to a condition favorable to health; its meaning is relative and must be defined for each application.

Disinfectant

a compound that kills microorganisms on inanimate objects.

Bacteriostatic

capable of preventing bacteria from multiplying. Many compounds are bacteriostatic and prevent bacterial replication, but do not directly kill microorganisms.

PHYSICAL METHODS OF MICROBIAL CONTROL

Moist Heat under Pressure

Over 90% of all medical and laboratory products are sterilized by steam under pressure. This procedure is accomplished in a pressure chamber called an *autoclave* (Figure 8-1). Steam may be generated within the chamber or introduced from an external source under pressure. As steam enters the chamber, air must be expelled through an escape valve. Once air is expelled, the escape valve is closed and the steam pressure is increased to 1.1 kg/cm^2 (15 lb/in.^{2}). Under these conditions the temperature rises to 121° C. At this temperature, with moisture, cell structures are completely disrupted; proteins and nucleic acids are denatured and cell membranes are broken. When using an autoclave, it is necessary to allow time for the temperature to penetrate through all the material and then remain at 121° C for 15 to 20 minutes. A large bundle of items such as surgical drapes or bandages may require exposure times of 30 to 60 minutes or even longer to ensure sterility throughout the package. Items like bandages or surgical instruments that must remain sterile should be wrapped in covers to prevent them from becoming contaminated after they are removed from the autoclave. Not all materials can be autoclaved. Moisture associated with autoclaving causes such products as dry powders to become soggy, and the heat involved may

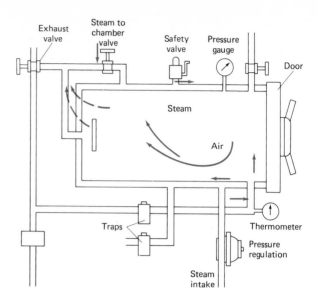

Figure 8-1   Schematic drawing of a steam autoclave.

Heat-sensitive
capable of being damaged or
destroyed by heat. Chemicals and
biological substances are
considered to be heat-sensitive if
they are damaged by temperatures
of 50°–60° C within 15–20 minutes.
Any material may be classified as
heat-sensitive if the temperature at
which it is destroyed is specified.

Botulism
a toxic disease caused by a
specific microorganism,
Clostridium botulinum. Also used
as a general term for food
poisoning.

damage many plastic products or electronic instruments used in
hospitals. Fluids that contain **heat-sensitive** components cannot
be sterilized by autoclaving. Containers of fluids to be sterilized
must not be tightly sealed, for such sealing may prevent the movement of steam to and from their contents; once sterilization is
achieved, autoclave pressure must be released slowly to prevent
excessive boiling and evaporation.

Various tests are used to determine if sterility has been attained. Papers impregnated with heat-sensitive chemicals that
change color when exposed to a critical temperature are useful but
not totally reliable indicators of sterility. The most reliable indicator is a *spore strip test.* Paper strips impregnated with bacterial
spores are placed in the center of the materials being autoclaved.
After the sterilization cycle is completed, the spore strip is placed
in a broth medium. If no growth occurs in the broth after incubation, the material is assumed to be sterile. The spore strips are
sometimes placed between wrapped bundles so that they can be
removed without unwrapping the sterilized materials. Conven-
ient-to-use spore strip test kits are commercially available (Figure
8-2).

Moist heat in the form of pressure cooking is used in home
canning and in the commercial canning industry. For nonacidic
foods, it is necessary to destroy all bacterial spores that may be
present before the foods are processed. This procedure is used to
protect consumers from **botulism.**

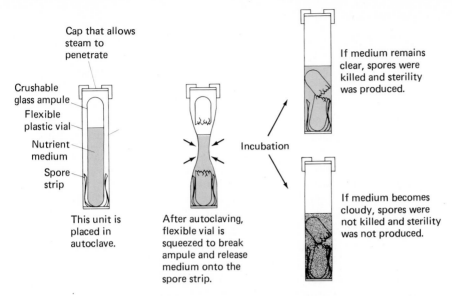

Cap that allows
steam to
penetrate

Crushable
glass ampule

Flexible
plastic vial

Nutrient
medium

Spore
strip

This unit is
placed in
autoclave.

After autoclaving,
flexible vial is
squeezed to break
ampule and release
medium onto the
spore strip.

Incubation

If medium remains
clear, spores were
killed and sterility
was produced.

If medium becomes
cloudy, spores were
not killed and sterility
was not produced.

Figure 8-2   A commercial-type spore strip for testing if the autoclave cycle produced sterility.

Moist Heat Not Under Pressure

Boiling and live steam, not under pressure, destroy most vegetative forms of bacteria in several minutes. Bacterial spores and certain viruses may survive boiling temperatures for several hours, however. The moderate heat of pasteurization is useful in treating some liquids, such as milk or beverages. Pasteurization occurs via either of two procedures: the *holding method* or the *flash method*. In the holding method, the liquid is heated to 62.8° C for 30 minutes; the flash method heats the fluid to 71.7° C for 15 seconds. Pasteurization does not sterilize, but does kill disease-producing bacteria that might be transmitted in the liquid. It also greatly reduces the number of other bacteria in the liquid and thus significantly retards the rate of spoilage of products like milk.

Dry Heat

Hot-air ovens are used as dry heat sterilizers but dry heat requires higher temperatures for longer periods than moist heat in order to achieve sterilization. Using dry heat, an exposure at 180° C for 2 hours is needed to kill bacterial spores. Dry heat is used for sterilizing such items as glassware, powders, and oils. Another form of dry-heat sterilization is the direct exposure of instruments or inoculating loops to open flames for brief periods, a procedure called *flaming*. Incineration of waste products readily destroys any contaminating microorganism that might be present.

Ultraviolet Light

Ultraviolet (UV) light is highly germicidal at wavelengths of 2600 Å. This wavelength of light is absorbed by DNA molecules and the increase in energy causes a rearrangement of some chemical bonds. In particular, new chemical bonds are formed between adjacent thymine bases on the same chain of the DNA molecule, which in turn renders the DNA of the UV-irradiated microorganism nonfunctional. If the UV-inactivated microorganisms are subsequently stored in the dark or are exposed to white light, the chemical bonds might be restored to their original positions and the microorganisms could again become viable.

Sunlight contains UV light; consequently, it has definite germicidal properties. UV light is also produced by mercury vapor lamps. When placed in air ducts or over surfaces, these lamps greatly reduce the number of viable microorganisms in the field of irradiation. UV light does not penetrate solids, a factor that has limited its use to disinfecting surfaces, clear liquids, and air. High-intensity UV lamps located in air-supply ducts to such critical areas as operating rooms, nurseries, and intensive care areas can greatly reduce the chance of infections being transmitted to these areas by the airborne route. Also, air leaving contaminated areas, such as isolation rooms, morgues, or laboratories, can be exposed to UV light to prevent the spread of disease-producing microorganisms from such sources. UV light is damaging to human tissue and direct exposure must be avoided.

Ionizing Radiation

Forms of ionizing radiation, such as x rays and gamma rays, are able to transmit much more energy than UV light, and have greater killing effects on microorganisms. Radiation with this much energy actually breaks one or both DNA strands, which may permanently interfere with DNA replication and therefore any subsequent cell multiplication. Ionizing radiations can penetrate such products as fabrics, plastics, liquids, and foods to produce sterilization. Currently, ionizing radiation is used to sterilize products like surgical sutures and disposable plastic items. Meats are effectively sterilized by ionizing radiation, have a shelf life comparable to that of heat-processed canned meats, and are much more nutritious and palatable. Such sterilized meats have been used by astronauts during space flights and some military food rations are preserved by ionizing radiation, but as yet this process has had only limited general use.

Filtration

Filtration is an effective means of removing most microorganisms from liquids and gases. Liquids, like serum, or solutions containing heat-sensitive materials can be freed of microbial cells by passing them through filters with pore sizes small enough to retain bacterial cells. Filters made of asbestos, fused glass fragments, or diatomaceous earth have been used for many years. Biologically inert, precisely produced cellulose ester membrane filters are widely used (Figure 8-3). Such filters are available in pore sizes as small as 0.025 μm. One with a pore size of 0.22 μm effectively removes all bacteria from a fluid, and use of filters with smaller pores will remove some viruses which may be found in solution. Filters of this type are also used to trap and concentrate bacteria that are dispersed in large volumes of liquids. This procedure is useful in bacterial testing of drinking water.

Airborne microorganisms can be effectively removed from air by filtration. Filters made of various fiber media are widely used in air ducts to remove both inert and microbial particles. Varying densities of filter media can remove the desired size and amounts of airborne particles. Special filters, referred to as *absolute* or *HEPA* (High-Efficacy Particulate Air) filters, consist of a tightly woven fiberglass medium and effectively remove 99.9% of all airborne particles down to the size of 0.3 μm. HEPA filters remove all types of airborne microorganisms. Even though viruses are as small as 0.02 μm, when airborne they are usually attached to larger particles of dust or dried mucus that are readily trapped by HEPA fil-

Figure 8-3   Placing of a membrane filter into a filter holder. After being assembled, the unit is covered and sterilized.

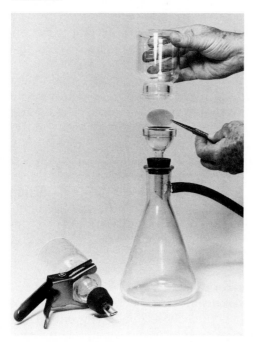

ters. Air filters are used in air-supply systems servicing such hospital areas as operating rooms, nurseries, and intensive care units.

CHEMICAL METHODS OF MICROBIAL CONTROL

Hospitals, clinics, and laboratories rely heavily on chemical antiseptics and disinfectants to reduce or eliminate harmful microorganisms on skin or inanimate objects. Thousands of different chemical formulations are commercially available as disinfectants and no single product is suitable for all applications. Several different chemical disinfectants are needed to accommodate the needs of most clinics or hospitals. Persons working in hospitals need to be aware of what disinfectant to use for each type of application. Even though thousands of commercial products are available, most disinfectants belong to one of the categories discussed in the following pages.

Factors Affecting Disinfectant Action

Disinfectants destroy or prevent the growth of microorganisms via generalized effects produced on the microbial cells. Some disinfectants are surface-active agents that disrupt the normal functioning of cytoplasmic membranes; others cause **denaturation** of proteins, such as enzymes, that are essential for cell growth and function. The action and uses of some common groups of disinfectants are shown in Table 8-1.

Denaturation
a change from a natural to an unnatural state. This term is often used to describe the process of alteration of the tertiary or secondary configuration of a protein.

The ability of a chemical disinfectant to act on a microorganism and the extent of that action depend on the following factors.

Time Not all microbes are killed at the same time after the addition of a disinfectant. Therefore the disinfectant must remain in contact with the contaminated material long enough to allow for the killing of all microbes (Figure 8-4). During most short applications, chemical agents do not sterilize; however, if the time is extended to periods of 12 to 24 hours, sterilization is often possible.

Temperature The killing effects of disinfectants are increased at higher temperatures. Most disinfecting procedures are standardized and carried out at room temperature. The time of exposure must be extended when materials are disinfected at low temperatures.

pH The acidity or alkalinity of the environment also influences the interaction of disinfectants with microorganisms and may increase or decrease the action, depending on the agents. Thus the effects of pH must be considered separately for each disinfectant.

Table 8-1　Mode of Action, Uses, and Properties of Major Categories of Chemical Disinfectants

Agents	Major Action	Common Uses	Other Properties	Use Dilution (%)
Alcohols	Lipid solvents Denatures proteins	Skin antiseptics Surface disinfectants	Rapid action Flammable Dries skin	70
Mercurials	Inactivates proteins	Skin antiseptics Surface disinfectants	Weak cidal activity Inactivated by organic matter	0.1
Silver nitrate	Denatures proteins	Antiseptic for eyes and burns	Inactivated by organic matter Limited range of microbes affected	1
Phenolic compounds	Disrupts cell membranes Inactivates proteins	In antiseptic skin washes Disinfect inanimate objects	Not inactivated by organic matter Stable Some objectionable odors	0.5–5
Iodine	Inactivates proteins	Skin antiseptic	Soluble in alcohol Rapid action Mixes with soaps	2
Chlorine compounds	Oxidation of enzymes	Water treatment Disinfect inanimate objects	Inactivated by organic matter Flash action Corrosive Irritates skin	5 (as bleach)
Quaternary ammonium compounds	Surface active Disrupts cell membranes Denatures proteins	Skin antiseptic Disinfect inanimate objects	Neutralized by soap Odorless Nonirritating	Less than 1
Glutaraldehyde	Inactivates proteins	Cool sterilizing agent for heat-sensitive instruments	Unstable Toxic High activity in alkaline range	1–2

171

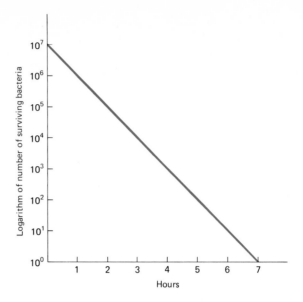

Figure 8-4   An example of the death rate of a bacterium when treated with a constant concentration of disinfection at a constant temperature and pH, and plotted logarithmically.

Types of microorganisms   Some variations in susceptibility between species of microbes occur. Microbes are sometimes grouped as to their susceptibility to disinfectants into the following three groups:

- *Group A,* the vegetative forms of most bacteria and enveloped viruses that are easily killed by disinfectants
- *Group B,* the more difficult to kill tubercle bacillus and nonenveloped viruses
- *Group C,* the highly resistant bacterial spores and viruses, such as those that cause hepatitis.

Presence of extraneous matter   The presence of materials like soil, blood, and pus may react with some disinfectants and reduce their ability to react with microbes. For this reason, it is strongly recommended that surfaces and materials to be disinfected be thoroughly cleaned before treatment with the disinfectant.

Proper exposure   Care must be taken to ensure proper exposure of all parts of the object to the disinfectant. Tightly packaged material or closed containers, for instance, may not allow complete penetration or contact with the disinfectant.

Concentration of disinfectant Generally the more concentrated the disinfectant, the shorter is the killing time. At low concentrations the compound may be only bacteriostatic whereas at higher concentrations it may be bactericidal. The concentration needed to kill microorganisms varies from microbe to microbe and from disinfectant to disinfectant.

Groups of Chemical Disinfectants

Organic solvents Compounds of the organic solvent group include *chloroform, toluene,* and *alcohols.* Their action is to disrupt the structure and function of plasma membranes and to denature proteins. Chloroform and toluene are most often used as additives to solutions that must be kept free from microbial growth. The widely used alcohols are among the most useful disinfectants or antiseptics. They are highly effective against vegetative bacterial cells, including the tubercle bacillus, but are less effective against spores. Alcohol is very useful as a skin disinfectant because it effectively kills bacteria, has a cleansing effect by removing accumulated lipids, and evaporates without leaving a residue. Ethyl and isopropyl alcohol are equally effective and concentrations of 70% should be used. Concentrations below 70% begin to lose some effectiveness. Isopropyl alcohol is most often used, for it does not come under the governmental regulations placed on alcohols used in beverages.

Heavy metals

MERCURIALS Various mercury-containing compounds, called *mercurials,* were widely used as disinfectants in the past. One such compound, *mercuric chloride,* is quite toxic to humans and is now rarely used. Other mercurial preparations known as *mercurochrome, merthiolate, metaphen,* and *mercresin* are less toxic. Merthiolate is sometimes used as a preservative for vaccines and metaphen may be used to irrigate the urethra. These metal compounds combine with active chemical (sulfhydryl) groups on proteins including enzymes. The result of such interaction is the inactivation of these enzymes and ultimately cell death. The mercurials, however, are not as effective as many other preparations and are usually corrosive to metallic instruments. In general, other disinfectants are preferred over the mercurials.

SILVER COMPOUNDS Some silver compounds are useful disinfectants, the most common being *silver nitrate.* A 1% silver nitrate solution is used in the routine irrigation of eyes of newborn babies to prevent gonorrheal infections. This procedure is required by law in all 50 states. Dressings applied to burns are sometimes soaked in a 0.5% solution of silver nitrate to help control bacterial infections. Colloidal silver compounds that slowly release silver ions are used in some antiseptics and in some filters for water purification.

COPPER COMPOUNDS Copper ions can also inhibit the growth of microorganisms. Dilute solutions of compounds such as *copper sulphate* are sometimes used in aquaria to reduce algal and fungal growth.

Phenol and phenol derivatives The natural product *phenol*, also called *carbolic acid*, is fairly toxic to tissues, is corrosive, and has a disagreeable odor; yet historically it has served as an important disinfectant. Pasteur recognized the ability of phenol to prevent decomposition of organic matter. This observation prompted Lister to use the product to prevent infections of surgical wounds. Carbolic acid in dilute solution is an effective skin disinfectant and will not cause tissue injury if exposure is limited to less than an hour. Various phenol derivatives, called *phenolics*, have been developed that are effective disinfectants and yet do not have many of the objectionable traits of phenol. Although phenol is rarely used today, three phenolic compounds are common: *cresols, hexachlorophene,* and *chlorhexidine.*

CRESOLS Cresols are obtained from coal tars, are less toxic than phenol, and have strong germicidal actions. Cresols can be mixed with soaps without losing germicidal activity. For many years a mixture of 2% cresol and liquid soap was sold under the trade name of Lysol. This old-type Lysol had a characteristic cresol odor that was familiar to most persons living before the 1940s. In later years mixtures of soaps and improved phenolic compounds with less odor have been marketed under the trade name of Lysol. They are effective products for disinfecting inanimate objects or organic wastes.

HEXACHLOROPHENE This phenolic compound is especially effective against staphylococci and streptococci and can be used against many other microbes as well. Hexachlorophene retains its antimicrobial effectiveness when mixed with soaps or detergents, is nonirritating to skin, and leaves a protective film after application. It is bactericidal at high concentrations and bacteriostatic at lower concentrations. During the 1960s, hexachlorophene had many medical and nonmedical applications. Newborn infants were routinely bathed in mild solutions of hexachlorophene, a procedure that greatly reduced bacterial colonization and subsequent infection by staphylococci. In the early 1970s, however, evidence from animal studies suggested that hexachlorophene may be absorbed into the blood and cause brain damage. And even though no evidence exists for its toxic effects on newborn humans, restrictions have been placed on its use. Many hospitals stopped using hexachlorophene in newborn care only to see an increase in the number of staphylococcal infections. Today most hospitals use hexachlorophene in smaller amounts when treating newborns and are still able to control staphylococcal infections effectively. Hexachlorophene, however, is no longer allowed in over-the-counter products, such as deodorants and cleansing agents. A 3% concentration is mixed with soaps, detergents, and lotions to form effective antiseptic skin-cleaning products for medical applications. Phisoderm, Phisohex, and Hexagerm are examples of hexachlorophene-containing products. These products are widely used in hospitals and clinics for routine washing and disinfection of hands, surgical scrubs, and preoperative cleansing of skin. In addition to the immediate effect when applied, hexachlorophene leaves a protective film on the skin for several days. Used with discretion, hexachlorophene is a valuable product in controlling microorganisms in the medical environment.

CHLORHEXIDINE A 4% concentration of *chlorhexidine gluconate* mixed with detergent and 4% alcohol is now being widely used as a surgical handscrub, cleanser for superficial skin wounds, and handwashing agent. It is highly effective against both Gram-positive and Gram-negative bacteria and fungi. It leaves a protective film on skin and no irritation to skin has resulted from extensive use. Hibiclens is an example of a chlorhexidine-containing product.

Halogens The halogens *iodine* and *chlorine* are among the most useful chemical disinfectants. Chlorine is widely used in treating water. If free chlorine is added directly to water, a reaction occurs to form hypochlorous acid (HOCl), an active disinfectant. Chlorine compounds, such as *hypochlorites,* that slowly release free chlorine are also effective disinfectants of water. Hypochlorites are the common household bleach agents, such as Clorox and Purex. Chlorine compounds are routinely used to sanitize food- and dairy-processing equipment and to treat swimming pools. Chlorine bleaches are useful household disinfectants and can be used on dishes, utensils, toilets, or other noncorrodible materials. Chlorine compounds should not be used on skin or open lesions; moreover, they are corrosive to metals. Chlorine is readily inactivated by organic matter and dilute solutions easily lose their effectiveness when excessive organic matter is present in solutions or on surfaces.

Iodine is among the most effective skin antiseptics. A preparation known as **tincture** of iodine, a 2% concentration of iodine dissolved in alcohol, is widely used as a skin antiseptic and to treat minor wounds. A 2% solution of iodine in water is also an

Tincture
an alcoholic solution. Thus tincture of iodine is a solution of alcohol that contains iodine.

Detergent

a compound similar to soap, but not made from fats. Detergents are used as cleaning agents because of their ability to emulsify dirt. Detergents are not disinfectants.

effective antiseptic. Iodine forms complexes with soaps and **detergents** without losing its antiseptic qualities; such products are called *iodophors*. Iodophors are soluble in water and gradually release the iodine. They are not as active as tincture of iodine but have the advantage of being less irritating and nonstaining. They also have the cleansing effect of soap or detergent. Iodophors are used as antiseptic soaps, preoperative skin disinfectants, and general disinfectants in medical and industrial environments.

Halogens are effective because they oxidize (remove hydrogen from) sulfur-containing amino acids. These are the same active areas of protein that combine with heavy metals (see above). Because free, reduced sulfhydryl groups are needed throughout the cell, disinfection with heavy metals or halogens is very effective.

Surface-active agents Various surface-active compounds have detergentlike characteristics and cause the destruction of microbial membranes. The *quaternary ammonium compounds*, often referred to as *quats*, are *cationic detergents* and are the only surface-active agents with effective antibacterial activity. These agents are effective against a wide range of vegetative bacteria. They are not effective against spores, some vegetative bacteria, and the more stable viruses. These compounds are used for disinfecting floors, walls, furniture, and other inanimate objects. They have the advantages of being odorless, colorless, tasteless, inexpensive, nontoxic, soluble in water, and active in low concentrations.

Common detergents and soaps are *anionic detergents* and are excellent cleaning agents, but are not antimicrobial. Such surface-active agents can effectively clean large numbers of microorganisms from skin or other surfaces, but are essentially nontoxic to microorganisms. As a rule, thorough washing with such agents removes in excess of 90% of the microbes present.

Formaldehyde Formaldehyde is a gas that acts as a fumigant and a gaseous disinfectant. It dissolves in water to make a 37% solution, which is then called *formalin*. Solutions containing 5% to 10% formalin are widely used for preserving and **fixing** tissue specimens. Animals dissected in biology classes are fixed in formalin; and as most students in these classes can attest, formalin has a disagreeable odor and is irritating to tissues. Because of these objectionable properties, it has limited use as a disinfectant in clinics and patient-related activities.

Fixing

stopping degenerative changes in tissues or biological specimens. Fixatives are chemicals that are used to preserve biological specimens for future examination.

Glutaraldehyde Glutaraldehyde is related to formaldehyde and is germicidal against a wide range of microorganisms. It is used as a cold sterilizing agent for many items that would be damaged by heat. It is widely used for sterilizing dental equipment, pieces of equipment used in inhalation therapy, and equipment with optical lenses. Glutaraldehyde is most germicidal in the alkaline pH range and so a 0.3% sodium bicarbonate solution is added to a 2% glutaraldehyde solution just before it is to be used. An alkaline pH results and the solution is then said to be activated. Activated glutaraldehyde retains its potency as a disinfectant for about 4 weeks. Materials to be sterilized must be clean and completely immersed in 2% activated glutaraldehyde for 12 hours. Glutaraldehyde is irritating to tissues and has a mildly disagreeable odor; thus its use is limited to inanimate objects.

Hydrogen peroxide   A 3% solution of hydrogen peroxide (H_2O_2) is sometimes used to clean wounds. It is nonirritating to the tissues and has only a brief, mild disinfecting action due to its rapid breakdown to water and oxygen. Hydrogen peroxide affects the cells much like the halogens, and inactivates essential protein structures by oxidizing reduced sulfur groups.

Ethylene oxide   Ethylene oxide vaporizes readily at room temperatures and is a highly effective sterilizing agent in the gaseous form. It is active against all microorganisms, including bacterial spores. The major advantage of ethylene oxide gas is its ability to sterilize at room temperature and without high levels of moisture. It is slow acting, however, and 12 hours are required to destroy spores at 70° C. Also, ethylene oxide is explosive when mixed with air; for this reason, it is always diluted with an inert gas, such as carbon dioxide. A 10% to 15% concentration of ethylene oxide is used for sterilization. Special chambers or especially adapted autoclaves are used for this form of gas sterilization. Such items as plastic ware, **catheters,** sutures, electronic instruments, and heart-lung machines that may be damaged by heat are sterilized with ethylene oxide. In the past few years this form of sterilization has become an essential procedure in most hospitals. Items sterilized with ethylene oxide must be well aerated to remove any residual gas.

Catheter
a tube, usually of rubber or plastic, that can be placed into a body cavity (e.g., urethra) or a blood vessel to allow easy drainage of body fluids or the placement of medications into the body.

Other disinfectants   Acids and alkalies have antimicrobial activities due primarily to the free hydrogen or hydroxyl ions. Such acids as *benzoic* or *propionic* acid, or their salts, are added to foods to help retard spoilage. Some aniline and acridine dyes have bacteriostatic activities and are used in treating lesions on the skin and mucous membranes.

Evaluation of Chemical Disinfectants

The official method of evaluating a disinfectant is the *phenol coefficient method*. This method compares the effectiveness of the test disinfectants to that of phenol against bacterial strains of *Salmonella cholerasuis, Staphylococcus aureus*, and *Pseudomonas aeruginosa.*

Sterilization, Disinfection, Housekeeping, and Waste Disposal to Prevent Transmission of HTLV-HIV

Sterilization and disinfection procedures currently recommended for use in health care and dental facilities are adequate to sterilize or disinfect instruments, devices, or other items contaminated with the blood or other body fluids from individuals infected with HIV (AIDS virus). Instruments or other nondisposable items that enter normally sterile tissue or the vascular system or through which blood flows should be sterilized before reuse. Surgical instruments used on all patients should be decontaminated after use rather than just rinsed with water. Decontamination can be accomplished by machine or by hand cleaning by trained personnel wearing appropriate protective attire and using appropriate chemical germicides. Instruments or other nondisposable items that touch intact mucous membranes should receive high-level disinfection.

Several liquid chemical germicides commonly used in laboratories and health care facilities have been shown to kill HIV at concentrations much lower than are used in practice. When decontaminating instruments or medical devices, chemical germicides that are registered with and approved by the U.S. Environmental Protection Agency (EPA) as "sterilants" can be used either for sterilization or for high-level disinfection depending on contact time; germicides that are approved for use as "hospital disinfectants" and are mycobactericidal when used at appropriate dilutions can also be used for high-level disinfection of devices and instruments. Germicides that are mycobactericidal are preferred because mycobacteria represent one of the most resistant groups of microorganisms; therefore, germicides that are effective against mycobacteria are also effective against other bacterial and viral pathogens. When chemical germicides are used, instruments or devices to be sterilized or disinfected should be thoroughly cleaned before exposure to the germicide, and the manufacturer's instructions for use of the germicide should be followed.

Laundry and dishwashing cycles commonly used in hospitals are adequate to decontaminate linens, dishes, glassware, and utensils. When cleaning environmental surfaces, housekeeping procedures commonly used in hospitals are adequate; surfaces exposed to blood and body fluids should be cleaned with a detergent followed by decontamination using an EPA-approved hospital disinfectant that is mycobactericidal. Individuals cleaning up such spills should wear disposable gloves. Information on specific label claims of commercial germicides can be obtained by writing to the Disinfectants Branch, Office of Pesticides, Environmental Protection Agency, 401 M Street, S.W., Washington, D.C., 20460.

In addition to hospital disinfectants, a freshly prepared solution of sodium hypochlorite (household bleach) is an inexpensive and very effective germicide. Concentrations ranging from 5000 ppm (a 1:10 dilution of household bleach) to 500 ppm (a 1:100 dilution) sodium hypochlorite are effective, depending on the amount of organic material (e.g., blood, mucus, etc.) present on the surface to be cleaned and disinfected.

Sharp items should be considered as potentially infective and should be handled and disposed of with extraordinary care to prevent accidental injuries. Other potentially infective waste should be contained and transported in clearly identified impervious plastic bags. If the outside of the bag is contaminated with blood or other body fluids, a second outer bag should be used. Recommended practices for disposal of infective waste are adequate for disposal of waste contaminated by HIV. Blood and other body fluids may be carefully poured down a drain connected to a sanitary sewer (*MMWR* 34:573, 1985).

The time required to kill these bacteria by using dilutions of the test disinfectants compared to dilutions of phenol gives the comparative strength of the two compounds. By comparing all disinfectants to phenol, it is possible to gain a comparison of their relative potency. The phenol coefficient method does not give information on the dilution of a given disinfectant that might be suitable for a given object or surface. A second test, called the *use-dilution method*, is now officially used to determine the concentration of a disinfectant that is needed to kill bacteria effectively. In this test ten small stainless cylinders contaminated with the test bacteria are placed in the test dilutions of the disinfectants and left for 10 minutes. If all bacteria are killed on all ten cylinders, the dilution of disinfectant is considered suitable for use.

CONCEPT SUMMARY

1. The removal of all living microorganisms from an environment (sterilization) or the removal of most pathogens (disinfection) is usually accomplished by physical or chemical means. Heat, radiation, and filtration are most commonly used to obtain sterile conditions whereas the bactericidal actions of alcohols, phenols, halogens, and aldehydes are frequently applied for disinfection. Both industrial and household uses of these procedures are intended to reduce the number of microorganisms in our environment so that health and safety are maintained.

2. There are a finite number of ways by which bacteria are destroyed by sterilizing and disinfecting agents: membrane disruption, protein denaturation, enzyme inhibition, or nucleic acid (DNA) alteration.

STUDY SUMMARY

1. Make a table that classifies each of the disinfectants into a category based on their mode of action.

2. What feature of bacteria makes it necessary to heat materials above the boiling temperature to ensure sterility?

3. A solution of phenol kills all the bacteria in a suspension in 10 minutes. In similar suspensions a solution of a disinfectant A also kills all the bacteria in 10 minutes, but it takes disinfectant B 20 minutes to kill all the bacteria. Calculate the phenol coefficient of A and of B.

REFERENCES FOR FURTHER STUDY

1. *Disinfection, Sterilization and Preservation,* 2nd ed. S. Block, 1972, Lea and Febiger.
2. Chemical Disinfectants. *Annual Review of Microbiology.* 12:525, 1958.
3. *Principles and Methods of Sterilization in Health Sciences,* 2nd ed., J. Perkins, 1982. Charles C Thomas.
4. *Manual for Clinical Microbiology,* 4th ed., E. Lennette, 1985. American Society for Microbiology.

chapter 9

CHEMOTHERAPEUTIC AGENTS

Antimicrobial chemotherapeutic agents are chemicals that can selectively interfere with the growth of microorganisms and yet not interfere significantly with the functions of the cells of the infected animal host. This type of activity is known as **selective toxicity.** Generally, diseases caused by bacteria are more effectively controlled by chemotherapeutic agents than are diseases caused by fungi, protozoa, or viruses. A primary reason for this difference is that bacteria are procaryotic cells and possess some structures and metabolic processes that often differ greatly from those of the eucaryotic cells of the animal host. Based on these cellular differences, it is possible to develop chemicals that specifically interfere with procaryotic cell functions but not with the activity of eucaryotic cells. On the other hand, it has been difficult to find chemicals that selectively inhibit one type of eucaryotic cell, such as fungi, without interfering with animal cells as well. The development of antiviral agents has been more difficult because viruses use host cell functions to carry out their replication activities, and as yet few chemical agents can interfere selectively with viral activity but not with the functions of the host cells. Early historical developments of chemotherapeutic agents were covered in Chapter 1. The continued development of new chemotherapeutic agents over the past 40 years is one of the most important achievements of medical science and has resulted in saving millions of lives and alleviating untold suffering.

An ideal chemotherapeutic agent should possess as many of the following characteristics as possible:

1. Be highly toxic to a large number of pathogens
2. Have no toxicity to the host
3. Not induce the development of **antibiotic resistance** in mutant microbes
4. Not induce **hypersensitivities** in the host
5. Not interfere with the normal host defense mechanisms

Antimicrobial
capable of killing or stopping the growth of a microbe. Antibiotics are antimicrobial materials.

Selective toxicity
the quality possessed by a substance that can damage or destroy a living organism in the presence of another organism that remains unaffected.

Antibiotic resistance
a condition in which a microbe is unaffected by the presence of a compound used for antimicrobial therapy.

Unfortunately, the ideal chemotherapeutic agent has not yet been found. Most have some toxicity to the host and induce varying degrees of hypersensitivity or allow the development of resistant mutant microbes. Thus, some tradeoff is given for all applications of chemotherapeutic agents, and benefits to the patient must be weighed against possible adverse side effects.

Only those antimicrobial agents that are the natural products of microorganisms are called *antibiotics*. Antimicrobial compounds that are made in the laboratory but not produced by living organisms are referred to as *synthetic* agents. Because the word *chemotherapy* has been extensively used in connection with tumor therapy, the term *antimicrobial* is often preferred over *chemotherapeutic* when discussing infectious disease.

SYNTHETIC AGENTS

Hypersensitivity
an immune response that causes an individual to overreact to the presence of an antigen resulting in an allergic condition.

Chemotherapeutic agents may act by mimicking essential components needed in normal cellular reactions. When present, the chemotherapeutic agent is taken into a cellular reaction in place of the normal component. Once integrated, the chemotherapeutic agent prevents the cell from functioning or developing in a normal manner. Extensive efforts have been carried out to develop synthetic chemicals that would interfere with specific microbial functions, yet relatively few useful compounds have been developed. Most useful synthetic antibacterial agents are related to the *sulfonamides*.

Sulfonamides

Since their discovery in the mid-1930s, the sulfonamides have been important agents in treating a variety of bacterial infections. Sulfonamides, sometimes simply called *sulfa drugs*, are various derivatives of a molecule called *para-aminobenzene-sulfonamide* or just *sulfonamide* (Figure 9-1).

Competitive inhibitor
a compound that competes with a substrate for position at the active site on an enzyme, but which cannot be changed by the enzyme. These compounds prevent normal essential enzyme function.

Mechanism of action The sulfonamides are structurally similar to *para-aminobenzoic acid* (PABA) and function as **competitive inhibitors** of this compound. PABA is an essential component in the synthesis of *folic acid*, which is an essential metabolite for both mammalian and procaryotic cells. Mammalian cells, however, depend on preformed folic acid obtained in their diet whereas procaryotic cells synthesize their own using PABA. This difference in the source of folic acid allows sulfonamides to function as effective chemotherapeutic agents. In bacteria, the sulfonamide molecule

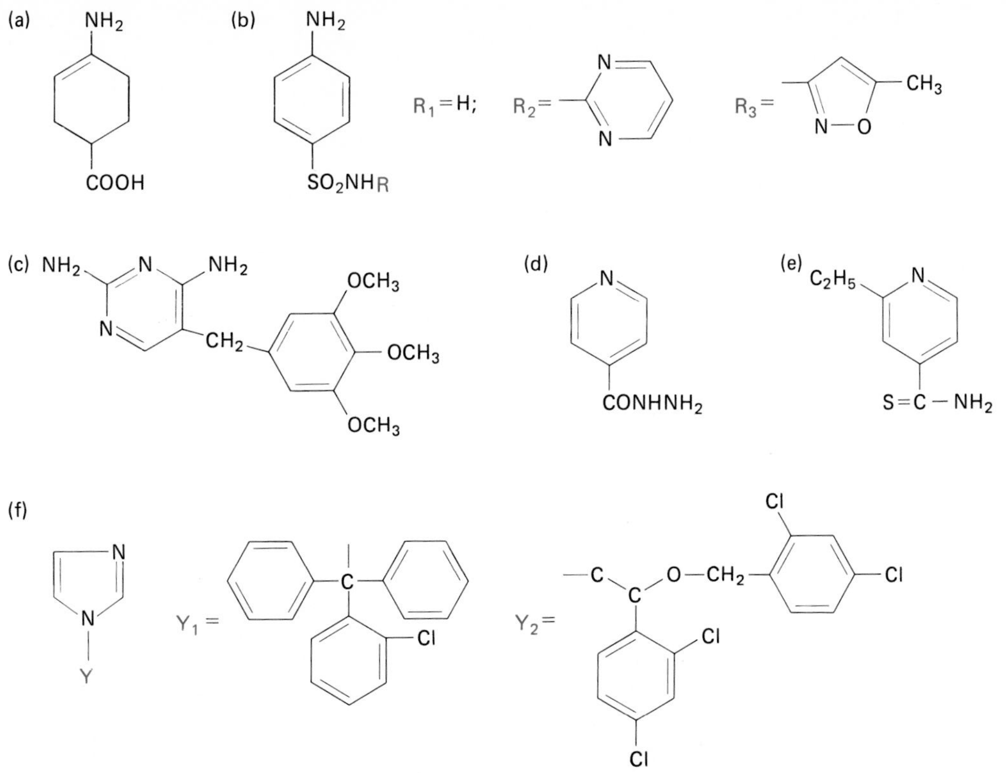

Figure 9-1 Structure of some synthetic antimicrobial agents: (a) p-animobenzoic acid, a bacterial metabolite. (b) Sulfonamide, an analog of p-aminobenzoic acid. Chemically modified at position "R," the sulfonamide becomes a "sulfa drug," e.g., R_1 = sulfonamide, R_2 = sulfadiazine, R_3 = sulfamethoxazole. (c) Trimethoprim, most commonly used in fixed combination with sulfamethoxazole. (d) Isoniazid and (e) Ethionamide which are used almost exclusively as therapy against tuberculosis. (f) The imidazole nucleus, modifications of which produce antifungal agents, e.g., Y_1 = clotrimazole, Y_2 = Miconazole.

is able to substitute for PABA during the synthesis of folic acid and this results in nonfunctional folic acid.

The enzymes that convert PABA to to folic acid are unable to distinguish between PABA and sulfonamide. If only a small amount of a sulfa drug is present, most of the enzyme continues to interact with PABA and the cell continues to grow but at a reduced rate; as the concentration of sulfa increases, there is a greater and greater possibility that the enzyme will find only the sulfa drug to interact with and the cell will stop growing. Such chemical interactions, which depend on the relative concentration of the inhibitor and the normal substrate, are known as *competitive inhibition* reactions (Figure 9-2). That is, there is competition between the two substrates for the active site on the enzyme molecule.

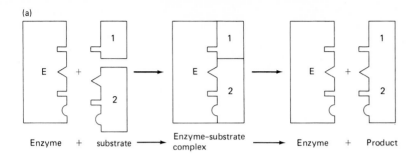

(a)

Enzyme + substrate ⟶ Enzyme-substrate complex ⟶ Enzyme + Product

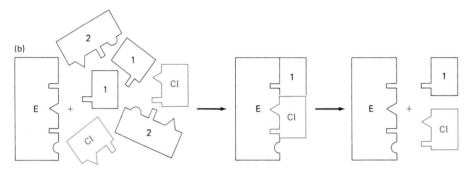

(b)

Figure 9-2 Representation of competitive inhibition of enzyme function by a substrate analog. (a) Normal enzyme substrate interaction leading to product formation. (b) The addition of a competitive inhibitor to the reaction results in competition for active site on the enzyme. (In this example the competition is between C1 and 2.) The successful formation of product depends on the relative concentrations of C1 and 2.

In bacteria, just as in humans, the short-term absence of a necessary metabolite does not result in death. However, for a single cell, such a condition results in the cessation of growth. If the needed metabolite is again made available to the cell within a reasonable time, it will once more begin to grow. Such a condition is analogous to placing a culture of bacteria in the refrigerator; although the cells do not immediately die, the cold reduces their rate of metabolism to a point where growth is essentially stopped. When the culture is again placed in the incubator, growth soon returns to normal. This condition of suspended growth is known as *bacteriostasis* and antimicrobial drugs that lead to such a reversible growth state are called *bacteriostatic* agents. Sulfonamides are an example of a bacteriostatic drug. The mode of action of several classes of antimicrobials is shown in Table 9-1.

Clinical applications Because of the extensive use of sulfonamides during the late 1930s and throughout the intervening years, numerous bacteria are now resistant to these antimicrobial drugs

Table 9-1   Mode of Action of Antimicrobial Agents

Antibiotic Class	Representative	Action
Penicillins	Ampicillin	Inhibits peptidoglycan synthesis; inactivates autolytic enzymes
Cephalosporins	Cephalothin	Inactivates peptidoglycan synthesis
Tetracycline	Doxycycline	Inhibits protein synthesis by inhibiting aminoacyl-tRNA binding to 30-S ribosomal subunit
Chloramphenicol	Chloramphenicol	Blocks protein synthesis by inhibiting peptidyl transferase
Macrolides	Erythmomycin	Inhibits protein synthesis by blocking translocation reaction
Vancomycin	Vancomycin	Blocks early cell wall synthesis
Quinolones	Ciprofloxacin	Inhibits DNA gyrase enzyme; prevents unfolding and refolding of DNA
Polymyxins	Polymyxin B	Prevents membrane transport functions
Aminoglycosines	Amikacin	Prevents protein synthesis by interfering with 30-S ribosome function

at concentrations normally achieved in patients. For this reason, in spite of the relatively low level of toxicity due to these agents, antibiotics are preferred over sulfa drugs in most clinical treatments today. The major exception is in the treatment of urinary tract infections; sulfonamides can reach high levels of concentration in the urine and are generally effective as therapeutic agents. Combinations of antibiotics and sulfonamides have also been used to suppress the number of bacteria in the intestinal tract prior to surgery. The major toxicity problems associated with sulfonamide use are due to some hypersensitivity reactions and the tendency of sulfonamides to crystallize in the kidney with resulting damage to the renal tubules.

One of the newer sulfonamide drugs is actually a combination of a sulfonamide (sulfamethoxazole) and a similar compound (trimethoprim) that also competitively inhibits an enzymatic reaction in the biosynthesis of folic acid. This compound, *tri-methoprim-sulfamethoxazole*, is sold by several names, such as Bactrim or Septra, and has increased application in a number of serious disease conditions caused by organisms of the genera *Shigella*, *Haemophilus*, and *Pseudomonas*.

Other Synthetic Agents

Several synthetic agents are widely used in treating tuberculosis and leprosy. The *sulfones* are a group of compounds, related to the sulfonamides, that are effective against infections caused by the acid-fast bacilli. Their use today is limited almost entirely to the treatment of leprosy. *Para-aminosalicylic acid* (PAS), an analog of PABA, is an effective bacteriostatic agent for the treatment of tuberculosis but has limited effectiveness against other diseases. *Isoniazid* (INH) is effective and the most widely used agent in the treatment of tuberculosis. It is often used in combination with other antituberculosis agents. The exact mode of action of INH is not known. *Ethambutol* (Embutal or EMB) is another effective antituberculosis agent that is always used in combination with PAS or INH. In fact, therapy for active tuberculous disease should always include multiple antituberculous agents. A number of these agents are listed in Table 9-2. The structures of several sulfonamides and related synthetic chemotherapeutic agents as well as para-aminobenzoic acid are shown in Figure 9-1.

ANTIBIOTICS

Penicillins

Penicillin is a term applied to a group of closely related compounds produced by various fungi of the genus *Penicillium*. Some penicillins are the natural product; others have been chemically altered in the laboratory. Penicillin, the first antibiotic discovered, has been the most useful. During the late 1930s and early 1940s, when penicillin was first used, it became known as the miracle drug because it could often cure otherwise fatal diseases rapidly. The most dramatic effects of penicillin use were seen on some major killer diseases, such as pneumonia, scarlet fever, staphylococcal diseases, and the venereal diseases gonorrhea and syphilis. The

Table 9-2   Agents Used to Treat Tuberculosis

Major or Primary Compounds	Minor or Secondary Compounds
Ethambutol (EMB)	Capreomycin
Isoniazid (IHN)	Cycloserine
p-aminosalicylic acid (PAS)	Ethionamide
Rifampin	Kanamycin
Streptomycin	Pyrazinamide
	Thiacetazone
	Viomycin

natural penicillins are primarily effective against Gram-positive bacteria, Gram-negative cocci, and the syphilis spirochete. Because of its great success, there was a strong tendency during the late 1940s and 1950s to use penicillin in treating a wide variety of infections. This widespread and often indiscriminate use, particularly in the hospital environment, led to the emergence of many penicillin-resistant staphylococci. By the late 1950s the effectiveness of penicillin in treating staphylococcal infections had greatly diminished. At this time it was discovered that the basic central structure of the penicillin molecule could be produced by *Penicillium* molds under special controlled conditions. Various chemical side chains could then be added to this basic structure to modify its action (Figure 9-3). Through extensive, empirical investigations and testing, a series of altered or semisynthetic penicillins were found that have enhanced antimicrobial activities. Several are able to kill bacteria that are resistant to the natural penicillin; others are effective against a wider range of bacteria. A list of some semisynthetic penicillins and their uses is given in Table 9-3. Figure 9-4 is a diagrammatic representation of the development of many available penicillin compounds.

The action of penicillin is to interfere specifically with new bacterial cell wall synthesis during cell division. The cross-linkages of the peptidoglycan strands are prevented from forming. Without a complete cell wall, the high internal osmotic pressure of the bacterial cell results in rapid cell lysis. Because mammalian cells have no cell walls, penicillin is generally nontoxic to these

Figure 9-3   The structure of penicillin. The common portion of all penicillins is 6-APA. This molecule may be modified at "R" to produce a wide variety of "synthetic" penicillins, as exemplified by R_1 = penicillin G, R_2 = Methicillin, R_3 = ampicillin.

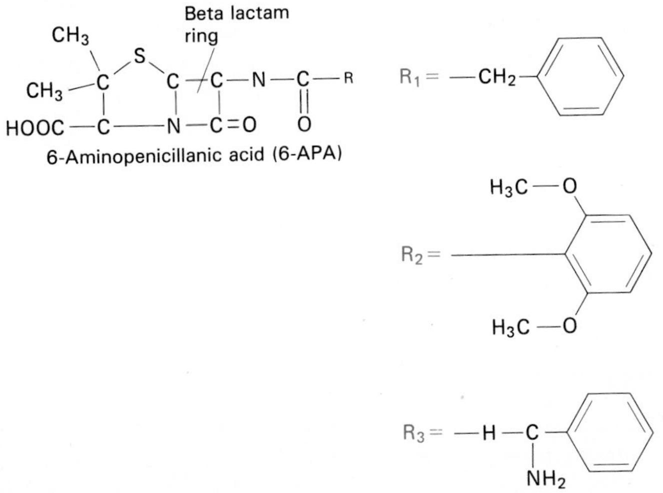

Table 9-3   Penicillins Commonly Used in Treatment of Bacterial Infection

Name	Source	Common Uses
1. Penicillin G (Benzylpenicillin)	Natural	
2. Penicillin V	Natural	Oral penicillin (acid stable).
3. Methicillin	Semisynthetic	Nos. 3 through 6 used in treatment of infections caused by penicillinase-producing staphylococci. Cloxacillin can be given orally.
4. Oxacillin	Semisynthetic	
5. Nafcillin	Semisynthetic	
6. Cloxacillin	Semisynthetic	
7. Ampicillin	Semisynthetic	A broad-spectrum penicillin used against Gram-negative bacteria and for patients with endocarditis.
8. Carbenicillin	Semisynthetic	Nos. 8 and 9 are specific-use penicillins, used to treat *Pseudomonas* infections.
9. Ticarcillin	Semisynthetic	
10. Piperacillin	Semisynthetic	A new penicillin used in treatment of Gram-negative bacterial infections.

cells and can be used in relatively large concentrations. Complications do occasionally result in persons who are allergic to penicillin, however.

Bacterial resistance to the penicillins results mostly from bacterial production of enzymes called *penicillinases*. Penicillinase splits the beta-lactam ring of the penicillin, producing an inactive molecule (Figure 9-5). Some penicillins, such as penicillin G, are unstable in stomach acid and cannot be taken orally whereas others, such as penicillin V, are acid stable and can be absorbed intact from the gut. Penicillin is the treatment of choice when susceptible bacteria are causing infection because it is both less toxic to the host than other antibiotics and, in general, less expensive. It should not, of course, be used in persons who are hypersensitive to penicillin. The appropriate semisynthetic penicillins, such as *methicillin, nafcillin,* or *oxacillin,* are the agents of choice in treating penicillin-resistant staphylococcal infections. When a broader spectrum of activity is needed, *ampicillin, carbenicillin,* or *ticarcillin* might be used.

Aminoglycosides

The aminoglycosides include *streptomycin* and antibiotics with a similar chemical structure. Streptomycin (Figure 9-6) is bactericidal against various Gram-positive and Gram-negative bacteria

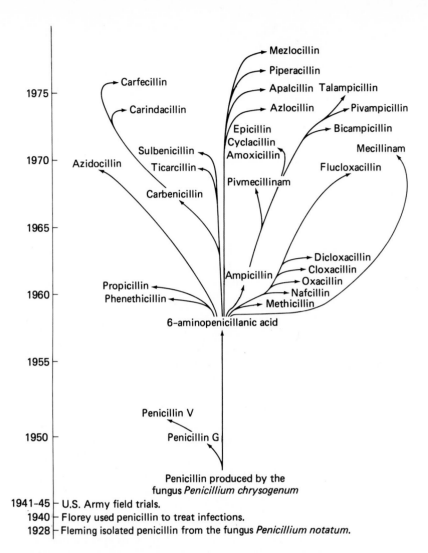

Figure 9-4 A schematic representation showing the approximate historical date and genesis of many of today's penicillins. This diagram shows the relatedness among penicillins.

Figure 9-5 Inactivation of penicillin by beta-lactamase enzyme.

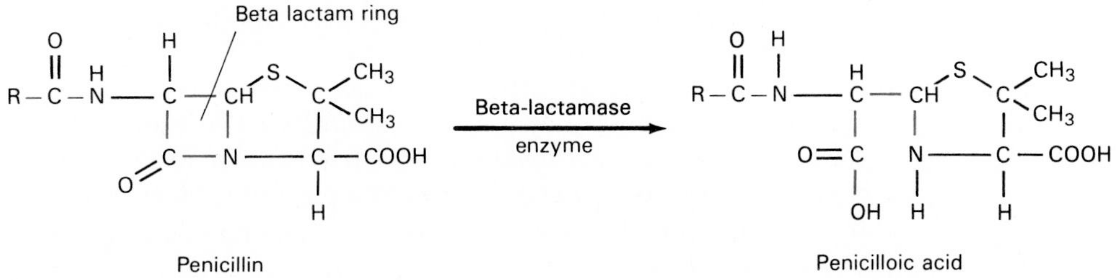

Penicillin

Beta-lactamase enzyme →

Penicilloic acid

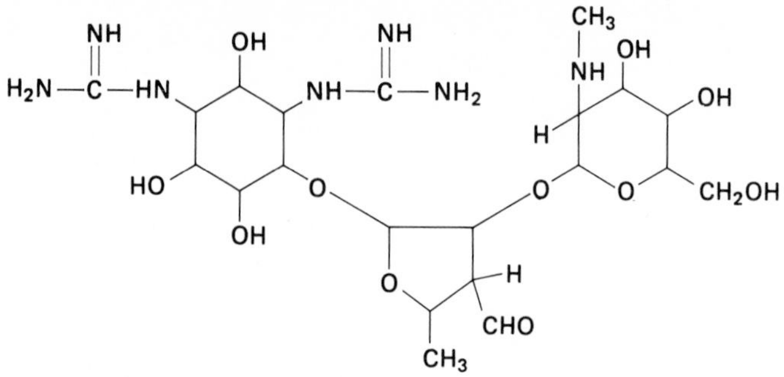

Figure 9-6 Chemical structure of streptomycin, first of the aminoglycoside antibiotics to have wide clinical application.

as well as the tubercle bacillus. It was the first major antibiotic developed after penicillin. When it became available in the mid-1940s, it was effective against many Gram-negative bacteria that were not susceptible to penicillin as well as against tuberculosis. It was the first effective antituberculosis agent to be developed. These antibiotics function by attaching to the small 30-S component of the 70-S procaryotic ribosomes. Such attachment interferes with the proper initiation of protein synthesis. The 80-S ribosomes of eucaryotic cells are not readily affected. Resistant mutant bacteria develop when the site of attachment on the ribosomal component is altered. Organisms such as anaerobes and streptococci are resistant because the cells are impermeable to the aminoglycosides. Some cells become resistant when they are infected with plasmids carrying genes that direct the synthesis of enzymes that modify and inactivate the antibiotics.

Aminoglycosides are among the most toxic of the commonly used antibiotics. Toxicity may lead to kidney damage, hearing loss, or other physical impairments. Since aminoglycosides cannot be given orally, patients usually must be hospitalized for **parenteral** administration. In order to prevent the excesssive accumulation of antibiotics in patients receiving aminoglycosides, it is necessary to monitor the concentration of the compound present in the body fluids. Such determinations, called *antibiotic assays,* are usually performed on the blood of patients receiving these or other toxic antibiotics. Using this technique, it is possible to monitor the amount of antibiotic given the patient and to maintain levels below the toxic concentrations.

Several widely used aminoglycoside antibiotics are *amikacin, neomycin, kanamycin, netilmicin, gentamicin,* and *tobramycin.* These antibiotics have a broad antibacterial spectrum and are used to treat serious infections that do not respond well to other chemotherapeutic agents. *Spectinomycin,* which is similar to the aminoglycosides, has a very specific use in the United States. It is used in the therapy of gonorrhea caused by penicillinase-producing *Neisseria gonorrhoeae.*

Parenteral

given into the body. Many medicines cannot be given orally (by mouth) because they taste bad, are destroyed by stomach acid, or are not absorbed from the intestine. These compounds are given parenterally by injection or through a catheter.

Tetracyclines

The tetracyclines are a small group of closely related antibiotics that are bacteriostatic against a wide range of both Gram-positive and Gram-negative bacteria as well as rickettsiae, chlamydiae, and mycoplasma. Because of this wide range of activity, they are called *broad-spectrum* antibiotics. Tetracyclines inhibit protein synthesis of growing bacteria by combining with the 30-S ribosomes and interfering with the binding of tRNA to mRNA.

Some natural and semisynthetic tetracyclines are *chlortetracycline* (Aureomycin), *oxytetracycline* (Terramycin), *doxycycline* (Vibramycin), and *minocycline* (Minocin). Although differing in structure and name, these compounds are mostly effective against the same microorganisms. These antibiotics are very useful in treating infections that are not responsive to penicillins and they can be taken orally; however, they may produce such side reactions as irritation of the intestinal tract, liver damage, and discoloration of teeth when taken before permanent dentition is formed.

The use of tetracycline during the early years of the antibiotic era led scientists to the discovery of a phenomenon generally applicable to **broad-spectrum** antibiotics. When these compounds are used indiscriminately or for long periods of time, normal bacterial flora, as well as pathogens, are frequently destroyed. The loss of normal flora often allows bacteria that are resistant to the antibiotic to increase rapidly in numbers. The large increase in the number of these organisms frequently results in disease that will not respond to the antibiotic being used. Tetracycline is commonly used to reduce the effects of acne in young adult populations. Its use under these circumstances is relatively safe when directed by a physician.

Broad-spectrum
effective against more than one kind of bacterium; usually suggesting antibacterial activity against both Gram-positive and Gram-negative bacteria.

Chloramphenicol

Chloramphenicol is a broad-spectrum antibiotic that is effective against a wide range of bacteria as well as rickettsiae and chlamydiae. It is, however, quite toxic to humans and is generally used only when other antibiotics are not effective. It is the drug of choice under some circumstances, such as in typhoid fever, and is very effective against anaerobic bacteria. It is commonly used in combinations with other antibiotics as empiric therapy in cases of meningitis. Chloramphenicol binds specifically to the 70-S ribosomes of procaryotic cells and blocks protein synthesis by preventing the formation of peptide bonds.

Erythromycin

Erythromycin is the most active of a group of related antibiotics called *macrolides* (Figure 9-7). The spectrum of activity of the macrolides is similar to penicillin. Erythromycin binds to the 50-S ribo-

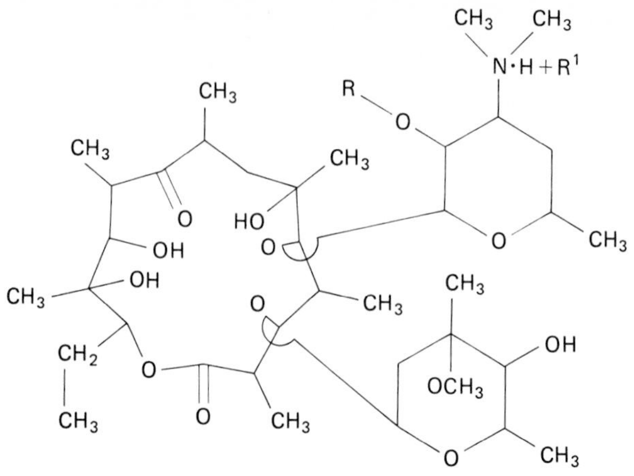

Figure 9-7   Structure of erythromycin, most commonly used of the macrolide antibiotics.

Bactericidal

capable of killing bacteria when used as a therapeutic or a disinfectant.

some subunit and may be either bacteriostatic or **bactericidal,** depending on the concentration. The mechanism of action is similar to that of chloramphenicol. This antibiotic is most often used as a substitute for penicillin in patients who are allergic to the latter drug. It has been used as therapy in severe cases of acne where tetracycline has not been effective. It is also the agent of choice in treating whooping cough, campylobacter and mycoplasma infections, and the relatively recently recognized Legionnaires' disease. Toxicity is usually not severe, but microbial resistance is common.

Lincomycin and Clindamycin

Lincomycin and clindamycin have a spectrum of activity similar to penicillin but their basic chemical structure differs from that of other antibiotics. They are very effective antistaphylococcal compounds with relatively low toxicity and are useful in treating patients who are allergic to penicillin. Their mechanism of action is similar to that of chloramphenicol and erythromycin. Clindamycin has been particularly useful in treating disease caused by Gram-negative anaerobic bacteria, and patients with toxic shock syndrome.

An increasing use of clindamycin has led to an important observation regarding undesirable reactions during or following antibiotic therapy. Certain patients who had been receiving clindamycin developed a severe, often fatal intestinal disease known as *pseudomembranous enterocolitis*. It was discovered that this antibiotic caused a severe loss of normal bowel flora except for several resistant bacteria, one of them an anaerobe known as *Clostridium difficile* (Chapter 20). Overgrowth by this organism resulted in the disease. It is now known that this condition can result following the use of almost any antimicrobial agent, and therapy involves both discontinuance of the inciting antibiotic and the reestablishment of normal bowel flora.

Rifampicin (Rifampin)

Rifampicin is a semisynthetic compound produced from the natural antibiotic rifamycin. It inhibits the growth of Gram-positive, Gram-negative, and acid-fast bacteria, can be taken orally, and is effective in low concentrations. It specifically blocks the transcription of mRNA. It has been particularly effective in treating tuberculosis and leprosy. Use of this drug usually results in the rapid selection of resistant bacteria, a feature that suggests using a therapeutic approach that will reduce the number of such resistant organisms. A customary approach when using rifampicin is to give it in combination with another antibiotic and give them simultaneously to the patient. The rationale for this **combination therapy** lies in an understanding of the genetics of mutation as discussed in Chapter 6. If, for any given phenotypic characteristic, the chance of developing a mutant organism that would be resistant to any given antimicrobial were 10^{-6}, and the chance of developing resistance to a second antibiotic were 10^{-7}, then, on the basis of probability, the likelihood that the organism would develop resistance to both antimicrobial agents at the same time would be 10^{-13}, a number so small that such resistance would probably not occur.

In spite of the selection of resistant bacteria, rifampicin is second only to vancomycin as a choice for treatment of infections due to methicillin-resistant *Staphylococcus aureus*, a particularly troublesome organism in many hospitals, and is the drug of choice in **prophylaxis** against infection by *Haemophilus influenzae*.

Cephalosporins

The structure and activity of cephalosporins resemble those of penicillin. They are effective against both Gram-positive and Gram-negative bacteria. Their advantage lies in their broad spectrum of activity as well as their relative resistance to some penicillinases.

Research and development in the area of antibiotics are proceeding rapidly with the cephalosporins, perhaps because it is relatively easy to alter the molecule chemically at several points (Figure 9-8), thus producing ''new'' antimicrobial agents. These modifications have produced a relatively large number of antibiotics.

Those cephalosporins that have activity primarily against

Combination therapy
treatment with more than one antibiotic at a time. Often used when there is doubt as to the cause of the disease, or when there is likelihood that a microorganism may be resistant to one antimicrobial if used alone.

Prophylaxis
use of an antimicrobial to prevent infection from occurring.

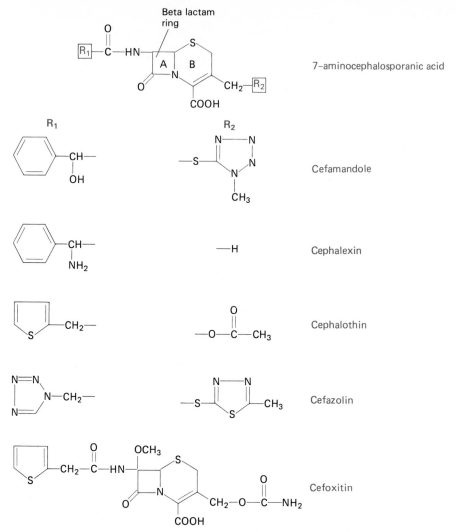

Figure 9-8   Chemical structure of some commonly used cephalosporin antibiotics. The 7-aminocephalosporanic acid molecule can be modified at R_1 and R_2 (as shown) to produce the indicated antibiotics. Cefoxitin, one of the newer cephalosporins, has a modification of the basic 7-aminocephalosporanic acid molecule in addition to R_1 and R_2.

Gram-positive bacteria are known as *first-generation* compounds; those active against *Enterobacteriaceae* are generally considered as *second-generation* cephalosporins, and those with exceptionally broad spectra that include organisms such as *Pseudomonas aeruginosa* (Chapter 25) are listed as *third-generation* cephalosporins. Although essentially nontoxic, these compounds cannot, with only rare exceptions, be taken orally and the newer antibiotics are extremely expensive. A number of these new agents, such as *ceftaxidime, cefoperazone, cefotaxime, cefoxitin,* and *cefamandole,* are presently in general clinical use.

Vancomycin

Vancomycin is a sugar-protein antibiotic that inhibits the completion of bacterial cell wall synthesis. This compound has been known for years, but its early use was associated with high levels of toxicity. More recent preparations do not have as many negative side effects, and the compound is presently used extensively in treatment of infections due to methicillin-resistant *Staphylococcus aureus* (Chapter 15). It is also effective against some causes of bacterial **endocarditis.**

Endocarditis
infection of the tissues lining the inside of the heart or valves in the heart.

Bacitracin

Bacitracin is a polypeptide that interferes with the development of the cell wall. It is effective against many Gram-positive bacteria. The high toxicity of this agent has primarily limited its use to topical ointments.

Polymyxins

The polymyxins are simple polypeptides that are quite toxic to humans. Their mode of action is to disrupt the functions of plasma membranes of Gram-negative bacteria. They are used to treat some of the more resistant Gram-negative bacilli, although toxicity severely restricts their use.

New Classes of Antibiotics

Of several "new" antibacterials, two classes appear to have the potential for extensive clinical use: the *quinolones* and the *penems*.

Quinolones   The quinolones are similar to an older, seldom-used compound known as *nalidixic acid*. They prevent unwinding of procaryotic DNA so that it cannot be transcribed. These compounds have a very broad spectrum and are used for systemic disease, diarrhea, and urinary tract infection. The best known of these agents are *ciprofloxacin* and *ofloxacin,* although many similar compounds are presently being studied (Figure 9-9).

Penems   The penems are remarkable compounds that almost meet the requirements for the "magic bullet" hoped for by Paul Ehrlich many years ago (Chapter 1). These compounds bind to bacterial penicillin-binding proteins in the periplasmic space. They are essentially nontoxic, have a very broad spectrum (only a few bacteria are resistant), and are very stable. They are effective at low concentration and come close to meeting the conditions of an ideal antibiotic noted earlier in the chapter (Figure 9-10).

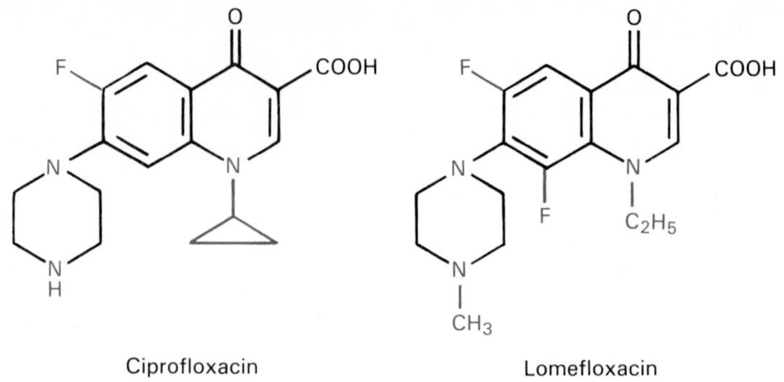

Figure 9-9 Two examples of quinolone antibiotics. These compounds interfere with coiling and uncoiling of DNA, resulting in cell death.

ANTIFUNGAL AGENTS

Polyenes

Polyenes specifically change the permeability of membranes of fungi and are useful as antifungal agents. *Nystatin* and *amphotericin B* are the major antifungal agents in this category. Nystatin is limited to topical applications because of its toxicity. Amphotericin B is a very toxic compound, but remains the only truly effective antifungal agent for serious systemic fungal infections.

Imidazoles

The imidazoles constitute a relatively new approach to fungal therapy. There are several such agents, *miconazole* and *ketoconazole* being perhaps the best known. These agents are a welcome addition to the rather limited antifungal therapeutic options. Their structure (Figure 9-11) is simple, and similar compounds have been used to treat diseases due to protozoa and helminths for several years. Their advantages are a limited toxicity and the fact that some can be taken orally. Fungal diseases of the skin as well as the deep, systemic mycotic diseases respond to these agents.

Figure 9-10 A new class of antimicrobial, the penem antibiotics.

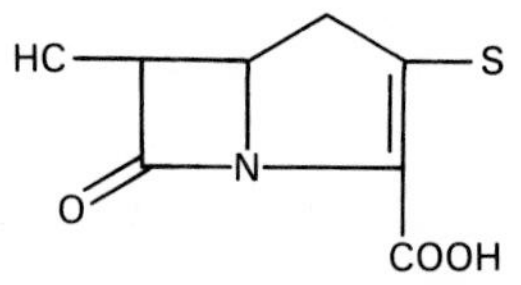

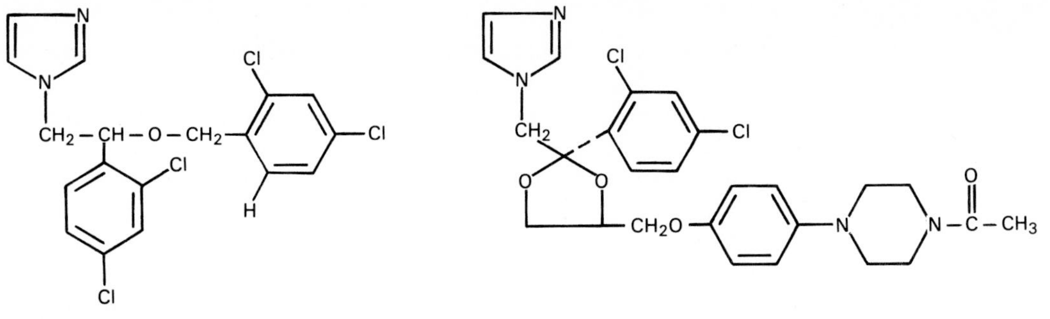

Miconazole

Ketoconazole

Figure 9-11   Representative imidazole anti-fungal antibiotics.

ANTIVIRAL AGENTS

As noted earlier, development of an antiviral agent is complicated by the fact that viruses do not have their own metabolic machinery. However, they have been discovered to induce the formation of several unique viral proteins by infected cells, and their nucleic acids are often somewhat different from those of their mammalian hosts. Scientists have capitalized on these very few differences in viral structure to develop several antiviral compounds, and further research in this area is being vigorously pursued. A list of presently available antiviral compounds is shown as Table 9-4.

Table 9-4   Antiviral Compounds

Compound	Virus Inhibited	Clinical Use
Amantadine hydrochloride	Influenza type A	Early treatment or prophylaxis of influenza
Idoxuridine	Herpes simplex	Topical for herpes keratitis
Cytarabine	Varicella-Zoster	Herpes keratitis, limited systemic zoster
Adenine arabinoside	Herpes simplex	Herpes keratitis and herpes encephalitis
Acyclovir	Herpes simplex type 2	Early treatment of genital herpes
Ribavirin	Respiratory syncytial virus	RSV pneumonia in infants
Methisazone	Variola	Smallpox

MICROBIAL RESISTANCE

A major problem associated with chemotherapy is the selection of resistant microorganisms. Microorganisms may spontaneously mutate against a given trait in their environment once in every 10^5 to 10^{10} cell divisions. Because of their rapid multiplication rates, the chance of microbial mutations against a given antimicrobial agent is quite probable. In this situation, the mutant may rapidly multiply in the presence of the antibiotic and produce many resistant progeny. In addition to spontaneous mutations, genetic resistance may be passed from one bacterium to another by small, circular extrachromosomal DNA fragments called *resistance plasmids* or *R factors*. A resistance plasmid may contain the genetic information that codes for resistance to one or several antibacterial agents; when the plasmid is passed to a new cell, the trait of antibiotic resistance is also passed.

Certain resistant mutants function by producing enzymes that destroy or alter the chemotherapeutic agent. Others become resistant from changes occurring on the receptor sites to which the chemotherapeutic agent binds. Still others may develop resistance by changes occurring in the permeability of the cell to the chemical agent.

TREATMENT

Empirical therapy
treatment given on the basis of experience, and not as a result of susceptibility testing.

The procedure used in treating a disease should be designed so that the chance of a cure is maximal and the chance of developing a resistant microbial mutant is minimal. To achieve these goals, it is first necessary to determine which chemotherapeutic agents are effective against the disease-causing microbe. This process requires isolating the bacterial cause of disease and testing for its susceptibility to different chemotherapeutic agents. The most commonly used method of determining antibiotic sensitivity is to place antibiotic-impregnated disks on a Mueller-Hinton agar surface that has been inoculated with a film of the test bacterium (Figure 9-12). A zone of inhibition of bacterial growth is produced around the disks that contain effective antibiotics. This type of testing requires up to 24 hours, however, and with critically ill patients it may be desirable to initiate treatment before such testing is possible. Such **empirical therapy** is commonly used in clinical situations where time may be critical to the patient, and where it is possible to make a logical choice of antibiotics based on previous experience. Table 9-5 lists those antibiotics that are presently susceptibility-tested against bacteria isolated from human infec-

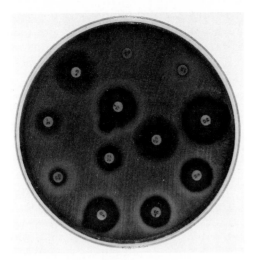

Figure 9-12   Antibiotic susceptibility test. The surface of the growth medium is inoculated such that the bacteria will grow as a confluent lawn. Paper disks containing the antibiotic are then placed on the inoculated surface. The susceptibility of the antibiotics is determined by measuring the diameter of the zone of bacterial growth inhibition.

Table 9-5   Antibiotics Suggested for Susceptibility-Testing Against Different Groups of Bacteria

Gram-Positive Cocci	Enterococcus	Pseudomonas	Enterobacteriaceae
Amikacin	Ampicillin	Amikacin	Amikacin
Cephalothin	Chloramphenicol	Carbenicillin	Ampicillin
Chloramphenicol	Erythromycin	Chloramphenicol	Cefamandole
Clindamycin	Penicillin G	Gentamicin	Cefoxitin
Erythromycin	Tetracycline	Polymyxin B	Cephalothin
Gentamicin		Sulfisoxazole	Chloramphenicol
Kanamycin		Tetracycline	Gentamicin
Penicillin G		Tobramycin	Polymyxin B
Methicillin			Tetracycline
Tetracycline			Tobramycin
Vancamycin			Trimethoprim-sulfamethoxazole

tions. More than one set of antibiotics is necessary for testing because not only is there considerable variation in the in vitro susceptibility of bacteria, but the concentration of antibiotic obtainable in the many body spaces also varies. Some antibiotics, for instance, can be used to treat a urinary tract infection in which the concentration of antibiotic can reach high levels, whereas those same antibiotics may not reach a high enough concentration in the lung to be useful in treating pneumonia. The several test sets of antibiotic agents also reflect the fact that a finite number of compounds can be conveniently tested at any one time. Rapid susceptibility tests, often requiring less than one day, are now available through automated systems using sensitive electronic instrumentation for reading results. Some of these rapid tests were described in Chapter 7.

When an effective antibiotic has been determined, treatment should be initiated as soon as possible or modified to appropriate antibiotics when empirical therapy was initiated. Antibiotics must be given in sufficiently high concentrations to result in a cure, and treatment should continue for some time after the symptoms of the infection have subsided. This procedure gives the best chance of a complete cure and minimizes the chance of selecting resistant mutant microorganisms. If low, rather than adequate, concentrations of antibiotics are given, it is much more probable that resistant mutants will develop. If treatment ends too soon, the infection may recur and further increase the probability of resistant mutants developing. Delay in initial treatment may allow the infection to penetrate to deeper body tissues where abscesses may develop and block the diffusion of the antibiotic to the site of the infecting microbe. If bacteria in an abscess are in the stationary-growth phase, antibiotics that are effective only against growing microbes will not work. In these situations, the abscess must be drained before effective treatment can be given.

COMPLICATIONS

Many antibiotics have direct toxic effects on humans and such effects must be considered and weighed against any possible antibiotic benefits. Allergies or hypersensitivities may develop against an antibiotic like penicillin, and patients should be questioned about such allergies before treatment is started. Unfortunately, there are few reliable tests to detect allergies to antibiotics.

Besides eliminating disease-causing microorganisms, antibiotics often destroy many bacteria of the normal flora of the body. A **superinfection** by an antibiotic-resistant, indigenous microorganism that is usually held in check by the normal flora may result.

Superinfection
a second infection that develops in addition to a previous infection; an infection that occurs as a result of antibiotic treatment.

Sentinel Surveillance System for Antimicrobial Resistance in Clinical Isolates of *Neisseria gonorrhoeae:* United States, 1986–87

Infections caused by strains of *Neisseria gonorrhoeae* that are resistant to recommended antimicrobials continue to be a growing public health problem. Over the past 3 years, the incidence of plasmid-mediated, penicillinase-producing *N. gonorrhoeae* (PPNG) has increased, and it now accounts for 2% of all reported gonococcal infections in the United States. However, the proportions of infections caused by organisms with chromosomally mediated resistance to penicillin, tetracycline, and spectinomycin and by gonococci with plasmid-mediated tetracycline resistance (TRNG) have been determined for only a limited number of localities.

The procedures for laboratory diagnosis and reporting of PPNG have been standardized, and over 90% of public health laboratories routinely test every gonococcal isolate for production of β-lactamase. However, ascertainment and reporting of other types of antimicrobial resistance have been inconsistent. Whereas PPNG can be detected by a rapid diagnostic test, laboratory diagnosis of chromosomally mediated resistance and TRNG requires relatively expensive antimicrobial susceptibility determination procedures on subcultures of primary isolates. Until recently, surveillance of these strains had been based on a passive reporting system; consequently, geographical areas performing more susceptibility tests than other areas may appear to have higher incidences of these strains.

Because recommendations for therapy should be based on accurate and timely surveillance of antimicrobial resistance in *N. gonorrhoeae,* the Division of Sexually Transmitted Diseases, Center for Prevention Services, CDC, in cooperation with the Sexually Transmitted Diseases Laboratory Program, Center for Infectious Diseases, CDC, and state and local health departments, has organized the Gonococcal Isolate Surveillance Project (GISP).

In this project, each of four regionally based laboratories chosen for their expertise in performing antimicrobial susceptibility determinations processes a prospective consecutive sample of isolates from five sexually transmitted disease clinics. Each month, the first 25 urethral isolates from male patients in each clinic are submitted to the regional laboratories where a test for β-lactamase is performed and minimum inhibitory concentrations (MICs) to penicillin, tetracycline, spectinomycin, cefoxitin, and ceftriaxone are determined. Classification of the isolates is based on the CDC surveillance definitions of plasmid-mediated resistance (PPNG, TRNG) and chromosomally mediated resistance. This report summarizes the results from the first 15 participating clinics.

Between August 1986 and July 1987, 1420 gonococcal isolates were evaluated. Nineteen isolates (1%) were PPNG, and 64 (5%) were TRNG. Forty-five of the TRNG isolates were reported from Baltimore, where TRNG accounted for 15% (45/300) of gonococcal isolates. For the 1337 non-PPNG, non-TRNG isolates, the geometric mean MIC to penicillin was 0.19 µg/ml; to tetracycline, it was 0.66 µg/ml; to cefoxitin, 0.33 µg/ml; to spectinomycin, 16.5 µg/ml, and to ceftriaxone, 0.003 µg/ml. Thirteen percent of the isolates without plasmid-mediated resistance were chromosomally resistant to penicillin, and 48% of them were chromosomally resistant to tetracycline. No isolates were resistant to spectinomycin or ceftriaxone (*MMWR* 36:585, 1987).

Such conditions frequently occur in the intestinal tract of persons on antibiotic therapy and mild intestinal disturbances are sometimes considered a necessary tradeoff for the successful treatment of a more serious infection.

CONCEPT SUMMARY

1. The concept of selective inhibition is the principle underlying the application of chemotherapy to microbial infections. Careful study of microbial structure, physiology, and metabolism has led to the development of a wide variety of antimicrobial agents useful in combating the infectious diseases of both humans and animals.

2. Both bacteriostatic and bactericidal antimicrobial agents are available. Their action is aimed primarily at the inhibition of essential metabolic activity, interruption of cell wall synthesis, disruption of cell membrane integrity, or suppression of nucleic acid function. Use of these agents has provided a surprising advantage to humans in their quest for good health.

3. A wide variety of antibacterial agents are available for treatment of infectious diseases. However, because the metabolism of parasitic eucaryotes is very similar to human metabolism and viruses depend entirely on host cell metabolic functions, only a few antifungal, antiviral, and antiprotozoal drugs have been effective in clinical practice.

STUDY SUMMARY

1. What explanation can you give for the very large number of antibacterial compounds available for therapy as compared to the small number of antiviral agents?

2. Describe the concept of selective inhibition.

3. Indicate the mode of action for the following classes of antimicrobial components: (a) sulfonamides, (b) penicillins, (c) tetracyclines, (d) aminoglycosides, (e) quinolones, and (f) cephalosporins.

4. Distinguish among the following terms: antibiotic, chemotherapeutic, antimicrobial, bactericidal, and bacteriostatic.

5. Which antibiotic is frequently used as a substitute for penicillin in patients who are allergic to penicillin?

6. Explain why the penicillins are a favored antibiotic under most conditions where they are effective.

REFERENCES FOR FURTHER READING

1. *Chemotherapy of infection,* W. Pratt, 1977. Oxford.
2. *The Antimicrobial Agents Annual,* vol. 1, P. Peterson, 1986. Elsevier.
3. *The Biologic and Clinical Basis of Infectious Diseases,* G. Youmans, 1985. Saunders.
4. *Antimicrobial Therapy,* B. Kagan, 1980. Saunders.
5. Quinolones. *Reviews of Infectious Diseases* 10, Suppl. 1, 1988.
6. Antibiotic Use and Resistance. *Reviews of Infectious Diseases* 9, Suppl. 3, 1987.
7. Antiviral Chemotherapy. *Infectious Disease Clinics of North America* 1:2, 1987.
8. Studies on Antibiotics and Enzyme Inhibitors. *Reviews of Infectious Diseases* 9:147, 1987.

chapter 10

HOST-MICROORGANISM INTERACTIONS

Host

an individual that provides a home
and nutritional support for a
microorganism.

HOST-PARASITE RELATIONSHIPS

Interactions between human **hosts** and microorganisms are complex and are influenced by many factors. This textbook deals with human diseases and human interactions with microbes, but the principles apply in a large degree to all animals. In fact, much of what we know about human disease and interactions with microorganisms has evolved through research on lower animal species.

Over the years various terms have been used to describe and categorize microbes into different groups relative to their interaction with human or other hosts. Some of these terms need to be introduced at this time. The beginning student should bear in mind that it is difficult to categorize biological phenomena neatly without some overlapping, particularly when attempting to categorize the complex interactions between microbes and human hosts. The concern here is not with the many indirect beneficial or detrimental effects of microorganisms on humans in the general biological cycles in nature, such as nitrogen fixation or spoilage of food, but with those situations in which the microbes are present in or on the tissues of humans or are involved in human diseases.

The term *pathogen* refers to a microorganism that is able to produce disease; *pathogenic* is used as an adjective when referring to such microorganisms. *Nonpathogens* are microbes that are not able to cause disease. It will become apparent that the dividing line between pathogens and nonpathogens is not distinct, and a large gray area exists in which microbes may be either pathogenic or nonpathogenic depending on the interactions of many traits of both the microbe and the host. For a further understanding of the concept of a pathogen, it is necessary to introduce the term *virulence*, which means disease-producing powers or potency of a pathogen. When referring to the disease-producing capabilities of a microorganism, it is sometimes more convenient to refer to them as having high, moderate, low, or no virulence. The word *pathogenicity* is frequently used interchangeably with the term virulence. The term *pathogenesis* means the development of a disease and is used when referring to the mechanisms, sequence of changes, and processes that occur in the development of a disease.

The terms *infection* and *disease* are often used interchangeably; however, by technical definition an infection occurs when a microbe is able to overcome the defense barriers and live inside the host; tissue damage may or may not result. Disease refers to those conditions where the host's tissues are damaged or their function is altered by the microorganisms. When referring to infections, it is often convenient to use the term *clinical* or *apparent* infection when signs and symptoms of the disease are apparent and *subclinical* or *inapparent* infection when no apparent signs or symptoms are produced. The term *colonization* is used when referring to the ability of a microorganism to establish itself on a body surface (Figure 10-1).

Another term that helps describe interactions between a host and microorganisms is *parasitism*. A *parasite* is an organism that lives in or on the host and derives its sustenance from the host. If this parasitic relationship is beneficial to both the host and the parasite, the relationship is called *mutualism*. If the parasite causes no damage to the host, it is referred to as a *commensal*. Of course, a parasite that causes disease is a pathogen. It is possible for a

Figure 10-1   A strain of the bacterium *E. coli* specifically adhering to and colonizing the intestinal epithelium, at the tip of a villous in the ileum, of a pig. Scanning electron micrograph; bar equals 10 μm. (Courtesy B. Nagy, *Inf. Imm. 13:*1214–1220)

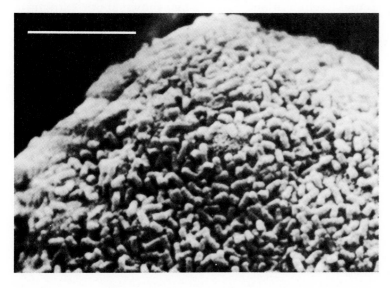

parasitic microbe to change from the commensal to the pathogenic relationship and vice versa. When the host's defense mechanisms are weakened, a commensal organism of moderate or low virulence that is normally unable to cause disease in a healthy person may then be able to multiply at a faster rate or gain access to deeper tissues and cause a clinical disease; under such conditions the microbe is referred to as an *opportunist*. Under other conditions, the balance between the host and a potentially virulent microbe may be such that the microbe is able to multiply and persist in the host as a commensal; yet when this microbe is transmitted to a new host a clinical disease may result. In such cases, the first host is called a *carrier*. Most microorganisms found in nature are not parasites and are able to use nonliving materials as nutrients; these microbes are called *saprophytes*. Most saprophytes are non-virulent; some, however, are able to cause diseases in humans.

The outcome of an infection is a result of the integrity of the host's defense mechanisms (discussed in subsequent chapters), the number of microorganisms, and the virulence of the invading microorganisms. The defense mechanisms may be stimulated to greatly increased effectiveness by immunization to a given pathogen. Perhaps of greater concern in clinical medicine today is the host (patient) whose natural defense mechanisms have been impaired or suppressed by other illnesses, genetic defects, stresses, or medical treatments; such a person is referred to as a *compromised host*. In most cases, for a microorganism to be a successful pathogen, it must possess those qualities that will allow it to enter the tissues, resist the host's defense mechanisms, multiply, and cause damage to or malfunction of tissues of the host.

The relationships between microorganisms and the host are presented in Figure 10-2. The varying levels of the host's defense mechanisms are shown at the left with the immunized host, resistant to highly virulent microorganisms, shown at one extreme and the compromised host, highly susceptible to low-virulence microorganisms, shown at the opposite extreme. The varying levels of microbial virulence are shown at the bottom of Figure 10-2. The high degree of resistance of the immunized host is normally specific only against the type of microorganism against which it was immunized. A normal, unimmunized host may have a variety of responses to microorganisms of high and moderate virulence, and a high degree of resistance toward infections by microbes of low virulence.

An additional dimension, along with the virulence of the microbe and levels of resistance of the host, is the number of microbes. This added dimension is shown in the following conceptual formula:

$$ID = \frac{N \times V}{HF}$$

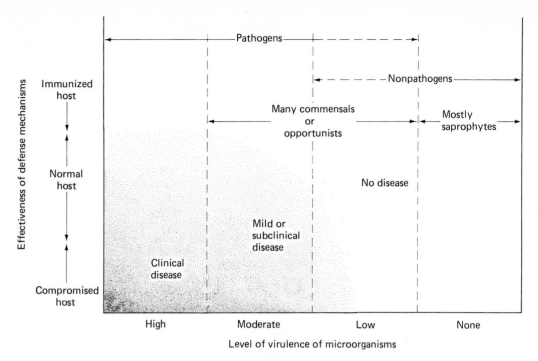

Figure 10-2   The interaction of microorganisms of varying levels of virulence with hosts of varying levels of resistance, and the resultant clinical outcome (the density of the dots represents the approximate severity of the disease).

where ID means infectious disease, V is the virulence of the microorganism, N is the number of microorganisms, and HF stands for host factors or the level of effectiveness of the host's defense mechanisms. Based on the interrelationships presented in this formula, the following examples could be postulated. Moderate to small numbers of low-virulence microorganisms would not produce disease in a normal host, but they may be able to produce disease in a host with impaired defense mechanisms; however, a large number of such organisms may be able to produce disease in a normal host. In the case of compromised patients, the "host factors" component of the formula is reduced, causing these individuals to become more susceptible to infections. The problem of the compromised patient is of increasing concern today. Many newer medical treatments and procedures, while providing significant improvements in many medical conditions, interfere with the normal defenses of the patient against microbial infections. An example is the treatment of a cancer patient with drugs that both slow down or stop the growth of the cancer cells and interfere with the ability of white blood cells to fight infections. Although the compromised patient may be given many meaningful years of added life by these new products, the patient's balance with microbes in his or her environment has been altered and this factor must be considered in the overall management of the case. Many infections encountered in medical practices today result from low-virulence microorganisms that are normally found on the tissues of the host (normal flora) but are able to cause infections due to the compromised conditions of a person's defense mechanisms.

NORMAL MICROBIAL FLORA OF HUMANS

The term *normal microbial flora* refers to those microorganisms that are the usual inhabitants of healthy individuals. Most would be considered harmless commensal microorganisms; yet some are potential pathogens—that is, opportunists—and do cause diseases when the balance between them and the host is altered. Under normal conditions, however, humans are able to live in healthy balance with the microorganisms that constitute their normal flora. In fact, some microbes that make up the normal flora may be beneficial to the host by interfering with the growth or attachment of pathogenic microbes.

The common types of microorganisms normally found on different parts of the body are mentioned in this section. The names of many microorganisms referred to here will be unfamiliar to most beginning students, but are being introduced at this time so that this section may serve as a reference source. Many microbes that are part of the normal flora but that are also able to cause specific disease **syndromes** will be discussed in greater detail in subsequent chapters.

Bacterial Sites

Skin The type and number of bacteria vary from one area of skin to another. The superficial layers of the skin (squamous epithelium) contain many dead cells that are colonized with a bacterium of low virulence called *Staphylococcus epidermidis*. This part of the skin may also contain small numbers of the more virulent *Staphylococcus aureus*. Low numbers of *Streptococcus* and some Gram-negative bacilli may also be present. Gram-positive bacilli, referred to as *diphtheroids,* are of very low virulence and are widespread as a normal inhabitant of the skin. An anaerobic bacterium called *Propionibacterium acnes* inhabits the **sebaceous glands** and is not destroyed by most methods used to disinfect the skin. This bacterium is a common contaminant in blood or other tissue samples collected by passing a needle through the skin. Fortunately, it is a very low grade pathogen, but it may work **synergistically** with other bacteria in the development of pimples.

Syndrome
a number of symptoms occurring together that characterize a specific disease.

Sebaceous glands
small glands located in the skin that secrete oils to the surface of the skin.

Synergistic
capable of working together. Two organisms are synergistic when they are able to produce a host response greater than the sum of the effects they produce when acting alone. Often used in connection with antimicrobial therapy.

Respiratory tract   The nares may contain large numbers of such bacteria as *Staphylococcus epidermidis*, *Staphylococcus aureus*, and diphtheroids. A Gram-negative coccus called *Branhamella catarrhalis* and an opportunistic pathogen called *Haemophilus influenzae* are periodically present. Large numbers of diphtheroids and *Branhamella catarrhalis* also inhabit the pharynx. The pathogenic bacteria *Streptococcus pyogenes*, viridans streptococci, *Streptococcus pneumoniae*, *Neisseria meningitidis*, and *Haemophilis influenzae* may periodically be carried in the pharynx. As a result of effective defense mechanisms that rapidly remove contaminating microorganisms (see Chapter 11), the trachea, bronchi, bronchioles, and alveoli are usually free of microorganisms in healthy persons.

Mouth   The mouth contains large numbers of diverse types of bacteria, and marked variations, kinds, and numbers are associated with the presence or absence of teeth or tooth decay. Some bacteria are of low virulence but may cause troublesome infections if introduced into deeper tissues—for example, from a bite. Other bacteria are able to cause tooth decay, and many are nonvirulent. Several types of microorganisms commonly found in the mouth are listed in Table 10-1. When clinical specimens are being collected from the throat or lower respiratory tract, care should be taken to minimize contamination of the swab or aspirate with oral secretions, for the large number of bacteria in the mouth will often obscure the pathogen being sought.

Stomach   The high acid content of the human stomach keeps the number of viable microorganisms in this organ low. Certain microbes, however, are able to survive passage through the stomach.

Intestines   The microbial content of the small intestines changes drastically from relatively few bacteria in the upper portion to massive numbers in the lower section. The contents of the colon provide an ideal environment for the growth of many species of microorganisms. It has been estimated that over 100 different species of bacteria may be common inhabitants of the colon. Their

Table 10-1   Genera of Bacteria Most Commonly Found in the Human Oral Cavity

Anaerobic	Facultative Anaerobic
Actinomyces	*Haemophilus*
Bacteroides	*Lactobacillus*
Peptostreptococcus	*Neisseria*
Veillonella	*Staphylococcus*
	Streptococcus

concentration may reach 10^{11} cells per gram of fecal material, which represents about a third of its total weight. Intestinal flora become established early in life and generally humans live in healthy balance with these microorganisms. Such microorganisms may offer several benefits to humans by producing certain vitamins, by aiding in food digestion, and by stimulation of the immune responses of the host. These masses of common bacteria may also help suppress the growth or block the attachment of pathogens that might enter the intestinal tract.

The common bacteria of the colon can be categorized as either *facultative* or *obligate* anaerobes. The facultative anaerobes include the Gram-negative bacilli commonly called the *enteric bacilli*, which include such genera as *Escherichia, Klebsiella, Enterobacter,* and *Proteus.* Also present are staphylococci and streptococci. The yeast, *Candida albicans*, is frequently present. For many years it was assumed that the facultative anaerobes were the major inhabitants of the colon. However, the use of improved anaerobic culture methods has shown that over 99% of the colon bacteria are obligate anaerobes. They include various species of the genera *Bacteroides, Fusobacterium, Clostridium, Peptostreptococcus,* and *Eubacterium.*

Genitourinary tract   Some bacteria are found in the lower portion of both the male and female urethra. Normal bladders, ureters, and kidneys are free of microorganisms. The female genital tract has a complex and varying microbial flora. With menarche the vaginal and cervical tissues become populated with lactobacilli that produce lactic acid and maintain the pH of these tissues at 4.4 to 4.6. This acid environment inhibits the growth of the Gram-negative enteric bacteria but allows growth of such microorganisms as bacteroides, diphtheroids, staphylococci, enterococci, and *Candida albicans*. The microflora of the vaginal canal undergo some cyclic fluctuations with hormonal variation.

TRANSMISSION OF MICROORGANISMS

Contagious disease results from the ability of a pathogenic microorganism to multiply in a host, to exit from that host, be transmitted to one or more secondary hosts, and enter and cause disease in the secondary hosts. The term *communicable* is also used in describing such diseases. It should be noted however, that not all infectious diseases (caused by a living organism) are communicable. There are many (e.g., tetanus) that cannot be transmitted directly to a second host.

Exit of Microorganisms from the Host

Microorganisms found in the mouth and respiratory tract are expelled to some extent during normal speech and breathing. Singing and shouting expel larger numbers and coughing and sneezing expel massive numbers. Many microorganisms are dispersed on small airborne bits of mucus and saliva known as **aerosols**. The moisture evaporates within a very brief period and the remaining particle is called a *droplet nucleus*. These microbe-laden particles may remain suspended in air currents to be carried to new hosts. In addition to being aerosolized, saliva may serve as a **vehicle** for microbial transmissions by kissing or expectoration. Bacteria attached to the skin scales are continually being shed from the body. Massive numbers of microorganisms are present in feces and are readily spread to new hosts living under conditions of poor sanitation. Urine and other secretions of the urinogenital tract may contain some microorganisms, but host-to-host transmission from these tissues usually results only from direct contact. Blood from a healthy person is free of microorganisms; however, blood from persons with certain diseases contains pathogenic microorganisms that may be taken up and transmitted by bloodsucking **arthropods** or by blood transfusions. Milk may act as a vehicle for the microorganisms shed from a lactating female with infection of the mammary gland. The routes of exit of microorganisms from the body are shown in Figure 10-3.

Aerosol

an airborne suspension of particles. A microbial aerosol may pose a serious health hazard.

Vehicle

any object or substance that can carry microorganisms from one host to another.

Arthropods

a large group of invertebrate animals, many of which have biting or sucking mouthparts such as the mosquito and other insects.

Figure 10-3   Possible routes of exit of microorganisms from the body.

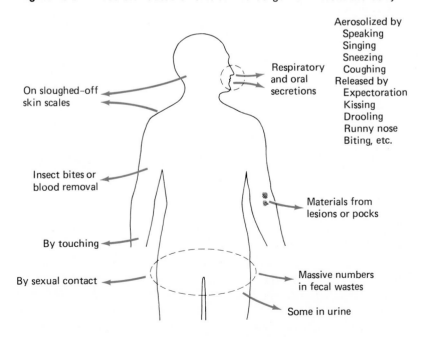

Routes of Transmission and Entry of Microorganisms into the Host

Most microorganisms (normal flora) shed from a healthy person will be the same as those found in persons about them; thus the exchange of these microorganisms is of little consequence. If a person is a carrier of a pathogen or has an active infection, however, the spread of that persons's microorganisms may cause infection in a new host. Some pathogens are transmitted to humans from animals or birds and, in the case of some fungal infections, the infectious spores are carried from the soil to humans by airborne route. Various modes of transmission are shown in Figure 10-4 and possible routes of microorganism entry into the body are shown in Figure 10-5.

Airborne transmission   A majority of the infectious diseases of humans are of the respiratory tract and most of them are transmitted through the air. Microorganisms are vigorously aerosolized due to the increased coughing, sneezing, and secretion of mucus

Figure 10-4   Possible routes of transmission of microorganisms to humans.

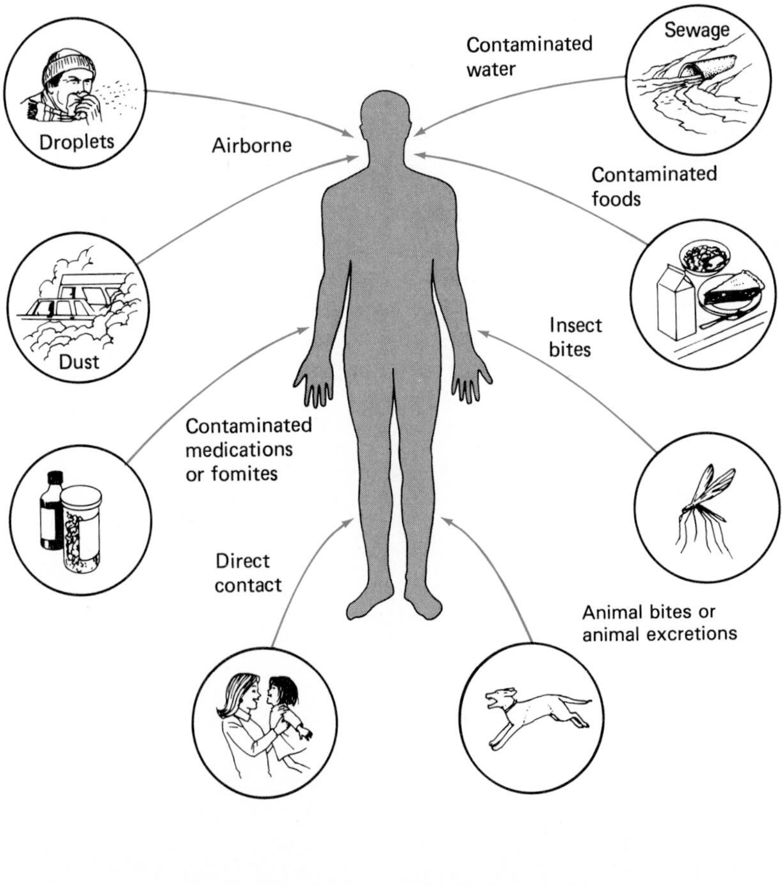

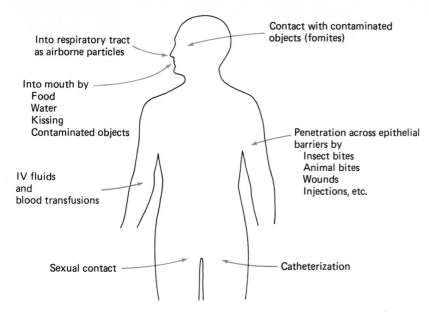

Figure 10-5   Possible routes of entry of microorganisms into the body.

associated with a respiratory infection. Many aerosolized microbes become associated with droplet nuclei whereas others are deposited on such surfaces as floors, clothing, and bedding. The microorganisms present on various objects may become aerosolized on dust particles due to physical movement or air currents and may be inhaled by persons in the area. This form of transmission is most efficient in enclosed, crowded buildings and is an important source of infections in hospitals. Airborne bacteria may also cause infections by settling onto open wounds during surgery or when bandages are changed.

Mouth   Many microorganisms enter the body by the ingestion of contaminated foods or water, by kissing, or by placing contaminated objects in the mouth.

Bites   A significant number of infectious agents are transmitted from host to host by biting insects. Some insects transmit the pathogen mechanically by first feeding on an infected host and then feeding on a new host with its contaminated mouth parts. However, in most instances, after the insect has ingested contaminated fluids from an infected host, the pathogen proliferates in the insect. When such an insect bites a new host, large numbers of the pathogen may be inoculated into the body tissue or defecated onto the skin. This material is then rubbed into the skin when a person scratches the irritation caused by the insect bite.

Some infections, such as rabies, are transmitted by the bites

Acanthamoeba Keratitis in Soft-Contact-Lens Wearers: United States, 1985–86

Within a 9-month period from mid-1985 to February 1986, CDC received reports of 24 cases of *Acanthamoeba* keratitis, a much higher number than previously reported during similar time periods. Twenty (83%) of the patients wore contact lenses. Of these, 2 wore hard lenses (1 hard, the other rigid gas-permeable); 4 wore extended-wear lenses; and 14 wore daily-wear soft lenses. Between July and October 1986, CDC performed a case-control study of soft-contact-lens wearers to identify the risk factors associated with *Acanthamoeba* keratitis.

Patients were selected for the study from persons with *Acanthamoeba* keratitis reported to CDC before August 1986 and who wore soft contact lenses, had onset of keratitis symptoms after June 1985, and had species of *Acanthamoeba* isolated from corneal smears or biopsy and/or demonstrated in stained corneal scrapings or tissue. Controls were selected from the files of the ophthalmologist or optometrist originally prescribing contact lenses for the patient and were matched with the patient by general contact-lens type (daily-wear soft contact lenses [DWSL] or extended-wear soft contact lenses [EWSL]), age (+5 years), and city of residence.

CDC personnel used a standardized telephone questionnaire to obtain information from patients and controls on the specific brands of contact lenses and associated solutions they used, their routine lens-cleaning procedures, and their behavioral activities. To study the prevalence of *Acanthamoeba* and other microbial contaminants, investigators asked controls to submit contact-lens solutions and lens-care hardware to CDC to be examined for contamination with *Acanthamoeba*, bacteria, and fungi. Similar materials were not available from patients because they had not been wearing their lenses for as long as 12 months.

Twenty-seven patients with *Acanthamoeba* keratitis and 81 uninfected, matched controls were interviewed. The 27 patients resided in 12 states. All of the patients had onsets of symptoms between June 1985 and June 1986, with no seasonal predilection. Twenty patients (74%) and 59 controls (73%) wore DWSL. The remainder in both groups wore EWSL. There was a significantly higher proportion of males among patients than among controls (14/27 [52%] compared with 14/81 [17%], odds ratio [OR] = 7.29, 95% confidence interval [CI] = 2.53–20.76).

of mammals. Because of the large and varied numbers of microorganisms in mouths, troublesome infection may result from bites, particularly human bites.

Contact Although some preceding modes of transmission are by contact, it is desirable to expand this concept further because of its significance in routine medical care. *Direct contact* entails the touching of infected tissues with uninfected tissues. Some pathogens require intimate contact for their successful transmission and are most effectively passed from person to person by sexual

Patients were significantly more likely than controls not to disinfect their lenses as frequently as recommended by lens manufacturers (18/25 [72%] compared with 26/81 [32%], OR = 5.83, CI = 2.22–15.32). Significantly more patients than controls used homemade saline solutions instead of commercially prepared saline solutions (21/27 [78%] compared with 14/81 [17%], OR = ∞, CI = ∞–∞. Because most persons using homemade solutions used them for several purposes, no distinction could be made as to whether a particular usage was more likely to be associated with infection than other usages. No association was noted between any of the commercially prepared contact-lens solutions or contact lenses and infection.

Patients were significantly more likely than controls to wear their lenses while swimming (17/27 [63%] compared with 24/81 [30%], OR = 6.24, CI = 1.90–20.46). This association remained statistically significant after controlling for sex. Patients were not more likely than controls to place their lenses in their mouths, wear their lenses in a hot tub, or report an injury to the eye.

Seventy-two (89%) controls submitted at least one specimen for microbiologic study. All solutions and hardware had been previously opened and used by the participant. All of the 11 homemade saline specimens submitted were colonized with bacteria and fungi. Eight (73%) showed relatively high levels of contamination ($\geq 10^5$ colony-forming units [CFU] of bacteria and fungi per milliliter). Acanthamoebae were isolated from two of these: *A. hatchetti*, from one, and *A. polyphaga*, from another. In contrast, only one (2%) of the 59 commercially prepared saline specimens was contaminated with bacteria or fungi, and none were contaminated with *Acanthamoeba*. Fluid samples from 56 (69%) of the 81 specimens of lens-care hardware had positive bacterial/fungal assays; 46 (57%) had titers between 10^5 and 10^8 CFU/ml. Acanthamoebae were isolated from three specimens. No disinfectants, daily cleaners, or eye drops/lubricants were contaminated with bacteria, fungi, or *Acanthamoeba* (*MMWR* 36:397, 1987).

intercourse or kissing. A person with an infected skin lesion may readily transmit the infection by direct contact. This mode of transmission is of special concern to medical personnel, for they may inadvertently transmit such an infection to patients; conversely a patient may transmit an infection to attending personnel. *Indirect contact* requires intermediate objects, called *fomites*, to transmit the pathogen. The fomites become contaminated by coming in contact with pathogens from an infected patient. Then, at some later time, the pathogen may be transferred to a second person who comes in contact with the contaminated fomite. In medical practice such items as hands, clothing, instruments, toys, and books may serve as fomites in transferring infections between patients. Disposable items, proper handwashing, gloving and gowning, and similar procedures to prevent transmission of infections in hospitals or clinics should receive continual emphasis. Water and food are the most commonly involved fomites in our everyday environment.

Endogenous spread   The preceding examples describe the *exogenous* spread of microbes—that is, microbes coming from a source outside the host. It is also possible for microbes to spread from one part of a host to another, a process called *endogenous* spread. Many opportunistic pathogens found in the upper respiratory tract, mouth, or intestinal tract may be spread to open lesions or other tissues and cause serious infections. Some common examples are the spreading of intestinal bacteria into the urethra to cause a urinary tract infection, the "leakage" of intestinal bacteria across the intestinal mucosa into the blood and lymphatic systems, and the spread of oral microbes to eyes by moistening contact lenses with saliva or to wounds by licking. Possible routes of endogenous spread of microorganisms are shown in Figure 10-6.

Figure 10-6   Possible routes of endogenous spread of microorganisms.

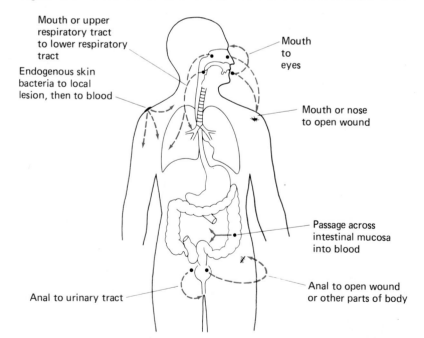

CONCEPT SUMMARY

1. The interaction between a host such as a human and the microbial world can best be viewed as a seesaw where the fulcrum is moved in favor of one or the other as the balance of normality is altered. Thus classic nonpathogens can become pathogens to a host suffering from environmental pressures whereas a virulent microorganism may at best coexist with a host that is well adapted to its environment.

2. All life forms, humans included, are endowed with a contingent of microorganisms collectively referred to as *normal flora*. These organisms, although capable of producing disease, frequently provide a beneficial component to life and participate in maintaining a normal environment for their hosts.

3. Microorganisms are transferred from one host to another through a variety of mechanisms, including food and water, human or animal bites, contact, and aerosols.

STUDY SUMMARY

1. Distinguish between the following terms: (a) pathogen and nonpathogen, (b) virulent and avirulent, (c) infection and disease, (d) parasite and saprophyte, and (e) carrier and case.

2. What roles (positive or negative) are played by normal microbial flora?

3. Why are the human mucosal surfaces inhabited by such large numbers of ''normal flora''?

4. The use of public health and personal sanitation methods has had its greatest effect on reduction of infectious agents that are transmitted by what means?

5. Because of proximity requirements for transmission, agents of disease that are transmitted by direct contact are somewhat unique. Control of these infections seems to depend less on public health procedures and more on _____?

REFERENCES FOR FURTHER STUDY

1. *The Biologic and Clinical Basis of Infectious Diseases,* G. Youmans, 1985. Saunders.

2. *Microbes, Man and Animals,* A. Linton, 1982. Wiley.

3. *Medical Microbiology,* J. Sherris, 1984. Elsevier.

4. *Review of Medical Microbiology,* 17th ed., E. Jawitz, 1987. Appleton & Lange.

5. Mechanisms of Bacterial Virulence. *Annual Review of Microbiology* 39:21, 1985.

chapter 11

NONSPECIFIC HOST DEFENSE MECHANISMS

Humans are endowed with a wide variety of mechanisms that help protect them from the many microorganisms encountered during their lives. These mechanisms include the external tissues that act as a first line of defense to help prevent microorganisms from penetrating into the deeper body tissues. If microbes do penetrate the external barriers, however, they encounter a second line of defense that includes internal mechanisms like phagocytosis, antimicrobial fluids, and inflammation. These mechanisms, referred to as *nonspecific defense mechanisms*, are an innate part of the body and will function immediately against any microorganism or particulate material that might land on or enter the body tissues. Nonspecific defense mechanisms are the subject of this chapter.

Antibodies are important additional defense mechanisms, sometimes called the third line of defense, that are acquired only after the first exposure of the host to an invading microorganism or its virulence factors. Antibodies are specific because they will only react against the type of microorganisms that originally stimulated their formation. The protection afforded by antibodies is called *acquired immunity* and will be discussed in the following two chapters.

The term *immunity* generally refers to resistance to a disease as a result of acquiring antibodies. In the broader usage, however, the term may encompass all forms of resistance to diseases. *Nonspecific immunity,* for example, is often used to refer to the resistance resulting from mechanisms other than antibodies, and **innate immunity,** also called racial, *natural,* or *inherent immunity,* refers to resistance to a given disease as a result of genetic traits of the host.

Innate immunity
inborn or natural immunity; mechanisms of resistance to infection that are not acquired after birth.

NONSPECIFIC EXTERNAL DEFENSE MECHANISMS

The external defense mechanism consists of those components of the body that prevent microorganisms from attaching to body tissues or penetrating into the deeper, more susceptible tissues. The actions of various host defense mechanisms are listed in Table 11-1.

Bacterial Interference

Often the attachment site for a given pathogen is very specific and if the attachment site on a tissue is already occupied by one bacterium, it cannot be readily occupied by a second bacteriuim. In this regard, we are becoming increasingly aware that many bacteria that make up the normal flora of the host occupy many of these tissue receptor sites. They thus interfere with the attachment of many potentially harmful pathogens and perform a valuable service in helping to protect the host. Also, the normal microbial flora may compete with the invading pathogen for available nutrients and hence suppress their growth. In addition, some bacterial species of the normal flora secrete proteins called *bacteriocins* that specifically inhibit the growth of some invading pathogenic bacteria.

Physical Barriers and Chemical Agents

The resident and transient microbial flora of the tissues and organs described are generally incapable of producing disease if the physical integrity of the tissue barriers remains intact. The intact epithelial membranes, both epidermis and mucous membranes, are the most important defense mechanisms that humans possess against microbial invasion. The parts of the body exposed to the

Table 11-1   Host Natural Defense Mechanisms

Defense System	Action
Epithelial surface	Physical barrier prevents pathogen entry
Mucosal surfaces	Traps bacteria
Lysozyme	Dissolves peptidoglycan
Phagocytic cells	Ingests and destroys pathogens
Ciliated cells	Moves pathogens away from body
Fatty acids	Prevents bacterial growth
Stomach acid	Destruction of ingested pathogens
Normal bacterial flora	Competes with pathogens
Urine excretion	Removes pathogens from body
Complement system	Mediates phagocyte function

external environment are endowed with a variety of mechanisms to prevent microorganisms from penetrating to the more susceptible internal tissues. The more important mechanisms are described next.

Skin Intact skin provides a barrier that cannot be penetrated by most microorganisms. Most pathogenic bacteria are unable to survive on clean healthy skin for any length of time, partly because of the acid pH of the skin, which is inhibitory to most pathogenic bacteria, and partly because of bactericidal acids secreted in the sebaceous glands in the skin. An exception is the bacterium *Staphylococcus aureus,* which is able to persist on the skin and is a frequent source of infection when the integrity of the skin is altered.

Mucous membranes Body cavities such as the vagina, bowel, and respiratory tract are lined with mucosal membranes that consist of one or more layers of living cells. The cells are bathed in **mucus,** a viscid film that helps remove microbes. These surfaces, however, while offering a valuable protective barrier against most microorganisms, are more easily penetrated by some microorganisms than is the intact outer epidermis.

Mucus
a thick secretion produced by mucous cells that covers mucosal membranes. Mucus contains a polysaccharide called *mucin* along with a variety of cells and salts.

Eyes Along with the barrier effect of the intact tissues, the secretion of tears and the movement of eyelids provide a continuous flushing action that disposes of contaminant microorganisms. Tears also contain an enzyme called *lysozyme* that destroys certain Gram-positive bacteria.

Outer ear canal The surface of the outer ear canal is lubricated with a waxy deposit that contains effective antibacterial components.

Alimentary canal The physical integrity of the mucosal **epithelium** is extremely important in preventing the spread into the blood or deeper tissues of the massive numbers of bacteria found in the mouth and lower intestinal tract. Along with this barrier effect, the flow of saliva and the act of swallowing continually dilute bacteria in the mouth. Stomach acid destroys large numbers of microorganisms that are swallowed. Secretion of mucus along the intestinal tract aids in trapping and removing microorganisms. The mucous secretion contains some antibacterial substance and antibodies to help further reduce the numbers of microorganisms.

Epithelium
the nonvascular (having no blood vessels) cellular layer covering internal and external body surfaces.

Genitourinary tract The intact epithelium presents a physical barrier and the flushing action of urine keeps most microorganisms restricted to the lower portion of the urethra. The protective role of the acid pH of the female genital tissues was discussed in Chapter 10.

Respiratory tract   The respiratory tract is endowed with a unique series of defense mechanisms against the continuous onslaught it experiences from a wide variety of airborne microorganisms. The positions of various defense mechanisms are shown in Figure 11-1. Nasal hairs are of some value by inducing turbulence of the inhaled air and by acting as very crude filters. The *nasal turbinates* provide a large exposure surface and cause increased impaction of the larger airborne particles against the surface of the turbinates.

Much of the surface of the nasal cavity is lined with *ciliated eipthelium.* Ciliated epithelium contains large numbers of ciliated cells. Each ciliated cell contains several hundred cilia (hairlike structures) that are rapidly and continuously beating. Inter-

Figure 11-1   Defense mechanisms of the respiratory tract.

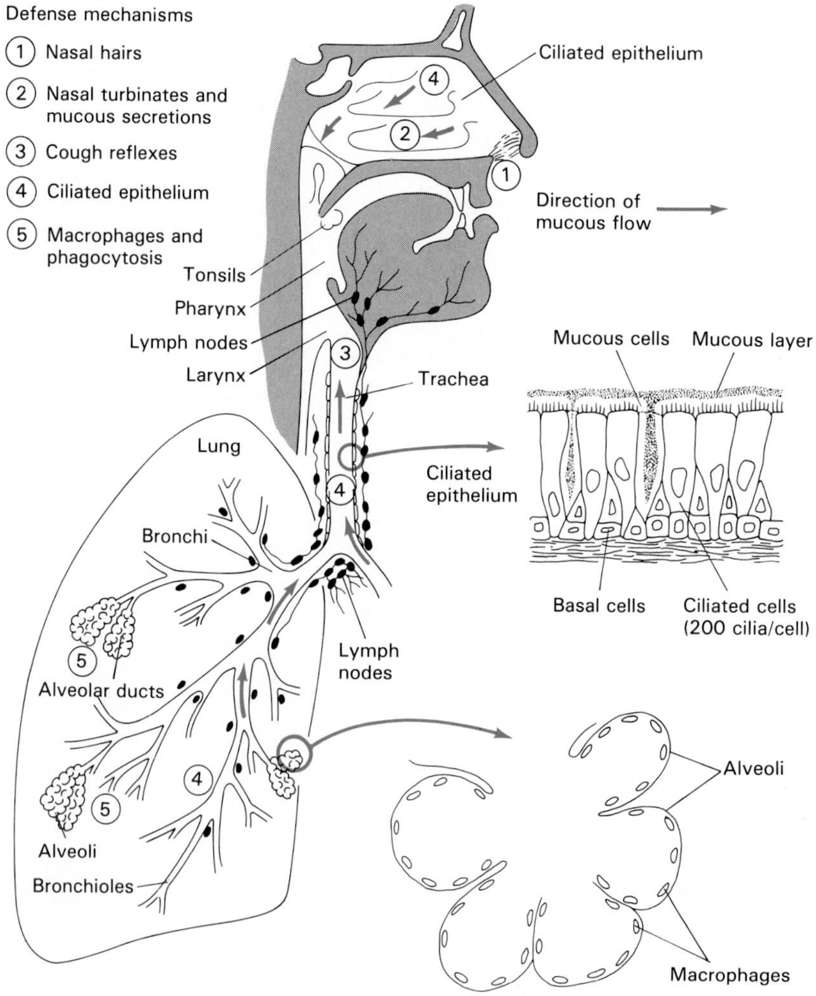

spersed between every four to five ciliated cills is a mucus-secreting cell. A film of mucus forms on top of the ciliated epithelium and serves as a sticky surface to trap the airborne particles impacted onto it. Mucus also contains antimicrobial substances. The rhythmic movement of the cilia moves this mucous film, with the entrapped particles, into the pharyngeal area where the mucus can be disposed of, usually by swallowing. A significant portion of the larger airborne particles is removed by these mechanisms of the upper respiratory tract.

The smaller airborne particles are carried into the trachea, bronchi, and bronchioles where many are impacted onto the ciliated epithelium that completely lines these passages. The direction of mucous flow is from the lungs to the opening of the trachea. As mucus accumulates at the top of the trachea, it is removed by ''clearing the throat'' and disposed of by swallowing. When mucus begins to accumulate or particles become trapped along this ciliated epithelium, the cough reflex is triggered and coughing aids in dislodging and removing these materials from air passageways. Only the smallest microbe-containing airborne particles (those between 5 and 10 µm) are able to penetrate into the air sacs (alveoli) of the lungs. Large numbers of phagocytic white blood cells, called *alveolar macrophages,* are located in the air sacs and are able to ingest and destroy most microorganisms deposited in healthy lungs. Overall the mechanisms of the respiratory tract, when functioning properly, effectively protect the host against many potential airborne pathogens.

NONSPECIFIC INTERNAL DEFENSE MECHANISMS

After a pathogenic microbe has become attached to the tissues of the host, it may be able to pass into the cell because of its own invasive mechanisms or it may be introduced into the deeper, more susceptible tissues through sections of epithelium that have been injured. Once beyond the protective outer barrier of the body, the invading microorganisms encounter a series of internal host defense mechanisms. Because these mechanisms are closely associated with the activities of the *white blood cells* (WBCs), also referred to as *leukocytes,* the structure and function of these cells, as well as other components of the blood, are discussed next.

White Blood Cells

White blood cells can be divided into three categories: *granulocytes, monocytes,* and *lymphocytes.* Specialized types of cells are found within each category. The WBCs are involved in such host

Phagocytosis
a process by which cells ingest particulate matter (such as microbes) from their environment. When this process is carried out by specific host cells it provides a valuable defense against infection.

defense activities as **phagocytosis** (the ingesting of foreign particles), inflammation, and antibody formation. Often different types of WBCs will function in a cooperative effort to produce the final result. These interactions are discussed in the following sections. The development of the different types of WBCs is outlined in Figure 11-2.

Granulocytes Granulocytes get their name from the large number of granules present in their cytoplasm. These granules may contain chemicals that act as stimulators of certain body responses or they may contain enzymes that aid in the digestion of microorganisms and other materials. The granulocytes have lobular nuclei and are 9 to 12 μm in diameter. Because of the extreme variable nature of their nuclei, they are also called *polymorphonuclear leukocytes* or simply PMNs. These cells are formed and mature in the bone marrow and are continually being released into the blood. They circulate for several hours and then pass into the tissue

Figure 11-2   Development of the different types of white blood cells.

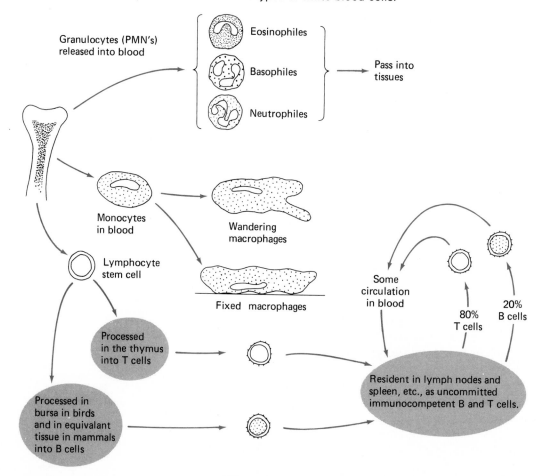

Granulocytes (PMN's) released into blood

Eosinophiles

Basophiles

Neutrophiles

Pass into tissues

Monocytes in blood

Wandering macrophages

Lymphocyte stem cell

Fixed macrophages

Some circulation in blood

80% T cells

20% B cells

Processed in the thymus into T cells

Processed in bursa in birds and in equivalant tissue in mammals into B cells

Resident in lymph nodes and spleen, etc., as uncommitted immunocompetent B and T cells.

spaces, where they remain for a few days and then die. These cells do not divide after leaving the bone marrow and the body is required to produce about 10^{11} new cells per day. Many granulocytes are held in reserve in the spleen and bone marrow; when an inflammation occurs, large numbers are released into the blood and the rate of production of new cells is accelerated. Normal blood contains from 5000 to 9000 WBCs per cubic millimeter and 70% to 75% of them are granulocytes. When inflammation occurs in the body, the increased output of granulocytes may increase the total number of WBCs well above the normal level. This increased WBC count is one of the valuable signs used to diagnose the presence of inflammation in a patient. The different types of granulocytes are *eosinophils, basophils,* and *neutrophils,* names derived from their staining characteristics. The full range of functions of the eosinophils is not understood. They seem to be involved with some allergic responses and parasitic infections. They constitute only 2% to 4% of the total WBCs found in the blood. The basophils make up less than 1% of the WBCs. They contain granules of histamine and may be involved in controlling the movement of body fluids involved in the inflammatory response. Neutrophils are the most numerous WBCs, constituting 65% to 70% of the total, and are active phagocytes. Large numbers are involved in the early phases of the inflammatory response.

Monocytes   The monocytes are those cells that possess a large smooth nucleus and a large area of cytoplasm. These cells are formed in the bone marrow. When they are released into the blood, they are from 14 to 20 μm in diameter. Circulating monocytes make up 1% to 6% of the total WBCs. Monocytes collect in or pass into many different body tissues and become known as *macrophages.* Whether all different types of macrophages come from the same type of monocyte is not known. In the transformation from monocyte to macrophage the cell increases in size to 25–50 μm. Some macrophages are motile and are called *wandering macrophages.* These wandering cells move by ameboid action and are found throughout all tissues and cavities of the body. Other macrophages become attached to the walls of blood capillaries and sinusoids and are known as *fixed macrophages.* All macrophages are active phagocytic cells. They live for months after leaving the bone marrow. Under an appropriate stimulus macrophages may divide or become ''activated'' in that their phagocytic and antimicrobial capabilities are considerably increased.

Lymphocytes   Lymphocytes make up 20% to 25% of the WBCs. Some are small, about 6 μm in diameter; others are about 12 μm in diameter. They are round with a large, smooth nucleus and a small amount of cytoplasm. Lymphocytes develop from *stem cells* that are originally produced in the bone marrow. These cells are

Thymus
an endocrine gland located behind the breastbone near the throat. It is large in childhood and decreases in size in adults.

released from the bone marrow and develop into two different types of lymphocytes, *B cells* and *T cells.* The stem cells that become T cells first pass to the **thymus,** where they are influenced by thymic hormones to become T cells. Many T cells circulate throughout the body and constitute about 60% to 80% of the lymphocytes found in the blood. Moreover, many are found in the lymph nodes and spleen. The organ or hormone that influences the stem cells to change into B cells has not yet been identified in humans but is currently thought to reside in the bone marrow. The influencing organ in birds is the *bursa of Fabricius.* A majority of the B cells are found in lymph nodes and the spleen. The T cells and B cells are involved in the production of cell-mediated immunity and the production of antibodies (Chapter 12).

Other Blood Components

Red blood cells (RBCs), which constitute 45% of the blood volume, will not be discussed, for they have no apparent direct role in fighting invading microorganisms.

A brief introduction into the fluid components of blood will be useful in understanding concepts presented later. When blood is collected and substances are added to prevent clotting, the blood cells can be separated from the fluid by settling out. The remaining fluid is called the *blood plasma.* If blood is allowed to clot, a clear yellowish fluid called *serum* remains. The major difference between plasma and serum is that plasma still contains fibrinogen and other essential components for blood clotting. Both fluids are rich in other proteins. The serum proteins can be separated into two major types called *albumin* and **globulin.** The globulin proteins can be further separated into three types called *alpha, beta,* and *gamma.* Most antibodies that form against microorganisms are found in the gamma globulin fraction of the blood serum and are called *immunoglobulins.* Figure 11-3 shows the formation of blood plasma and serum as well as the separation of serum into its different classes of proteins based on their rate of migration through an electrical field (electrophoresis).

Globulins
a group of proteins found in human serum. The gamma globulins are antibody proteins and are produced by B lymphocytes.

Phagocytosis

Neutrophils and macrophages are the major cells involved in the phagocytosis and destruction of microorganisms (Figure 11-4). Phagocytosis is perhaps the most important defense mechanism of the host once the pathogen has penetrated beyond the epithelial and mucosal barriers. The first step in phagocytosis requires the attachment of the foreign particle to the cell membrane. Some bacteria readily attach to phagocytes and so are readily phagocytized whereas others will not attach and are thus difficult to phago-

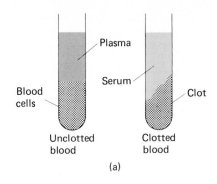

(a)

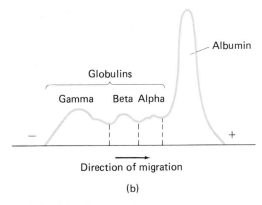

(b)

Figure 11-3   (a) The source of blood plasma and blood serum. (b) The separation of blood serum into major types of proteins based on the rate of migration through an electrical field.

Figure 11-4   Scanning electron micrograph showing a branch-shaped bacterium (*Nocardia asteroides*) being phagocytized by a macrophage. Arrow points to the area where the bacterium is being enfulged. (Courtesy B. L. Beaman, *Inf. Imm. 15:*925–937)

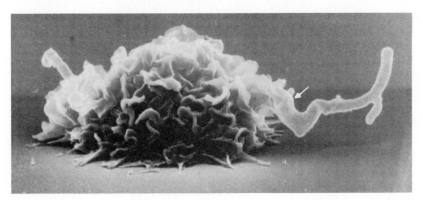

cytize. Phagocytosis is facilitated if the phagocyte is able to trap the bacterium against a rough surface; in this case, phagocytosis can occur without attachment. Attachment and phagocytosis are much more effective if the microorganisms are coated with specific antibodies.

Once attachment of the microbe has occurred, the cell membrane extends around the particle and fuses to form an intracellular membrane-bound vacule containing the microbe. This vacule is called a *phagosome.* The phagosome next fuses with the lysosomes, thereby causing the release of digestive enzymes into the phagosome. This combined structure is called a *phagolysosome.* These enzymes, along with the hydrogen peroxide that is also produced by the phagocytic cell, readily destroy most microorganisms or break down other particles of organic material. The phagocytosis and intracellular digestion of a bacterium are shown in Figure 11-5.

Lymphatic System

The lymphatic system consists of a complex network of thin-walled ducts (lymphatic vessels), strategically located filtering bodies called *lymph nodes,* and concentrations of large numbers of lymphocytic cells in various organs or tissues. The lymphatic ves-

Figure 11-5   Mechanisms of phagocytosis and destruction of bacteria of a macrophage.

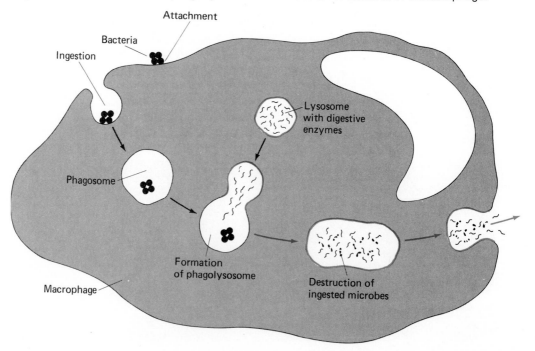

sels are widespread and generally parallel to the blood vessels. They are particularly plentiful in the skin and along the respiratory and intestinal tracts. A major function of the lymphatic vessels is to serve as return ducts for the fluid that is continually diffusing out of the blood capillaries into the body tissues. Before the lymph fluid is returned to the blood, it must first pass through several lymph nodes. The major concentrations of lymph nodes that filter fluid coming from the lymphatic vessels of the skin are located in the neck, inguinal, and axillary regions (Figure 11-6). Deeper lymph nodes are located along the respiratory and intestinal tracts—that is, in areas where microorganisms are most likely to invade the deeper body tissues. The lymph fluid flowing out of the lymph nodes flows into large collecting ducts that eventually drain into the thoracic duct, which, in turn, empties into the bloodstream. The lymph nodes contain a series of narrow passageways, called **sinusoids,** that are lined with macrophages. The phagocytic activity of these macrophages removes extraneous par-

Sinusoid

a small open cavity through which body fluids travel. Sinusoids greatly increase the space available for fluid, causing the fluid to go slowly through these areas.

Figure 11-6   (a) The superficial lymphatic ducts and nodes. (b) Cross section of a lymph node. The fluid filters through the sinuses of the node where large numbers of macrophages are located. The germinal centers contain the antibody-producing cells.

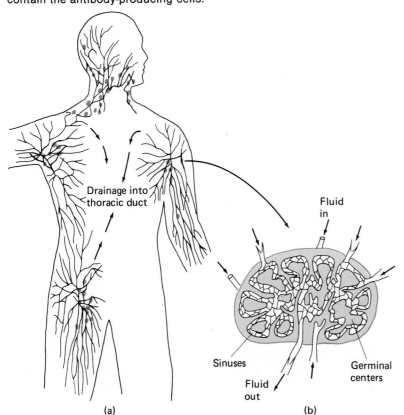

Drainage into thoracic duct

Fluid in

Sinuses

Fluid out

Germinal centers

(a)

(b)

ticulate matter, including most microbes, that may be carried in the lymphatic fluid. Under normal conditions the lymph nodes successfully prevent invading microorganisms from reaching the bloodstream. When large numbers of bacteria become trapped or multiply in the lymph nodes, inflammation may occur with accompanying swelling and tenderness. The presence of swollen lymph nodes is a useful clinical sign for the diagnosis of an infection in the tissues being drained into that node. Lymph nodes also serve as a storage organ for the lymphocytes and are initiating sites for antibody responses.

Reticuloendothelial System (RES)

Reticuloendothelial system is a composite name given to those tissues and organs that contain the mononuclear phagocytic cells; this system has also been referred to as the *mononuclear phagocyte system*. Many macrophages are found in the loose connective tissue fibers called *reticulum* and are fixed to the endothelial cells that line the sinusoids of such organs as the lymph nodes, liver, spleen, and bone marrow. Both fixed and wandering macrophages, as well as circulating monocytes, are part of the RES. Most microorganisms that find their way into the lymphatic system or into the blood or other tissues of the RES are generally disposed of within a few minutes by phagocytosis.

Inflammation

When tissue injury occurs, whether by physical trauma or the multiplication of microorganisms, a series of reactions is set in motion to remove or contain the offending agents and repair the damage. This series of events is referred to as the *inflammatory response* and is outlined in Figure 11-7. The inflammatory response is initiated by the release of such chemicals as histamine, serotonin, kinins, and prostaglandins. These chemicals are contained in certain tissues and WBCs and are released in response to trauma to the tissues. Histamine is one of the most important chemical mediators and is found in high concentrations in circulating basophils and *mast cells*. Mast cells resemble basophils but are scattered throughout various body tissues, with the largest concentration being in the mucosal tissues. These chemical mediators, often called *vasoactive agents,* can rapidly affect the flow of blood and the permeability of blood vessels in the immediate area. Their release causes the blood vessels in the surrounding area to dilate, which brings an increased flow of blood to the injured tissues. This process occurs within several minutes and is accompanied by an increased permeability of the walls of the blood vessels, which allows an increased amount of plasma and PMNs to move from

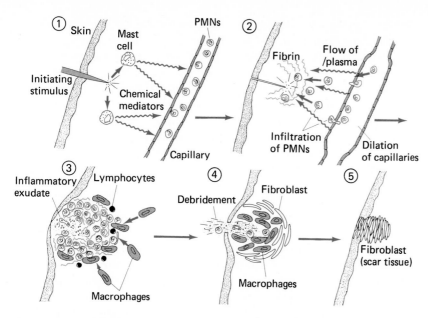

Figure 11-7   The progression of an inflammatory response from the initial stimulation to abscess formation, to healing with the formation of scar tissue.

the vessels into the area of injury. The chemical mediators of inflammation appear to have an attractive influence for PMNs that draws these WBCs to the inflammatory site; this process is called **chemotaxis.** After several hours of the inflammatory response the tissue will be reddened, warm, swollen, and painful due to the increased blood and plasma flow into the area. If the stimulus that initiates the inflammatory response is the growth of microorganisms in the tissues, the PMNs begin collecting in large numbers and will phagocytize and destroy many microbes. Plasma flowing into the area carries clotting factors, including fibrinogen, which begins to form a network of fibrin strands around the injured area. The fibrin and PMNs continue to build up over several days and are joined by other cells to form a barrier, called the *inflammatory barrier,* around the injured area. The center of the area becomes the battleground in which large numbers of dead bacteria and dead PMNs begin to accumulate in pools of fluids; this fluid is called the *inflammatory exudate* or, more commonly, *pus.* This accumulation of pus circumscribed by the inflammatory barrier is called an *abscess.* As the inflammatory process continues, other types of white blood cells enter the area. Increased numbers of lymphocytes appear and are thought to attract and stimulate macrophages. Macrophages next begin to appear in large numbers to aid further in walling off the injured area, to clear up debris

Chemotaxis
movement of a cell toward a chemical influence. Protective phagocytic cells are attracted by chemicals released by damaged body cells.

through phagocytosis, and to help in repair. If the abscess has formed in superficial tissue, the inflammatory barrier and skin may break and allow the pus to be expelled. Expelling of the pus, if not accompanied by damage to the inflammatory barrier between the abscess and deeper tissues, may help accelerate healing of the lesion. A pimple or boil is an example of such a skin abscess. If the abscess is in deeper tissues and the inflammatory exudate cannot be expelled, healing is much slower. A standoff may be reached in an abscess in that the bacteria are in an environmental niche of dead tissue that affords them protection from host defense mechanisms and, at the same time, they may be in a metabolically inactive state so that antibiotics may not affect them. Often surgical drainage is needed at this time to clean out the debris or pus. The last phase of the inflammatory response is the growth of repair cells called *fibroblasts*. The fibroblasts are long, slender cells that form a wall of scar tissue around the injured area. They continue to form scar tissue until the void where the normal cells were destroyed has been filled. It may be several weeks from the beginning of the response until complete healing has occurred. Scar tissue formation is basically a beneficial response; however, excessive scar tissue formation in vital organs may result in impaired function, and excessive scarring is undesirable on exposed areas of the body for cosmetic reasons. The inflammatory response occurs with most injuries; if microbial infection is not present, healing occurs without pus formation.

CONCEPT SUMMARY

1. Each individual is endowed with a number of barriers to infection that function without respect to the kind of possible disease-producing agent. These barriers are called *nonspecific host defense mechanisms.*

2. Nonspecific host defense mechanisms often function in sequence such that a breach in one barrier leads to the action of the next. These barriers are anatomical (e.g., the skin), mechanical (e.g., ciliary movement), chemical (e.g., lysozyme in tears), and cellular (e.g., granulocytes and macrophages).

3. The reticuloendothelial system has a major responsibility in maintaining body defense against invading microorganisms. Cells and body fluids from this system are primarily responsible for the beneficial inflammatory response associated with many types of infections.

STUDY SUMMARY

1. Why is an intact epithelium the most significant nonspecific protection against infectious disease?
2. What function do ciliated epithelial cells have in nonspecific disease resistance?
3. What is the fundamental functional difference between granulocytes and monocytes?
4. Would the function of lymphocytes be associated with primary or secondary defense mechanisms?
5. Construct a table or diagram that shows the interrelationships among the phagocyte system, lymphatic system, and reticuloendothelial system.
6. List, in order of occurrence, five functional steps of the inflammatory process.

REFERENCES FOR ADDITIONAL STUDY

1. *Immunology III*, J. Bellanti, 1985. Saunders.
2. The T Cell and Its Receptor. *Scientific American* 254:36, 1986.
3. *Medical Microbiology*, J. Sherris, 1984. Elsevier.

chapter 12

ACQUIRED IMMUNE RESPONSES

Lymphocyte
a type of white blood cell that is
involved in the immune response.

Acquired immunity refers to the resistance of a host resulting from the formation of antibodies or antibodylike responses. The acquired immune response is a dual system. One part of this dual system is called the *humoral antibody response* and includes those responses that lead to the formation of antibody molecules that circulate with the body fluids. The other part is called the *cell-mediated immune response* and involves the production of special types of **lymphocytes** that possess specific reactive sites on their outer surface.

Much new information about mechanisms of the immune responses and characteristics of antibodies has become available in recent years, but a detailed description is beyond the scope of this textbook. Our coverage here and in Chapter 13 is limited to an overall view of the formation and functions of antibodies and the cell-mediated immune response, how these phenomena can be manipulated by the use of vaccines to prevent diseases, and how acquiring these responses can be used to help in the diagnosis of diseases. Some detrimental effects of immune responses on the host are also discussed.

ANTIGENS

The basic concept of the immune responses centers around the ability of the body to react against certain types of foreign chemical substances. Any foreign substance that stimulates a host immune response is called an *antigen.* Antigens are usually proteins or carbohydrates of over 10,000 Daltons molecular weight; some lipid complexes, however, may also function as antigens. A common immune response is the development of an antibody. Once an antibody is formed, it will specifically combine only with the type of antigen that stimulated its production. Moreover, the antibody is not formed against the entire antigen but only against certain chemical groups of the antigen called *antigenic determinants,* or epitopes. An antigenic determinant that is separated from the remainder of the antigen is normally not able to stimulate antibody formation because of its small size, but it can react with antibodies that are already formed. Under these conditions the antigenic determinant is called a *hapten.* Protein antigens and their antigenic determinants that may make up part of a bacterium are diagrammatically represented in Figure 12-1.

ACQUIRED IMMUNE RESPONSES

Development of the acquired immune response depends on the interaction of at least three specific types of cells. Each of these cells is derived from stem (precursor) cells which are most often found in the bone marrow. Once formed, these juvenile cells are subject to a variety of maturation processes which lead them to differentiate into specific lymphoid or reticuloendothelial cells. In this process, some of the juvenile cells mature to become macrophage cells (refer to Chapter 11); others come under the influence of the thymus gland and mature as thymus-derived lymphocytes **(T-cells)**; a second class of lymphocyte **(B-cell)** also develops, although the exact source of maturation influence is not known.

Development of specific acquired immunity relies upon the antigen processing and presenting capabilities of macrophages or other cells with similar functions, T-cells which produce chemicals that regulate the growth and development of both B-cells and

T-cell
a lymphocytic cell responsible for regulation of the immune response by both B-cells and T-cells involved in cell-mediated immunity.

B-cell
a lymphocytic cell programmed to produce specific antibodies.

Figure 12-1   Antigens associated with bacterial cells. A single cell may contain a number of different antigens. Antigenic determinants are the smaller segments (dark areas) of the antigens.

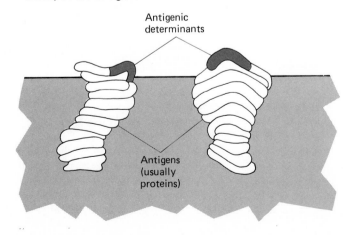

Antigenic determinants

Antigens (usually proteins)

other T-cells, and B-cells which are capable of becoming antibody-producing plasma cells. The actions of these cells in an immune response are further discussed in this chapter and are outlined in Figures 12-2 and 12-3.

When the body is exposed to the complex antigens associated with invading microorganisms, both humoral (B-cell) and cell-mediated (T-cell) immune responses may be stimulated. The acquired immune responses are usually beneficial to the host in that they offer added protection against invading microorganisms; these responses, however, may sometimes react against the host or produce certain types of antibodies that cause undesirable side reactions. These undesirable reactions are called **allergies** or *hypersensitivities*. The immune responses are discussed under three general categories: (1) formation of circulating or humoral antibodies, (2) formation of cell-mediated immunity, and (3) allergies and hypersensitivities.

Allergy

a hypersensitivity response.

Figure 12-2   Theorized sequence of events that are involved in the production of circulating antibodies.

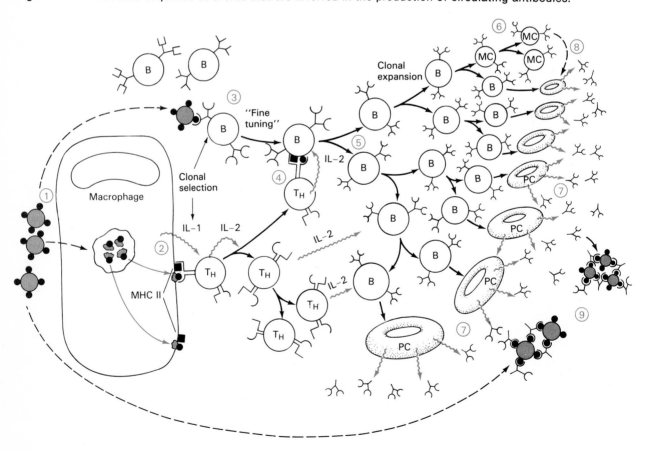

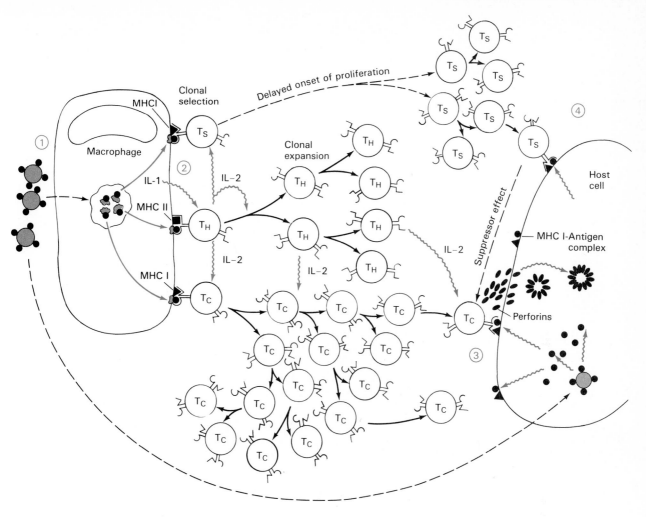

Figure 12-3   Theorized sequence of events that are involved in the cell-mediated immune response.

HUMORAL ANTIBODY RESPONSE

Humoral antibodies are released into the blood and are found in most tissue fluids. The antigens associated with microorganisms and foreign proteins, in general, are excellent simulators of this antibody response. These antibodies are effective in helping destroy invading microorganisms or in neutralizing toxins.

When foreign antigens enter the body tissues a sequence of events occurs that involves interactions between macrophages, B-cells, and T-cells. Some of the details of these interactions are still not fully understood; the following presentation is a simplified interpretation of current theories regarding these events. When a foreign antigen enters the body much of it is phagocytized by macrophages and some remains circulating free in the blood for some time. The phagocytized antigen is processed by the macrophage and the antigenic determinants are presented on the surface membrane of the macrophage. This presented antigen will selectively combine with an immature *helper T-cell.* This combining stimulates the macrophage to release a hormonelike protein called *interleukin 1.* Interleukin 1 stimulates the selected T-cell to multiply and differentiate into mature helper T-cells. These events play an important role in the cell-mediated immune response as well as the antibody response and will be described in more detail when we examine cell-mediated immunity.

Meanwhile, some of the circulating antigen combines with a specific protein receptor on a B-cell. A very close fit needs to exist between the antigenic determinant of an antigen and the protein receptor of a B-cell before the two can combine. Within the body, B-cells are found with receptor proteins having millions of different configurations. However, a single B-cell has receptors of only a single configuration. For the B-cells to have the genetic information to produce these millions of variations in the protein molecules of the receptor, millions of different sequences of DNA would have to be present in the genes that direct the production of these receptors. It had been difficult to explain how B-cells, which all come from common **stem cells,** could have such diverse genetic composition. This dilemma was resolved by the work of Dr. S. Tonegawa, which demonstrated that the sections of DNA that control the variable region of the receptor proteins are made up of segments of DNA that are able to be rearranged into millions of different sequences. This rearrangement apparently occurs after a stem cell has been committed to become a B-cell. When an antigen enters the body, a B-cell with a close-fitting receptor will attach to its antigenic determinant. This is called *clonal selection.* Once the B-cell has been selected by attachment to the antigen, it can then be directed to change into antibody-producing cells (plasma cells). Part of this process involves "fine tuning" of the genes that control the makeup and configuration of the B-cell receptor by altering the sequence of some individual nucleotide bases; this results in receptors with an exact fit to the antigenic determinant, and later allows highly specific antibodies to be made against that antigenic determinant. Also, B-cells ingest and process antigens in a manner similar to macrophages and present the processed antigens on their outer membrane. A mature receptor-specific helper T-cell now combines with the antigen on the B-cell. This stimulates the T-cell to release *interleukin 2.* Interleukin 2 first activates the fine-tuned B-cell to divide into many identical B-cells, a process called *clonal expansion;* it then stimulates most B-

Stem cell

a cell, usually found in bone marrow, that is a precursor to the more fully differentiated T- and B-cells.

cells to differentiate into *plasma cells* while a few remain as **memory B-cells.** The plasma cells contain increased amounts of cytoplasm, endoplasmic reticulum, and ribosomes, which equip them to produce large amounts of proteins. The main proteins produced by the plasma cells are the circulating antibodies, which are called **immunoglobulins** (Ig). These antibodies contain receptor sites that are produced under the direction of the fine-tuned genes that were developed in the B-cell. The memory B-cells remain in the body for many years and become involved in the secondary antibody response, which is discussed below.

Memory B-cell

a B-cell that has been directed to produce a specific antibody, and is programmed to reproduce other B-cells that make the same antibody when it responds to a signal from the specific antigen.

Immunoglobulin

antibody.

Classes and Structure of Antibodies

Five different classes of circulating antibodies, or immunoglobulins, have been identified and are designated IgG, IgM, IgA, IgD, and IgE. The properties of these immunoglobulins are shown in Table 12-1. The basic unit of an antibody, as typified by IgG, consists of two heavy and two light polypeptide chains connected in a Y-type arrangement (Figure 12-4). The arrangements of amino acids at the top of the four chains of the Y are variable and form the specific receptor sites of the antibody. These specific receptor sites, called *variable regions,* will combine only with an antigenic determinant that is the same as that of the original antigen that initiated the antibody response. The remainder of the antibody molecule does not vary and is called the *constant region.*

IgG antibodies are the major type present in the circulation; most are in the blood, but lesser amounts are found in other fluids, such as lymph, synovial, and spinal fluids. IgG is an important long-term antibody that helps protect the host against infections. This antibody is able to cross the placenta in humans in the transfer of passive immunity to the newborn.

IgM antibodies consist of clusters (polymers) of five Y-shaped immunoglobulin basic structures. These antibodies appear

Table 12-1   Properties of Four Classes of Human Immunoglobulins

Property	IgG	IgM	IgA	IgE	IgD
No. of Y-shaped units	1	5	2	1	1
Molecular weight	145,000	850,000	385,000	200,000	180,000
How transferred to offspring	Via placenta	Not transferred	Via milk	Not transferred	Not transferred
Half-life (days)	25	5	6	2	3
Where found in body	40 in blood, 60% in extracellular fluid	90% in blood, 10% in extracellular fluid	Mostly in secretions	Attached to PMNs or mast cells	Attached to B-cells

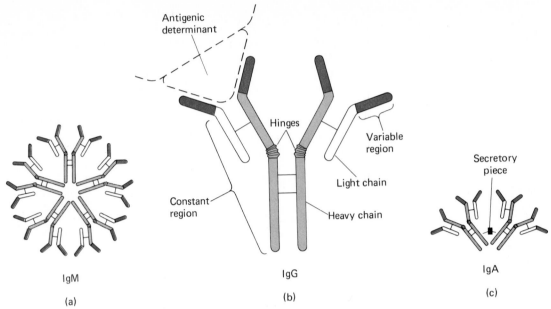

Figure 12-4 The structures of immunoglobulins. (a) Structure of IgM showing pentamer arrangement of the basic immunoglobulin Y-shaped units. (b) Details of the IgG structure (scale enlarged). (c) Dimer arrangement of IgA.

earlier in the infection than the other classes of immunoglobulins, and offer valuable assistance to the host during the critical early stages of an infection. IgM is found mostly in blood fluids but disappears from the body soon after the onset of the infection and does not cross the placenta.

IgA antibodies are made up of two (dimer) Y-shaped basic structures. These immunoglobulins are readily secreted and, besides being found in the blood, are also found in tears, saliva, mucosal secretions, and similar fluids. IgA offers valuable protection against infections of the superficial tissues, such as the mucosal surfaces of the respiratory, intestinal, and genitourinary tracts.

IgD is found only in low concentrations and seems identical to the specific receptor sites on B-cells. IgE is associated with allergies and will be discussed later.

Primary and Secondary Humoral Antibody Responses

After exposure to an antigen, small amounts of antibody first appear in a few days, but readily measured amounts usually cannot be detected until about a week after stimulation. A steady rise in antibody concentrations occurs over the next 2 weeks until the maximum level is attained at about 3 weeks. The level of antibodies then slowly decreases over the ensuing years. A given IgG antibody will remain in the body for only a few months after it is formed; therefore the prolonged persistence of antibodies must result from the continual activity of specific antibody-producing cells.

If a person has experienced a primary antibody response to a given antigen and is reexposed at some later date to the same antigen, a rapid antibody response is stimulated and high levels of antibodies are produced within a few days instead of a few weeks. This is called the *anamnestic, booster,* or *secondary response* and is associated with the memory B-cells that were produced as part of the primary response. These memory B-cells are long-lived and some will remain in the body for years. These cells are preprogrammed such that when they encounter the same type of antigen that stimulated the primary response, they rapidly change into antibody-producing plasma cells. This mechanism allows the body to replenish its antibody supply before the invading microorganism has had a chance to cause a clinical disease, and in many cases confers lifelong immunity to the host. The primary and secondary responses of IgG and IgM are shown in Figure 12-5.

Effect of Humoral Antibodies on Microorganisms

When a microorganism such as a bacterium enters the body tissues, antibodies may be formed against many cellular components such as internal proteins, toxins, capsular antigens, or flagella, as well as different antigenic determinants on the cell surface. Thus, the antigen-antibody reactions may involve various components of the microorganism with varied effects. Also, antibodies often work in conjunction with other components of the host's defense

Figure 12-5   Primary and secondary responses of IgG and IgM antibodies.

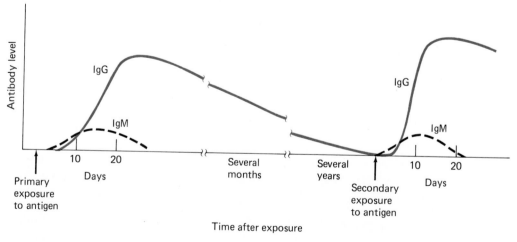

mechanisms, such as phagocytic cells, or complement, to protect the host from disease. The following categories cover the most common ways that antibodies function against microorganisms.

Promotion of phagocytosis Antibodies which combine with surface antigens may bind the microbes into clumps by forming antibody bridges between cells. This is called an **agglutination** reaction. These clumps of microbes are much more readily phagocytized than are single cells. In addition, some antibodies may first attach to the antigen with their receptor sites, and the opposite end (the constant region) of the antibody molecule may specifically attach to the phagocytic cell. This step binds the microbe to the phagocytic cell, which greatly facilitates the process of phagocytosis. Antibodies that render microorganisms more susceptible to phagocytosis are called *opsonins*.

Interference with attachment Antibodies may combine over the surface of the microbes and prevent any undesirable attachment to host cells. They are called *neutralizing* antibodies because they neutralize the ability of the microbe to cause infection.

Neutralization of toxins Antibodies may neutralize the toxins produced by microorganisms. Such antibodies are called *antitoxins*.

Activation of the complement system The complement (C′) system is a group of nine or more protein components found in normal serum and designated C1, C2, C3, C4, and so on. When this system is activated, different components of the system stimulate and amplify such host defense mechanisms as inflammation, chemotaxis, and phagocytosis and cause lysis (breaking up) of certain microorganisms or other cells. The complement system becomes activated when an antigen-antibody reaction occurs and forms a complex with and activates the first component of complement. A few molecules of the activated first component, in turn, activate many more molecules of one of the other components of complement (C4) which, in turn, activates yet a larger number of molecules of the next component (C2), and so on through the other components. The components of the complement system were numbered as they were discovered and not in their order of action in the complement cascade. In fact, it is possible for certain chemical signals to activate the complement system by first interacting with components other than C1. This activation system is referred to as the alternate pathway. The expanding effect, as the reactions cascade through the complement system, allows a small number of antigen-antibody reactions to trigger a greatly amplified protective effect as a result of the host defense mechanisms that are stimulated by the activated components of complement.

Agglutination

a process by which small particles or cells hold together in a group (clump). Some antibodies can cause agglutination of their specific antigens.

CELL-MEDIATED IMMUNE RESPONSE

The cell-mediated immune response involves the T-cell–type lymphocytes. This immune response causes destruction of host cells that have become altered by such events as infection by invading microorganisms or transformation to cancerous cells. T-cells are thought to contain a section of DNA (similar to that found in B-cells) that can be rearranged into millions of different sequences. This section of rearrangeable DNA contains the genes that control the configuration of receptor proteins that project out of the plasma membrane of T-cells. All receptors on a single T-cell are of the same configuration. These T-cell receptors are made up of two polypeptides, called the *alpha* and *beta chains.* Among the millions of configurations that naturally exist on the receptors of T-cells are some that will specifically combine with antigenic determinants of most any foreign antigen. In addition, part of the T-cell receptor is programmed to specifically combine with proteins found on the plasma membrane of the host's cells (Figure 12-3). These host-cell proteins are called the *major histocompatibility complex* (MHC). There are two classes of MHC, called *class I* and *class II.* Class I MHC protein is found on the plasma membrane of all cells of the body while class II MHC protein is present only on the membranes of macrophages, B-cells, and related immune cells. To function, the receptors of T-cells must simultaneously recognize both the foreign antigen and the MHC protein. Thus, most T-cells can only mobilize an immune response against foreign antigens that are associated with host-cell membranes. The main T-cell lymphocytes are of two general kinds. The first possesses a protein antigen on its surface called the *T4 antigen* (also called the *CD4 antigen*); these are referred to as the *T4 lymphocytes* or helper cells and will recognize only the class II MHC proteins. The second kind of lymphocytes have a *T8 antigen* (also called *CD8*) on their membranes and are called *T8 lymphocytes.* T8 lymphocytes recognize only the class I MHC proteins.

A simplified overview of the events that occur in the cell-mediated immune response is shown in Figure 12-3. The initial stages of this response are the same as those that were outlined for the antibody response. The invading antigen is first processed by the macrophage and then presented on the surface of the macrophage in a complex with class II MHC protein. A T4 lymphocyte, called a *helper T-cell,* that has a receptor that is complementary to the antigen-MHC complex attaches to the macrophage-antigen complex (clonal selection). This induces the macrophage to secrete *interleukin 1* that in turn stimulates the selected immature helper T-cell to become a mature helper T-cell. The mature helper T-cell secretes *interleukin 2* and is stimulated to divide into a clone of many identical cells (clonal expansion). This clone of selected helper T-cells now orchestrates the immune response against the invading antigen. T-4 helper cells are the primary target of the human immune deficiency virus (HIV) which causes acquired immune deficiency syndrome (AIDS). HIV kills the infected T-4 cells and prevents them from completing their critical role of stimulating the immune response. In the meantime, a T8 lymphocyte, called a *cytotoxic T-cell,* attaches to the same antigen that has complexed with the class I MHC protein and is stimulated by interleukin 2 to proliferate into many identical progeny cells (clonal expansion). These cytotoxic T-cells circulate throughout the body and, when they encounter the original foreign antigen-MHC complex on the surface of a host cell, they attach to this complex. Once attached, the cytotoxic T-cell releases, among other proteins, a protein called *perforin* that inserts into the plasma membrane of the host cell and causes holes to form in this membrane. This leads to the destruction of the altered host cell. In addition, various of the stimulated immune cells release one or more of a group of *lymphokines.* These lymphokines induce a variety of responses such as attraction of macrophages to the site of the antigen–cytotoxic T-cell interaction, activation of macrophages, and other responses that aid in the destruction of the cells being attacked. (Table 12-2). An inflammatory response is often part of this reaction and may lead to the formation of scar tissue around the antigen. The cell-mediated immune response is sometimes referred to as *delayed* hypersensitivity, for it requires several days for the first phase of this reaction to be seen after an antigen is injected into the tissues of a sensitized host; this phenomenon is the basis of skin tests that are used in the diagnosis of such diseases as tuberculosis (see Chapter 22).

Once the specific immune responses have reached a high level and have fulfilled their main functions, a third type of T-cell,

Table 12-2   Major Lymphokines Released by Killer T-Cells and the Responses They Mediate

Lymphokine	Response or Action
Cytotoxic factor	Kills foreign cells and adjacent host cells
Transfer factor	Stimulates nonsensitized lymphocytes at the site of the antigen to change into sensitized T cells and aid in intensifying the response
Macrophage chemotactic factor	Attracts macrophages to the site of the antigen
Migration-inhibitory factor	Immobilizes macrophages to keep them from leaving the area of the antigen
Macrophage-activating factor	Greatly increases phagocytic activity and the ability of microphages to kill foreign cells and break down ingested materials

called a *suppressor T-cell,* is stimulated to proliferate. Suppressor T-cells are also under the influence of helper T-cells and their function is to dampen and eventually slow down the immune reponse.

Some of the selected T-cells are long-lived and continue to circulate in the host as memory T-cells. Should the host be reexposed to the same antigen at a later time, these memory cells would recognize that antigen and rapidly remobilize the full cell-mediated immune response. A substance called *interferon* is also released by killer T-cells and has inhibitory effects on the growth of some cancer cells and on the multiplication of viruses. Interferons are also produced by cells that are infected with viruses and are important defense mechanisms against new viral infections. Interferons will be discussed in more detail in the chapters on viruses.

Additional types of white blood cells, called *natural killer cells,* are a normal component of the host's defense mechanisms. They appear to be able to attack virus-infected cells and tumor cells spontaneously without the necessity of being preprogrammed against a specific antigen. Also, they do not seem to be influenced by helper T-cells. Natural killer cells are thought to kill infected or altered host cells by mechanisms similiar to those used by cytotoxic T-cells. The action of natural killer cells seems to be enhanced by interferons.

HYPERSENSITIVITIES AND HARMFUL EFFECTS OF ANTIBODIES

Sometimes immune responses are harmful to the host because they react against host tissues or stimulate the release of excessive amounts of chemical mediators. Such reactions are referred to as *hypersensitivities* and *allergies.*

These harmful reactions depend on various interacting factors, such as nature and dose of antigen, route of injection, and the physiological conditions of the host. They may involve either the humoral or the cell-mediated immune systems. Still, the more typical allergic reaction involves a different type of an immune response that produces antibodies of the immunoglobulin E class (Figure 12-6).

Hypersensitivity

Antigens that induce allergies are called *allergens.* Many different substances are capable of functioning as allergens. Some of the more common allergens are plant pollens, animal hairs, and food.

(a) First exposure to allergen

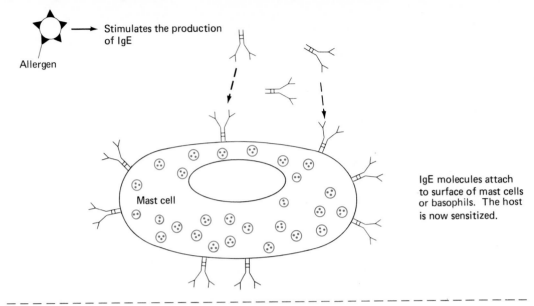

Allergen

Stimulates the production
of IgE

Mast cell

IgE molecules attach
to surface of mast cells
or basophils. The host
is now sensitized.

(b) Subsequent exposures
to the same allergen

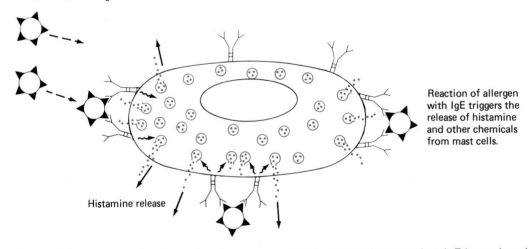

Histamine release

Reaction of allergen
with IgE triggers the
release of histamine
and other chemicals
from mast cells.

Figure 12-6 An immediate type allergic response. (a) No reaction is seen when IgE is produced and attaches to mast cells by their constant region. (b) Reaction is seen after subsequent exposures to allergen as a result of the release of histamine, etc.

Mast cells

cells containing certain high-concentration chemicals that can produce severe systemic reactions when released into the circulation.

The mechanism of stimulation and formation of IgE is not well understood but appears to be similar to the mechanisms used to produce the other immunoglobulins. Once formed, IgE molecules do not remain free in the circulation but rapidly attach to either **mast cells** or *basophils*. This attachment involves the constant region of IgE and is such that the antibody reactive sites of IgE molecules are pointing out from the cells and are still free to react with the antigen. Once this sequence of events occurs, the host is sensitized to the specific allergen. When the host is subsequently exposed to the allergen, the allergen specifically attaches to the reactive sites of the IgE antibodies that are already attached to the mast cells. This antigen-antibody reaction triggers the release of *histamine* and other related substances from the mast cells. Histamine has immediate effects on the surrounding tissues, such as dilation and increased permeability of blood vessels, contraction of smooth muscles, and increased mucous secretions. If this reaction occurs along the mucosal lining of the upper respiratory tract, the symptoms are the familiar runny nose, watery eyes, itching, and sneezing of hay fever. If the reaction occurs through contact of allergens with mast cells located in the skin, hives (urticaria) may result. Reactions along the intestinal tract may result in such symptoms as vomiting, abdominal pain, and diarrhea. If the reaction between the allergen and sensitized mast cells or sensitized basophils is of sufficient magnitude, as would occur with the injection of the allergen into the body, systemic *anaphylactic shock* may occur. This situation involves a massive shift of blood flow from some vital organs and may result in the death of the patient within a few minutes after the injection. An injection of epinephrine may counter the effects of systemic anaphylactic shock.

Allergy testing   Skin testing can be used to determine the type of substance to which a person is allergic. Extracts of suspected allergens are injected intradermally (between the layers of skin) or a drop of the extract is placed on an area of skin that has been lightly scratched. If the person is hypersensitive, an immediate (within minutes) reaction of reddening and swelling will occur at the site of contact with allergen. Often a person will be tested simultaneously for sensitivity to different allergens by injecting extracts of each into different areas of skin.

Control of allergies   Once the specific allergen is identified, a person can take the necessary precautions to avoid the substance. Food allergies are most easily avoided, but people can also move from a geographic area where an allergen of plant origin is present or can avoid a certain species of animal and so on.

A person may become *desensitized* by receiving injections of extracts of an allergen. When introduced into the deeper tissues by injection, the allergen is thought to stimulate the formation of IgG antibodies. These antibodies are then able to react with the allergen on subsequent natural exposures and neutralize its ability to react with the IgE antibodies attached to the mast cells. Thus no allergic reaction occurs.

Perhaps the most popular but least effective method of relieving allergy symptoms is the use of various medications. *Antihistamines* are widely used and have the direct effect of neutralizing the action of histamine. Other substances that act as decongestants, expectorants, or suppressants of pain and so on may be used in conjunction with antihistamines to bring added symptomatic relief. *Corticosteroids* may also be effective in treating some allergies but should be used with proper medical discretion, for they have a suppressive effect on the entire immune system and may render the recipient more susceptible to infectious diseases in general.

Delayed Hypersensitivity

Allergies involving cell-mediated immunity occur after exposure to certain types of antigens. Exposure to poison ivy is a familiar example. No visible reaction is seen on first exposure; however, a typical T-cell–mediated immune response is stimulated. On subsequent skin contact with poison ivy, the sensitized T-cells react with the poison and induce a gradual localized reaction of reddening and swelling that reaches a peak response about two days after exposure. Some infectious disease agents cause the patient to develop a T-cell–mediated immunity. In these patients the delayed hypersensitivity response can be used as a diagnostic tool. Small amounts of the antigen are injected intradermally or placed on the skin of a suspected patient. If the person has become hypersensitive to the antigen because of earlier infection, an inflammation reaction occurrs at the site of antigen placement. This reaction is the basis of the tuberculin skin test used in the diagnosis of tuberculosis.

CONCEPT SUMMARY

1. The acquired immune response results from antigenic stimulation of lymphocytic cells in the body. These lymphocytes are of two general types: B cells and T cells.

2. The humoral immune response is characterized by the production of specific immunoglobulins, called antibodies, produced by B lymphocytes in response to antigenic stimuli. These antibodies are found in one or more of five classes of immunoglobulins. Each type of immunoglobulin acts uniquely in disease limitation by serving as agglutinins, neutralizing toxins, opsonins, and inhibitors of pathogen attachment.

3. Acquired cell-mediated immunity is largely a function of the T cells. These cells are activated by the presence of antigen so that they fulfill numerous functions in the process of disease control.

4. Some individuals overreact or react in an altered way to the

presence of antigen in their environment. Such overactivity is known as *hypersensitivity.* Hypersensitivity reactions are often damaging to the host and may require considerable effort and expense to control.

STUDY SUMMARY

1. Describe the role in the immune response of each of the following cell types: (a) macrophages, (b) T-helper and T-suppressor cells, (c) B cells, and (d) plasma cells.

2. Explain how each of the following participates in the immune response: (a) interleukins, (b) immunoglobulins, (c) complement, (d) lymphokines, and (e) interferon.

3. Draw a diagram that can be used to explain the concept of antigenic memory.

4. How did the work of Tonegawa help to explain the clonal selection theory?

5. Describe the functional differences between the variable and the constant regions of the immune globulins.

6. Diagram the cellular processes that lead to immune hypersensitivity.

REFERENCES FOR FURTHER STUDY

1. Anti-Idiotypes and Immunity. *Scientific American* 255:38, 1986.

2. The T-Cell and Its Receptor. *Scientific American* 254:36, 1986.

3. The Molecules of the Immune System. *Scientific American* 253:122, 1985.

4. How Killer Cells Kill. *Scientific American* 253:84, 1985.

5. The Immune System in AIDS. *Scientific American* 253:84, 1985.

6. Immunity in Infective Diseases. *Reviews of Infectious Diseases* 10:223, 1988.

chapter 13

APPLICATIONS OF THE IMMUNE RESPONSE

Acquired immunity resulting from the production of circulating antibodies or cell-mediated immunity may offer protection for prolonged periods or even for the lifetime of the host. It is called *active immunity,* as the host actively produces its own antibodies, and it may be stimulated either by natural infections or by artificial exposure to antigens in the form of vaccines.

It is also possible to confer a short-lived immunity by the transfer of antibodies from one host to another. This type is called *passive immunity* and occurs *naturally* when antibodies are passed from mother to offspring or *artificially* by the injection of antisera.

TYPES OF IMMUNITY

Traditionally the types of antibody-induced acquired immunity are divided into four categories:

1. Natural active immunity
2. Artificial active immunity
3. Natural passive immunity
4. Artificial passive immunity

Natural Active Immunity

Natural active immunity develops after recovery from a naturally acquired infectious disease. During the process of the infection large amounts of microbial antigens stimulate the production of a maximum amount of antibody. Usually both humoral antibodies and cell-associated immunity are stimulated. These antibodies remain in the body for years. During this time any reexposure to the same pathogen results in rapid destruction of the invading microbe. Even if the time between the first exposure and reexposure has been so long that most of the original antibodies have disappeared, memory cells, which are responsible for the recall or anamnestic response, rapidly stimulate the production of new antibodies before the invading microbe is able to cause a serious or even a clinically evident disease. Immunity of this type is more effective against diseases in which the microorganisms must pass through the blood or into deeper tissues compared to infections of such superficial tissues as the respiratory or intestinal mucosa. But even when complete immunity is not maintained, reinfections are generally much less severe than the original infection. This basic immune response is shown in Figure 12-5.

Artificial Active Immunity

The immune mechanism of the body can be stimulated to produce antibodies when antigens are introduced by artificial means—that is, in the form of a vaccine. Three general categories of vaccines are used: *killed, toxoid,* and *attenuated.*

Killed vaccines   Killed vaccines are made by culturing large numbers of a pathogenic microorganism and then subjecting them to treatment by heat or chemicals. When just the right amount of treatment has been given, the components of the microbe that are necessary for multiplication are destroyed, but the antigens are not altered. If these killed microbes are injected into the tissues of the host, they can be phagocytized by macrophages and passed to the lymphatic tissues, where specific antibodies will be produced. With one injection it is usually not possible to get enough antigen into the tissues to produce a maximum stimulation of antibodies. In order to obtain the maximum antibody stimulation, the immunization must be repeated about every other week for a total of three or four injections. The effectiveness of this type of vaccine may be enhanced by mixing the killed microbes with such materials as mineral oils or alum. These materials are called *adjuvants* and slow down the clearance of the vaccine from the tissues, thereby providing a longer exposure to the antigen. Generally adjuvants are not used in vaccines for humans, for they may cause some discomfort. Some vaccines are purified fractions of the microbe rather than the entire microbial cells. Several newer vaccines, for example, use only the capsule of the bacteria as the immunizing agent. Such fractionated vaccines help reduce undesirable side reactions caused by endotoxins and other materials found in the intact microbial cells. A new generation of purified antigen vaccines produced by genetic engineering is being developed. Such vaccines will contain only the antigens that stimulate protective antibodies and this factor will help reduce adverse side reactions. This technology is particularly useful in providing purified viral antigens that cannot be produced economically by conventional methods.

The immunity induced by a killed vaccine does not persist as long as the immunity induced by a natural infection. Often the immunity has disappeared or is greatly reduced after several years. Then if a single dose of the vaccine, called a **booster** dose, is given, the anamnestic reaction is stimulated and high levels of antibodies are produced in just a few days. If booster doses are given every few years, an immune state can be maintained continuously.

Toxoid vaccines Diseases like diphtheria and tetanus are caused by exotoxins. The antibodies formed against exotoxins are called *antitoxins* and are able to prevent such diseases. Vaccines against such toxin-caused diseases contain inactivated toxins, called **toxoids**, rather than killed microbial cells. Toxins are converted into toxoids by the addition of chemicals or by exposure to heat. The antibody response to toxoids is similar to that produced by killed vaccines in that a series of primary doses and periodic booster doses are needed for maximum and continued protection.

Living attenuated vaccines *Attenuated* means "weakened" or "reduced in force." These vaccines contain microorganisms with a low virulence. Under most conditions they produce only a mild or subclinical disease. These attenuated microbes proliferate in the tissue to yield a mass of antigens similar to the amount produced by the natural disease; thus a single dose stimulates a high antibody level that lasts for a prolonged period. In some cases, the living vaccine can be given by a natural route of infection—for example, the oral administration of the living polio vaccine. Such vaccines are easier to administer than those that must be given by hypodermic injection.

A disadvantage of living vaccines is that an occasional mild or even an active infection may result from the vaccine itself. This factor is of particular concern in persons with defective or suppressed immune mechanisms and such persons should not receive living vaccines. Similarly, pregnant females should avoid receiving living vaccines because the attenuated microbes may cause infection of the developing fetus. The most commonly used vaccines and their recommended administration schedules are listed in Table 13-1.

Natural Passive Immunity

The newborn of many species receive antibodies from their mothers. This antibody gives them valuable protection during the critical early phase of life. Some mammals, such as calves and pigs,

Booster
a second or subsequent dose of antigen given to increase the level of immunity.

Toxoid
a modified toxin that has lost its toxic properties but retains its antigenic properties.

Table 13-1 Currently Available Vaccines

Vaccine	Type of Immunogen		Recommended Schedules
Commonly recommended immunizations			
DPT	Diphtheria and tetanus toxoid with killed *B. pertussis*	P.[a] B.[b]	3 doses 2, 4, 6 months 18 months, 6 years
Polio	Live attenuated oral, trivalent (types 1, 2, and 3)	P. B.	2 doses, 2, 4, months 14 months, 6 years
MMR	Live attenuated measles, mumps, and rubella	P.	1 dose, 15–18 months
Influenza	Formalin inactivated virus	P. B.	All during epidemic years; persons at high risk Annual
HIB	Type b polysaccharide	P.	2 years/no booster
Immunizations recommended for specified circumstances			
Pneumococcus	Capsular polysaccharide of most common types	P. B.	Persons over 2 years at high risk Unknown
Cholera	Phenol inactivated *Vibrio cholerae*	P. B.	Travel to cholera area 6 months
BCG	Attenuated *Mycobacterium bovis*	P. B.	Persons at increased risk Not recommended
Typhoid	Killed *Salmonella typhi*	P. B.	Persons at high risk 3 years
Rabies	Killed attenuated virus	P. B.	Preexposure, persons at high risk Postexposure, all persons Under some conditions
Smallpox	Live attenuated vaccinia virus	P.	Not recommended
Yellow fever	Live attenuated virus	P. B.	Travel to endemic areas 10 years
Hepatitis B	Inactivated Dane particles	P. B.	3 doses, high-risk persons Unknown
Meningococcal	Polysaccharide (types A, C, Y, W-135)	P.	Persons at increased risk

[a]*P = primary immunization schedule.*
[b]*B = booster immunizations.*

obtain the passed antibodies in a substance called *colostrum,* which is present in their mother's milk during the first week after delivery. With humans and many other mammals, much of the passive transfer of antibodies occurs across the placental barrier; these are IgG antibodies and at birth the infant has a full complement of the same antibodies found in its mother. The role of colostrum and the passage of antibodies to the infant in human milk are not clearly understood. Some IgA antibodies appear to be passed by this means and may offer protection to the mucosal surfaces of the intestinal tract. Natural passive immunity lasts from 3 to 6 months in humans.

Pertussis Vaccine

General use of standardized pertussis vaccine has resulted in a substantial reduction in cases and deaths from pertussis disease. However, the annual number of reported cases has changed relatively little during the last 10 years, when annual averages of 1835 cases and ten fatalities have occurred. in 1983, 2463 cases were reported; in 1981, the latest year for which final national mortality statistics are available from the National Center for Health Statistics, six deaths were recorded. More precise data do not exist, since many cases go unrecognized or unreported, and diagnostic tests for *Bordetella pertussis*—culture and direct-immunofluorescence assay (DFA)—may be unavailable, difficult to perform, or incorrectly interpreted.

For 1982 and 1983, 53% of reported illnesses from *B. pertussis* occurred among children under 1 year of age, and 78%, among children under 5 years of age; 13 of 15 deaths reported to CDC occurred among children under 1 year old. Before widespread use of DTP (diphtheria, pertussis, tetanus) vaccine, about 20% of cases and 50% of pertussis-related deaths occurred among children under 1 year old.

Pertussis is highly communicable (attack rates of over 90% have been reported in unimmunized household contacts) and can cause severe disease, particularly in very young children. Of patients under 1 year of age reported to CDC during 1982 and 1983, 75% were hospitalized, approximately 22% had pneumonia, 2% had one or more seizures, and 0.7% died. Because of the substantial risks of complications of the disease, completion of a primary series of DTP early in life is essential.

In older children and adults—including, in some instances, those previously immunized—infection may result in nonspecific symptoms of bronchitis or an upper respiratory tract infection, and pertussis may not be diagnosed because classic signs, especially the inspiratory whoop, may be absent. Older preschool-aged children and school-aged siblings who are not fully immunized and develop pertussis can be important sources of infection for young infants, the group at highest risk of disease and disease severity. The importance of the infected adult in overall transmission remains to be defined.

Controversy regarding use of pertussis vaccine led to a formal reevaluation of the benefits and risks of this vaccine. The analysis indicated

Artificial Passive Immunity

Under certain circumstances a person may receive a supply of preformed antibodies taken from another host and injected into the person needing antibodies. This artificially passed immunity only lasts for several weeks. Before the development of antibiotics, it was a common practice to produce high levels of antibodies in horses or cows, for instance, and then collect their serum and use it as *antiserum* to treat various infectious diseases of humans. Although this procedure had some value, serious side reactions often occurred due to hypersensitivities that developed against the animal serum. Antiserum therapy is still used against some

that the benefits of the vaccine continue to outweigh its risks.

Because the incidence rate and severity of pertussis decrease with age, and because the vaccine may cause side effects and adverse reactions, pertussis immunization is not recommended for children after the seventh birthday, except under unusual circumstances.

Preparations used for immunization. Pertussis vaccine is a suspension of inactivated *B. pertussis* cells. Potency is assayed by comparison with the U.S. Standard Pertussis Vaccine in the intracerebral mouse protection test. The protective efficacy of pertussis vaccines in humans has been shown to correlate with the potency of vaccines.

Absolute contraindications. If any of the following adverse events occur after DTP or single-antigen pertussis vaccination, further vaccination with a vaccine containing pertussis antigen is contraindicated.

1. Allergic hypersensitivity.
2. Fever of 40.5°C (105°F), or greater within 48 hours.
3. Collapse or shocklike state (hypotonic-hyporesponsive episode) within 48 hours.
4. Persisting, inconsolable crying lasting 3 hours or more or an unusual, high-pitched cry occurring within 48 hours.
5. Convulsion(s) with or without fever occurring within 3 days. (All children with convulsions, especially those with convulsions occurring within 4–7 days of receipt of DTP, should be fully evaluated to clarify their medical and neurologic status before a decision is made on initiating or continuing vaccination with DTP).
6. Encephalopathy occurring within 7 days; this includes severe alterations in consciousness with generalized or focal neurologic signs. (A small but significantly increased risk of encephalopathy has been shown only within the 3-day period following DTP receipt. However, most authorities believe that an encephalopathy occurring within 7 days of DTP should be considered a contraindication to further doses of DTP.) (*MMWR* 36:168 1987.)

infectious diseases, but it is more effective in treating diseases caused by toxins. Whenever possible, human antiserum, particularly the gamma globulin fraction, is used because it concentrates the antibodies and reduces the chance of hypersensitivity. Antisera effectively treat such diseases as diphtheria, tetanus, and botulism poisoning caused by toxins. In addition, antisera can be produced against various venoms and then used in treating victims of bites by venomous animals. Passive immunity may also be used as a prophylactic (preventive) measure for high-risk persons who may have recently been exposed to an infection.

MEASUREMENT OF ANTIBODIES
AS A DIAGNOSTIC TOOL

The presence of humoral antibodies in someone's serum indicates that the person has either had a specific disease or has been immunized against that disease. Furthermore, the level of antibodies may give some indication as to how recently this person was exposed to the disease.

An analysis of the levels of specific antibodies present in the serum of a patient is an important diagnostic tool. In diagnosing an infectious disease, it is important to obtain a serum sample from the patient as early as possible, preferably during the first few days of illness. Called the *acute phase* serum, this sample should contain no or only low levels of antibodies against the microorganism causing the disease. Several weeks later a second serum sample should be taken. This is called a *convalescent phase* serum and should contain higher levels of antibodies against the disease-producing microorganisms (Figure 13-1). If the increase in antibody levels between the acute and the convalescent phase is significant, usually fourfold or greater, it is assumed that the disease was caused by the microorganism against which the antibodies were formed. Before this diagnostic test can be run, a pathogenic microorganism is needed to serve as the test antigen. Ideally this microorganism is isolated from the patient during the illness. If the signs and symptoms of the disease are compatible with the type of disease caused by the isolated pathogen, the diagnosis of the disease based on this evidence alone is fairly certain. If a specific rise in antibodies occurred against this pathogen, the diagnosis is confirmed. If no specific pathogen was isolated from the patient, however, the signs and symptoms of the disease might be consistent with a disease caused by any one of several different

Figure 13-1   The relationship between the period of illness and the time to collect acute and convalescent phase serum samples.

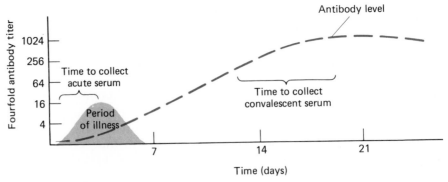

pathogens. Because diagnostic laboratories generally have commercially prepared antigens obtained from the more commonly encountered pathogens, a laboratory could be asked to determine the levels of antibodies in the acute and convalescent phase sera against many of the suspected pathogens. The pathogen against which a significant rise in antibody level is seen is assumed to cause the disease.

In other situations, it may be desirable to know if a person had previously had a specific disease. A woman in the early stages of pregnancy, for example, may have been exposed to rubella—a disease known to pose a serious threat to the developing fetus should the expectant mother become infected. It would be useful to know if the expectant mother had antibody immunity to rubella. In this case, the serum of the expectant mother could be tested for antibodies against rubella and then the course of action determined.

The analysis of amounts and types of antibodies has many applications in diagnostic medicine, epidemiology, and research work. The study of antigen and antibody reactions in vitro (in test tubes) is called *serology*. Some more commonly used methods of detecting and measuring antibodies and antigens are discussed in the following pages.

SEROLOGIC TESTS

Either a known antigen or a known antibody is needed for most serologic tests. Many routinely used antigens or antibodies (antisera) are available from commercial sources. If a known antigen is used, the serum samples can be tested to determine if they contain specific antibodies against this antigen. On other occasions, it may be necessary to identify an unknown antigen. Generally the antigen to be identified is a microorganism that cannot be completely identified by its physiologic or morphologic characteristics. This unknown microorganism is tested against known selected antisera; when specific reactions occur, a specific identification can be made.

The relative amount of antibodies in a serum sample is measured by determining the extent to which the serum can be diluted and still produce an observable antigen-antibody reaction. The term **titer** refers to this relative amount of antibodies. It is common to use either two-, four-, eight-, or ten-fold dilutions of serum in determining the antibody titer. If the last tube in which a detectable antigen-antibody reaction occurred was a dilution of 1:2456, for instance, then the antibody titer would be reported as 256.

Titer
the concentration of specific antibody present in the serum of an individual.

Agglutination Tests

Agglutination tests use whole cells or particles about the size of cells as antigens. When antibodies attach to the antigenic determinants on these cells or particles, they form bridges that result in aggregates of interconnected particles. Such aggregates or agglutinations are visible to the naked eye (Figure 13-2). Agglutination tests are used to detect antibodies against bacterial cells, to determine red blood cell types, and are also used in various artificially constructed tests. In the artificial tests, known antibodies or antigens are attached to small particles of latex or to tanned red blood cells. Such treated particles may then be used in agglutination tests to detect the corresponding antigen or antibody in test specimens.

Figure 13-2 Agglutination reactions.
(a) Agglutination of bacterial cells by IgG type antibodies. (b) Tube (top) and slide (bottom) agglutination reactions in four-fold dilutions of serum. The reaction is positive through a dilution of 1:256, therefore the titer is 256.

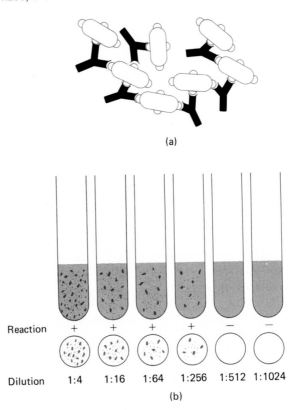

(a)

Reaction	+	+	+	+	−	−
Dilution	1:4	1:16	1:64	1:256	1:512	1:1024

(b)

Precipitation Tests

Precipitation tests use soluble antigens. The interaction of proper ratios of these antigens with specific antibodies results in a precipitation reaction. This reaction can best be visualized as a faint line that appears at the interface of a solution of antibodies and antigens. These tests are carried out in small-diameter tubes, known as **capillary tubes,** in which the antigen is layered over the antiserum. A ring of precipitation will be seen at the interface of the two solutions if specific antibodies and antigens are present. These tests are called *ring tests* and *capillary tube tests* (Figure 13-3a).

A convenient and widely used method of demonstrating precipitation reactions is by *immunodiffusion,* a procedure that is also called the *Ouchterlony* method (named after its discoverer). Solutions of specific antigens and antibodies are placed in adjacent wells that are formed in an agar gel. A line of precipitation occurs where the diffusing antigen and antibodies come together. This precipitated antigen-antibody complex becomes fixed in the agar and is readily visualized (Figures 13-3b, and c).

Capillary tube
a glass tube with a very small opening running through the tube. The opening is usually less than 1 mm in diameter.

Neutralization Tests

Neutralization tests use living microorganisms that are exposed to antibodies in test tubes. After the antibodies have had a chance to react with the antigens on the microbe—usually for a period of an hour or two—the mixture is inoculated into a suitable experi-

Figure 13-3   Precipitation (ppt.) reactions between antigens (Ag) and antibodies (Ab). (a) A precipitation reaction in a small diameter test tube. (b) Precipitation reaction in an agar gel. (c) Use of the agar gel method to identify unknown antigens that will react with a known antibody; in this case, antigen "C" is identified as the specific antigen.

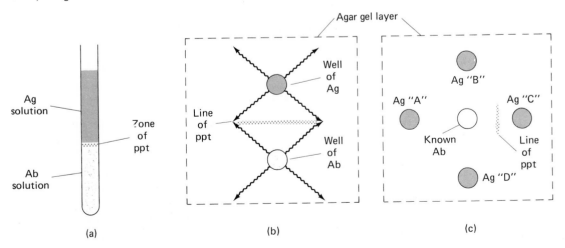

mental host. If the microorganism has reacted with specific antibodies, it will be unable to multiply in the host; that is, it is neutralized. This test is often used to identify viruses.

Complement Fixation Tests

Earlier it was noted that complement enters into a complex with certain antigen-antibody reactions (Chapter 12). Once complement has entered into this complex, it is not free to enter into a second reaction; that is, it is fixed. By finding out if the complement has become fixed, it is possible to determine if an antigen-antibody reaction has taken place. The steps of a complement fixation test are outlined in Figure 13-4.

If a serum sample is being analyzed by the complement fixation test for antibodies against a known antigen, it is first heated to 56° C for 30 minutes to destroy any residual complement that might be present. Next, the known antigen and a standard amount of complement are added to the serum. If the serum contains specific antibodies to the antigen, a complex of complement-antigen-antibody will form and the complement will be fixed. This reaction is not visible, however. Therefore an indicator system is used to tell if the reaction has occurred. The indicator system uses both a known antigen and a known antiserum. The antigen is sheep red blood cells and the antiserum contains antibodies against the sheep red blood cells. The sheep red blood cells and antiserum are added to the original test system; if a specific reaction did not occur in the original test, the complement is still available to complex with the indicator system, which results in the lysis (dissolving) of the red blood cells. This reaction is readily visible. If the sheep red blood cells do not lyse, it is assumed that the original reaction fixed the complement and so specific antibodies must have been present in the original serum. This is an indirect test for antibodies and adequate controls are needed to show that all components are working properly before any assumption can be made.

Fluorescent Antibody (FA) Tests

It is possible to conjugate (attach) certain fluorescent dyes to known antibodies. The antibodies can then be mixed with test microorganisms; if a specific reaction occurs, the antibodies, along with the fluorescent dye, will attach to the microbial antigens. This reaction is carried out on a microscope slide. When it is placed under a fluorescence microscope (Chapter 2), the areas where specific antigen-antibody reactions have occurred will fluoresce. Using this method (Figure 13-5), it is possible to identify a specific type of microbe in a mixed microbial population.

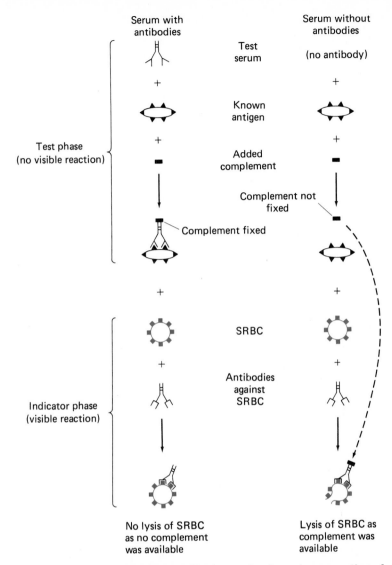

Figure 13-4   Complement [▬] fixation test using a known antigen [◁▷] to test serum for the presence of antibodies [人] against this Ag. This test shows the response of serum samples with and without specific Ab. The indicator phase of this test uses sheep red blood cells (SRBC). When complement becomes fixed in the test phase, it is then not available to form a complex with and cause lysis of the SRBC in the indicator phase of the test. Thus no lysis means the test is positive for the presence of antibodies in the original serum.

Hemagglutination Inhibition (HI) Tests

Hemagglutination inhibition tests, which are relatively simple to conduct, are useful in detecting antibodies against certain types of viral infections. Some viruses specifically attach to red blood

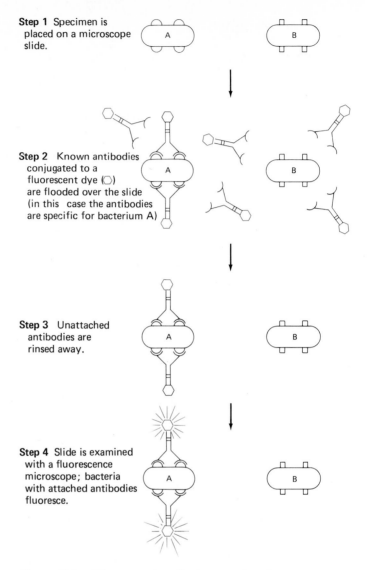

Step 1 Specimen is placed on a microscope slide.

Step 2 Known antibodies conjugated to a fluorescent dye (○) are flooded over the slide (in this case the antibodies are specific for bacterium A)

Step 3 Unattached antibodies are rinsed away.

Step 4 Slide is examined with a fluorescence microscope; bacteria with attached antibodies fluoresce.

Figure 13-5 Fluorescent antibody procedure for identification of a bacterium in a clinical specimen.

cells and cause the cells to agglutinate. This process is called *hemagglutination* and is a useful method for detecting the presence of such viruses. If coated with antibodies, the virus cannot cause hemagglutination. Thus, in the hemagglutination inhibition test the serum is reacted with a known virus and then the red blood cells are added. If specific antibodies are present in the serum, they will coat the virus and inhibit the occurrence of hemagglutination. If hemagglutination does not occur, the presence of antibodies is indicated.

Radioimmunoassay (RIA)

The RIA is a highly sensitive test that uses radioactive materials to detect small amounts of antigens and determine the quantitative amount of antigen in tissues, body fluids, or blood. Its primary use is in detecting hepatitis B antigens in blood collected for transfusion (Chapter 36). Although a very useful test, it does suffer from certain disadvantages: it is complex, requires expensive equipment, and uses radioactive materials. Specially equipped laboratories are usually required to run this test.

Enzyme-Linked Immunosorbent Assay (ELISA)

The ELISA test is nearly as sensitive as the RIA test, but it does not require radioactive materials and can be done with less elaborate equipment. It can be used to measure the amounts of either antigens or antibodies in a test sample. The procedure for detecting antibodies is shown in Figure 13-6. Here known antigen is ab-

Figure 13-6   Indirect ELISA test to detect antibodies in human serum.

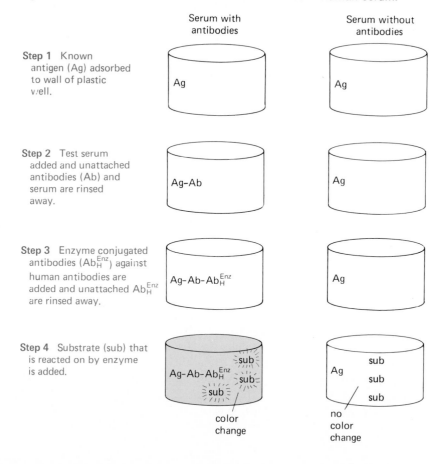

Serum with antibodies   Serum without antibodies

Step 1 Known antigen (Ag) adsorbed to wall of plastic well.

Ag   Ag

Step 2 Test serum added and unattached antibodies (Ab) and serum are rinsed away.

Ag–Ab   Ag

Step 3 Enzyme conjugated antibodies (Ab_H^{Enz}) against human antibodies are added and unattached Ab_H^{Enz} are rinsed away.

$Ag–Ab–Ab_H^{Enz}$ Ag

Step 4 Substrate (sub) that is reacted on by enzyme is added.

$Ag–Ab–Ab_H^{Enz}$ sub sub sub

color change

Ag sub sub sub

no color change

Conjugated

attached. Proteins to which a specific substance or molecule has been attached are said to be conjugated to the added molecule or substance.

sorbed onto the wall of wells in special plastic plates. Then serum to be tested for antibodies is added to the wells. If specific antibodies are present, they will attach to the absorbed antigen; the wells are then rinsed to remove all components of the serum except the attached antibodies. If the test serum is from humans, the next step would be to add specially prepared antibodies against human gamma globulin; these antibodies are produced in an animal such as a goat or rabbit. The antihuman antibodies are **conjugated** to an enzyme. These conjugated antibodies will react with the human antibodies that are attached to the absorbed antigen. The wells are again rinsed to remove any unattached enzyme-conjugated antibodies. Next, a substrate is added that will be acted on by the enzyme in such a way that a color is produced. The intensity of the color can be measured by a spectrophotometer or, less accurately, by the eye and is proportional to the amount of antibody that attached to the antigen. When all reagents are prepared, the ELISA test can be carried out in less than one hour. This test is very useful in applications where a rapid detection of antigens or antibodies is needed and it is adaptable to most routine serologic tests. It is used as the primary screening technique for diagnosis of AIDS.

MONOCLONAL ANTIBODIES

Monoclonal antibody

an antibody derived from a hybridoma clone of cells, which produces only one type of epitope.

Monoclonal antibodies are preparations of antibodies that are all specific for the same antigenic determinant (epitope). Such pure antibody preparations have many useful applications in various areas of medicine and research. It is not possible to produce preparations of pure antibodies in intact animals, for animals are invariably exposed to a variety of antigens and most antigens contain a variety of antigenic determinants. Thus animal serum will always contain a mixture of antibodies. Monoclonal antibodies are produced by cells growing in test tube (in vitro) cultures, using a unique procedure developed in the mid-1970s at Britain's Medical Research Council by Cesar Milstein and Georges Köhler. These researchers were able to fuse two types of cells together into a single cell called a **hybridoma.** The hybridoma cells are able to express properties of both parent cells. The two cells used to make monoclonal antibodies are a mouse tumor cell, called a *myeloma cell,* and an activated B cell from the spleen of an immunized mouse. The myeloma cell has the ability to grow indefinitely in a test tube but is not able to produce specific antibodies. The activated B cell can produce specific antibodies against a single antigenic determinant but cannot grow in a test tube; however, the myeloma–B cell hybridoma is able to grow indefinitely in test

Hybridoma

a cell that results from combining two cells together (hybrid). For preparation of monoclonal antibodies, one of the cells is a myeloma cell and the other is an activated B cell.

tubes and to produce antibodies. Once a hybridoma that is secreting antibodies against a known antigen is produced, massive cultures of this cell can be propagated and will, in turn, produce large amounts of the pure or monoclonal antibody. Often it is necessary to screen many hybridoma cells to find the one that is producing the desired specific antibody (Figure 13-7).

Figure 13-7   A schematic outline of a method used to produce monoclonal antibodies.

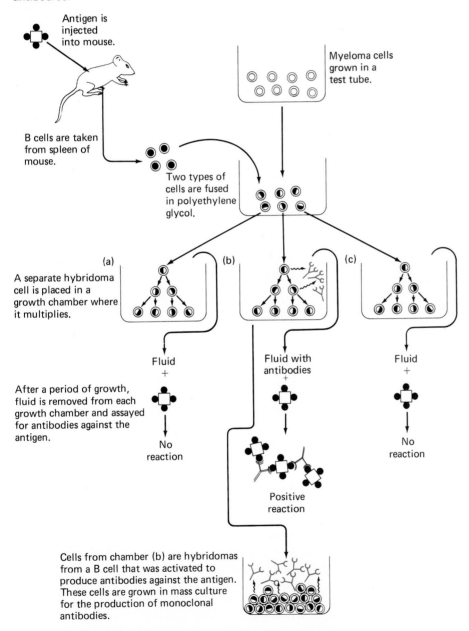

Antigen is injected into mouse.

Myeloma cells grown in a test tube.

B cells are taken from spleen of mouse.

Two types of cells are fused in polyethylene glycol.

(a)

(b)

(c)

A separate hybridoma cell is placed in a growth chamber where it multiplies.

After a period of growth, fluid is removed from each growth chamber and assayed for antibodies against the antigen.

Fluid
+

No reaction

Fluid with antibodies
+

Positive reaction

Fluid
+

No reaction

Cells from chamber (b) are hybridomas from a B cell that was activated to produce antibodies against the antigen. These cells are grown in mass culture for the production of monoclonal antibodies.

Immunization Practices in Colleges: United States, 1984–86

Outbreaks of vaccine-preventable diseases continue to occur in colleges. In 1985, 354 measles cases were reported on 26 college campuses. In 1986, the United States had a provisional total of 6273 measles cases; 174 (2.8%) of these occurred on 21 campuses. Despite longstanding primary school immunization requirements, 5% to 20% of college students still do not have documented immunity to measles and/or rubella.

In May 1983, the American College Health Association (ACHA) adopted a Preadmission Immunization Policy, recommending that, by September 1985, colleges and universities require all students to present documentation of immunity to measles, rubella, and other vaccine-preventable diseases as a prerequisite to matriculation or registration. Likewise, since 1980, the Immunization Practices Advisory Committee has recommended that college and university administrations strongly consider establishing such requirements. To evaluate implementation of these recommendations, a survey of 3606 colleges and universities was conducted jointly by the CDC and ACHA in the fall of 1984. The 1984 survey was conducted by state and local immunization program personnel in the ten Public Health Service regions. In eight of these regions,

data were obtained from more than 50% of colleges. In order to assess further progress, ACHA conducted a follow-up survey in the spring of 1986. For this survey, a questionnaire was mailed to the 3210 U.S. colleges and universities registered with ACHA or the American Council of Education.

In 1984, 16% of 1861 responding institutions required measles and rubella immunizations as a condition for attendance. Of the 3210 colleges surveyed in 1986, 1085 (34%) responded. Of those responding, 601 (55%) reported having a preadmission immunization requirement (PIR); 499 (45%) included both measles and rubella. In both surveys, there was considerable variation by region.

The 1984 survey did not collect information regarding enforcement of existing requirements; however, the 1986 survey did. Of the 601 colleges reporting a PIR, 305 (51%) placed a hold on first or second semester registration for noncompliers. Another 21% reported other sanctions including fines, withholding grades, suspension, and letters to the students or their parents from the Student Health Office or Dean's Office. Some prohibited dormitory residence, use of stu-

Because of their specificity for a single antigenic determinant, reactions between monoclonal antibodies and antigens are much more precise than those produced from the antisera of intact animals. Thus monoclonal antibodies are widely used in diagnostic kits to identify isolated microorganisms or detect antigens. Monoclonal antibodies are also useful for specific antiserum therapy against infectious diseases, toxins, and possibly some forms of cancer. In some applications, monoclonal antibodies are attached to specific drugs; when injected into a patient, the antibodies spe-

dent health services, or participation in clinical work by students training in health professions.

Colleges without a PIR were asked whether they considered such a program important and why they did not have one. Of 403 schools responding, 253 (63%) felt that a PIR was important. The majority (62%) cited their general policy of not instituting special entrance requirements as their reason for not having a PIR. Twenty-six percent replied that they did not have adequate personnel to administer a program. Lack of access to a computerized data storage system was mentioned by 27%. The major barriers to implementation seemed to involve procedures rather than disagreement concerning the importance of the recommendation.

In the 1986 survey, colleges and universities were also asked about their policy regarding education and vaccination against hepatitis B infection. Twenty-four percent of respondents had a policy recommending hepatitis B vaccine for certain high-risk groups. These high-risk groups included male homosexuals, nursing students, dental students, other health care students, and foreign students from endemic areas. The survey did not assess the overall representation of these groups in the responding colleges. In general, in the majority (> 90%) of responding institutions, all categories of students had to bear the cost of the vaccine.

Editorial note: During the past decade there has been a shift in focus at colleges and universities regarding the necessary content of a PIR. At first, the emphasis was on tetanus and diphtheria prophylaxis as well as tuberculosis skin testing. As campuses continued to experience measles and rubella outbreaks with their potential for significant morbidity and even mortality, colleges began requiring documentation of immunity to measles and rubella, as well as to mumps, diphtheria, tetanus, and poliomyelitis. The recent emphasis on hepatitis B infection and acquired immunodeficiency syndrome (AIDS) has led many health care professionals to recommend that colleges require hepatitis B vaccination for those at risk and provide students with information on AIDS. On May 30, 1986, the ACHA Council of Delegates passed a resolution recommending that colleges educate their students at high risk for hepatitis B concerning their need to be vaccinated (*MMWR* 36:209, 1987).

cifically attach to the pathogen or target tissue, which concentrates the effect of the drug against the target and minimizes its effect on normal tissues. Monoclonal antibodies are used in research work in which specific identification of components can be made by immune reactions. They are also used as "handles" to pluck a specific substance out of a mixture of chemicals. Today, monoclonal antibody procedures are being applied in many areas of medicine, research, and industry and represent a highly useful new technology.

CONCEPT SUMMARY

1. Several types of immunity are known and can generally be classified as either active or passive forms of immunity. Active immunity is the result of the individual's own production of antibody whereas passive immunity is based on the receipt of antibody produced by some other human or animal.

2. Numerous types of vaccine can be used to stimulate active immunity in humans. These vaccines depend on the presence of complete antigens found in the normal unaltered pathogen. The degree of immunity and the length of the immune state depend on the kind of vaccine used and the type of immunity made available.

3. The presence of antibody is determined by laboratory procedures known collectively as *serology*. There are many serologic tests. These tests are useful in determining the degree of immunity maintained by an individual. They are also helpful in determining the presence or absence of some disease states.

STUDY SUMMARY

1. The quality and length of immunity is usually much greater for natural active immunity than for other categories. What feature of this type of immunity accounts for this observation?

2. What developments in disease control have reduced the need for clinical use of artificial passive immunity?

3. Upon what premise is it possible to state that a rise in antibody titer to a specific microorganism correlates with diagnosis of a specific disease?

4. All of the serologic tests for antibody are similar in that they either test for the presence of antibody or antigen. These tests are possible because the reaction between antigens and antibodies is _____.

5. Explain why it is possible to use antibody to sheep red blood cells as an indicator of antigen-antibody interaction in the complement fixation test.

6. What is the function of the myeloma cell in developing monoclonal antibodies?

REFERENCES FOR FURTHER STUDY

1. *Microbiology,* B. Davis, 1969. Harper & Row.
2. *Basic Immunology and Its Medical Applications,* J. Barrett, 1980. Mosby.
3. *Microbiology for the Allied Health Professions,* A. Delaat, 1973. Lea & Febiger.
4. Vaccines against Encapsulated Bacteria. *Reviews of Infectious Diseases.* 9:176, 1987.

INTRODUCTION TO INFECTIOUS DISEASES

Disease reservoir
a natural source of a disease agent. Such reservoirs may be sick patients, asymptomatic carriers, recovered patients, or environmental sources.

V arious defense mechanisms of the host were described in preceding chapters. When functioning properly, these mechanisms are important in determining the outcome of the interactions between pathogenic microorganisms and the host. Some mechanisms that allow certain microorganisms to overcome or circumvent these defenses and then cause tissue damage are discussed in this chapter. The methods used to determine if a specific microbe is the cause of a disease are also discussed, and the format used in the following chapters for presenting the various infectious diseases of humans is introduced.

MICROBIAL PATHOGENICITY AND VIRULENCE

A great majority of the microorganisms found in nature are unable to grow in the human body and so cannot produce disease; they are the *saprophytic* microbes. Some microbes, however, possess mechanisms that enable them to produce disease; they are the *pathogens.* Some microbes cause diseases indirectly by producing *toxins* (poisons). These toxins may be produced by bacteria in foods that are eaten by the host. Most microbial diseases are categorized as *communicable (infectious),* which means that the microbe itself must be transmitted to the host. The source of the microbe may be another host or some nonliving **disease reservoir.** In order to be a successful pathogen of a communicable disease, a microorganism must be able to:

1. Survive passage from one host to another or from the reservoir to the host

2. Attach to or penetrate into the host's tissues

Table 14-1   Some Bacterial Virulence Factors

Virulence Factor	Characteristics	Bacteria or Example
Toxin	Endotoxin, lipopolysaccharide Gram-negative cell wall, heat-stable, pyrogenic	Gram-negative bacteria
	Exotoxin, polypeptide, antigenic highly toxic, toxoids formed	Diphtheria toxin
		Staphylococcal enterotoxin
		Tetanus neurotoxin
Enzyme	Protein, specific activity	Collagenase: *Clostridium*
		Coagulase: *Staphylococcus*
		Hyaluronidase: *Streptococcus*
Capsule	Polysacharide or polypeptide, antiphagocytic	*Haemophilus influenzae*
		Streptococcus pneumoniae
		Bacillus anthracis
Pili/Fimbriae	Attachment to host cells	*Neisseria gonorrhoeae*

3. Withstand (for a period of time) the host's defense mechanisms

4. Induce damage to or malfunction of the host's tissues

In some cases, the mechanisms of pathogenicity and virulence possessed by a pathogen are well characterized; at other times the processes by which a microbe causes disease are not well understood. Certain microbes vary in their ability to cause disease. Those with strong capabilities are highly virulent whereas those with weak capabilities are pathogens of low virulence. Table 14-1 lists some of the better known microbial virulence factors.

Microbial pathogenicity is a result of the functioning of one or more of the mechanisms discussed in the following pages.

Attachment

In order to infect a host, most microbes must first attach to a specific receptor site on a tissue of the host. Most microbes that lack the chemical groups that take part in this specific attachment are flushed or otherwise expelled from the body. This specificity, which is also called *trophism,* is determined by traits of both the host and the pathogen. The specificity of receptor sites may vary from organ to organ within the body of the host and from one host species to another. Thus, one infectious disease may involve only specific tissues or organs of the body whereas another dis-

Attachment site

the position at which an organism attaches itself to host tissues. This is usually determined by specific receptor sites on the host cell and pathogen.

ease may involve different tissues. Similarly, some animal species are highly susceptible to a given pathogen whereas another species is completely refractory to that same pathogen. The significance of specific **attachment sites** for the initiation of viral infections has been recognized for many years. Today it is recognized that specific tissue attachment is also important for the initiation of many bacterial infections.

Circumvention of Defense Mechanisms

Various mechanisms present in some bacteria increase their survival time in the host. One such mechanism is the ability to decrease the rate at which pathogens are phagocytized. Many bacteria possess *capsules* that block the attachment of the bacterial cell to phagocytic cells and thus interfere with phagocytosis; some pathogenic strains of staphylococci and streptococci secrete a substance called *leukocidin* that kills white blood cells before they can phagocytize the bacteria. Certain microbes are readily phagocytized but are able to withstand the destructive mechanisms functioning in nonstimulated macrophages: these microbes survive and may continue to multiply while inside the phagocyte. They may also be transported by the phagocyte to other tissues while being protected from antibodies and other antimicrobial substances in the body fluids.

An enzyme called *hyaluronidase* that breaks down hyaluronic acid is secreted by some pathogens. Hyaluronic acid is a substance that binds host cells together; therefore the production of hyaluronidase may aid the spread of the bacteria between cells of a tissue. Some bacteria possess enzymes called *fibrinolysins* that dissolve the fibrin clots that form part of the barrier of the inflammatory response. Such bacteria are less readily contained by the inflammatory reaction.

Most strains of *Staphylococcus aureus* possess a surface protein called *protein A.* Protein A interacts with the constant region of IgG molecules thereby pointing the reactive (variable) ends of the antibody molecules away from the bacterium which minimizes the effects of antibody immunity against staphylococci.

Induction of Tissue Damage or Malfunction

Stimulation of inflammatory responses   Certain bacteria stimulate vigorous inflammatory responses that, in turn, alter the function of the normal host tissues. *Streptococcus pneumoniae,* for example, a major cause of bacterial pneumonia, induces an acute inflammatory response in the lungs that results in a rapid accumulation of fluid **exudate.** These fluids interfere with the normal functions of the lungs. The tubercle bacillus induces a strong cell-mediated immune response that results in the formation of nod-

Exudate

a secretion from vessels that collects in body tissues and spaces, or from the tissues that is discharged outside the body.

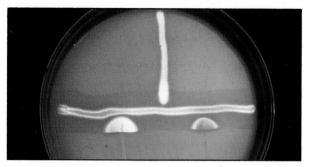

37. Positive (bottom) and negative (top) CAMP test (see Chap. 16). (Courtesy J. M. Matsen)

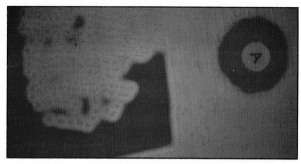

38. Positive bacitracin disk test for identification of group A *Streptococcus* (see Chap. 16). (Courtesy J. M. Matsen)

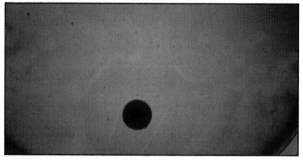

39. Positive optachin disk test for identification of *Streptococcus* pneumonia. (Courtesy J. M. Matsen)

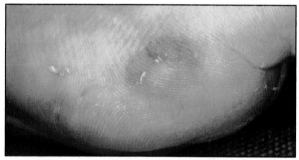

40. Streptococcal cellulitis of the foot. (Courtesy J. M. Matsen)

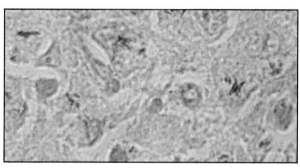

41. Acid fast bacilli (see Chap. 22) in the liver of patient with AIDS.

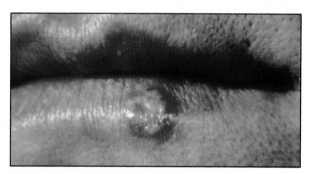

42. Herpes lesion (fever blister) on lip of patient (see Chap. 35).

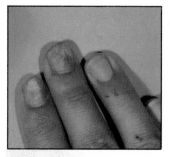

43. Fungal infection of fingernails.

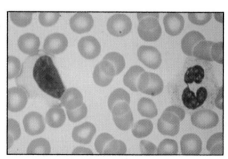

44. A typical lymphocyte in blood of patient with infectious mononucleosis (Wright's stain) (see Chap. 35).

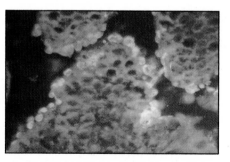

45. Positive indirect immunofluorescence test for antibodies to *Cryptosporidium* in infected mouse ileum (see Chap. 31). (Courtesy of P. N. Campbell and W. L. Current)

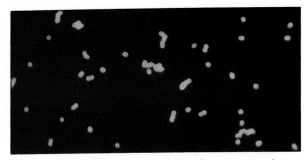

46. Fluorescent antibody test positive for streptococci.

47. Fluorescent antibody test for *Chlamydia* (see Chap. 28). Green particles are elementary bodies; infected cells are bright green.

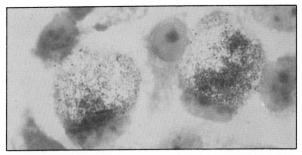

48. Giemsa stain of cells infected with *Chlamydia trachomatis* (see Chap. 28).

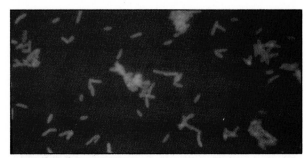

49. Fluorescent antibody test positive for *Legionella pneumophila*.

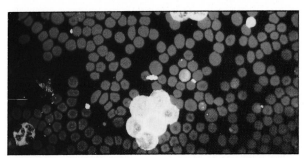

50. Immunofluorescent antibody test for feline leukemia virus antigens in white blood cells of cat. Feline leukemia is a retrovirus similar to human immune deficiency virus (see Chap. 41). (Courtesy W. Hardy, Jr.)

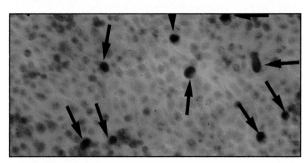

51. Iodine stained inclusion bodies produced in cells infected with *Chlamydia trachomatis*.

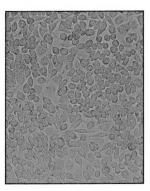

52. Hamster cells in culture.

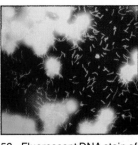

53. Fluorescent DNA stain of a spiral-shaped *Mycoplasma (Spiroplasma)* (see Chap. 27). (Courtesy G. J. McGarrity and T. Steiner)

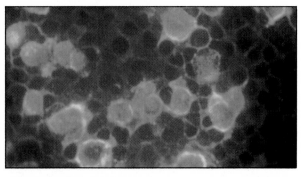

54. Immunofluorescent stain of virus infected cells in cell culture (see Chap. 32).

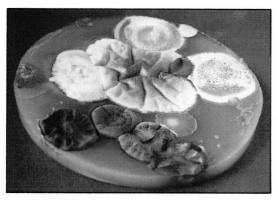

55. Unidentified fungi and actinomycete colonies growing on nutrient agar. (Courtesy K. F. Bott)

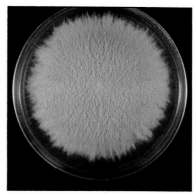

56. Colony of dermatophyte mold (see Chap. 30).

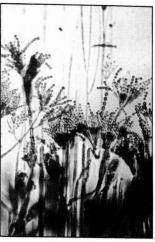

57. Photomicrograph of *Penicillium* species (see Chap. 30). (Courtesy *Laboratory Medicine*, vol. 18, no. 3)

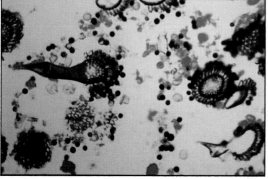

58. Silver stain of lung tissue infected with *Aspergillus* (see Chap. 30). (Courtesy of *Laboratory Medicine*, vol. 17, no. 2)

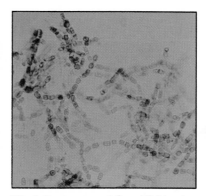

59. Arthrospores of *Coccidioides immitis* (see Chap. 30).

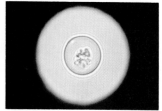

60. *Cryptococcus neoformans* (see Chap. 30) from an India ink preparation.

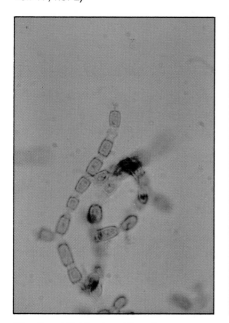

61. *Coccidioides immitis* arthrospores.

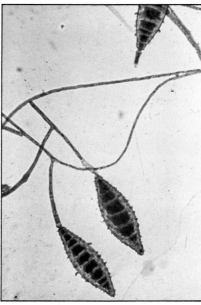

62. Macroconidia of mold dermatophyte.

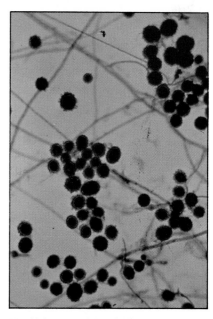

63. Unique conidia of *Histoplasma capsulatum* (see Chap. 30).

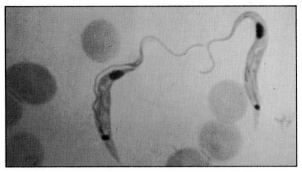

64. Giemsa stain of *Trypanosoma brucei* (see Chap. 31). (Courtesy American Society for Microbiology)

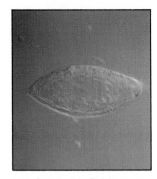

65. Ovum of *Schistosoma haematobium* from urine of infected patient. (Courtesy R. Barlow and T. Minnick)

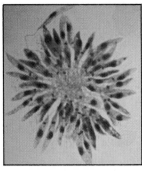

66. Aging *peishmania tropica* (see Chap. 31) grown in artificial culture. (Courtesy R. Barlow and T. Minnick)

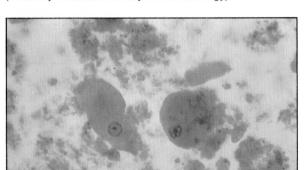

67. Trichrome stain of fecal specimen containing *Entamoeba histolytica* (see Chap. 31).

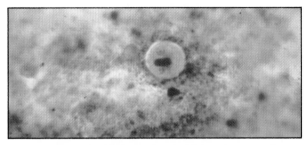

68. *Entamoeba histolytica* stained with iron hematoxylin.

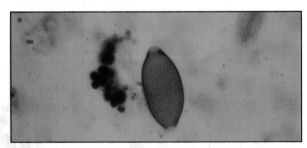

69. Iodine stain of fecal specimen containing egg of *Trichuris trichiura*.

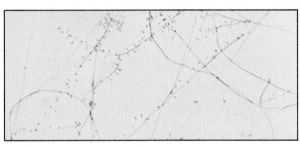

70. Microconidia along hyphae of safranin stained mold.

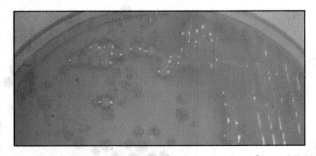

71. *Klebsiella* colonies on MacConkey agar (see Chap. 24).

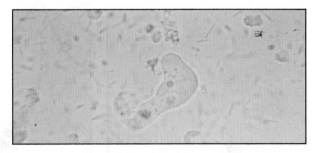

72. Wet, unstained fecal preparation containing *Entamoeba histolytica* trophuzoite.

(We are most appreciative to the Centers for Disease Control Atlanta, for use of the following figures: 3, 5, 9, 11, 12, 15, 19, 25–33, 42, 47, 49, 51, 54, 56, 59, 61–63, 67–70, 72.)

ules of scar tissue and eventually causes the destruction of normal lung tissue.

Secretion of enzymes   Various enzymes secreted by certain pathogenic bacteria are thought to contribute to the disease process by destroying tissues. *Collagenase* and *lecithinase* are enzymes produced by the bacteria that cause gas gangrene. These enzymes break down tissue fibers and cell membranes and probably contribute to the cell destruction associated with gangrene. *Hemolysins* are enzymes that destroy red blood cells. They are produced by several different pathogenic bacteria. The direct contribution of hemolysin, lipase, or nuclease, if any, to pathogenicity is not known. *Lipases* and *nucleases* are bacterial enzymes that break down fats and nucleic acids.

Production of toxins   Some microbes produce toxins that are important mechanisms in the production of diseases. There are two general categories of toxins, *exotoxins* and *endotoxins*. Exotoxins are proteins that are secreted from the bacterial cell into the surrounding medium. Endotoxins are part of the cell wall and only small amounts may escape into surrounding fluids from living bacteria. Greater amounts of endotoxin are released when the bacteria die and their cell walls disintegrate. The two types of toxins differ markedly in potency and functions.

Exotoxins are extremely powerful biological poisons. The botulism food-poisoning toxin is the most powerful chemical toxin known. It has been estimated that 1 mg of purified tetanus toxin could kill 100 million mice. The action of exotoxins on the host is highly specific, often involving a single essential chemical reaction in the host's tissues. Examples of this specificity are the botulism and tetanus toxins that specifically interfere with the transmission of nerve impulses, and diphtheria toxin that specifically inhibits protein synthesis by preventing the elongation of the polypeptide chain during the process of translation. The actions of the exotoxins are covered in greater detail later in this text when the specific diseases are discussed. Exotoxins can be converted into toxoids that are used as vaccines to stimulate specific antitoxin immunity against the toxin. These **antitoxins** readily neutralize the toxins and play an important role in recovery, treatment, and immunity against diseases caused by exotoxins. Fortunately, most exotoxins are readily destroyed by heat, an important factor in reducing the number of outbreaks of botulism food poisoning.

Endotoxins possess characteristics that differ considerably from those of the exotoxins. Endotoxins are less potent and larger amounts are needed to induce disease symptoms. Their effects on the host are general, producing such clinical signs and symptoms as fever, diarrhea, and circulatory disturbances, including **shock.** Endotoxins are composed of complexes of proteins, polysaccha-

Antitoxin
antibody produced in response to a toxin or toxoid. Antitoxin-toxin interactions usually inactivate the toxin.

Shock
a marked, sudden depression of physiologic function, such as blood pressure, that is often life-threatening.

Table 14-2   Comparison of Characteristics of Exotoxins and Endotoxins

Characteristics	Exotoxins	Endotoxins
Potency	High	Low
Effects on cells	Specific	Nonspecific
Stability to heat	Labile (inactivated at 60° to 80° C)	Stable (resists 120° C for 1 hour)
Forms toxoids	Yes	No
Composition	Proteins	Protein lipopolysaccharide complexes

rides, and phospholipids. They cannot be converted into toxoids and are highly resistant to inactivation by heat. The endotoxins are found primarily in the cell walls of Gram-negative bacteria whereas exotoxins are produced by both Gram-positive and Gram-negative bacteria.

Exotoxins can cause disease even when the producing bacterium is restricted to a relatively superficial tissue, such as mucosal epithelium. Or, as in the case of food poisoning, exotoxin production may occur remote from the host. In contrast, endotoxins generally affect the host when they are released following the death and destruction of large numbers of Gram-negative bacilli that may be infecting the tissues. Endotoxins undoubtedly contribute significantly to the pathogenesis of many diseases caused by Gram-negative bacteria. It is possible to reproduce some disease symptoms in a host by injecting purified endotoxins. Occasionally endotoxin-contaminated intravenous fluids have inadvertently been infused into a patient, resulting in serious reactions, including shock. This situation can even occur in fluids that have been sterilized in an autoclave, for endotoxins are not readily destroyed by heat. Exotoxin and endotoxin characteristics are summarized in Table 14-2.

DETERMINING THE ETIOLOGIC AGENT

The mere presence of a microorganism in a lesion or diseased tissue is not sufficient to prove that this microbe is the cause (etiologic agent) of the disease. This problem was recognized early in the study of infectious diseases by Robert Koch, who developed criteria to be used to incriminate a suspected microbe as the etiologic agent of a given disease. These criteria, known as *Koch's postulates*, are as follows:

1. The suspected microorganism must be found routinely in hosts with the disease.

2. The microorganism must be isolated from the host and grown in pure culture.

3. When microbes from the pure culture are inoculated into a healthy susceptible host, they must be able to cause the same disease.

4. The microorganism must next be recovered from the experimentally infected host.

Koch's postulates have served as useful criteria in establishing the etiology of many distinct infectious diseases. Nevertheless, the etiologic role of certain microbes in more subtle diseases—particularly those caused by the synergistic reaction of several microbes or factors and those produced in compromised hosts by opportunist microbes—has not been as readily demonstrated by these criteria.

HOST FACTORS

This chapter has primarily focused on the microorganism as a cause of infectious diseases, while Chapters 11 and 12 focused on the response (immunologic processes) of the host to challenges from its environment. It should be self-evident that whether or not a microorganism is able to infect or cause disease in any host depends on a balance reflecting all host protective mechanisms and all organism virulence factors. If this balance favors the host, infection may not occur or, if it does, the ultimate outcome will favor the host. On the other hand, if the balance favors the microorganism, disease is assured and death may be an outcome.

The miracles of modern medicine have had profound effect on the host-parasite relationship. The great plagues of the past such as cholera, diphtheria, dysentery, and tuberculosis have largely yielded to the efforts of medical science. Improvements in diagnosis, therapy, and prevention have relegated many former leading causes of death such as smallpox, yellow fever, and plague to historical interest. Although some of these diseases still occur, the frequency of occurrence is rare and the outcome is usually favorable. The question might be asked, If science has had such great success in preventing and curing microbial disease, what need is there for a continuing interest in medical microbiology?

The answer to this question is not so much in terms of the microbe, as in terms of the human host. Today by far the majority of serious infectious diseases are nosocomial (hospital-associated). These diseases often occur in patients who have, by past medical standards, undergone heroic medical procedures. While such procedures have preserved the lives of many patients, they have also

Toxic Shock Syndrome Following Influenza: Oregon, 1986
Update on Influenza Activity: United States, 1986

Oregon. A case of toxic shock syndrome (TSS) following influenza has been reported.

On December 11, 1986, a 13-year-old white female with fever, hypotension, and acute respiratory failure was seen at an Oregon hospial. Pertinent findings on physical examination yielded a temperature of 39° C (102° F); blood pressure of 60/0; evidence of upper airway obstruction; and conjunctival, palatal, and lingual hyperemia. A chest radiograph at the time of admission showed a bilateral increase in lung markings consistent with a diagnosis of early adult respiratory distress syndrome.

During the 24 hours following admission, the patient developed a diffuse, erythematous, sunburnlike rash and watery diarrhea. She required both intravenous fluids and vasopressors and treatment of severe hypotension. A diagnosis of toxic shock syndrome was considered and was supported by laboratory findings of thrombocytopenia (70,000/mm^3), renal insuffiency (creatinine level = 2.8 mg/dl, urea nitrogen level = 40 mg/dl), hypocalcemia (Ca = mg/dl), and elevated levels of creatine kinase (12,000 U/L) and aspartate aminotransse (367 U/L). *Staphylococcus aureus* was isolated from two tracheal aspirates obtained the day of admission. Other studies, including vaginal cultures, blood cultures, and urine oxygen testing, were negative for pathogenic organisms.

Although the patient's menstrual cycle had begun 6 days before admission, she had not used tampons or other intravaginal devices and was not sexually active. However, she had a history of a 4-day prodrome of an influenzalike illness consisting of fever (temperature = 40° C [104° F]), malaise, myalgias, sore throat, and substernal chest discomfort.

The patient was discharged following a 10-day hospitalization. On a follow-up examination 20 days after admission, full thickness desquamation of the palms and soles was noted. Testing of acute- and convalescent-phase sera revealed a rise in hemagglutination-inhibition antibody titer to influenza A (H1N1) from 32 on December 13 to 1024 at the time of her follow-up examination on December 31.

United States. Outbreaks of type A (H1N1) influenza activity are continuing. For the week ending January 31, six western states and Puerto Rico reported widespread outbreaks of influenzalike illness, and 19 states and the District of Columbia reported regional outbreaks of influenzalike illness. This is the sixth week with more than 20 states reporting outbreak activity. The level of current activity is below the peak of the previous winter when 37 states reported outbreaks for 1 week in February.

Editorial note: This 13-year-old girl's illness meets the case definition for TSS, which is caused by toxin-producing *S. aureus* in a susceptible host. The temporal relation between the child's illness and menstruation is most likely coincidental since no *S. aureus* was isolated from the vagina. The *S. aureus* isolated from the tracheal aspirates is the most likely cause of TSS in this patient. TSS associated with *S. aureus* respiratory infections has been reported previously. TSS following influenza was first reported last year during an epidemic of influenza type B. This is the first case of TSS following influenza reported to CDC this year and the first case reported following influenza type A (H1N1).

The occurrence of TSS following influenza may be coincidental, but *S. aureus* pneumonia as a complication of influenza is well documented. Physicians are encouraged to obtain cultures and serologies for influenza in cases of TSS following influenzalike illness or during influenza epidemics (*MMWR* 36:64, 1987).

left the patients highly vulnerable to infection by the microflora of the hospital environment. Such infections (pneumonia, wound and urinary tract infection, and bacteremia) would likely not have occurred without attendant compromise of host defenses. In addition to these nosocomial infections, there have been a variety of community-acquired infectious diseases that are based on changes in the normal host immune state—diseases such as *Pneumocystis* pneumonia, Legionnaires' disease, AIDS, *Mycobacterium avium* infections, tuberculosis, and diarrhea due to crytosporidium. These appear to be the plagues of the present and future. They are the diseases that have filled the void left by their departed predecessors and for which we again turn to the science of microbiology in hopes of finding a cure.

A STUDY OF INFECTIOUS DISEASES

The following chapters present an overall view of many diseases of humans that are caused by microorganisms. The various diseases are discussed according to the taxonomic categories of the causative microorganism. It is felt that this approach provides a concise coverage of the subject. Diseases caused by bacteria are described first, followed by fungal, protozoal, and viral diseases. The section on bacterial diseases starts with diseases caused by the Gram-positive cocci, followed by the diseases caused by Gram-negative cocci, spirochetes, acid-fast bacilli, and Gram-positive and Gram-negative bacilli. DNA-containing viruses appear first in the section on viral diseases and are followed by the RNA-containing viruses. In the discussions of infectious diseases, emphasis is given to the mechanisms of disease production (pathogenesis), clinical characteristics, and modes of transmission, treatment, and prevention—that is, those concepts of greatest concern to paramedical personnel who are directly involved in patient care. Less emphasis is given to the detailed methods used by microbiologists in the diagnostic laboratory.

Each of the following chapters covers the diseases caused by a single genus or by a group of related microorganisms. The coverage of most diseases includes the following general sections:

1. *Causative microbe.* This section contains a brief description of some general morphological and physiological properties of the microorganisms, along with information on classification when appropriate.

2. *Pathogenesis and clinical diseases.* This section includes a discussion of the mechanisms whereby the microbe is able to cause diseases and the types of clinical diseases resulting from the infection.

3. *Transmission and epidemiology.* In this section the mode of transmission and the relationship of various factors in influencing the distribution and frequency of diseases in various human populations are discussed.

4. *Diagnosis.* This section describes the general procedures used to identify a given disease in a patient.

5. *Treatment.* The responses of the infection to the various chemotherapeutic agents, antitoxins, or other medications are discussed here.

6. *Prevention and control.* This section describes the various methods used to prevent or reduce the amount of contact with infectious agents. The use of vaccines and preventive (prophylactic) treatments where applicable is also discussed.

7. *Clinical notes.* Following the discussion of many topics throughout the text, a report on an actual occurrence of a specific medical problem is given. These notes are largely taken from the U.S. Department of Health, Education and Welfare/Public Health Service publication called the *Morbidity and Mortality Weekly Report (MMWR).* This document is published weekly by the Centers for Disease Control (CDC) in Atlanta, Georgia. Along with the selected case reports, *MMWR* gives a weekly update on the rate of various diseases in the different states. The clinical notes presented in this textbook were selected to demonstrate current problems encountered with infectious diseases. They are also selected to help amplify and show applications of some concepts related to the epidemiology, treatment, diagnosis, or control of these diseases. In some cases, the reports have been modified from the original in order to make them more understandable to the introductory student or simply to reduce their length. Some of the clinical notes in the early chapters were written by the authors and relate to clinical application of microbial concepts and practice.

CONCEPT SUMMARY

1. Characteristics that endow a microorganism with virulence and facilitate its survival in the host, leading to pathogenicity, are those characteristics that permit the organism to withstand the host defenses, maintain residence in the host, and produce factors damaging to host tissue.

2. Bacterial virulence factors include the production of exotoxins, endotoxins, and enzymes. These substances circumvent

the host defense mechanisms and produce tissue damage, resulting in disease.

3. The application of Koch's postulates has resulted in the determination of the etiology of infectious diseases.

STUDY SUMMARY

1. Prepare a list of characteristics that are known to increase microbial virulence.

2. Why are antitoxins effective in protecting against exotoxic diseases, but have little role in protection against endotoxin?

3. Write a paragraph that explains the rationale for acceptance of Koch's postulates.

4. Describe the relationships between a potential host and its microbial environment.

REFERENCES FOR FURTHER STUDY

1. *Microbes, Man and Animals,* A. Linton, 1982. Wiley.

2. *The Biologic and Clinical Basis of Infectious Diseases,* 3rd ed., G. Youmans, 1985. Saunders.

3. *Principles and Practice of Infectious Diseases,* G. Mandell, 1985. Wiley.

4. The Role of Immune Complexes in the Pathogenesis of Bacterial Infections. *Annual Review of Microbiology* 39:475, 1985.

STAPHYLOCOCCI

Blood agar
agar to which blood was added
before the agar solidified.

S taphylococci are perhaps the best examples of parasites that have great pathogenic potential, yet are able to live in symbiotic balance with their hosts. In spite of their ability to produce serious, life-threatening diseases, pathogenic staphylococci are present on the skin or mucous membranes of all humans. Generally they act as opportunists, causing infections only in damaged tissues. These infections may be serious, and hospital-acquired staphylococcal diseases are recognized as a major problem. The prevention and control of these infections depend on the combined efforts of all hospital personnel.

BACTERIA

The spherical-shaped bacterium called *staphylococcus aureus* is the causative agent of a wide variety of human infections. Many strains, with varying degrees of virulence, exist and are frequently carried on the skin, in the nose, and around the rectum of healthy persons. These bacterial cells are about 1 μm in diameter, and usually occur in grapelike clusters (Figure 15-1), a characteristic that provided the basis for their name (Greek *staphyle* = bunch of grapes). This bacterium is facultatively anaerobic, non-spore-forming, and some strains have notable capsules. **Blood agar** is the medium generally used for its isolation from infected tissues; however, most common media will support its growth. *S. aureus* produces round, raised, opaque colonies that often have a golden-yellow (aureus) color. The golden color is the result of the production of a lipid pigment contained in the organism. The morphology of staphylococci is shown in Figure 15-1. *S. aureus* is differentiated from other staphylococci by its ability to clot plasma; this species secretes an enzyme called *coagulase*, which activates the clotting mechanism of normal plasma. Staphylococci that do not secrete coagulase are of low virulence and are currently classified into 19 species. The most ubiquitous coagu-

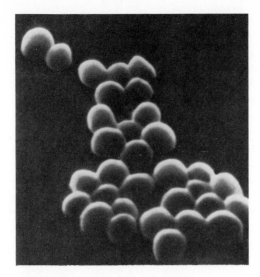

Figure 15-1   Scanning electron micrograph of a staphylococcus showing the characteristic cluster arrangement (magnification 8000×). (A. S. Klainer and I Gies, *Agents of Bacterial Disease.* Harper & Row: Hagerstown, MD, 1973. Figure 12a, p. 18.)

lase-negative species is *S. epidermidis,* a common human skin commensal. Two of the coagulase-negative staphylococci, *S. epidermidis* and *S. saprophyticus,* are responsible for human disease.

STAPHYLOCOCCAL DISEASES

Pathogenesis and Clinical Diseases

Several features contribute to the difficulty often encountered in controlling and treating staphylococcal infections. *S. aureus* is widespread, being found on the tissues of many healthy individuals (from 30% to 50% of the population at any given time). It is very stable, surviving for months when dried in pus or other body fluids, and it is more resistant to common disinfectants than most other vegetative bacteria. Genetic traits are readily transferred between strains of *S. aureus* by plasmids and phages (Chapter 6). This has led to the emergence of many strains that are resistant to commonly used antibiotics.

Although most strains of *S. aureus* are of relatively low virulence and usually harmless when restricted to the superficial layers of intact skin, they are often able to cause infection once they

Suppuration

an accumulation of white blood cells resulting in the formation of pus.

Enterotoxins

exotoxins produced by a variety of bacteria that are absorbed through the intestinal mucosa. Most such toxins cause nausea, vomiting, and/or diarrhea.

gain entry into damaged skin or deeper body tissues. The staphylococci are prime examples of *pyogenic* (pus-producing) bacteria. Infections due to these organisms are characterized by **suppuration** and localized inflammation. *Staphylococcus* is the first of four such groups of pyogenic cocci including *Streptococcus pyogenes, S. pneumoniae* and *Neisseria* that will be presented. The pathogenicity of *S. aureus* appears to be associated with the production of various enzymes and toxins and includes such substances as hemolysins, coagulase, leukocidin, hyaluronidase, and a fibrinolysin. Some *S. aureus* secrete a toxin called *exfoliatin* that causes the peeling of superficial skin layers of infected persons. About 50% of the strains of *S. aureus* may secrete any of several **enterotoxins** that cause acute intestinal symptoms (food poisoning) when ingested in contaminated foods. The presence of protein A on virulent staphylococci may protect them from antibodies. The sites of the major staphylococcal infections of humans are shown in Figure 15-2.

Figure 15-2   The sites of the major staphylococcal infections of humans.

A— Tissues where *S. Aureus* are often found but do not normally cause disease

Diseases that may be caused by *S. Aureus* are:
B— Pimples and impetigo
C— Boils and carbuncles on any surface area
D— Wound infections and abscesses
E— Spread to lymph nodes and to blood (septicemia), resulting in widespread seeding
F— Osteomyelitis
G— Endocarditis
H— Meningitis
I— Enteritis and enterotoxin (food poisoning)
J— Nephritis
K— Respiratory infections:
  Pharyngitis
  Laryngitis
  Bronchitis
  Pneumonia

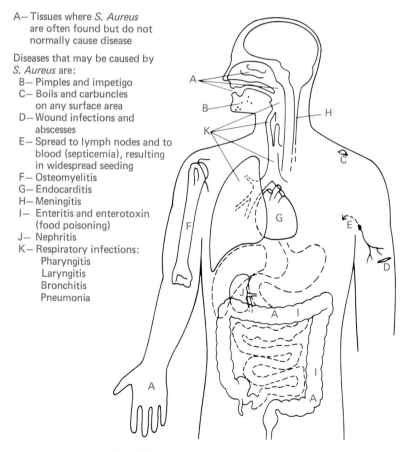

Superficial infections   Even though staphylococci are able to infect all tissues of the body, the most common infections are of the superficial tissues. *S. aureus* is a common cause of boils, carbuncles, impetigo (Figure 15-3), and infections of surgical or accidental wounds and burns. Characteristically these infections form an abscess, a localized lesion with a cavity of destroyed (necrotic) tissue filled with pus (suppuration). Scar tissue forms on healing. These infections are usually treated with topical antibiotics or, if abscesses are present, by surgical drainage of the pus. In otherwise healthy individuals, these infections tend to resolve without serious consequences.

Systemic infections   Various forms of trauma resulting around a superficial abscess, such as squeezing a boil, may force large numbers of staphylococci into the blood where they are carried to many tissues of the body, thus causing **systemic** infection. If this situation occurs, the body's natural defenses may not be able to cope with the bacteria, and abscesses may develop in various deep organs, such as the liver, lung, or brain tissue. Such infections are always serious and are often life-threatening. The presence of bacteria in the blood is called *bacteremia* or, more commonly, blood poisoning, and is a condition associated with a high mortality. *S. aureus* may settle in the lungs to cause **pneumonia,** or in the pelvis of the kidneys to cause pyelonephritis. In young children the staphylococci have a tendency to infect the bone, causing *osteomyelitis.* Osteomyelitis is frequently a long-term chronic disease. If

Systemic
pertaining to the whole body. Systemic infections are not localized to one area of the body but are carried throughout the host, usually through the bloodstream.

Pneumonia
a condition in which a fluid exudate collects in the air spaces of the lung.

Figure 15-3   Impetigo caused by a staphylococcus. This is an infection of the skin most often occurring in children. (Courtesy Centers for Disease Control, Atlanta)

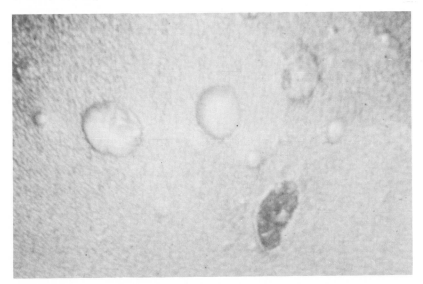

untreated it may lead to loss of bone function or even death. When present in bone joint spaces the disease is *septic arthritis*. When staphylococci infect the heart chambers or valves, the disease is called *endocarditis*. When they infect the meningeal tissues that line the central nervous system, it is called *meningitis*, and so on. Both endocarditis and meningitis are serious life-threatening infections.

Toxic Shock syndrome and scalded skin syndrome   *Toxic shock syndrome* usually begins suddenly with high fever, vomiting, and diarrhea. In some cases, sore throat, headache, muscle aches, shock, kidney failure, and a red skin rash may be seen. Patients frequently shed the skin from their hands and feet after recovery. Without prompt supportive treatment, death may result. This syndrome was first recognized when a sharp increase in the number of cases was reported in the late 1970s and 1980. Intensive epidemiologic studies demonstrated that most cases occurred in females during or immediately after their menstrual period, and that most cases (99%) were assocaited with the use of superabsorbent tampons. Staphylococci that produced the enterotoxin TSST-1 were found in high concentrations in the vaginal canal of affected females. It is now theorized that the introduction of superabsorbent tampons in the late 1970s created a condition in a small percentage of users that permitted the excessive growth of toxin-producing staphylococci. Once this association was recognized, the use of such tampons was discouraged and the number of cases of toxic shock syndrome greatly decreased (Figure 15-4). Some nonvaginal cases occur in both men and women. The organisms involved are characteristic of other staphylococci but are also noted to have slower growth rates and to produce small colonies. The toxin has been well studied and is now referred to as toxic shock syndrome toxin-1 (TSST-1).

Infections of infants or young children with exfoliatin-producing strains of *S. aureus* may cause a condition termed *scalded skin syndrome*. Wide areas of skin become denuded and have the appearance of scalded skin; this syndrome may be fatal, but is usually benign. Most patients are only moderately ill and recover uneventfully.

Food poisoning   Food poisoning is not an infection but an intoxication resulting from the ingestion of food containing preformed staphylococcal enterotoxin. During the preparation of foods it is very easy for the food handler to seed the food with staphylococci from his nose or from a skin lesion. If this food is not properly cooled and refrigerated at 4°C, the staphylococci may multiply and release enterotoxin. Enough enterotoxin may be produced in 2 to 6 hours to cause severe symptoms. Foods that are not cooked after preparation—for example, potato salads and cream pies—are

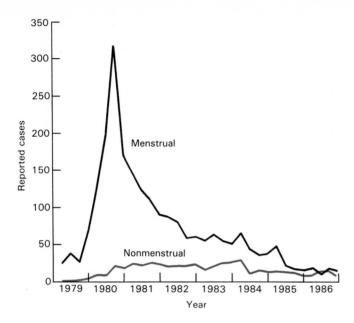

Figure 15-4   Reported cases of toxic-shock syndrome in the United States, 1979 to 1987.

common sources of this type of food poisoning. Staphylococci also reproduce rapidly in cooked meats. Their ability to grow at relatively high (9%) salt concentrations makes cured and salted meats, such as ham, special concerns. Enterotoxin is fairly stable to heat and is not destroyed in foods that are cooked at moderate temperatures after the toxin has been formed. Such symptoms as severe nausea, vomiting, abdominal pain, diarrhea, and prostration may begin to occur as early as 2 hours after ingesting the toxin. Complete recovery generally occurs within a day or two. A number of enterotoxins are produced by *S. aureus*. These are designated A through E and produce similar symptoms. Enterotoxin F has been shown to be TSST-1, the toxin responsible for toxic shock syndrome.

Other staphylococcal infections   The coagulase-negative staphylococci are not as virulent as *S. aureus* and are responsible for many fewer infections. However, two of these organisms, *S. epidermidis* and *S. saprophyticus* are becoming increasingly common causes of human infection. *S. epidermidis* is the most common cause of infections in patients with implanted **prosthetic** (artificial) devices such as heart valves and artificial joints. It is also commonly found in intravenous catheters and feeding lines used in seriously ill patients. *S. saprophyticus* looks very much like *S. epidermidis* but is resistant to the antibiotic, novobiocin. This organism has become a relatively frequent cause of urinary tract infection in sexually active young women.

Prosthetic device

a manufactured substitute for a failed body structure, e.g. artificial knee joint, or heart valve. Other long-term artificial materials that may be implanted for a variety of reasons are also referred to as prosthetic devices.

Transmission and Epidemiology

Because all humans are intermittent carriers of *S. aureus,* sources of infections are often difficult to determine. In many cases, the source may be autogenous; that is, it originates with the patient. A burn on the hand, for example, could become infected from bacteria carried on the patient's own skin or in his nose. Spreading from person to person may occur by direct or indirect contact. Medical personnel who work with patients with staphylococcal infections must use good aseptic procedures to avoid transmitting staphylococci to other patients. Nurses or physicians who are carriers or who have skin lesions may unwittingly infect patients. Care must be taken that the hands of medical personnel or that contaminated instruments do not spread *S. aureus* from one patient to another.

Because many strains of staphylococci are widespread, specific identification methods are needed to distinguish among different strains when tracing the route of transmission of an infection. A laboratory procedure called *phage typing* is used to make this distinction (Figure 15-5). **Phages** are viruses that attack and destroy only specific host strains of bacteria (Chapter 32). By using

Phage
a bacterial virus. Bacterial viruses require specific host cell receptors.

Figure 15-5 Phage typing of *Staphylococcus aureus.* The agar plate was first inoculated with a pure culture of *S. aureus* so as to form a complete layer of bacteria. A suspension of each test phage was dropped on its designated location (indicated by number). Clearing resulted where the phage destroyed the bacterium. In this example, the test bacterium was susceptible to phages, 6, 47, 53, 81, and 83. (Courtesy Centers for Disease Control, Atlanta)

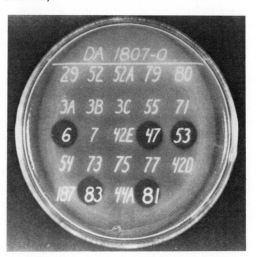

a series of staphylococcal phages against the staphylococci isolated from a given environment, it is possible to determine which staphylococci are identical to or different from the strain isolated from a lesion or from foods. Different staphylococcal strains have different patterns of resistance and susceptibility to the phages used (see clinical notes). Some isolates of *S. aureus* cannot be typed by this procedure, and none of the coagulase-negative staphylococci are susceptible to the phages used.

Diagnosis

Diagnosis of staphylococcal infection is generally based on the isolation of the organism from a lesion or other site of infection. *S. aureus* on blood agar plates will produce a zone of clear **hemolysis** around its typical golden-yellow colony; *S. epidermidis* and *S. saprophyticus* are rarely hemolytic and produce white colonies. The pathogenic strains of *S. aureus* are coagulase-positive. These characteristics of *S. aureus,* along with its ability to ferment mannitol, are used to differentiate it from the ever-present coagulase-negative staphylococci. Some *S. aureus* produce white colonies; thus colony pigmentation is not a dependable characteristic for identifying this bacterium.

Hemolysis
the breaking of blood cells. Staphylococci often cause hemolysis of the cells in blood agar.

Treatment

One of the cardinal features of *S. aureus* is its ability to develop resistance against chemotherapeutic agents. During the 1950s most hospitals and hospital personnel (up to 90%) became colonized with strains that had developed resistance to penicillin. New antibiotics have since been developed and are still relatively effective. The emergence of resistant strains against these new antibiotics has been slowed by avoiding abuses in antibiotic therapy (see Chapter 9). Before treatment of staphylococcal infections is initiated, the most effective antimicrobial agents should first be determined by sensitivity testing and then vigorously administered until the infection is cured.

Of recent concern has been the development of staphylococcal resistance to penicillinase-resistant antibiotics. These organisms are termed **methicillin-resistant,** and they pose a serious treatment problem. The number of staphylococcal infections due to methicillin-resistant strains has risen from a few isolated cases in the 1970s to more than 10% of cases by 1988.

In addition to antibiotic therapy, surgical treatment is frequently necessary to effect a cure from staphylococcal infection. Abscesses should be drained, when possible, to remove inflammatory debris that may block the diffusion of antimicrobial agents to the site of the bacteria; surgical debridement of the osteomyelitis and removal of infected prosthetic devices may be essential

Methicillin-resistant
resistant to methicillin, a penicillinase-resistant antibiotic. Methicillin-resistant organisms create a difficult treatment problem because of the limited number of antibiotics that can be selected from for use.

Staphylococcus aureus Bacteremia: Great Britain, 1975

An analysis of the 140 reports of bacteremia due to *Staphylococcus aureus* received in the first three months of 1975, by the public health laboratory in Great Britain, illustrates both the severity of the infection (16% of the reports concerned patients who died) and the variety of clinical conditions with which it is associated. The infections were distributed among all age groups, and the greatest number of patients, 26, presented with fever of unknown origin, and clinical septicemia with no apparent source of infection; such patients appear to be at particular risk since 7 (27%) died. Twenty-two (16%) of the patients were children and no deaths were reported. A further 20 patients (14%)—7 of whom were children—had septic arthritis; one of these patients, a 65-year-old man, died.

Infected blood clots in blood vessels resulted in bacteremia in 16 patients, of whom 11 had infected intravenous catheter sites and 4 were heroin addicts. The 13 postoperative cases were mostly secondary to surgical wound infection and included 1 fatality. Staphylococcal infection was believed to have contributed to the 3 reported deaths among 11 patients with cancer or other serious debilitating illness. Bacteremia was secondary to staphylococcal pneumonia in 12 patients; the severity of this condition is reflected in the death of 7 of the 10 patients for whom the outcome was reported. Endocarditis was reported in 8 patients, 3 of whom died; 1 of the 8 patients had an aortic valve prosthesis, but the remaining patients had infections apparently unrelated to cardiac surgery (*MMWR* 24:268, 1975).

Staphylococcal Food Poisoning on a Cruise Ship: Caribbean, 1983

In February 1983, an outbreak of staphylococcal food poisoning occurred on a Caribbean cruise ship sailing from the United States. The probable source was cream pastries served during two separate meals.

The overall attack rate of acute gastroenteritis

components of treatment in these diseases. In these instances, surgical drainage may remove an environmental niche where the staphylococci are in a metabolically inactive stage and would thus not be affected by the chemotherapeutic agent. Also, such accumulations of pus or debris may serve to protect the infecting organism from the normal host cellular defenses.

Prevention and Control

Most individuals seem to develop antibodies against staphylococci early in life. These antibodies may contribute substantially to the resistance that most healthy individuals have against this bacte-

on board, estimated from the 56 passengers who responded to a 10% systematic survey of the 715 passengers, was 32%. Ninety-four percent of patients filling out questionnaires complained of nausea and/or vomiting, 82% reported diarrhea, and 60% reported abdominal cramps. Symptoms usually subsided within 12 hours, although 36% of patients indicated illness lasted at least 2 days. The incubation period ranged from 1 to 8 hours (median 5 hours).

When plotted by time of onset, the number of cases peaked twice, corresponding to meals served 2 days apart. Forty-six (95.8%) of 48 patients and 20 (58.8%) of 34 well passengers ate the cream pastry served for dessert on the evening of February 22 ($p < .001$). Seven (70%) of 10 patients and 4 (13.5%) of 30 controls are a similar pastry item for lunch on February 24 ($p < .001$).

Staphylococcus aureus, phage type 85/+, was isolated from the stools of 5 (38.4%) of 13 patients cultured and from none of 9 controls. The same staphylococcal phage type was grown from a perirectal swab, an anterior nares culture, and a swab of a forearm lesion from 3 of the 7 crew members who made pastry. Pastries from the implicated meals were not available for culture because the pastry kitchen routinely disposed of leftovers.

Investigation of the ship's pastry kitchen did not reveal any improper food handling in the preparation of the pastry items. Refrigeration temperatures were adequate, and the food handlers were free of pustular skin lesions. However, because the pastry was prepared in large quantities in several steps by a number of food handers, opportunities could have existed for the introduction of staphylococci into the pastry, with adequate time for incubation of the enterotoxin.

Editorial note: Although *Staphylococcus* remains the second most common etiologic agent (after *Salmonella*) in food-borne outbreaks in the United States, this is the first well-documented outbreak of staphylococcal food poisoning on a cruise ship sailing from the United States. This outbreak emphasizes the importance of extreme care in adequately refrigerating perishable food items prepared in large kitchens. The elaboration of staphylococcal enterotoxin requires incubation at temperatures above 6.7° C (44° F). The investigation also shows the value of phage typing to support epidemiologic evidence on the probable source of an outbreak, despite the inability to culture the implicated food item (*MMWR* 32:294, 1983).

rium; however, in injured tissues or in compromised patients this immunity is often not sufficient to prevent infection. No successful vaccines are available against *S. aureus*.

Prevention of staphylococcal infection is primarily a function of good **aseptic** techniques in hospitals and clinics where both infectious and susceptible patients congregate. Methods must be used to minimize the spread of microorganisms in critical areas. First, patients with open infected wounds should be isolated (see Chapter 43). Secondly, personnel who work in critical areas, such as operating rooms or newborn nurseries, should be screened to determine if they are carriers of drug-resistant strains. Those who

Aseptic
germ-free.

are carriers should be restricted from these areas until their condition is cleared up. Any type of infected lesion on hospital personnel should be promptly treated and precaution should be taken to protect patients from infection from this source.

The newborn nursery presents special problems in that about 90% of infants become carriers of *S. aureus* during the first 10 days of life. It is important that they do not become colonized with the virulent drug-resistant strains prevalent in hospitals. Skin disinfectants, especially hexachlorophene, are useful in decreasing the staphylococcal carrier rate in infants. The practice of immersing (bathing) newborns in hexachlorophene solutions has been discontinued to reduce the chance of any toxic reaction, but discrete washing of the skin with this disinfectant is appropriate and effective. In some cases, it has been beneficial to deliberately colonize infants with a nonvirulent strain of *S. aureus*. This step seems to interfere with subsequent colonization by virulent strains.

Air-handling systems should be designed to carry patient-generated airborne bacteria away from other patients or hospital personnel and to prevent any recirculation of these microorganisms to other areas of the hospital.

CONCEPT SUMMARY

1. Staphylococci are ubiquitous Gram-positive cocci not infrequently associated with infections of both humans and animals.

2. Of the several species of Staphylococcus, *S. aureus* is the most virulent and most commonly isolated from human infections. This organism is typical of other pyogenic cocci in that infections are characterized by the production of pus.

3. Numerous disease conditions may occur due to the staphylococci, ranging from food poisoning through osteomyelitis and pneumonia to the relatively recently described toxic shock syndrome. Treatment of many of these infections requires surgical intervention along with aggressive antibiotic therapy.

STUDY SUMMARY

1. List five characteristics of staphylococci that are related to virulence of these organisms.

2. What features of toxic shock syndrome and scalded skin syndrome are shared in common?

3. With what kinds of infection are coagulase-negative staphylococci commonly associated?

4. What feature of *S. aureus* has made therapy of infections due to this organism particularly difficult during the past few years?

5. What characteristic of coagulase-negative staphylococci has made control of infection very difficult?

REFERENCES FOR FURTHER STUDY

1. *Microbiology—1986*, L. Leive, 1986. American Society for Microbiology.

2. *Manual of Clinical Microbiology*, E. Lennette, 1985. American Society for Microbiology.

3. *Diagnostic Microbiology*, S. Finegold, 1986. Mosby.

4. A New Staphylococcal Enterotoxin, Enterotoxin F, Associated with Toxic Shock Syndrome. *Lancet* 1:1017, 1981.

5. The Disease Spectrum: Epidemiology and Etiology of Toxic Shock Syndrome. *Annual Review of Microbiology* 38:315. 1984.

6. Prospective Study of 114 Consecutive Episodes of *Staphylococcus aureus* Bacteremia. *Reviews of Infectious Diseases* 9:891, 1987.

chapter 16

STREPTOCOCCI

Both pathogenic and nonpathogenic species of streptococci are found associated with humans and animals. The pathogenic species produce a wide variety of toxins and cause a wide variety of lesions and diseases. Historically, some streptococcal diseases have been among the most serious diseases of humans. Fortunately, these bacteria are easily destroyed by chemotherapeutic agent. And as a result, even though streptococcal infections are still common, their impact on illness and death today is only a small fraction of what it was prior to the 1930s.

BACTERIA

Streptococci are Gram-positive, coccal-shaped bacteria that usually appear in chains of various lengths (Figure 16-1). These bacteria are moderately resistant to environmental factors; that is, they may remain living for days to weeks after being expelled from the body. Streptococci are readily killed by common disinfectants and most are highly susceptible to a wide range of chemotherapeutic agents, including penicillin. Bacterial species of the genus *Streptococcus* are widespread in nature and are part of the normal bacterial flora of the skin, nose, mouth, and mucosal surfaces (including the gut) of humans and animals. It is often difficult to distinguish clearly between many streptococcal species, which has made a precise classification of these bacterial difficult. Streptococci grow well on blood agar plates and many species secrete *hemolysins* (enzymes that dissolve RBCs) that produce different patterns of hemolytic zones around the colonies. These hemolytic patterns are used to make a preliminary identification of streptococcal groups. A clear zone surrounding the colony is called *beta*-hemolysis, a zone with an opaque greenish color is called *alpha*-hemolysis, and some species produce no hemolysis.

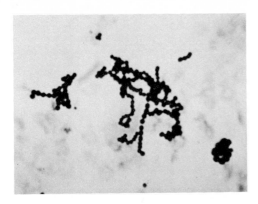

Figure 16-1
Photomicrograph of streptococcal cells.

The most usable classification system, the **Lancefield system,** used differences in carbohydrate antigens located in the cell wall of beta-hemolytic streptococci. Under this system, streptococci have been divided into 18 major groups, designated A through V. The most important streptococcal infections of humans are caused by the species *Streptococcus pyogenes,* which are mostly of Lancefield group A. Group A can be further subdivided into some 60 types based on differences in an antigen called the **M-protein.** This M-protein is important, because it is responsible for virulence; antibodies formed against it give protection to the host (Figure 16-2). The other groups or categories of streptococci include some species that are also associated with human infections and are listed in Table 16-1. The major emphasis of this chapter is on the diseases caused by *S. pyogenes* with a brief summary of diseases caused by some other streptococci. A bacterium previously called *Diplococcus pneumoniae* has been reclassified as a streptococcus and is now called *Streptococcus pneumoniae;* this bacterium is a major cause of pneumonia and is discussed separately in Chapter 17.

Lancefield classification

a classification of beta-hemolytic streptococci based on the carbohydrate antigens present in the wall of the cell. Serogroups A through V have been identified.

M-protein

a major virulence factor of streptococci. Located on the cell surface this antigen can be used to separate group A streptococci into over 60 serotypes.

Figure 16-2   Cross-section of surface structures of streptococci. The wall is a unit structure composed of mucopeptide, group carbohydrate, and protein antigens.

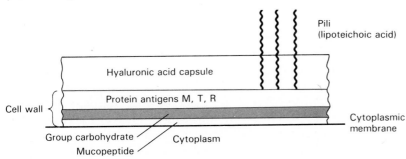

Table 16-1   Non–Group A Straptococci That Cause Disease in Humans

Organisms	Diseases
Group B streptococci	Neonatal meningitis, sepsis
Streptococcus groups C, G	Occasional wound infection, pharyngitis
Group D—enterococci	Urinary tract infection, bacteremia, endocarditis
Viridans streptococci	Endocarditis, rare meningitis or cystitis
Streptococcus pneumoniae	Pneumonia, wound infections, sepsis meningitis

DISEASES CAUSED BY *STREPTOCOCCUS PYOGENES*

Pathogenesis and Clinical Diseases

Various extracellular and intracellular substances produced by *S. pyogenes* contribute to the ability of this species to withstand the body's defense mechanisms and cause tissue damage. Several more prominent substances and their effects are as follows:

1. *Capsule,* which helps retard phagocytosis.
2. *M-protein,* which both retards phagocytosis and helps the bacteria adhere to mucosal epithelium.
3. *Erythrogenic toxin,* which produces the fever and rash associated with scarlet fever and is produced under the genetic control of plasmid DNA.
4. *Streptolysin O* and *streptolysin S,* two separate hemolysins that lyse red blood cells and damage various host cells. Streptolysin O is oxygen-labile; streptolysin S is stable in oxygen.
5. *Streptokinase,* a fibrinolysin that digests fibrin in the inflammatory barrier.
6. *Hyaluronidase,* the spreading factor. Hyaluronidase is an enzyme that breaks down hyaluronic acid, which acts as an intracellular glue.

In addition, various other cellular substances may also contribute to the pathogenicity and/or virulence of *S. pyogenes.* The major types of clinical conditions associated with group A streptococci are shown in Figure 16-3 and are discussed next.

Sore throat (pharyngitis)   Streptococcal **pharyngitis,** referred to as "strep throat," is very common. Children up to 15 years of age average about one infection per year. Each infection is caused by a different M type, as antibody immunity will generally offer pro-

Pharyngitis
infection of the pharynx. The pharynx is the upper portion of the throat. This disease is usually accompanied by enlarged lymph nodes, erythema, and soreness.

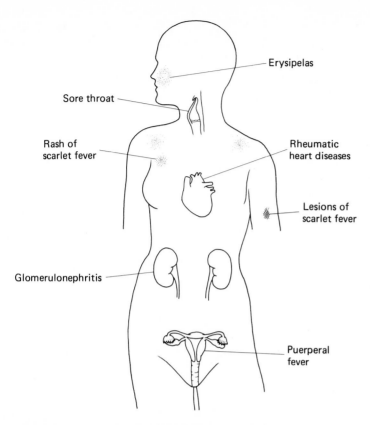

- Erysipelas
- Sore throat
- Rash of scarlet fever
- Rheumatic heart diseases
- Lesions of scarlet fever
- Glomerulonephritis
- Puerperal fever

Figure 16-3   Some of the prominent clinical diseases associated with Group A streptococcal infections.

tection for some time against repeated infections with the same type. This infection is not life-threatening; however, strains vary in virulence, and infections with highly virulent bacteria may cause a severe sore throat with fever, headache, swollen cervical lymph nodes, and **purulent** exudate in the throat. Infections in older children and adults tend to be milder and less frequent, due in part to the antibody immunity that has developed against many strains encountered in earlier childhood. The infection may also spread from the throat directly into the lungs to cause pneumonia or may penetrate into the pleural cavity, causing severe inflammation (pleuritis). It is important to seek therapy for streptococcal pharyngitis in order to prevent subsequent **sequelae** such as rheumatic fever.

Scarlet fever   Scarlet fever may result simply from the production of erythrogenic toxin by the streptococci that are causing pharyngitis or other relatively benign streptococcal infections. This toxin diffuses into the blood and is carried to the skin, where it causes a diffuse reddish rash. The more virulent erythrogenic toxin-

Purulent
associated with the production of pus.

Sequela
a condition or illness directly relating to an earlier condition but which develops some time after the first illness.

producing strains are quite invasive and are able to spread through the lymphatic system and into the blood. They may then be carried throughout the body, resulting in infections of the joints, bones, endocardium, skin, and so on. This form of scarlet fever is quite severe and was not an uncommon cause of death in the era before penicillin. The outer layers of affected skin are frequently sloughed during recovery from scarlet fever (Figure 16-4).

Puerperal fever   Puerperal fever, also known as *childbed fever,* is a group A streptococcal infection of the uterus that may occur in women shortly after childbirth (postpartum). The streptococci often spread rapidly from the inflamed uterus to the blood and the resulting widespread infection may cause death. This disease captured the interest of Semmelweis (see Chapter 1), and was one of the first examples of human-to-human transmission of infection.

Infections of the skin   *S. pyogenes,* like *Staphylococcus aureus,* is able to cause lesions on the skin where prior injuries, such as insect bites, wounds, and burns, have occurred. *Impetigo* is commonly caused by streptococci and *erysipelas* is a specific type of streptococcal skin lesion. Impetigo is a relatively common, usually benign, superficial infection of the skin. Lesions may occur anyplace on the body and are characterized as blisters that break and dry with crusty scabs. Children are the most common victims of this disease, which is relatively easily treated with topical antibiotics (Figure 16-5).

Erysipelas often occurs on the face and probably starts from streptococci coming from the throat or nose and entering a skin abrasion. The lesion spreads outward, causing marked reddening,

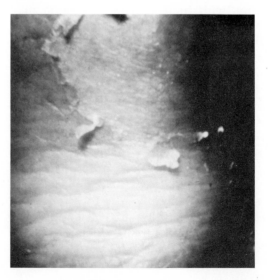

Figure 16-4   Skin peeling from scarlet fever patient. (Courtesy J. M. Matsen, University of Utah)

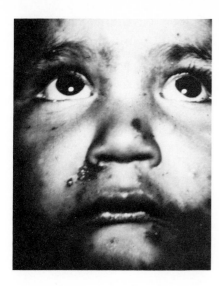

Figure 16-5 Streptococcal impetigo. (Courtesy J. M. Matsen, University of Utah)

or **erythema**, and swelling (edema) of the skin with a sharply defined advancing edge. Recovery usually takes a week or longer; if no treatment is given, this condition may be fatal in some patients.

Poststreptococcal diseases The poststreptococcal diseases are *glomerulonephritis* and *rheumatic fever*, and have their onset from 1 to 4 weeks after an **acute** streptococcal infection. These two conditions are not infections, but occur as a direct result of previously untreated streptococcal pharyngitis or **pyoderma**. Today these two diseases are the most serious problems associated with group A streptococcal infection. In spite of much research, the mechanisms and pathogenesis of these diseases are not well understood. Some evidence indicates that they are immune complex diseases, which means that there is an interaction between antibodies and tissue-associated antigens, which, in turn, induces an inflammatory response. The inflammatory response results in the formation of scar tissue, which replaces some of the normal body tissue. The antibodies involved in these two diseases are those produced in response to the streptococcal infection.

Glomerulonephritis involves the basement (filtering) membrane of the glomeruli of the kidneys. The inflammation and scarring of these membranes may result in severe kidney malfunctions and, in some cases, death. This disease is most commonly induced by streptococcal type 12 of group A, and may result following infection of the skin or other tissues. Other streptococcal types may occasionally cause this disease. Primary infections with type 12 streptococci are infrequent, and only about 0.5% of individuals with streptococcal disease go on to develop poststreptococcal glomerulonephritis. About 80% to 90% of the cases undergo slow

Erythema
redness of the skin resulting from dilation of the capillaries.

Acute
a current, rapid, short manifestation of disease symptoms.

Pyoderma
infection of the skin by a pus-producing (pyogenic) bacterium.

spontaneous healing whereas the others develop a chronic form of the disease. Recurrent attacks are rare.

Rheumatic fever develops as a sequela in fewer than 0.05% of cases of acute streptococcal pharyngitis but may be caused by almost any one of the group A strains, and usually develops in children 5 to 15 years of age. Some signs and symptoms are fever, malaise, inflamed and aching joints (arthritis), subcutaneous lesions, and heart lesions. These complications may occur alone or in various combinations. However, about half the cases may be mild and go undiagnosed. Injury to the heart (rheumatic heart disease) is the most serious effect of rheumatic fever and currently is the most common cause of permanent heart valve damage in children. Subsequent infections with group A streptococci may aggravate and cause recurrences of this disease. Because many different strains of streptococci cause rheumatic fever, persons who have had one attack must guard against reinfection and often use penicillin as a prophylactic.

Transmission and Epidemiology

The various strains of *S. pyogenes* are widespread in humans, many of whom are asymptomatic carriers. These bacteria are found in the respiratory tract, mouth, intestines, or on the skin of about 5% of the general population in the summer and around 10% in the winter. The carrier rate is generally higher in children between 1 and 15 years of age. Because of this high carrier rate, streptococci are readily transmitted when large numbers of persons share common environments. Persons with acute infections are an obvious source of infection and transmission can readily occur from these individuals via respiratory droplets or by direct or indirect contact. When highly virulent strains are carried into elementary schools, sharp outbreaks of pharyngitis and scarlet fever may occur. Due to the accumulative buildup of antibodies to many different types, outbreaks among adults are less likely.

Diagnosis

Diagnosis of a streptococcal infection is based on both clinical and laboratory findings. The basic laboratory procedure is to swab the site of infection and either culture the material from the swab on a blood agar plate or use a rapid streptococcal antigen detection test. Cultures are examined after 24 hours of incubation for the presence of beta-hemolytic colonies, which, if present, are further studied to determine if they are group A streptococci. The antigen detection tests are commonly employed in physicians' offices and medical clinics. These procedures afford rapid (less than 2 hours) results and are a fairly sensitive method for detection of group A streptococci from cases of pharyngitis.

On the basis of clinical examination only, staphylococcal infections may be difficult to distinguish from some streptococcal infections. To differentiate between the two types of bacteria following culture, a *catalase test* is used. This test is done by placing a small amount of growth from a colony in hydrogen peroxide; if the catalase enzyme is present, bubbles of oxygen are released. Staphylococci are positive for catalase and streptococci are negative. *S. pyogenes* can be distinguished from other beta-hemolytic streptococci by placing a paper disk containing a low concentration of the antibiotic bacitracin onto a freshly swabbed agar plate; growth of *S. pyogenes* will be inhibited by the bacitracin whereas the other streptococci will not.

Glomerulonephritis and rheumatic fever are diagnosed primarily on the basis of clinical and serologic findings. These are postinfection sequelae and attempts to culture streptococci are not successful. However, because they follow streptococcal infection, the patient should be expected to have a high antibody titer to streptococcal antigens. The most useful tests measure antibody to either streptolysin-O or DNAse B antigens. A high titer to either of these antigens suggests a recent group A streptococcal infection.

Treatment

The beta-hemolytic streptococci are highly susceptible to most antimicrobial agents. Penicillin is effective in more than 90% of cases and is the antibiotic of choice. Other antibiotics can be used in patients who are allergic to penicillin. Erythromycin is generally recommended. Because streptococci tend to develop resistance to tetracyclines and sulfa drugs, these agents should not be used.

Penicillin therapy will usually produce a rapid cure of most acute infections. Symptoms usually resolve within 24 hours of treatment, and destruction of the bacteria is usually complete within 10 days. Treatment should be started as soon as practical in order to reduce the chance of the subsequent development of rheumatic fever. Prompt diagnosis and treatment are particularly important in children, for they have the greatest predisposition to rheumatic fever. Early treatment is also important in helping to reduce the chance of transmitting the infection. Moreover, therapy can be used to try to clear streptococci from known carriers; this factor is particularly important for medical personnel who work with highly susceptible patients.

Prevention and Control

Vaccines are not available for the preceding streptococcal diseases; and because of the large numbers of serotypes, the development of vaccines is considered unfeasible.

The best control measure is to use basic medical procedures

Hospital Outbreak of Streptococcal Wound Infection: Utah, 1976

Seven cases of group A beta-hemolytic streptococcal wound infections, six culture-proven and one presumptive, occurred from January 30 to February 15, 1976, among postsurgery patients at a 135-bed community hospital in northern Utah. Five patients had culture-proven wound infections, a sixth had a wound infection with Gram-positive cocci in the exudate, and a seventh had culture-proven bacteremia and meningitis. All cases occurred less than 48 hours after surgery.

Initial review of the patients' charts revealed that major surgery was the only experience shared by all. The 6 culture-confirmed cases were then compared to the 34 other patients who had operations on the same days as the cases.

Exposures to one anesthesiologist and to one surgeon were the only factors significantly associated with subsequent infection.

Cultures of throat and anus were obtained from all operating room personnel. The same anesthesiologist was found to carry the epidemic organism; he had asymptomatic anal carriage.

The operating room was closed on February 17. The anesthesiologist withdrew from surgery and was treated with benzathine penicillin. Repeat throat and anal cultures 3 days after initiation of treatment and 10 days after completion were negative. Increased surveillance by infection control committee members revealed no further wound infections or colonization by group A streptococci (*MMWR* 25:141,1976).

Outbreak of Scarlet Fever: California, 1977

An outbreak of scarlet fever and poststreptococcal acute glomerulonephritis (AGN) occurred among residents of Santa Catalina Island, California, from March through July 1977. The epidemic organism, M2T2 SOR+ group A streptococcus, was previously implicated in outbreaks

to prevent the transmission of infection. Individuals with a known infection should be isolated; for instance, a child with untreated pharyngitis should not attend school, and an infected patient in a hospital should be isolated from other patients. Medical personnel have a special responsibility to follow standard aseptic procedures to avoid transmitting these organisms between patients. Care should be used in delivery rooms and in working with recently delivered mothers to prevent transmission to their highly susceptible uterine tissues.

The best means to prevent rheumatic fever and glomerulonephritis involves early diagnosis and treatment of children who have acute streptococcal infections. The recurrence of rheumatic fever is prevented by prophylactic (preventive) penicillin treatment—that is, daily doses of penicillin. Often persons who reof scarlet fever and AGN occurring in Los Angeles and Mexico City.

Since the end of March, 65 cases of streptococcal pharyngitis (53 of them with scarlet fever) were identified by physician reports and a school survey. Symptoms among all patients with streptococcal disease consisted of fever (in 93%), sore throat (89%), rash or desquamation (82%), vomiting (62%), headache (59%), and enlarged lymph nodes in neck (44%).

Six cases were diagnosed between the end of March and the end of May, but the incidence increased dramatically in June, peaked in the third week, and declined after school recessed June 18. Sporadic cases continued to occur in July; the most recent onset was July 23. Distribution of cases over the 4-month period suggested person-to-person transmission. Except for 7 adults and 10 preschoolers, illness was confined to a single school (grades K–12) but involved only grades K–6; fifth-graders experienced the highest attack rate (14/23, 61%). The teacher in that class was also affected and the attack rate for children sitting at the front of that classroom was higher than for those in the back. The secondary attack rate in family members who did not attend the elementary school or a local preschool was 12.2%.

All cases were screened for signs and symptoms of AGN. Diagnosis showed three definite and three probable cases of nephritis, based on hematuria, cylinduria, and hypocomplementemia. Only one child had symptoms of nephritis; the others were asymptomatic and would not have been identified without screening efforts. Streptococci from 31 to 32 ill persons from whom the isolate was available for typing were identified as belonging to the epidemic strain M2T2 SOR+ group A streptococcus.

The first two cases in the outbreak were in a preschool child and his mother who had recently returned from an area of Mexico in which scarlet fever was prevalent. The organism may have been introduced to the island at this point, although there was ample opportunity for transmission from elsewhere on the mainland (*MMWR* 26:311, 1977).

ceived severe heart damage from the first attack of rheumatic fever must be given penicillin therapy for years or for their lifetime. In many of these cases, it is often difficult to resolve the balance between benefits and abuses of such long-term penicillin therapy.

OTHER STREPTOCOCCAL INFECTIONS

Group B

Lancefields group B streptococci (*S. agalactiae*) are commonly found in the genital and intestinal tracts of normal persons. They are also widely (2% to 40%) found in the vagina of pregnant

Serotype

a strain of bacteria with a unique antigen such that it induces antibody specific for that organism.

Sepsis

the presence of bacteria in the blood stream. Bacteremia and septicemia are often used as synonyms for sepsis.

women. There are five capsular **serotypes** of *S. agalactiae* (1a, 1b, 1c, II and III). Type III is most frequently responsible for human disease. Although group B streptococci may cause urinary tract, ear, and wound infections, they are most important as a cause of neonatal (newborn) infection. Newborn infants may become colonized during passage through an infected birth canal. These children may (1.3 to 3 per 1000 live births) develop serious **sepsis** (bacterial in the bloodstream) and pneumonia with a mortality rate of about 55%. This "early onset" form of the disease is often associated with deliveries that are complicated or premature. Another form of the disease, "late onset," affects infants more than 7 days of age (average 24 days). These patients are infected after birth, they most commonly have meningitis, and their mortality rate (23%) is lower.

Group C

Occasionally species of group C streptococci have been implicated as the cause of such infections as impetigo, abscesses, pneumonia, and pharyngitis.

Group D

Group D streptococci are significant human pathogens, causing endocarditis, sepsis, and urinary tract infection. Three species (*S. durans, S. faecalis, S. faecium*) of this group are designated as *enterococci*, and are separated from other group D organisms because of their ability to grow in media containing 6.5% NaC1. These organisms are normal inhabitants of the human gut and are resistant to a broad range of antibiotics. Recent proposals have recommended that this group of organisms be placed in their own genus, to be known as *Enterococcus*. Their resistance to antimicrobial therapy along with the serious nature of endocarditis infections due to these organisms (mortality rates range from 30% to 60%) make them of special interest in the medical community.

Viridans Group

At least ten species of non-beta-hemolytic streptococci are designated as viridans streptococci. They are the primary cause of up to 70% of all cases of bacterial endocarditis and are sometimes isolated from patients with deep wound infections, abdominal abscesses, and septicemia. These organisms are present in the human mouth and pharynx, and they are thought to be a contributing cause of tooth decay. Persons whose heart valves have been damaged by rheumatic fever should be given prophylactic antibiotics before oral or genital surgery to reduce the risk of subsequent endocarditis from these organisms.

CONCEPT SUMMARY

1. The genus *Streptococcus* includes a large number of primarily commensalistic bacteria. These organisms are often found as normal flora in both animals and humans. They are Gram-positive, and diseases produced by these organisms are suppurative.

2. The pathogenic streptococci are classified on the basis of a polysaccharide capsular antigen. The group A organisms are of particular concern to humans, although human infections are also caused by members of the other groups, notably groups B and D.

3. The relatively benign disease, streptococcal sore throat, is of importance primarily because of the delayed sequela associated with such infections. Most streptococcal diseases are readily treated with penicillin.

STUDY SUMMARY

1. What component of the streptococcal cell is used as an antigen in determining serologic classification?

2. Streptococcal pharyngitis is a relatively benign disease without mortality. What feature of this disease makes it important for patients to receive antibiotic therapy?

3. What is the usual source of group A streptococci that is transmitted from person to person?

4. Name the primary clinical concerns (diseases) associated with each of the following streptococci: (a) group A, (b) group B, (c) group D, and (d) viridans.

5. What is the present theory as to the basis of rheumatic fever?

REFERENCES FOR FURTHER STUDY

1. Genetic Studies of the M-Protein of Group A Streptococci. In *Microbiology—1986*, p. 30. American Society for Microbiology.

2. Bacterial Adherence: The Attachment of Group A Streptococci to Mucosal Surfaces. *Reviews of Infectious Diseases* 9:S 475. 1987.

3. Group B Streptococcal Bacteremia in Men. *Reviews of Infectious Diseases* 8:912,1986.

4. *Medical Microbiology*, J. Sherris, 1984. Elsevier.

5. *Diagnostic Microbiology*, 7th ed., S. Finegold, 1986. Mosby.

chapter 17

STREPTOCOCCUS PNEUMONIAE

Diplococcus
cocci that occur as pairs such that two cells are normally present together.

Pneumococcal infections rank among the important causes of human illness. Before the era of antibiotics, pneumococcal pneumonia was the leading cause of human death. Even with the use of antibiotics, it is still responsible for significant mortality and the only infectious disease to have the dubious distinction of still being in the "top ten" causes of death in the United States. Pneumococcal pneumonia is a potential threat to every hospital patient or person with a compromised host defense mechanism. Medical personnel must be continually alerted to the possible occurrence of this disease in the care of all patients. For many years *Streptococcus pneumoniae* was classed as a separate genus called **Diplococcus.** Research has demonstrated close similarities to the streptococci, however, and so the diplococci were reclassified as a species of the genus *Streptococcus.* They are routinely referred to as *pneumococci.*

BACTERIUM

S. pneumoniae is a Gram-positive coccus that characteristically occurs in pairs or short chains (Figure 17-1). The virulent strains possess a prominent capsule that plays an important role in the pathogenesis of pneumococcal diseases by retarding the rate of phagocytosis. The capsular material is composed of polysaccharide and is antigenic. These antigens have been used to subdivide the pneumococci into more than 80 types. Protection against infection is type-specific and depends upon antibody to the capsular polysaccharide. The organism can be cultivated on enriched media supplemented with 5% blood. *S. pneumoniae* produces alpha-type hemolysis, which may cause it to be mistakenly identified as a viridans streptococcus. Pneumococci are traditionally highly susceptible to penicillin as well as other antibiotics; however, some penicillin-resistant strains are now emerging. These orga-

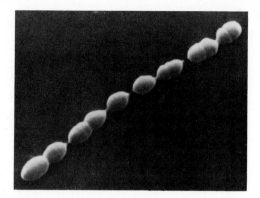

Figure 17-1 Scanning electron micrograph of *Streptococcus pneumoniae* showing the chain arrangement and the tendency to form pairs of cocci (diplococci) (magnification 10,000×). (A. S. Klainer and I Gies, *Agents of Bacterial Disease.* Harper & Row: Hagerstown, MD, 1973. Figure 5-3, p. 69.)

nisms do not survive long outside the body and are readily destroyed by disinfectants.

PNEUMOCOCCAL INFECTIONS

Pathogenesis and Clinical Diseases

S. pneumoniae is widespread in the general population. From fewer than 10% to over 60% of healthy persons may be carrying this bacterium in their respiratory tract. The higher **carrier rates** are seen during the winter and correlate with increased occurrence of *pneumococcal pneumonia*. This bacterium does not possess any apparent enzymes or toxins associated with invasiveness; the major mechanism of virulence is the prominent capsule that impedes phagocytosis. In a healthy active person the macrophages are usually able to control any pneumococci that may enter the lower respiratory tract. Only when the defense mechanisms of a host become suppressed are the pneumococci able to multiply and establish a focus of infection. As the pneumococci begin to multiply, they induce an acute inflammatory reaction with a rapid infiltration of edematous fluid. This fluid nourishes the bacteria, which in turn increase their rate of multiplication and stimulate a greater inflow of fluids. The initial accumulation of fluids also impedes phagocytosis and may impede the infiltration of antimicrobial agents into the lesion. The infiltrated fluids, which contain

Carrier rate

the number of individual carriers in a specific population who are infected by a microorganism.

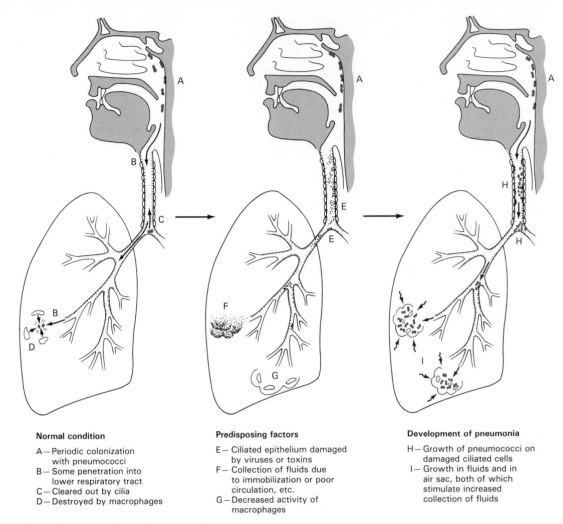

Normal condition

A — Periodic colonization
    with pneumococci
B — Some penetration into
    lower respiratory tract
C — Cleared out by cilia
D — Destroyed by macrophages

Predisposing factors

E — Ciliated epithelium damaged
    by viruses or toxins
F — Collection of fluids due
    to immobilization or poor
    circulation, etc.
G — Decreased activity of
    macrophages

Development of pneumonia

H — Growth of pneumococci on
    damaged ciliated cells
I — Growth in fluids and in
    air sac, both of which
    stimulate increased
    collection of fluids

Figure 17-2   Predisposition to and the development of pneumococcal pneumonia.

many PMNs and RBCs may rapidly fill the infected lung causing areas of *consolidation*. This fluid takes on the characteristics of typical inflammatory exudate. In most less serious cases, the increased number of PMNs, along with the macrophages, are able to contain the pneumococci; the infiltrated fluid then disperses and the lung tissue is restored to its original condition without permanent damage. When given early, antibiotics greatly accelerate the recovery process.

In more serious pneumonias, the accumulation of fluid continues and spreads from one lobe to another and areas of consolidation develop in which the pneumococci are less susceptible to phagocytosis and antibiotics. The pneumococci may spread from the lungs into the pleural cavity or pericardium and cause abscesses in these areas. The infection in the pleural space is called *pleurisy*. Such infections may continue to expand, resulting in the death of the patient. On the other hand, if specific antibodies develop in time, a crisis may be reached, followed by recovery.

The symptoms of classical pneumonia begin with the rapid onset of shaking chills and fever between 38.8° and 41.4° C. Severe chest pains are often present. A cough develops and the sputum is purulent and rust colored (contains RBCs). In many untreated cases, the crisis is reached in about 5 to 10 days, followed by recovery. Overall the death rate in untreated cases is 30% compared to 5% in treated cases. The outcome is greatly influenced by the age and underlying predisposing conditions of the patient. The stages in the development of pneumococcal pneumonia are outlines in Figure 17-2.

Other infectious processes associated with *S. pneumoniae* include *otitis media* (inner ear infection), septicemia, wound infections, and meningitis. Mortality from pneumococcal disease is highest for meningitis (up to 55%) and septicemia (40%) in spite of appropriate antibiotic therapy. Otitis media, while painful, is relatively benign and most commonly occurs in young children. Infection may also spread via the blood or by direct extension to other body tissues. Septicemia and meningitis are common outcomes when the pneumococci spread beyond the respiratory tract; currently pneumococci are one of the most frequent causes of these infections in young children.

Transmission and Epidemiology

In most cases, the source of infection is endogenous—that is, from the pneumococci already present in the respiratory tract. Person-to-person transmission of the pneumococci readily occurs, but the disease occurs only in those with predisposing conditions. The most common predisposing factors include viral infections of the respiratory tract (Figure 17-3); physical injury to the respiratory tract from inhaling toxic or irritating substances including anesthetic gases, prolonged immobilization in bed which may result in accumulation of fluids in the lungs, alcoholism, increasing age, diabetes; and immunodeficiency diseases such as Hodgkin's or sickle cell anemia.

Pneumonia is most often seen in infants, elderly persons, alcoholics, or persons with chronic diseases. An estimated 500,000 persons in the United States will contract pneumonia each year and about 50,000 deaths will result. The seasonal variations and increased number of cases of all types of pneumonia occurring during influenza epidemics are shown in Figure 17-4. About 25% of the pneumonia in adults is caused by pneumococci and 75% of these cases are due to only 9 of the 83 different pneumococcal

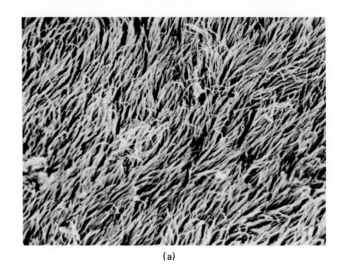

(a)

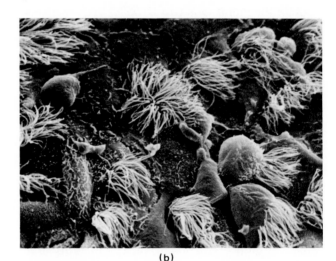

(b)

Figure 17-3 (a) Scanning electron micrograph of normal ciliated epithelium showing a continuous protective blanket of cilia. (b) Ciliated epithelium damaged by a viral infection which renders the respiratory tract much more susceptible to secondary bacterial infections. (S. E. Reed and A. Boyd, *Inf. Imm.* 6:68–76, Figures 1 and 4, with permission from ASM)

serotypes. More pneumonia is seen in the winter and generally parallels the incidence of viral respiratory infections.

Diagnosis

Typical cases are usually diagnosed on the bases of physical examination and lung x -rays. Laboratory diagnosis entails demonstrating the pneumococci in the **sputum**, blood, or **cerebral spinal fluid** (CSF), by direct microscopic examination and by culturing on artificial media. If specific antiserum is added to a suspension of a pneumococcus, it will cause the bacterial capsules to become visible. This reaction is called the *quellung reaction* and is useful in

Sputum
a collection of mucus, host, and parasite cells coughed up from the lung in cases of pneumonia or bronchitis.

Cerebral spinal fluid (CSF)
a watery fluid that is produced in the brain and forms a cushion surrounding the central nervous system.

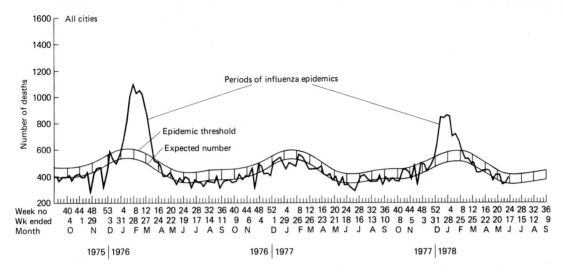

Figure 17-4 The reported number of deaths from pneumonia in 121 selected cities in the United States, September 1975 to June 1978. The sharp increases result from persons being predisposed to pneumonia as a result of influenzal infections (*MMWR 27:*422, 1978).

determining the specific pneumonococcal serotype. Differentiation of the pneumococci from viridans streptococci is often necessary, because they produce the same reaction on blood agar plates. The pneumococci are distinguished from the viridans streptococci by their bile solubility. For this test, pneumococci are added to solutions containing bile salts and the cells dissolve, whereas in a similar test the viridans cells do not dissolve. Alternatively, the optochin disk test may be used; for this test, a paper disk containing a chemical called *optochin* is placed on an agar plate that has been seeded with the test bacterium. Optochin inhibits the growth of pneumococci but not of viridans streptococci. Various serologic tests are available to detect the presence of pneumococcal antibodies or antigens in the serum of the patient.

Treatment

Most pneumococci (97%) are still susceptible to penicillin; only occasionally is a resistant strain isolated (see clinical note). Treatment with penicillin should be started as soon as pneumococcal pneumonia is suspected. The longer treatment is delayed, the more difficult it is to cure the disease. The response to penicillin, when initiated early, is often dramatic and bacteria are cleared from the system in a few hours. The effects of both sulfa drugs and penicillin on pneumonia helped justify the title of ''wonder drugs'' that was applied to these agents shortly after their discovery. For the first time in history, the number one killer of humans could often be cured with relative ease and rapidity. When penicil-

Multiple-Resistant Pneumococcus: Denver, Colorado, 1980

In November 1980, a multiply-resistant strain of *Streptococcus pneumoniae*, serotype 6B, was isolated from the cerebrospinal fluid (CSF) of an 11-month-old infant with meningitis. The isolate was found to be resistant to penicillin G, chloramphenicol, and tetracycline; this is the first instance reported in the United States of a pneumococcus resistant to all three drugs.

The minimum inhibitory concentration (MIC) for penicillin G was 1 μg/ml. The organism was sensitive to rifampin, and the child, who had responded poorly to penicillin, recovered after treatment with ampicillin, chloramphenicol, and rifampin.

Since the child had regularly attended a day-care center with approximately 55 other children, a survey was conducted at the day-care center to detect carriage of the resistant isolate. Throat cultures from 4 of 14 children (29%) in the toddler room (under age 2 years) were positive for the multiply-resistant pneumococcus (MRP); in the preschool area, 4 of 37 children (11%) and 1 of 10 adult employees (10%) were positive. A total of 125 children and staff members in six other day-care centers in the metropolitan area had negative throat cultures for MRP. To date, no other cases of invasive disease with this MRP have been recognized.

Editorial note: The first report of penicillin-resistant pneumococci appeared in 1967. Since then, relatively resistant and resistant strains have been reported from many parts of the world. The prevalence of relative resistance reported in clinical isolates has varied from 1% to as high as 16%, but most studies show a prevalence of approximately 2%.

In 1977, multiply-resistant pneumococci appeared in South Africa, and since then have been recognized in the United Kingdom, Australia, New Guinea, and the United States. This report of penicillin-resistant pneumococci and other reports describing relative penicillin resistance in the United States emphasize the need to screen all clinically significant pneumococcal isolates for penicillin sensitivity (*MMWR* 30:197, 1981).

lin cannot be used because of allergic reactions, some broad-spectrum antibiotics are appropriate.

Prevention and Control

Prophylactic treatment
therapy used to prevent infection or disease.

Endogenous bacteria
those bacteria which are part of the normal bacterial flora of the host. These bacteria pose a threat to their host only if the host becomes immunocompromised.

Good nursing and medical management practices are effective in minimizing or preventing the development of pneumonia in compromised hospital patients. **Prophylactic treatment** with penicillin might be warranted in high-risk patients with viral respiratory disease or other conditions that might predispose the tissues to pneumococcal infections. Even though pneumonia is often caused by **endogenous bacteria,** exogenous transmission may also be important in a hospital or nursing home environment, and compromised patients should be isolated from pneumonia patients in par-

Table 17-1   Purified Capsular Polysaccharide Antigens Contained in *Streptococcus pneumoniae* Vaccine

Types			
1	9	22	54
2	12	23	56
3	14	26	57
4	17	34	68
5	19	43	70
8	20	51	

ticular. In extreme cases, such as highly immunosuppressed organ transplant patients, protective isolation from all persons is necessary. Elective surgery should not be performed on a person with a respiratory infection. Hospitalized or confined patients should be required, if possible, to sit up and get out of bed periodically to prevent the pooling of fluids in the lungs. Maintaining good circulation and healthy ''dry'' lungs is the best preventive measure against nosocomial pneumococcal pneumonia.

Before the development of effective antibiotics, vaccines against pneumonia were used with some effect. Because of the increased death rates from pneumonia in elderly persons and compromised patients in recent years, plus the difficulty of treating pneumonia in many of these persons, renewed interest in antipneumococcal vaccines has been stimulated. A pneumococcal vaccine has been available in the United States since 1978. This vaccine contains the capsular antigens from 23 of the most commonly encountered serotypes. Although data regarding its usefulness is varied, the vaccine is still recommended for young children, elderly persons, and others such as persons without a functional spleen or with health conditions that would predispose them to serious pneumococcal disease. Table 17-1 lists the pneumococcal antigens presently included in the vaccine.

CONCEPT SUMMARY

Streptococcus pneumoniae has historically been of primary importance as a human disease agent. It is still a common cause of serious pneumonia, particularly in compromised patients. Therapy with penicillin has greatly reduced the fear of this organism and a multivalent vaccine that greatly reduces the incidence of this disease is now available.

STUDY SUMMARY

1. What feature of *Streptococcus pneumoniae* led to its classification for many years as *Diplococcus pneumoniae*?

2. *Streptococcus pneumoniae* gets its name because it is so frequently the cause of human pneumonia. List four other clinical conditions (diseases) commonly caused by this organism.

3. What is the reservoir of *S. pneumoniae*?

4. In the clinical laboratory *S. pneumoniae* is easily confused with what other organism?

5. What feature of host resistance is most responsible for immunity to *S. pneumoniae* infection?

REFERENCES FOR FURTHER STUDY

1. Pneumococcal Endocarditis: *Reviews of Infectious Diseases* 8:786, 1986.

2. *The Biologic and Clinical Basis of Infectious Diseases*, 3rd ed., G. Youmans, 1985. Saunders.

3. *Principles and Practices of Infectious Diseases*, 2nd ed., G. Mandell, 1985. Wiley.

4. Invasive Pneumococcal Infections: Incidence, Predisposing Factors and Prognosis. *Reviews of Infectious Diseases* 7:133, 1985.

chapter 18

Neisseria

acteria of the genus *Neisseria* are the fourth of the major pyogenic cocci to be presented. These organisms differ from the other pyogenic cocci both in their fundamental properties (they are Gram-negative), and in the specific nature of the diseases they produce. There are several species of *Neisseria*; two of them have taken their species names from the disease they produce. *N. meningitidis* is the leading cause of young adult meningitis, and *N. gonorrhoeae* is the cause of the most frequently reported sexually transmitted disease, gonorrhea. Although these two species are similar in structural and physiological makeup, the diseases they cause are clinically quite different and will be discussed separately.

BACTERIA

The *Neisseria* are Gram-negative diplococci (paired cocci; Figure 18-1), which usually have a common flattened or concave side. They are a little less than 1 μm in diameter and are nonmotile. The pathogenic strains are **fermentive,** but others often fail to ferment glucose (Table 18-1).

These organisms are environmentally fragile and are readily inactivated by exposure to drying, chilling, sunlight, acids, and alkalies. They can be cultivated on laboratory media if special care is taken to prevent inactivation. Growth occurs best on blood or chocolate agar (a medium enriched with blood and heated, which turns the blood a chocolate color), in a CO_2-enriched environment. The two species can be differentiated on the basis of sugar fermentation tests. Most *N. meningitidis* strains produce apparent capsules whereas *N. gonorrhoeae* strains produce very slight capsules. Fimbriae are present on *N. gonorrhoeae*. Even though the *Neisseria* possess typical Gram-negative-type cell walls, they are susceptible to penicillin. *N. meningitidis* is commonly referred to as the *menin-*

Fermentive
organisms which are capable of producing relatively large amounts of acid from a carbohydrate.

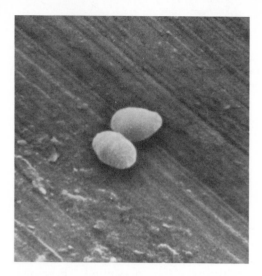

Figure 18-1   Scanning electron micrograph of *Neisseria gonorrhoeae* showing the typical diplococcal arrangement of the "bean-shaped" cocci (magnification 10,000×). (A. S. Klainer and I. Gies, *Agents of Bacterial Disease.* Harper & Row: Hagerstown, MD, 1973. Figure 7-1, p. 83.)

gococcus and the *N. gonorrhoeae* as the *gonococcus*. Nonpathogenic strains are found on the mucosal surfaces of the human alimentary tract.

MENINGOCOCCAL INFECTIONS

Pathogenesis and Clinical Diseases

Based on a polysaccharide capsule, *N. meningitidis* can be divided into 13 different serogroups. Group A (sometimes called the *epidemic strain*) is most often the cause of meningococcal disease throughout the world, but in the United States groups B, C, Y, and W–135 are most often involved. The main mechanisms of pathgenicity and virulence appear to be the capsule that helps retard phagocytosis and cell wall endotoxin that is thought to be responsible for most of the toxic effects of the disease. The meningococci are widespread in the general population and are readily transmitted via the airborne route. They multiply in the nasopharyngeal area without causing any disease; an infected individual

Table 18-1   Biochemical Identification of *Neisseria* Species

Species	Acid from			
	Glucose	Maltose	Sucrose	Lactose
N. meningitidis	+	+	−	−
N. gonorrhoeae	+	−	−	−
N. lactamica	+	+	−	+
N. sicca	+	+	+	−
N. cinerea	−	−	−	−

may carry these organisms for many months. Such a **carrier** state may induce an immune response in the person and cause resistance to the given serogroup with which that person is colonized. This carrier, however, serves as a reservoir from which the bacteria may be transmitted to those who live in close contact with the person. The carrier rate varies in different populations. The rate is 3% to 30% in a general population in which no clinical disease is present compared to a rate of 15% to 50% in persons who live or work around patients with clinical meningococcal diseases and may reach 80% during an epidemic. The carrier rate in military personnel is generally higher than in other populations.

Once meningococci are colonized in the respiratory membranes, the person may experience mild sore throat and fever. Meningococci may be carried into the lymphatic system and then into the blood. If the host is unable to contain the infection at this point—and no information is available as to how many infected persons progress to this point without symptoms developing—the bacteria become deposited in various tissues, such as skin, **meninges**, joints, and lungs. In a few days lesions may develop in these tissues with the manifestation of signs and symptoms of the disease. In the disseminated infections, **hemorrhagic** lesions may occur in the involved tissue, along with high fever and prostration. Subcutaneous hemorrhagic lesions sometimes occur, giving the person a spotted appearance.

The disease *spinal meningitis*, more properly called *meningococcal meningitis*, is a relatively rare outcome of the much more common meningococcal infections. Meningitis is accompanied by various **neurologic** symptoms; the death rate in untreated cases may be as high as 85%. With treatment, however, the overall death rate is 10% to 15%. *Disseminated meningococcal disease* may also occur without meningitis and has a high death rate as well.

The presence of specific antibodies in the serum offers protection against the disseminated disease but apparently does not cure the carrier stage in the nasopharyngeal tissues. Most adults have acquired antibody immunity against meningococci due to previous subclinical infections, whereas most infants have passive

Carrier
a living host that is infected by an organism but does not have clinical symptoms of disease. Carriers may have asymptomatic infections or may be individuals who have recovered from the disease but continue to shed the causative agent into the environment.

Meninges
membrane coverings of the brain, and spinal cord. Inflammation of this membrane is referred to as *meningitis*. Meningitis may be either septic (bacterial) or aseptic (nonbacterial). Aseptic meningitis is often caused by virus infection.

Hemorrhagic
associated with bleeding. Hemorrhagic lesions of the skin often appear as red spots or blemishes. These lesions frequently become dark blue or black in color and may involve large areas of the skin.

Neurologic
pertaining to the nervous system, either central (brain and spinal cord; CNS) or peripheral (nerves extending from the CNS to other body tissues).

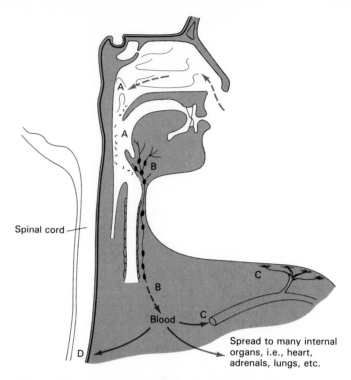

Figure 18-2 The pathogenesis of meningococcal infections. Stages of infection: A. Bacteria may be implanted in the nasopharynx. This phase of the infection is often asymptomatic, but in some cases may cause a sore throat. B. Bacteria may pass into the blood stream via the lymphatic system. C. Septicemia with inflammation of blood vessels and areas of hemorrhaging in the skin. Much of the damage is caused by endotoxins. The disease may range from mild to rapidly fatal. D. Meningitis, with headache, fever, and signs of meningeal irritation (rash may or may not be present).

immunity during the first months of life. The pathogenesis of this disease is outlined in Figure 18-2.

Transmission and Epidemiology

Transmission of meningococci is usually via the airborne route; because of the large number of carriers in the general population, transmission may occur at any time. Transmission is more efficient from a person with a clinical infection, however, and a significantly higher number of cases occur in a patient's household contacts than in the general population. Children are frequently exposed early in life and a higher incidence of disseminated dis-

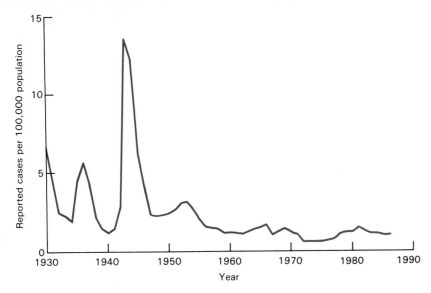

Figure 18-3 Reported cases of meningococcal infection per year in the United States between 1930 and 1988. (Courtesy Centers for Disease Control, Atlanta)

ease is seen in the 6- to 24-month age range. This represents the period between loss of passive immunity and acquisition of active immunity. For less obvious reasons, the next age group that is most susceptible are the 10- to 20-year-olds. More than two-thirds of all cases occur in persons under 20 years of age. Many meningococcal disease outbreaks have been associated with military recruits. The higher number of cases in military recruits probably results from close personal contact in barracks, and the increased exposure due to the high carrier rate in military personnel.

Sporadic cases are seen in most areas; however, epidemic meningitis does occur periodically in areas throughout the world. The sporadic cases run about 3 per 100,000 in the general population per year whereas the rates during an epidemic may increase to several hundred per 100,000 per year. The annual case rate in the United States is presented in Figure 18-3.

Diagnosis

Direct microscopic examination of infected tissues or fluids may reveal the presence of the meningococci and provide a rapid diagnosis. Inoculation onto appropriate nutrient agar is also used to demonstrate the presence of meningococci. Cerebral spinal fluid and other body fluids can be rapidly tested for the presence of *N. meningitidis* antigens. This procedure may help to provide a guide to specify therapy against the disease.

Hospital-Acquired Meningococcemia: 1978

In February 1978 a nurse developed meningococcemia 3 days after assisting in the emergency room evaluation of a patient with meningococcemia and meningitis.

The index patient was a 25-year-old man who was seen in the emergency room with fever, malaise, myalgia, and a headache of 24-hour duration. A diagnostic lumbar puncture in the emergency room was unsuccessful because of the patient's lack of cooperation. He was taken to the postoperative recovery room, where he was given inhalation anesthesia and intubated; a lumbar puncture was then performed. The patient vomited several times in the emergency room and during intubation. Hospital personnel assisting with the anesthesia and lumbar puncture did not wear masks or follow other isolation precautions.

The patient's cerebrospinal fluid (CSF) had a protein level of 767 mg/dl, a glucose of 6 mg/dl, and a white blood cell count (WBC) of 20,7000/mm^3 with 98% neutrophils. Gram stain of the smear showed multiple Gram-negative diplococci that were both extracellular and intracellular. No pneumonia was seen on the chest x ray. Cultures of the blood and spinal fluid grew *Neisseria meningitidis*, subsequently identified as a sulfonamide-susceptible group B strain. Following diagnosis of the patient's disease, approximately 6 hours after his admission to the emergency room, he was placed in isolation.

Before he was placed in isolation, 24 medical personnel (physicians, nurses, orderlies, and others) had contact with the patient. These persons were informed of their possible exposure to meningococcal disease. Those with intimate contact with the patient were advised to take rifampin prophylactically for 2 days; 3 nurses and 2 orderlies received prophylaxis.

Three days after the index patient was admitted to the hospital a 39-year-old nurse developed headache, fever, and malaise. She had assisted with the intubation and suctioning of nasopharyngeal secretions from the index case at the time of his diagnostic lumbar puncture. Two days after onset of her symptoms she presented herself for examination and was noted to have scattered petechial lesions on her arms and legs. Her WBC was 17,400/mm^3 with 87% neutrophils. Lumbar puncture showed normal CSF; blood cultures were not obtained. Over the next several days she developed a more severe headache, more petechiae, and joint pains. Six days after her initial symptoms, she was admitted to the hospital and isolated with a presumptive diagnosis of meningococcemia. A repeat lumbar puncture was performed and revealed a WBC of 25/mm^3, mostly neutrophils, normal glucose and protein concentrations, and negative Gram stain and culture. A blood culture, however, grew group B *N. meningitidis* susceptible to sulfonamides.

On careful questioning, the nurse recalled that she had exposure to the nasopharyngeal secretions from the index patient, but afterward she had not received antibiotic prophylaxis. She had no other known contacts with persons with meningococcal disease or colonization and at the time of these two cases no other cases of meningococcal disease were occurring in the community.

Transmission of *N. meningitidis* to hospital personnel caring for a patient with meningococcemia or meningitis is rare and has been reported only when there is extensive contact with the infected individual. To minimize the risk of transmission of meningococcal infection to hospital personnel, a patient who has a disease compatible with meningococcal infection should be placed in respiratory isolation when the diagnosis is first suspected. Personnel who have had intimate contact with the patient's respiratory tract secretions should be given rifampin as chemoprophylaxis or a sulfonamide if the strain of *N. meningitidis* is known to be sensitive to sulfonamides (*MMWR* 27:358, 1978).

Treatment

Intravenous administration of large doses of penicillin is the most effective treatment. Broad-spectrum antibiotics such as chloramphenicol may be used in penicillin-allergic patients. The sulfonamids are effective if resistant strains are not causing the disease, although currently about one-half the isolates are resistant to the sulfonamides. Treatment is much more effective if started early in the infection. If meningitis is suspected in a young child, immediate treatment is essential, for the disease may progress rapidly and lead to death or permanent neurologic damage within less than 24 hours after the onset of severe symptoms.

Prevention and Control

Vaccines have been developed against serogroups A and C. These vaccines use purified capsular antigens and a single dose produces a good antibody response. Since 1971, over 500,000 military recruits have been vaccinated with serogroup C vaccine and 62,000 Egyptian school children have been vaccinated with serogroup A vaccine. No serious adverse reactions have occurred in those vaccinated, and serogroup C meningococcal meningitis has been virtually eliminated in military recruit populations. Before 1971, serogroup C was frequently the cause of meningitis in military recruits. Vaccines have been used in some cities where outbreaks of meningococcal meningitis occurred, but their use in civilian populations is still being evaluated. These vaccines do not seem to be effective in children under 2 years of age. The vaccine might also be used along with antibiotics in the prophylactic treatment of household contacts of meningococcal disease.

Household contacts and hospital personnel who are exposed to clinical cases should be given prophylactic doses of the antibiotic rifampin to reduce the chance of secondary cases occurring. Meningococcal patients in the hospital should be kept in isolation. Even though the risk to hospital personnel is low, the following clinical note illustrates the need for precaution in working with patients with meningococcal disease.

GONORRHEA

The term *gonorrhea* was introduced by the ancient physician Galen; it means the "flow of seed" and refers to the flow of pus from the urethra of infected persons. Diseases that may have been gonorrhea were described in ancient medical writings, and in the thirteenth century, gonorrhea was recognized as a *sexually transmitted disease*. Not until many years later, however, was a clear distinction made between gonorrhea and syphilis, because the two diseases often occurred simultaneously in the same person. Today, gonorrhea is among the most prevalent of the classical venereal diseases—or the sexually transmitted diseases as they are now called—and is the most frequent reportable disease in the United States.

Gonorrhea usually responds well to penicillin therapy; in fact, the availability of this drug in the 1940s made people believe that gonorrhea could be controlled or eliminated. Nevertheless, the liberalized sexual attitude of the 1960s–70s, together with the development and use of oral contraceptives, caused a marked upsurge in the number of cases of gonorrhea. At present, a worldwide pandemic of gonorrhea is occurring, with more than 1,000,000 cases reported each year in the United States. The development of penicillin resistance among some strains may make further control of this disease very difficult.

Antigens and Virulence

N. gonorrhoeae displays an interesting and somewhat confusing array of antigens. When first isolated from a symptomatic patient, the colonies are small (designated colony types 1 and 2) and may be either opaque or clear. On subsequent culture the colonies become larger (types 3 and 4) and are most often transparent. Colony types 1 and 2 are associated with a high level of infectivity and the presence of pili. Opaque colonies are associated with a cell surface protein known as protein II. Both protein II and pili appear to be involved in the attachment of gonococci to host cells. Such attachment is considered to be an important factor in the development of disease symptoms. Understanding of the significance of the antigenic colony type during disease is further complicated because it may vary from one type to another during the course of infection. Virulence factors other than those associated with bacterial attachment include the endotoxic lipopolysaccharide (LPS; Chapter 4) and the production of an enzyme that inactivates human IgA–1, one of the important immunoglobulins found on mucosal surfaces.

Pathogenesis and Clinical Diseases

The patterns of gonorrhea vary somewhat among the male, female, and the newborn. Therefore the clinical diseases are discussed separately for each group.

Gonorrhea in the male The gonococci are usually deposited in the lower portion of the urethra during sexual intercourse, and the bacteria attach to the surface cells of the urethra. The growing gonococci induce an acute inflammatory response in 2 to 8 days that may be accompanied by fever, a purulent discharge, and pain during urination. In most cases, the male experiences definite symptoms when infected. The infection may spread by direct extension along the ducts of the genitourinary tract with accompanying inflammation. The inflammation may close the urethra and prevent urination in 1% of the cases. The infection may also spread to the vas deferens (sperm ducts) and cause scarring and closure of this duct, which then results in infertility of the patient. In some cases, the bacteria spread into the blood and are carried to various internal organs or to bone joints, where inflammation (septic arthritis) may develop.

Gonorrhea in the female   Infection usually results from gonococci transmitted during sexual intercourse. The ensuing infection is of the cervix and often remains at a low level; in up to 80% of the infected females it is asymptomatic. Those patients with signs of the disease experience vaginal discharge, fever, a burning sensation, and abdominal pain. The abdominal pains are normally associated with spread of the infection to the fallopian tubes, a serious condition known as *salpingitis*. This form of gonorrhea may induce scarring with closure of the fallopian tubes in 20% of these women, which results in the loss of fertility. The fallopian tubes are also predisposed to secondary infections by other bacteria. Further extension of the infection into the lower abdomen occurs in 10% of the women with gonorrhea and is called **pelvic inflammatory disease** (**PID**). The duration of the asymptomatic infections is not known, but some evidence indicates that the infection may persist for months. Women using oral contraceptives are thought to be more susceptible to gonorrhea due to changes in the pH of the vaginal mucosa induced by birth control pills. The gonorrhea may spread into the blood and be carried to other organs in a small percentage of infected females. Renal gonorrhea is seen in about half the infected females and is common in homosexual males.

Pelvic inflammatory disease (PID) a serious intra-abdominal infection of females. PID usually follows vaginal or uterine infection, and is most often caused by one or more of the sexually transmitted disease agents. Reproductive sterility is a common outcome, but in some instances death may occur from PID.

Gonorrhea in children   Persons of all ages are susceptible to gonorrhea. The most common form of childhood gonorrhea is seen as an eye infection (gonococcal ophthalmia neonatorum) of the newborn. Contamination takes place during passage through the birth canal of a mother who has gonorrhea. If not treated, severe inflammation of the eyes and even blindness may result. The serious nature of gonococcal conjunctivitis in the newborn has led to the universally accepted practice of placing a few drops of dilute silver nitrate or penicillin directly onto the conjunctiva of the infant immediately following birth. Before routine disinfection of the eyes of newborns was required, gonococcal ophthalmia was the major cause of blindness in children.

Transmission and Epidemiology

Gonorrhea in adults is almost always transmitted by sexual contact. Increases and decreases in disease rates are directly related to major social changes associated with war or liberalized attitudes toward sex. The reported cases of gonorrhea are shown in Figure 18-4. Since the early 1960s, the rate of gonorrhea has increased steadily in most parts of the world and is now considered of epidemic proportions. Most cases of gonorrhea are seen in the ages and social groups that are most sexually active. The highest rate of disease is seen in the 15- to 30-year age groups with a peak rate in the 20- to 24-year age groups. High rates are also seen in such subpopulations as divorced persons and homosexuals. Over a million cases of gonorrhea are officially reported in the United States each year, but the actual number is thought to be three or four times greater. The number of cases of gonorrhea varies among the states and is shown in Figure 18-5.

Generally, immunity to gonorrhea infection does not develop and a person may be infected over and over again. The probability of a male becoming infected after sexual intercourse with an infected female is about 20%. The probability of the female contracting the disease from an infected male is thought to be greater; however, it is not as well determined because many females contract asymptomatic infections that go undetected.

Figure 18-4   Reported case rates of gonorrhea per year in U.S. civilians, 1941–1983. The leveling-off of reported cases since 1975 is thought to be the result of an increased government control program initiated in 1973 (modified from CDC annual summaries).

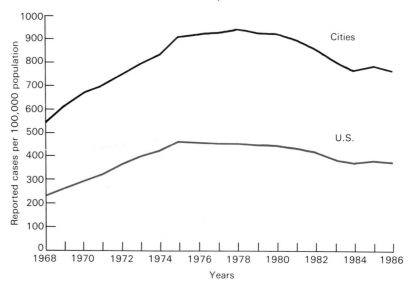

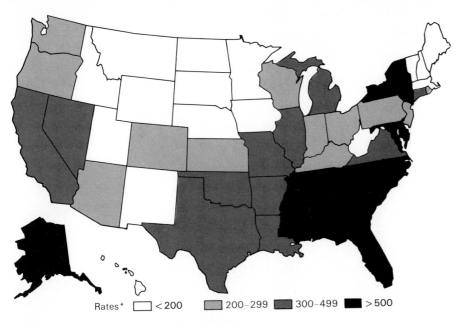

Rates* ☐ < 200   ▨ 200–299   ▩ 300–499   ■ > 500

*Based on reported cases per 100,000 population.

Figure 18-5   Occurrence of gonorrhea within states of the United States in 1986.
(Courtesy Centers for Disease Control, Atlanta)

Diagnosis

Diagnosis is much easier in males than females. The purulent discharge is examined with the microscope for the present of intracellular Gram-negative diplococci; if positive, the diagnosis is confirmed (Figure 18-6). If the microscopic test is negative, an attempt

Figure 18-6   Photomicrograph of pus from a patient with gonorrhea, showing a phagocytic cell filled with gonococci. (Courtesy Abbott Laboratories, Chicago)

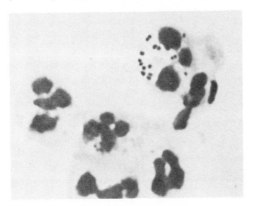

should be made to isolate the gonococcus on a culture medium to provide a positive diagnosis. It is much more difficult to observe gonococci microscopically in smears of exudate from infected females and this procedure is of limited diagnostic value in women. Cultures should be obtained from the cervix and anal canal and, if possible, inoculated directly onto a selective agar medium for gonococci, such as modified Thayer-Martin medium. If the specimen must be transported to the laboratory, special handling methods are required to prevent the inactivation of these delicate microorganisms. Because the diagnosis of asymptomatic infections in females is often difficult, there is currently a great need for a simple reliable test to detect these infections. Serologic tests are not well developed and are of limited value at present.

Treatment

In treating gonorrhea, penicillin is still the drug of choice. Over the years, however, gonococci have developed increased resistance to penicillin and currently a single injection of 4.8 million units is needed for most cures. Treatment with penicillin is usually dramatic and since the 1940s has functioned as a so-called wonder drug in curing gonorrhea. But in 1976 the first strain *N. gonorrhoeae* completely resistant to penicillin was discovered. Penicillin-resistant strains carry a plasmid that directs the formation of the enzyme β-**lactamase** (penicillinase) that is able to inactivate penicillin G, ampicillin, and cephalosporins. Penicillinase-resistant strains have been isolated from many countries through the world (Table 18-2).

Beta-lactamase
an enzyme capable of hydrolysing the beta-lactim structure of penicillin and cephalosporin antibiotics. This action renders the antibiotic ineffective.

After an initial increase, the number of cases of gonorrhea due to penicillinase-producing *Neisseria gonorrhea* (PPNG) began to decline. However, there has been a marked increase in the

Table 18-2   Locations with Identified Strains of β-Lactamase-Producing *Neisseria Gonorrhoeae* Through May 1981[a]

Africa	Americas	East Asia	Europe	South East Asia
Morocco	Canada	Philippines	France	Indonesia
Ghana	United States	Hong Kong	Belgium	Singapore
Mali	Mexico	Taiwan	Netherlands	Malaysia
Nigeria	Panama	Guam	United Kingdom	Thailand
Central African Republic	Argentina	Japan	West Germany	India
Gabon	Colombia	Republic of Korea	Denmark	Sri Lanka
Zaire		New Zealand	Poland	
Madagascar		New Hebrides	Switzerland	
Zambia		Australia	Sweden	
Senegal			Norway	
			Finland	

[a]*Information obtained through WHO Epidemiological Surveillance System; adapted from PAHO Epidemiologic Bulletin.*

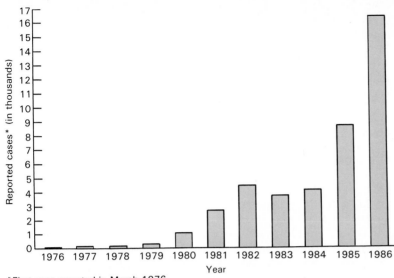

Figure 18-7 Reported cases, by quarter, of gonorrhea caused by penicillinase-producing *N. gonorrhoeae* in the United States, 1976 to 1981. The number of cases of gonorrhea caused by penicillin-resistant strains appear to be increasing (modified from CDC annual summaries).

number of recent isolates of PPNG, and it is feared that an epidemic of disease due to these organisms may be underway (Figure 18-7). Additional concern regarding penicillin resistance was raised by the recent discovery that some *N. gonorrhoeae* are resistant to penicillin because of a change in the bacterial chromosome. Although of considerable epidemiologic concern, penicillin resistance due to plasmids (PPNG) can be relatively easily detected, but chromosomal resistance will be both more difficult and expensive to determine. Persons with this resistant strain or who are sensitive to a penicillin can be cured with various other recommended treatment schedules (Table 18-3). The broad-spectrum antibiotics needed to treat the cases of gonorrhea caused by penicillin-resistant strains often have adverse side effects and are significantly

Table 18-3 Recommended Therapy for Gonorrhea

Infection	Primary Therapy	Alternative Therapy
Uncomplicated gonorrhea	Penicillin (4.8 million units)	Tetracycline (2.5 g/day)
Penicillin-resistant gonorrhea	Spectinomycin (2 g intramuscularly)	Cefoxitin with probenecid or Sulfamethoxazole/ trimethoprime (9 tablets/day)
Spectinomycin-resistant gonorrhea	Cefoxitin with probenecid (2 g and 1 g intramuscularly)	Cefotaxime (1 g intramuscularly)

CLINICAL NOTE

Disseminated Gonorrhea Caused by Penicillinase-Producing *Neisseria gonorrhoeae*: Wisconsin and Pennsylvania, 1986

During the period August–September 1986, CDC received four reports of disseminated gonococcal infection (DGI) caused by penicillinase-producing *Neisseria gonorrhoeae* (PPNG).

Cases 1 and 2: A 28-year-old woman (Patient 1) was admitted to a Racine hospital on August 4, 1986, with a 1-week history of arthritis of the left knee with effusion. Synovial and cervical cultures were both positive for PPNG. She was treated for 2 days with intravenous penicillin. When the culture results became known, her therapy was changed to ceftriaxone, 500 mg once daily. Despite the change in therapy, the knee remained swollen. Even though the dosage of ceftriaxone was increased to 1 g every 12 hours, the knee had to be surgically drained on August 14. The woman recovered rapidly and was discharged 1 week later.

The index patient's only recent sexual partner (Patient 2) was examined on August 8. He had had urethritis for 1 week and a swollen, painful left wrist for 2 weeks. Nine days earlier, he had been treated for the wrist symptoms with a nonsteroidal, anti-inflammatory agent. Upon examination, the patient had purulent urethritis and a tender, slightly swollen wrist. Urethral culture was positive for PPNG. The wrist was not cultured. He was treated intramuscularly with 2 g of spectinomycin and recovered completely.

Case 3: A 20-year-old woman seen in an emergency room in Philadelphia had had wrist pain for 1 week and pain in the right knee, left ankle, and the dorsum of the left hand for 3 days. On physical examination, she was febrile, had tenosynovitis of the extensor tendons of the left hand, and had effusion of the right knee and ankle. Arthrocentesis of the knee yielded purulent fluid which grew PPNG. A cervical culture was also positive for PPNG. Initially, she was treated intravenously with penicillin; therapy was changed to cefotaxime when culture results became available. She recovered completely.

Case 4: A 52-year-old woman seen in a Philadelphia emergency room had had pain in the right wrist and third finger of the left hand for 2 days. She was febrile, and the right wrist and proximal interphalangeal joint of the left third finger were swollen and tender. Arthrocentesis of the wrist yielded purulent fluid that grew PPNG. She was treated intravenously with penicillin. Therapy was changed to intravenous ceftriaxone when culture results became available. She recovered completely.

Antibiotic-susceptibility testing, auxotype, protein I serovar determination, and plasmid analysis of isolates from all patients were performed at CDC. All isolates were resistant to penicillin (minimum inhibitory concentration [MIC] 1–8 μg/ml), and all demonstrated moderate chromosomally mediated resistance to tetracycline (MIC range: 0.5–4.0 μ/ml) and to cefoxitin (MIC range: 0.5–2.0 μg/ml). All were sensitive to spectinomycin and ceftriaxone. All isolates were auxotype/serovar class Prov/IA-6, and all contained the 2.6 megaDalton (mDal) cryptic plasmid, the 3.2 mDal β-lactamase plasmid, and the 24.5 mDal conjugative plasmid. Despite the similarity of the isolates, suggestive of a clonal origin, no linkage could be demonstrated between the two Philadelphia patients or between either Philadelphia patient and the Wisconsin patients. (*MMWR* 36:161, 1987).

more expensive than penicillin. Should the penicillin-resistant strains become more widespread, the treatment and control of gonorrhea would become more difficult and expensive than it has been during the past 30 years.

No vaccines are currently available, although experimental data are being gathered for vaccine use. As was noted earlier, gonorrhea in the newborn is prevented by irrigating the eyes with a 1% solution of silver nitrate. This procedure is required by law in all states and has almost eliminated gonococcal ophthalmia in the newborn. Penicillin or erythromycin is sometimes used in place of silver nitrate. If a pregnant female has gonorrhea, she should be treated before delivery to further reduce the hazard to the newborn infant.

Prevention and control of gonorrhea is complicated by the **occult** nature of the infection in the female. Extensive studies involving more than 1.5 million women visiting a wide variety of medical services indicated that the rate of infection varied from 19.7% of those visiting a venereal disease clinic to 1.4% of women who were military dependents. Overall, the rate of infection was 5.7% of all females tested. Gonorrhea in adults is preventable by avoiding exposure to the disease. Still, history has clearly demonstrated that prevention will not be accomplished by this means. The risk of exposure can be reduced by using such devices as condoms. Reporting cases of gonorrhea to public health officials is helpful in that it aids in finding and treating persons who might be serving as sources of infection. Numerous education activities have been tried at various age levels in attempts to reduce the incidence of gonorrhea. But the increasing rate of gonorrheal infections shows that these programs have had limited success.

Occult
hidden or unknown.

CONCEPT SUMMARY

1. The Gram-negative diplococci (*Neisseria*) include two species of major clinical significance: *N. meningitidis*, the etiologic agent of epidemic meningitis, and *N. gonorrhoeae*, the causative agent of gonorrhea.

2. *N. meningitidis* is often found as normal body flora and yet is responsible for a fulminant infection that causes rapid mortality in its victims. The balance between a normal flora and disease due to this organism is not well understood.

3. Gonorrhea has become such a common disease that it is literally a household word. The epidemic state of this disease and the ease with which it is generally treated belie its potential for producing life-threatening infections.

STUDY SUMMARY

1. The *Neisseria* are pyogenic cocci, which means that they are _____.

2. What is the usual mode of transmission and the reservoir for (a) *N. meningitidis* and (b) *N. gonorrheae*?

3. What is the basis for protection against infections due to (a) *N. meningitidis* and (b) *N. gonorrheae*?

4. List two reasons why a microorganism of relatively low virulence such as *N. gonorrheae* is of such great medical concern.

5. Why is gonorrhea more easily diagnosed in males than females?

6. What are PPNG?

7. How can you account for a female infection rate due to *N. gonorrheae* of more than 5%, but a disease rate less than 0.1%?

REFERENCES FOR FURTHER STUDY

1. Acute Otitis Media Caused by *Branhamella catarrhalis*: Biology and Therapy. *Reviews of Infectious Diseases* 9:16, 1987.

2. Mixed Bacterial Meningitis. *Reviews of Infectious Diseases* 9:693, 1987.

3. Gonococcal Recidivision, Diversity and Ecology. *Reviews of Infectious Diseases* 9:846, 1987.

4. Gonococcal Infections. *Infectious Disease Clinics of North America* 1(no. 1):25, 1987.

5. *Manual of Clinical Microbiology*, 4th ed., A. Lennette, 1985. American Society for Microbiology.

chapter 19

SPIROCHETES

The spirochetes are members of the family *Spirochaetaceae*, which includes long, slender, coiled, motile microorganisms (Figure 19-1). Three genera of spirochetes contain species that are able to cause diseases in humans: *Treponema*, *Borrelia*, and *Leptospira*. The most important of these genera in human disease is *Treponema*, which includes the etiologic agent of syphilis (*Treponema pallidum*). Other syphilislike diseases such as yaws, pinta, and bejel are caused by bacteria either closely related to or identical with the syphilis spirochete. Two less common diseases, relapsing fever and leptospirosis, are produced by spirochetes of the genera *Borrelia* and *Leptospira*, respectively.

SYPHILIS

Bacterium

T. pallidum is a slender, tightly spiraled organism with a length of from 5 to 20 μm. The width of these organisms is only about 0.2 μm, which makes observation with a standard bright-field microscope difficult (Figure 19-2). The treponemas are highly motile and move through fluid in a twisting motion. When a fresh, wet-mounted specimen is viewed with a dark-field microscope, the motile spirochetes are easily seen. *T. pallidum* has not been grown on any artificial culture media and humans are the only natural host. Monkeys and rabbits, however, can be experimentally infected. The testes of rabbits support the growth of some syphilis spirochetes and are used to grow these bacteria for experimental and diagnostic tests. This bacterium can be kept alive and motile for up to 2 weeks if stored at 25°C under anaerobic conditions in a special medium. *T. pallidum* is quite fragile and only lives for a short period when shed from the body. It is readily killed by

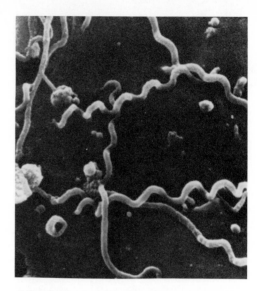

Figure 19-1 Scanning electron micrograph of the syphilis spirochete *T. pallidum* growing in rabbit testicular cells (N. S. Hayes, K. E. Muse, A. M. Collier, and J. B. Baseman, *Inf. Imm. 17:*174–186, Figure 3c, with permission from ASM).

disinfectants and is highly susceptible to penicillin and other antibiotics.

Pathogenesis and Clinical Disease

Among sexually transmitted diseases (Table 19-1), syphilis follows only gonorrhea in frequency of reporting. However, syphilis is potentially far more serious than gonorrhea and is a disease that,

Figure 19-2 Electron micrograph of *T. pallidum.* (Courtesy Centers for Disease Control, Atlanta)

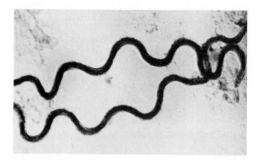

Table 19-1   Microbial Pathogens That Are Transmitted by Sexual Contact

Bacteria	Viruses	Fungi and Protozoa
Primarily transmitted by sexual contact		
Neisseria gonorrhoeae	Human Immune deficiency virus	Trichomonas vaginalis
Ureaplasma urealyticum	Herpes simplex II	
Gardnerella vaginalis	Papillomavirus	
Haemophilus ducreyi	Cytomegalovirus	
Calymmatobacterium granulomatis		
Chlamydia trachomatis		
Treponema pallidum		
Occasionally transmitted by sexual contact		
Group B streptococcus	Hepatitis B virus	Endamoeba histolytica
Campylobacter jejuni	Hepatitis A virus	Giardia lamblia
Shigella species	Molluscum contagiosum	Cryptosporidium
		Candida albicans

when untreated, may go through several stages over an extended period of time with varying clinical manifestations. The stages of syphilis in adults are primary, secondary, latent, and tertiary (Figure 19-3). Congenital syphilis also occurs when the disease is transferred in utero from an infected woman to her fetus. Syphilis is somewhat unusual in that both specific and nonspecific antibodies are formed against the infecting organism, but neither are protective against reinfection. In fact, it appears that many of the clinical symptoms produced in syphilitic patients are the result of the host immune response to the organism.

Primary syphilis   Sexual contact is almost always the mode of transmission of *T. pallidum*. The treponemas seem able to penetrate the mucosal tissues or gain entry through small lesions in the skin. The bacteria begin to multiply at the site of entry and are soon carried to the adjacent lymph nodes and eventually to the blood by which they are spread throughout the body. As a rule, after 10 to 30 days, but in some cases up to 70 days, a primary lesion appears at the site of infection. This lesion, which is usually genital, is called a *chancre*. The chancre is shallow, ulcerative, has a firm base, and is relatively painless. A chancre may reach more than 1 cm in diameter and is teeming with spirochetes (Figure 19-4). In some patients, often women, the chancre goes unnoticed due to its location in the deeper passages of the genital tract. With the appearance of the chancre, the disease is in the primary state

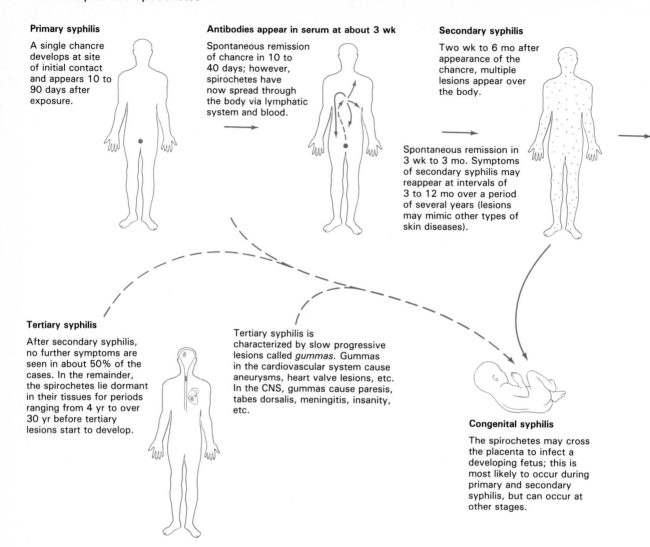

Primary syphilis

A single chancre develops at site of initial contact and appears 10 to 90 days after exposure.

Antibodies appear in serum at about 3 wk

Spontaneous remission of chancre in 10 to 40 days; however, spirochetes have now spread through the body via lymphatic system and blood.

Secondary syphilis

Two wk to 6 mo after appearance of the chancre, multiple lesions appear over the body.

Spontaneous remission in 3 wk to 3 mo. Symptoms of secondary syphilis may reappear at intervals of 3 to 12 mo over a period of several years (lesions may mimic other types of skin diseases).

Tertiary syphilis

After secondary syphilis, no further symptoms are seen in about 50% of the cases. In the remainder, the spirochetes lie dormant in their tissues for periods ranging from 4 yr to over 30 yr before tertiary lesions start to develop.

Tertiary syphilis is characterized by slow progressive lesions called *gummas.* Gummas in the cardiovascular system cause aneurysms, heart valve lesions, etc. In the CNS, gummas cause paresis, tabes dorsalis, meningitis, insanity, etc.

Congenital syphilis

The spirochetes may cross the placenta to infect a developing fetus; this is most likely to occur during primary and secondary syphilis, but can occur at other stages.

Figure 19-3   Stages in the pathogenesis of syphilis.

which lasts until the chancre goes away. The spontaneous disappearance of the chancre (usually within 3 to 6 weeks) may convince a naive patient to mistakenly believe that the disease is cured. The patient may then be without symptoms for a period ranging from 2 weeks to 6 months before the symptoms of secondary syphilis become evident.

Secondary syphilis   The spirochetes that spread through the body from the primary site of entry become deposited in many tissues, where they slowly multiply. Secondary syphilis is usually charac-

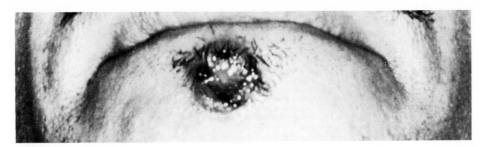

Figure 19-4   Primary syphilis with a chancre on the lower lip. (Courtesy Centers for Disease Control, Atlanta)

terized by the appearance of a generalized rash and lesions anywhere on the body (Figure 19-5). The lesions on the skin and mucous membranes may contain large numbers of spirochetes and are highly infectious. The patient may also experience such symptoms as headaches, fever, and sore throat. Lesions may also be present in bones, the central nervous system, or other organs. The skin lesions may be quite prominent; in earlier days this stage of the disease was called "great pox" to distinguish it from another common disease with smaller lesions—that is, smallpox. The secondary state gradually subsides. Complete recovery may be slow with

Figure 19-5   Secondary syphilis with rash-type lesions on the back. (Courtesy Centers for Disease Control, Atlanta)

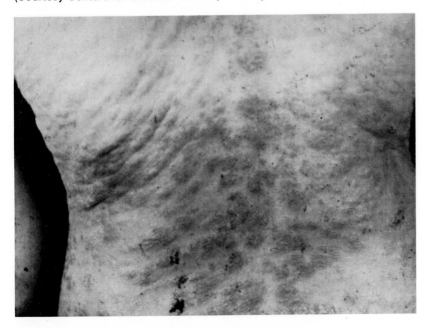

some signs remaining for several years. Any one of the following conditions may occur following this phase of the disease:

1. Complete remission with no further manifestations of the disease. This occurs in about 30% to 40% of untreated patients.

2. Recurrence of secondary lesions, often in modified forms. This may occur at 3- to 12-month intervals over the next several years. These recurring lesions may mimic other types of skin diseases.

3. Progression first into latent and then into tertiary syphilis.

Latent

unexpressed; similar to *occult*. This term is usually associated with diseases which have occurred but are in a "quiet" stage. The concept implied by this term suggests that some form of the disease will be expressed in the future.

Latent syphilis   A period of latency follows secondary syphilis. No symptoms of the disease are present during the latent period, but high levels of antibodies are in the serum. About half the patients who progress to the late latent phase have no further symptoms of syphilis. The others progress to the tertiary stage of the disease.

Tertiary syphilis   Signs of tertiary syphilis may appear any time from 3 to over 30 years following the secondary stage. However, in persons infected with *human immunodeficiency virus* (HIV, the etiologic agent of AIDS), symptoms of tertiary syphilis may develop rapidly and appear within only a few months following primary syphilis.

Lesions, called *gummas* (Figure 19-6), develop in various tissues of the body and may be due to a hypersensitivity reaction to the small number of spirochetes that have persisted in the body. Lesions may develop in the central nervous system, resulting in neurosyphilis, which may cause mental changes or resemble other neurologic diseases. Neurosyphilis is a major cause of insanity. The cardiovascular system is often involved, a common manifestation being the development of aneurysms in the aorta.

Congenital

associated with the fetal state. A congenital disease is one that is acquired by the fetus, usually as a result of a preceding maternal infection such that the infant is infected at birth.

Congenital syphilis   T. *pallidum* readily passes the placental barrier and a pregnant syphilitic woman may transmit the infection to the developing fetus. **Congenital** infection almost always occurs when the expectant mother develops primary syphilis, about 90% of the time if she has secondary syphilis, and around 30% of the time if the disease is latent. The fetus does not develop signs of congenital syphilis until the second trimester. The spirochetes become disseminated throughout the fetus and about 25% die in utero, resulting in a spontaneous abortion or stillbirth. Over half the syphilitic infants who are alive at birth show marked congenital defects, while some may appear normal at birth but develop symptoms at later periods. The manifestations of congenital syph-

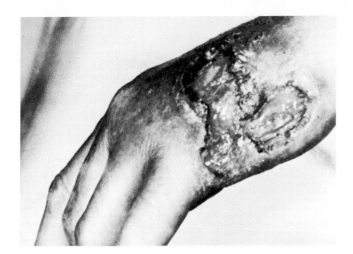

Figure 19-6   Tertiary syphilis with an ulcerative gumma on the hand. (Courtesy Centers for Disease Control, Atlanta)

ilis are variable but include such signs as skin lesions, enlarged spleens, anemia, pneumonia, eye damage, neurologic symptoms, mental retardation, and deformed bones, teeth, and cartilaginous tissues.

Transmission and Epidemiology

Generally transmission of syphilis is by sexual contact and persons most likely to contract this disease are those who have multiple sexual contacts. The epidemiologic patterns of primary and secondary syphilis are very similar to those seen with gonorrhea; that is, most cases occur in sexually active young adults. Overall, about 1 case of syphilis is reported to every 20 to 30 cases of gonorrhea. However, the rate of increase in the number of cases has been greater in recent years than for gonorrhea (Figure 19-7a,b). Although in the years just prior to 1986 the number of tertiary cases of syphilis had declined, this trend was reversed in 1986, and the number of tertiary cases nearly doubled in 1986 and 1987. The reason for this increase is not known.

Diagnosis

The appearance of a primary chancre or secondary lesions is suggestive of syphilis; these signs, however, may be confused with lesions or skin rashes caused by allergies or other infections. Diagnosis is first made by demonstrating the presence of the spiro-

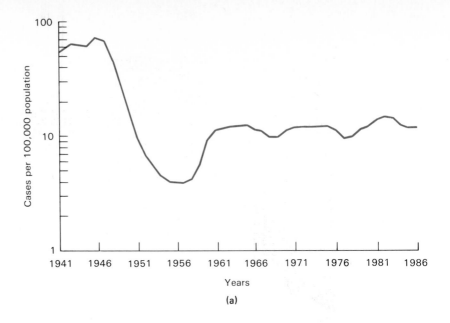

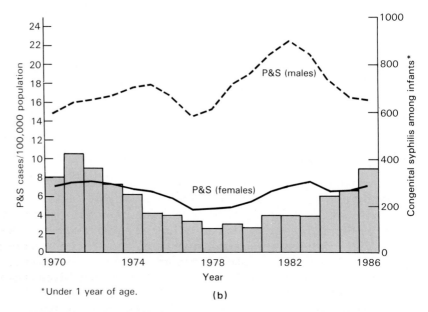

Figure 19-7 (a) Reported civilian cases of primary and secondary syphilis in the United States, 1941-1986. Syphilis is the third most frequently reported communicable disease in the United States. (b) Rate of occurrence of syphilis in males, females, and infants in the United States. (Courtesy Centers for Disease Control, Atlanta)

chetes in exudate from the lesion and then by serological tests. About 75% of cases can be diagnosed by direct dark-field microscopic examination of exudate from primary or secondary lesions. The exudate can also be fixed to a slide and stained with a specific fluorescent-labeled antibody for examination with a fluorescence microscope.

Various serological tests have been used over the past 70 years to detect syphilis antibodies. Antibodies appear several weeks after the primary lesion develops and remain in those persons who continue to harbor the spirochetes through the latent and tertiary stages. The serological tests for syphilis, often referred to as **STS**, are perhaps the most widely used of all serologic tests. They are often required of couples applying for marriage licenses, for some types of employment, for entrance into a military service, and as part of prenatal examinations. About 40 million such tests are run each year in the United States.

Two general types of serologic tests are used (Table 19-2). The first detects a nonspecific antibody, called *reagin*, that reacts with antigens from several sources and is produced by some disease other than syphilis. Among others, reagin reacts with a cardiolipin antigen that is extracted from beef hearts. Because the cardiolipin antigen is inexpensive, it is used in routine screening tests for syphilis. Flocculation tests, the chief tests used today, consist of adding the cardiolipin antigen to the test serum. Of these, the most used test is called the *VDRL* (Venereal Disease Research Laboratories) test and is positive when the cardiolipin forms into fine aggregates or floccules. Persons with a number of other diseases, such as hepatitis, diabetes, malaria, or other chronic diseases, may give a positive reaction to these screening tests for syphilis; such reactions are called *biological false positives*. All sera that are positive in the screening tests must be retested to confirm the results with a more specific serologic test that detects antibodies specific for *T. pallidum*. One such specific test is called the *fluorescent treponemal antibody* (FTA) test. The FTA test uses freeze-dried *T. pallidum* that are fixed to a glass slide. The test serum is added; if specific antibodies are present, they react with the *T. pallidum*. To determine

STS
serologic tests for syphilis. Serologic diagnosis of syphilis has been in use for many years. Nearly every known serologic procedure has been adapted to test for syphilis. Presently used STS are both highly specific and very sensitive.

Table 19-2 Serologic Tests for Syphilis (STS)

Nontreponemal Tests	Use
Flocculation tests	
VDRL (Venereal Disease Research Laboratory)	Screen and diagnosis
Reagin tests	
PCT (plasrnacrit)	Screen
USR (untreated serum reagin)	Screen
RPR (rapid plasma reagin)	Screen and diagnosis
Complement fixation tests	
Kolmer or Wasserman (complement fixation)	Rarely available

Treponemal Tests	Use
Immobilization	
TPI (treponema pallidum immobilication)	Diagnosis and research
Immunofluorescence	Diagnosis and screen
FTA-ABS (fluorescent treponemal antibody absorption)	
Hemmagglutination	
TPHA (treponema pallidum hemagglutination assay)	Diagnosis and screen

Specificity

the capacity of a diagnostic test to detect only truly positive specimens. A highly specific test would not have any false positive reactions. The following relationship is used to determine percent specificity of a test:

$$\frac{\text{true negative}}{\text{true negative + false positive}} \times 100$$

Sensitivity

the capacity of a diagnostic test to detect all positive specimens. A highly sensitive test would not have any false negative reactions. The following relationship is used to determine the percent sensitivity of a test:

$$\frac{\text{true positive}}{\text{true positive + false negative}} \times 100$$

if this reaction has taken place, the slide is rinsed to remove any unattached antibodies and then covered with fluorescent-labeled antibodies against human gamma globulin. If the test is positive, the spirochete–fluorescent antibody complex fluoresces when examined under a fluorescence microscope. Nonspecific antibodies must be removed from the patients sera before testing. This has given the name *absorbed* to the test, known as FTA-ABS.

Not all of the available tests have equal **specificity** and **sensitivity**. Careful consideration must be made regarding the circumstances of each patient in order to select the proper laboratory test for diagnosis.

Treatment

Penicillin is highly effective in treating syphilis and there is no evidence that resistant strains of *T. pallidum* are developing. Persons allergic to penicillin can be treated with erythromycin or tetracyclines. To treat primary or secondary syphilis successfully, penicillin must be maintained continuously in the system for 7 to 10 days. In the later stages of the disease, penicillin therapy should continue for at least 21 days. Treatment of syphilis at any stage before the onset of tertiary disease will block further progression of the disease. Treatment of pregnant syphilitic women early in pregnancy usually prevents congenital disease. Treatment later in pregnancy clears the infection in the fetus and prevents the occurrence of further tissue damage. Infants suspected of having congenital syphilis should receive treatment as soon as possible.

Prevention and Control

No syphilis vaccine is available. One widely used procedure to limit the spread of syphilis is to follow up and treat all persons who have had sexual contact with known syphilitic patients. This procedure, however, is often limited by a lack of public health personnel and operating funds. In addition, educational programs try to help people understand the mode of transmission, recognize symptoms, and how to receive treatment. Restricting one's sexual contact to a marriage partner is the most effective means of preventing syphilis and other sexually transmitted diseases.

OTHER TREPONEMAL INFECTIONS

Three similar diseases called *yaws*, *pinta*, and *bejel* result from treponemal spirochetes that are generally indistinguishable from *T. pallidum*. These diseases occur in people living under conditions of poor hygiene in the tropics or the Mideast. Transmission occurs by direct contact, not necessarily sexual, and primary infection usually happens in young children. Primary, secondary, and tertiary symptoms are seen. The exact relationship of these diseases to syphilis is not clear. It has been theorized that syphilis may have evolved from these diseases or vice versa. Yaws, pinta, and bejel are readily cured by penicillin. Infection rates decrease significantly when improvements are made in personal hygiene and living conditions.

RELAPSING FEVER

Sporadic cases of relapsing fever in humans are caused by spirochetes of the genus *Borrelia*. In contrast with *Treponema* species, the members of this genus stain with a variety of aniline dyes, and have been cultured in vitro. The most common species, *B. recurrentis* has an irregular, open spiral with several micrometers between turns. These organisms are frequently carried by ticks or lice and infection is transmitted to humans when they become infected and bitten by the insect vector. Tick-borne, or *endemic*, relapsing fever is seen occasionally in campers, for instance, who may spend time in tick-infested areas. The louse-borne, or *epidemic*, relapsing fever occurs most often in persons living in poverty or under crowded impoverished conditions associated with wars or other calamities.

The clinical disease is characterized by a sudden onset with accompanying fever, headache, and muscle pain. A rash may be seen in some patients. The infection may involve many tissues of the body. The first episode usually lasts 3 to 7 days, and climaxes with severe illness involving nausea, vomiting, and prostration. The patient quickly feels better and begins to gain strength. This afebrile period usually lasts up to 10 days, after which the patient relapses with symptoms similar to those of the initial period of illness. Patients often suffer 4–10 such relapses, usually with decreasing severity. The relapses are the result of the selection of antigenic variants of the organism, which then multiply and repeat the symptomatic process. The disease is treated with broad-spectrum antibiotics such as tetracycline and can be prevented by avoiding exposure to ticks or lice.

In recent years, a new human borrelial disease has been recognized. The organism, *B. burgdorferi*, precipitates an immunologic disease characterized by recurrent arthritic and neurologic problems including headache, **myalgia**, and fever. The disease is called *Lyme disease* after a small town in Connecticut where it was first characterized.

Myalgia
pain in the muscles.

Tick-borne Relapsing Fever: Colorado, 1977

Three cases of tick-borne relapsing fever were reported to the Colorado State Health Department during the late summer of 1977. The last case occurred in a 10-year-old Girl Scout from Denver, who spent 6 days (August 11–16) at a ranch about 8 miles west of Deckers, Colorado. During this time she slept on a mattress in a wooden-floored tent with 3 other girls. A total of 24 girls and 4 counselors were similarly housed in the immediate area. The patient reported an "insect bite" on the third day of camp and first became ill 6 days later on August 19 with a fever that lasted 4 days. A second recurrence of fever on August 30 prompted the taking of a thick blood smear, which showed the presence of spirochetes and confirmed the diagnosis of tick-borne relapsing fever. The patient was treated with tetracycline and showed immediate improvement.

No other illnesses occurred in the group or were reported from other Girl Scout units camping during July and August. The elevated platform tents used by Girl Scout campers were not conducive to rodent infestation. The general area has many natural harborages for chipmunks, however, and several nests, removed from decaying tree stumps within the camp, contained fleas and mites.

Editorial note: Although ticks were not found in association with this case, the vector probably was *Ornithodorus hermsi*, a nest tick of chipmunks and pine squirrels. No other relapsing fever vector is known to occur in the coniferous forest biome in North America.

The fact that no ticks were present in the rodent nests collected is not surprising. Normally *O. hermsi* ticks remain in the nest, where all life functions are accomplished and where the ticks can feed on their rodent hosts. If the rodent resident does not return, ticks eventually disperse from the nest in search of a blood meal. This dispersion could lead them to a human rather than a rodent host; however, ticks do not prefer a host-parasite relationship involving humans, so it tends to be of short duration (*MMWR* 26:357, 1977).

LEPTOSPIROSIS

The *Leptospira* are characterized by a very delicate, very tight coil. One end of the organism is characteristically bent into a hook shape (Figure 19-8). Only one species, *L. interrogans*, is a pathogen and it is found in a wide variety of wild and domestic animals. Among other tissues, the kidneys of the animals become infected and the leptospira are shed in the urine.

Humans become infected by direct of indirect contact with the urine from infected animals or with animal tissues. Leptospirosis is most often seen in persons who are frequently exposed to animals, such as veterinarians, farmers, abattoir workers, persons living in rodent-infested housing, and dog owners. Infections have also occurred from contact with contaminated water.

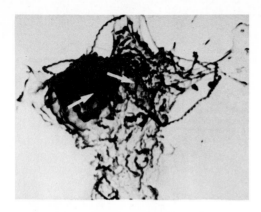

Figure 19-8 Electron micrograph showing *Leptospira Interrogans* in association with human polymorphonuclear leukocyte. Note tightly coiled leptospires. (Courtesy B. Wang et al, *Inf. Imm. 44*:459)

The portal of entry to the leptospira is probably through the mucous or breaks in the skin. The organisms spread through the blood and usually the kidneys become infected; other tissues are infected as well. A wide variety of symptoms may be seen. Less than 100 cases of human leptospirosis are confirmed by laboratory diagnosis each year in the United States (Figure 19-9), although it is thought that many more cases do occur but are not specifically diagnosed. It is possible both to isolate this spirochete on artificial

Figure 19-9 Cases of leptospirosis reported in the United States from 1955 to 1987. (Courtesy Centers for Disease Control, Atlanta)

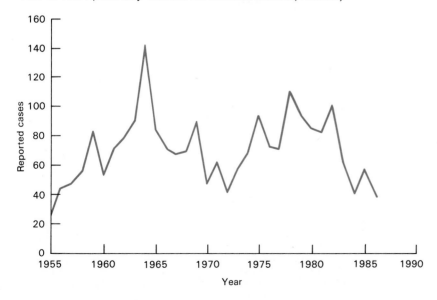

Leptospirosis: Tennessee, 1975

The first reported common-source outbreak of *Leptospira interrogans* in the United States occurred in Tennessee in August 1975.

An onset of illness struck seven children, four males and three females, ranging in age from 11 to 16 years, in the period of August 1 to 10. It was characterized by fever, headache, nausea, and/or vomiting, chills, myalgias, and abdominal pain. Hospitalization was needed in five of the seven cases; diagnoses included acute viral gastroenteritis, shigellosis, aseptic meningitis, and fever of unknown origin. The patient with the last diagnosis underwent laparotomy because of suspected appendicitis. A patient was treated as an outpatient for gastroenteritis and another did not consult a physician. The median duration of illness was 14 days and the mean hospital stay of the hospitalized patients was 6.6 days.

All seven patients had serologic evidence of recent infection with *L. interrogans.* Urine for culture was obtained from six patients 16 to 25 days after onset of illness; all were negative for leptospires.

All seven patients had swum in a local creek in the month preceding their illness. No other common source could be identified. A case-control study showed a definite association between acquiring leptospirosis and swimming in the creek. A questionnaire and serologic survey of 91 people who had swum in the creek during the summer of 1975 failed to detect any additional cases.

Samples of the creek water taken for culture and for animal inoculation 4 weeks after the outbreak did not yield the organism. Serum specimens were obtained from 50 cattle in five of seven herds pastured along the creek, but serologic testing did not implicate any herd. Wildlife was also considered as a possible source of contamination. Limited trapping was unsuccessful; no wild animals were obtained for testing. Because of the prominent gastrointestinal illness and because of failure to incriminate a bacterial pathogen, the outbreak was initially believed to have a viral etiology. Leptospirosis was considered only after the initial epidemiologic investigation incriminated swimming in the stream as the only common factor shared by all seven patients (*MMWR* 25:84, 1976).

---

media and to measure specific antibodies by various serologic tests. Isolation, however, is difficult and is infrequently accomplished.

Vaccines are used in veterinary medicine and are available to persons in high-risk occupations. Penicillin, streptomycin, and tetracyclines are effective if used early in the disease, but are generally not effective if given after about 4 days of illness.

CONCEPT SUMMARY

1. The spirochete of greatest medical concern is *Treponema pallidum*, the causative agent in syphilis. This disease occurs in several distinct stages with the last stage responsible for the

most serious pathology. It is a classic example of a sexually transmitted disease, although other means of transmission occur. No vaccine is available for control, but the disease responds well to antibiotic therapy.

2. Other spirochetal diseases, although relatively uncommon in the United States, can be severe and include leptospirosis, yaws, pinta, relapsing fever, and Lyme disease.

STUDY SUMMARY

1. Describe the features of the lesion associated with primary syphilis.

2. What structural (anatomical) features of the spirochetes are different from those common to a Gram-negative bacillus?

3. During which phase of syphilis is a patient most infectious for others?

4. How does tertiary syphilis differ from latent syphilis?

5. What are the advantages and disadvantages of the nontreponemal STS?

6. Which of the spirochetes can be cultured in vitro? Which can be visualized by staining with analine dyes?

7. What are the major sources of human infection by *Leptospira*?

REFERENCES FOR FURTHER STUDY

1. Ecology of Spirochetes. *Annual Review of Microbiology* 38:161, 1984.

2. Major Surface Proteins of the Lyme Disease *Borrelia* sp. In *Microbiology—1986*, p. 35. American Society for Microbiology.

3. Syphilis, Historical and Actual. *Reviews of Infectious Diseases* 8:1036, 1986.

4. Feasibility of Eradicating Yaws. *Reviews of Infectious Diseases* 7:S 335, 1985.

5. Endemic Non-Venereal Syphilis (Bejel) in Saudi Arabia. *British Journal of Venereal Disease* 60:293, 1984.

ANAEROBIC BACTERIA

T he anaerobic bacteria of medical interest are easily separated into two groups, those with and those without spores. The spore-forming anaerobes are all members of the genus *Clostridium*. They are Gram-positive bacilli, produce powerful exotoxins, and occur across a wide variety of habitats.

The non-spore-forming anaerobes are a group of diverse and incompletely characterized microorganisms. They form a significant proportion of the normal flora of the human body. Bacteria from this category constitute from 80% to 90% of the bacteria present on the skin, in the mouth, or in the upper respiratory tract, and about 99.9% of bacteria present in the intestinal tract. The non-spore-forming anaerobic bacteria include both Gram-negative and Gram-positive cocci and bacilli as well as spirochetes. Because these bacteria are more difficult to isolate and grow in pure culture than the aerobes, they have often been ignored or missed during routine bacteriological examinations of clinical specimens. These bacteria, however, are recognized as important opportunistic pathogens that produce a significant number of infections (Table 20-1). The two groups of anaerobic bacteria will be presented separately in this chapter.

CLOSTRIDIAL DISEASES

The genus *Clostridium* contains a large number of large, Gram-positive, spore-forming species, several of which are able to produce disease in humans. These anaerobic bacteria range in habitat from soil to the human mucosa; they are obligate anaerobes, many of which are killed by exposure to oxygen. They have a very active metabolism, ferment a variety of sugars, and have a very short generation time. Most clostridia produce one or a variety of very

Table 20-1   Infections Commonly Associated with Anaerobes

Infections	Percent of Positive Specimens Containing Anaerobes
Abscesses	
Abdominal	80–95
Brain	89
Cutaneous	60
Liver	52
Lung	85–93
Pelvic	88
Wounds	
Surgery colon	95
Decubitus ulcer	63
Sinusitis	50
Aspiration pneumonia	70–93
PID	25
Bacteremia	9

poisonous protein **toxins.** Representative species and the diseases produced by them will be presented.

Tetanus

Bacterium   *Clostridium tetani*, the causative agent of tetanus, is a large Gram-positive, spore-forming, motile, obligate anaerobic bacillus (Figure 20-1). It can be grown on blood agar or media containing meat. Various strains exist, but all produce the same exotoxin (tetanospasmin).

Pathogenesis and clinical disease   Because of the wide distribution of *C. tetani* (commonly found in soils and manures), wounds are often contaminated with these spores. However, the disease of tetanus does not develop in a great majority of cases. The condition of the wound must be such that an anaerobic environment exists with some dead tissue present. These conditions allow spores to germinate, bacteria to proliferate, and toxin to be produced. Such conditions are often seen in puncture wounds produced, for instance, by nails or splinters. Yet other types of wounds or conditions resulting in tissue damage may also offer a suitable environment for the growth of *C. tetani*. One frequently encountered form of tetanus occurring in underdeveloped countries is tetanus of the umbilicus of the infants born at home and treated with unsterile instruments.

Microbial toxin

any of a large number of protein or lipoprotein compounds produced by microbes which are poisonous to host tissues. The anaerobic bacteria produce a large variety of toxins.

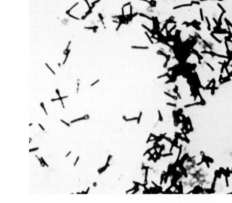

Figure 20-1
Photomicrograph of
Clostridum tetani. Many
have endospores at the
terminal end of the bacterial
cell. (Courtesy Centers for
Disease Control, Atlanta)

Synaptic
of the region where the nerve
impulse in a neuron is transmitted
to the responsive tissue (either
another neuron or a receptor cell).
These impulses are transmitted in
only one direction—neuron to
tissue.

Spasm
an involuntary contraction of a
muscle or muscle group.

The tetanus toxin is extremly potent. It is among the most
toxic substances known and a small amount is able to cause the
disease. The growth of *C. tetani* per se causes no tissue damage.
Usually signs and symptoms of the disease begin to occur 4 to
10 days after injury but may be delayed up to several months.
Symptoms are entirely the result of the toxin spreading through
the body. The toxin specifically affects the **synaptic** junction of
nerves by preventing the inhibition or erasing of nerve impulses
once they have crossed the synaptic junction. The nerve continues
to send impulses, a condition that results in spasmodic contrac-
tions (tetany) of the involved muscles. Early symptoms are muscle
stiffness with the muscles of the jaw often developing spasms
first. This condition gives the disease its common name of "lock-
jaw." As the disease progresses, **spasms** develop in other muscles. The spasms may be brief, but they can occur frequently and
cause great pain and exhaustion. In some cases, the spasms may
be powerful enough to cause bones to break. Respiratory complications are common and death rates high, especially in young children and elderly persons. In nonfatal cases, recovery takes several
weeks but is usually complete.

Transmission and epidemiology Transmission and epidemiology
of tetanus do not follow the pattern seen in many infectious diseases where the microbes are passed from host to host. Some situations are conducive to the development of tetanus, however.
Soils or materials in contact with animal wastes are usually heavily
contaminated with *C. tetani* and offer excellent sources of infection. Soil-contaminated wounds are the most frequent source of
infection. Before the development of an effective vaccine, tetanus
often resulted from wounds received in wars. Hundreds of thousands of cases of tetanus occurred during the Civil War, but only
12 cases were reported among U.S. troops during World War II.
About 100 cases per year are reported in the United States, 40%

of which result in death. The numbers of reported cases in this country are shown in Figure 20-2. Most of the cases (>70%) that occur in the United States are in adults 50 years of age or older (Figure 20-3). Older individuals are also more likely (52%) to die from tetanus than younger patients (13%). Large numbers of cases still occur in some underdeveloped tropical countries.

Diagnosis Diagnosis is made on the bases of the clinical disease. *C. tetani* is a common contaminant of wounds and may be found in patients who do not develop tetanus. Therefore the isolation of the bacterium from a patient may not be diagnostic.

Treatment As soon as clinical tetanus is suspected, steps should be taken to neutralize the existing toxin and prevent the formation of new toxin. Antitoxin, produced in humans, should be administered immediately. While antitoxin cannot reverse the toxic activity of the toxin bound to nerve tissue, it will inactivate toxins in the blood. Wounds should be debrided to remove dead tissues or foreign bodies, and large doses of penicillin or tetracycline should be given to prevent further growth of the bacterium. If muscle spasms occur, antispasmatic drugs should be used and respiration should be maintained by a positive-pressure breathing apparatus if necessary.

Prevention and control At present, the major involvement with *C. tetani* by most medical personnel in developed countries con-

Figure 20-2 Reported cases of tetanus by year in the United States, 1955-1983 (modified from CDC annual summaries).

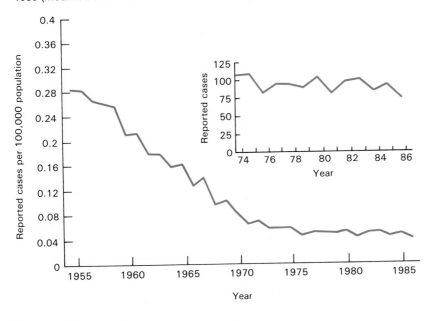

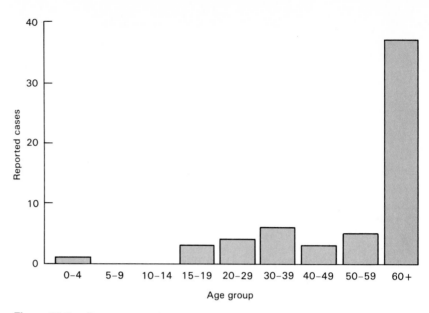

Figure 20-3   Occurrence of tetanus as a function of patient age.

cerns the prevention of this disease. Prevention through immunization has been extremely effective. In fact, approximately 95% of persons who develop tetanus have no record of immunization against the disease.

Immunization with tetanus toxoid should begin with infants 1 to 3 months old. The toxoid is usually given in combination with diphtheria toxoid and pertussis vaccine as the DPT vaccine. Three doses of DPT should be given several weeks apart. A booster dose should then be given 1 and 4 years later. After the age of 15, a tetanus booster should be given every 10 years. The vaccine given to adults is called *Td* (tetanus and diphtheria toxoid) and does not contain the pertussis antigen.

During the accident-prone years most young children are given booster doses with each new injury, a practice that is both unnecessary and unwise. Parents should keep an immunization record for their children so that such unnecessary immunizations can be avoided. When a person suffers an injury that is likely to result in tetanus and that person has no history of immunization, **passive immunization** with human antitoxin should be given as temporary protection. It should be followed by active immunization with the toxoid.

Neonatal umbilical cord tetanus can be prevented by actively immunizing pregnant females who have no history of previous immunizations. The newborn infant will then have natural passive immunity at the time of birth, which should reduce the chance of developing umbilical cord tetanus.

Passive Immunization
transfer of antibody to a susceptible host. The two types are natural (cross placental transfer) and artificial (gamma globulin given by injection.)

Neonatal Tetanus: Illinois, 1975

On May 6, 1975, a midwife delivered a male infant at home in a town across the Mexican border from Laredo, Texas. She reportedly cut the infant's umbilical cord with unsterilized scissors, tied it with a piece of string, and applied olive oil to the umbilical stump. The infant was adopted on the day of birth by a family from Chicago and appeared to be well until the third day of life when, en route to Chicago, he became irritable and ate poorly. When 5 days old, he could no longer nurse from a bottle. He was unable to open his mouth when crying and had several trembling spells associated with rigid flexion of his arms and extension of his legs. During these spells his head was kept in a neutral position; he perspired noticeably and was cyanotic. Each spell lasted approximately 10 minutes and occurred every 3 to 4 hours. The symptoms worsened and on the sixth day the infant was taken to the University of Chicago's Wyler Children's Hospital.

On admission it was noted that he had risus sardonicus (a grinning expression produced by spasms), opistotonus (difficulty in opening mouth), trismus (spasms with head and neck bent backward), and a temperature of 39.5° C. His umbilicus was inflamed and exuded a yellow purulent discharge. Laboratory evaluations at that time included a negative cerebrospinal fluid (CSF) examination and a normal serum calcium level. Gram stain of the umbilical discharge showed a mixed flora, including some large Gram-positive rods, which were thought by some observers to be compatible with *Clostridium tetani;* however, cultures grew only microaerophilic streptococci, peptostreptococci, and bacteroides. Neonatal tetanus was diagnosed on clinical grounds and the infant was given 1000 units of human tetanus immune globulin intramuscularly; antibiotic therapy with penicillin and gentamicin was begun. To control the muscle spasms, phenobarbitol and chlorpromazine were given and the infant was then rehydrated and maintained by continuous intravenous infusion.

Episodes of muscle spasm and periods of restricted respirations and cyanosis gradually decreased over the first 2 days of hospitalization; by the third day the infant could tolerate feeding and the administration of a sedative via a nasogastric tube. Gentamicin was discontinued on the third hospital day when admission blood and CSF cultures proved negative. When hypothermia of 35° C was noted on the fourth hospital day and attributed to chlorpromazine, diazapam was substituted for chlorpromazine and phenobarbitol to control muscle spasms. The infant's temperature returned to normal and the intensity of the muscle spasms decreased. But increasing tolerance to diazapam developed and the dose was increased over the next week to 10 mg/kg/day; for several days chlorpromazine was also given again in small doses. Penicillin was discontinued on the twelfth hospital day. On or about the thirteenth hospital day the tendency to have spasms began to decrease, and by the nineteenth day no symptoms related to tetanus toxin were discernible. On the twentieth hospital day bottle feedings were begun. Medications were gradually decreased as symptoms subsided and were discontinued by the thirty-fourth day with no apparent residual (*MMWR* 24:313, 1975).

Botulism

Bacterium C. botulinum is a large, Gram-positive, anaerobic bacillus that produces an exotoxin that causes food poisoning. Its spores are among the most heat-resistant and are able to withstand temperatures of 100° C for several hours. These spores will survive in heat-processed foods if the temperature does not reach the required level. Growth can occur in a wide variety of culture media as well as many types of food. Eight serotypes, based on the antigenic characteristic of the exotoxin, have been identified and are designated A through H. Cases due to type G have not been reported in humans.

Pathogenesis and clinical disease In most cases, botulism results from the ingestion of preformed toxin produced during the growth of *C. botulinum* in foods. Botulinum toxin is one of the most powerful known toxins and extremely small amounts (1–2 μg) are able to cause illness or death in humans. These toxins are destroyed by heating to 100° C for a brief period.

The toxin, generally type A, B, or E, is absorbed primarily from the small intestine, passes into the blood, and is carried to the peripheral nerves where it specifically reacts at the muscle-nerve junction. The toxin produces complete paralysis of the nerve impulse by preventing the release of **acetylcholine.** Death results from the paralysis of respiratory functions. Symptoms may appear as soon as 12 to 36 hours after ingesting contaminated food or may take as long as 8 days to appear. The first symptoms are often weakness and dizziness. Double vision (diplopia), difficulty in speaking (dipphonia) and swallowing (dysphagia), and dilated pupils usually occur. Some abdominal distress may be experienced. Fever is rare. Muscle weakness develops, leading to paralysis as the disease progresses. When paralysis of respiratory muscles occurs, death results. The mortality rate varies between 20% and 70% and is influenced by the amount and serotype of toxin consumed, as well as the time between ingestion and the initiation of antitoxin therapy.

In 1976 it was discovered that *C. botulinum* could grow in the intestines of infants and produce enough toxin to cause serious illness—infant botulism. The spore may be in various infant foods, but honey has been implicated in several cases. Not all infants appear to be susceptible and at present it is not known just which conditions allow the intestinal tracts of some infants to support the growth of *C. botulinum* (Figure 20-4). Signs of the disease in these patients may start with constipation, followed by weakness and then paralysis of the muscles of the head and neck. Paralysis may proceed to the arms and legs with death resulting from paralysis of the respiratory muscles. In cases that progress slowly, medical treatment can be applied in time to save the infant. In rapidly developing cases, death may result before significant signs are

Acetylcholine

a chemical messenger that functions to make a nerve-muscle junction. When this messenger is inhibited, the brain cannot signal the muscle to contract. This lack of muscle response is known as *flaccid paralysis.*

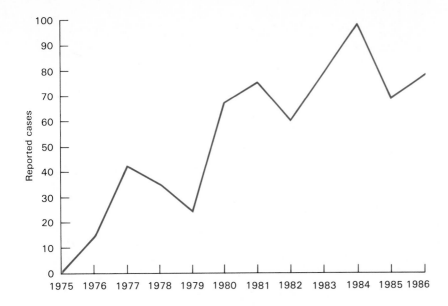

Figure 20-4 Cases of infant botulism in the United States between 1975 and 1986.

noted. Such death may be included under sudden infant death syndrome (sudden crib death), a problem that has long baffled medical investigators. It is now suspected that at least a percentage of sudden infant deaths is a result of infectious botulism.

Occasionally *C. botulinum* is able to grow in various environmental niches, such as animal feed, carcasses of dead animals or invertebrates, and sediments in lakes or ponds. Outbreaks of botulism poisoning occur when these contaminated materials are eaten by domestic or wild animals or birds. Under certain conditions outbreaks of botulism have occurred in wild ducks, resulting in the death of hundreds of thousands of the birds. Such wildlife epidemics are commonly due to botulinum toxin types C and D.

Transmission and epidemiology The *C. botulinum* spores are often present on food. Production of botulinum toxin results when the microorganism grows in an anaerobic environment in foods stored at room temperature. Alkaline foods favor the growth of *C. botulinum* and the development of the exotoxin.

Because botulism is a poisoning rather than an infectious disease, transmission from person to person does not occur. Circumscribed outbreaks, however, may result when a toxin-containing food is eaten by a number of people. Transmission of botulism generally involves home-canned foods; then the disease usually occurs only among family members. Outbreaks from improperly sterilized commercially canned food are quite rare. With commer-

Follow-up on Infant Botulism: United States, January 1978

Infant botulism, a disease apparently resulting from intraintestinal toxin production by *Clostridium botulinum,* was first recognized as a distinct clinical entity in late 1976. Since then, cases have been identified with increasing frequency (1, retrospectively, in 1975, 15 in 1976, 42 in 1977) and have been reported to the Centers for Disease Control from 15 states throughout the country: California (37), Pennsylvania (4), Utah (4), Washington (2), and (1 each) Arizona, Colorado, Montana, Nevada, New Jersey, New York, North Dakota, Oregon, Tennessee, Texas, and Wisconsin. Cases have occurred most frequently in the fall months, particularly in the past year; however, increased physician awareness may have accounted for this observation.

All patients identified thus far have had sufficient neuromuscular paralysis to require hospitalization. Constipation was the first symptom of illness in most cases, but frequently it was initially overlooked. A spectrum in the severity of symptoms has been noted. Some infants showed only lethargy, mild weakness, and slowed feeding whereas others became acutely ill with obvious feeding difficulty, severe generalized weakness, and hypotonia over a 1- to 3-day period, which, in some cases, progressed to respiratory insufficiency. A California and a Utah infant died following respiratory arrest.

Polyvalent antitoxin was administered to the first patient (1975) because the case was thought to be food-borne botulism. However, subsequent patients who received meticulous supportive care that focused on their nutritional and respiratory needs have been successfully managed.

In general, affected infants were the product of a normal gestation and delivery. They had no congenital abnormalities and were healthy until onset of illness. Of the 58 patients, 33 (57%) were males. The median age at onset was 10 weeks, the range 3 to 26 weeks.

No source of ingestible preformed botulinal toxin has been identified for any infant; neither did the patients share any exposure to a common food. Cases have occurred in exclusively breast-fed and exclusively formula-fed infants, although most infants had some exposure to food items other than milk. A potential source of *C. botulinum spores,* however, has been identified for six cases. Vacuum cleaner dust from the home of an infant with type A illness was found to contain *C. botulinum* type A whereas soil from the yard of an infant with type B illness yielded type B organisms. Three opened jars of honey taken from the homes of three infants with type B botulism who had been fed honey and water were found to contain type B organisms. Similarly, an unopened jar of honey of the same brand as that fed to an infant with type A illness was shown to harbor type A organisms. In contrast, *C. botulinum* was not found in 17 other commercial honey specimens, in 1 specimen from a private beekeeper, or in over 100 other foods tested, including cereals, baby food, formula, and breast milks; however, testing of foods and other potential sources of spores has not been done for all cases.

Editorial note: The identification of 57 of the 58 cases in only 24 months in 15 states located throughout the United States indicates that infant botulism occurs more commonly then previously realized. In California, Pennsylvania, and Utah some hospitals and physicians diagnosed subsequent cases shortly after identifying their first case. If cases are evenly distributed in the country, then by a conservative estimate at least 250 cases needing hospitalization may be occurring annually. Furthermore, because botulinal spores are found worldwide, there is no reason to suppose that cases are limited to the United States. Failure to identify cases in other countries may be explained by lack of physician awareness and limited laboratory facilities. Intensive case-finding is needed to provide sufficient data to elucidate the actual incidence, full clinical spectrum, mode of transmission, and other risk factors associated with this toxigenic disease.

Indications for the use of botulinal antitoxin or

oral antibiotics in the therapy of infant botulism are at present uncertain. It is not known whether administration of either will ameliorate the disease, shorten hospitalization, or diminish the risk of serious complications (*MMWR* 27:17, 1978).

Botulism and Commerical Pot Pie: California, 1982

On August 3, 1982, a 56-year-old woman residing in Los Angeles County, California, developed diplopia (double vision), weakness, difficulty breathing, and chest pain. She had respiratory arrest on admission to the hospital but was intubated, resuscitated, and placed in intensive care. Examination showed complete bilateral ptosis (drooping of eyelids), paralysis of eye muscles, facial weakness, and lack of reflexes. Cerebrospinal fluid was normal except for increased glucose. She had a past history of seizure disorder, diabetes mellitus, and organic brain syndrome. An infectious-disease consultant thought her subsequent fever was due to pneumonia secondary to aspiration, and he suspected botulism as the underlying cause of her illness.

The patient lived with her husband and grown son who both prepared meals for her and attempted a strict diet in consideration of her diabetes. When asked about the patient's food history before onset of illness, the husband and son named no likely suspects for botulism. No home-preserved foods had been served, and, with one exception, she had not eaten other foods that were not freshly prepared for her or were not also consumed by her husband and son. The exception was a commercial beef pot pie, which was accidently mishandled, then consumed by the patient one day before illness began.

The son had prepared the pot pie for an earlier evening meal. The frozen pie was baked in an oven for 40 to 45 minutes. As he was about to serve it to his mother, his father came home with some freshly cooked hamburgers just purchased at a take-out restaurant. The pot pie was put aside on an unrefrigerated shelf. Two and one-half days later, the son came home and found his mother had just consumed this pot pie without reheating it.

An uneaten portion of the pot pie, still in its metal plate, was retrieved by the family members. Type A botulism toxin was found in this pie by a mouse-inoculation test performed at a U.S. Department of Agriculture laboratory in Beltsville, Maryland, and type A toxin was also demonstrated in the patient's serum by the state's Microbial Disease Laboratory.

Editorial note: This is the third case of botulism associated with commercial pot pies reported from California; one other episode (involving two clinically diagnosed patients) was reported from Minnesota in 1960. Mishandling of the pot pies occurred in three of these episodes, and mishandling was also suspected in the fourth. The known mishandlings consisted of leaving the baked pot pie in the oven with the pilot light on, thereby maintaining "incubator" temperatures overnight. The pies were then eaten with no (or insufficient) reheating to destroy toxin. Or, as in the present case, the baked pie sat out at room temperature for over 2 days during hot weather—conditions that also could simulate an incubator.

In these situations, it is suspected that the original baking killed competing organisms in the pies and eliminated much of the oxygen. The heat-resistant, anaerobic *Clostridium botulinum,* which was evidently present and can be found in many fresh, frozen, and other food products, was then presumably able to germinate and produce toxin under the crust during storage at warm, incubatorlike temperatures. Products such as pot pies should be kept frozen before heating and ideally should be served hot after the first cooking. If any such product is to be saved, it should be quickly refrigerated, then reheated to hot temperatures. This would minimize any risk of botulinal poisoning (*MMWR* 32:39, 1983).

cially canned food, only four deaths from botulism poisoning have resulted in the United States in the past 45 years, whereas during this time more than 775 billion cans of food have been eaten. Yet the threat of botulism is always present, and continued monitoring of food-processing procedures and foods is needed to maintain this remarkable safety record. In general, from 20 to 30 cases a year are reported in the United States. Nevertheless, in 1977 several significant outbreaks of botulism food poisoning resulted when restaurants illegally used home-canned sauces and relishes and the total number of cases for that year increased to 114.

Diagnosis Because time is important in dealing with botulism food poisoning, a preliminary diagnosis must often be made on the basis of clinical and epidemiological evidence. A diagnosis based on clinical appearance is often difficult, for early symptoms are easily confused with other diseases. Furthermore, few physicians have personally seen patients with botulism and so would not easily recognize the symptoms. When isolated cases occur, there is little reason to suspect botulism. When botulism is suspected, specimens from serum, stool, and **gastric washing** should be collected and suspected foods obtained. The presence of toxin in these materials can be detected by injecting extracts into mice. If the toxins are present, the mice usually die within a few days.

Treatment Once botulism is suspected, antitoxin should be given as soon as possible. Because any one of the three most common toxin serotypes may cause the disease, a polyvalent antitoxin containing antitoxin to types A, B, and E is used. The antitoxin will not reverse the effects of toxin already affecting the nerves but will neutralize any circulating toxin. Supportive care, particularly in maintaining respiratory functions, is very important.

Prevention and control Proper procedures in preparing home-canned foods—that is, using **pressure cookers** to ensure destruction of spores—are the most important preventative measures. Before being served, home-canned foods should be boiled for several minutes to destroy any toxin that might be present.

Immunization with toxoids is effective but seldom used due to the rarity of botulism in the general public. With the current awareness of infant botulism—and if further research shows it to be a widespread problem—it might be desirable to vaccinate pregnant females so that passive immunity is present in the infant during the early months of life when it is most susceptible to this form of the disease.

Cellulitis and Gas Gangrene

Bacteria Various different species of the genus *Clostridium* are able to grow in the anaerobic environment of damaged body tissue. These bacteria may release toxins and enzymes that produce

Gastric washing
removal of stomach contents through a tube swallowed to allow washing of the stomach. This procedure can be used to obtain gastric samples for a variety of medical reasons.

Pressure cooker
a metal pan with a tight fitting lid in which water may be heated above the boiling temperature.

further tissue damage to the surrounding healthy tissue, causing anaerobic **cellulitus, myonecrosis,** or gas gangrene. *C. perfringens* is the most frequently involved *Clostridium* species producing these conditions. These clostridia are common inhabitants of the intestinal tracts of humans and animals and are found both on clothing and in the soil. *C. novyi* and *C. septicum,* along with other clostridia, are occasionally involved (Figure 20-5).

Pathogenesis and clinical disease   Numerous toxins and enzymes produced by clostridia (Table 20-2) are able to destroy tissues, particularly muscle fibers and connective tissues. Many wounds that occur in wartime or from automobile accidents become contaminated with various clostridia. When a niche of devitalized (dead or dying) tissue or foreign debris exists in a wound, it may create an anaerobic area in which the clostridia can proliferate. As the toxins and enzymes of the growing clostridia are released, the tissues adjacent to the wound are devitalized and the supply of oxygenated blood is stopped. This situation creates an expanded anaerobic area into which the clostridia can grow; the result is a further production of toxins, which again extends the area of tissue damage. Phagocytic cells of the host are essentially helpless against this infection, for the bacteria are sequestered in dead tissue out of reach of the defense mechanisms of the host.

Several forms of clostridial wound infections occur. The condition called *anaerobic cellulitis* is less severe than gas gangrene (myonecrosis) and does not involve the muscles. The infection spreads through subcutaneous tissues and between muscles. Gas is produced by the bacteria causing distention of the tissues. *Gas gangrene* is a more severe form of the infection with toxic destruction of adjacent muscle tissues and an ever-widening expansion of the lesion. The swollen tissues have a dark yellowish discoloration and produce a foul-smelling, dark fluid exudate. Gas is

Cellulitis
inflammation of connective tissues. These infections occur between muscles and are characterized by erythema and edema.

Myonecrosis
death and destruction of muscle cells. Myonecrosis is a serious clinical condition characteristic of gas gangrene and is fatal without proper rapid treatment.

Figure 20-5   Specimen from a patient with gas gangrene showing large Gram-positive bacilli (Clostridium), in a background of cellular debris. (Courtesy Centers for Disease Control, Atlanta)

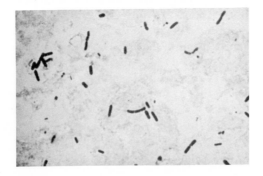

Table 20-2   Enzymes from *Clostridium* Associated with Pathogenesis

Enzyme	Toxin	Function
Lecithinase	Alpha toxin	Digests lecithin
Collagenase	—	Destroys connecting tissue
DNase	—	Disrupts DNA
Hemolysin	Theta toxin	Cardiac toxin, hemolysin

Shock

a condition in which there is a sharp decrease in blood pressure accompanied by depression of a number of physiologic parameters.

formed by the bacteria, causing some distention of the subcutaneous tissues and considerable pain. Symptoms of gas gangrene begin to appear 12 to 72 hours following injury. Along with the local tissue involvement, a generalized toxic reaction including fever, toxemia, and **shock** may be seen in the patient. Death results without proper treatment. Gas gangrene may develop in the uterus after mechanically induced abortion, and is seen more frequently following illegal abortions induced by nonmedical practitioners. Rapidly developing gas gangrene may occur in any section of the bowel that is deprived of a normal blood supply.

Transmission and epidemiology   As with the other clostridial diseases, person-to-person transmission is not a factor in the epidemiology. Disease results when host tissues are altered so that they allow the growth of the clostridia. Gas gangrene is a serious threat to persons with traumatic injuries, bowel obstructions, bowel surgery, reduced blood supply to given tissues, and so on. Elderly persons with poor circulation are prime candidates for this type of infection. Gas gangrene is a major problem in battlefield wounds when treatment is delayed.

Diagnosis   Laboratory diagnosis of clostridial wound infections is difficult and early diagnosis is made on clinical grounds.

Treatment   Removal of dead tissue from the wound is the first step in treatment. Penicillin or other antibiotics, along with antitoxins, should be given and are helpful if all dead tissue is removed. In many cases of gas gangrene, the spread of the infection cannot be stopped unless all infected tissue is removed; this often requires amputation of the involved limb, or extensive tissue removal. Hyperbaric oxygen (chambers of oxygen gas under 3 atmospheres of pressure to increase the amount of O_2 in the tissues) has been used with some limited beneficial effects in treating these anaerobic infections.

Prevention and control   Prompt cleaning and surgical debridement of wounds constitute the most important preventative measure. The rapid evacuation to field hospitals by helicopter of mili-

Food Poisoning: Tennessee, 1973

On November 2 and 3, 1973, an outbreak of gastrointestinal illness occurred among the 1100 employees of a large factory in Murfreesboro, Tennessee, following a special buffet meal served during all three work shifts on November 2. A questionnaire to determine the extent of illness was distributed to a random sample of 178 employees. A total of 146 individuals reported illness for an attack rate of 82%; their symptoms included diarrhea (89%), abdominal cramps (86%), nausea (48%) and vomiting (16%). Only 1 person was hospitalized. The median incubation period was 14 hours with a range of 1 to 25 hours. The attack rate was 75% for those on the night shift who ate first, 80% for the day shift, and 94% for the evening shift. Stool specimens were obtained from 20 ill persons; 17 yielded *Clostridium perfringens*, of which 16 were Hobb's type 5.

Further investigation revealed that the buffet meal consisted of turkey, dressing, gravy, green beans, potatoes, fruit salad, relish, rolls with butter, pies, coffee, and soft drinks. Food-specific attack rates implicated the turkey as the vehicle of infection (p < .01). Cultures of the leftover turkey subsequently yielded 330,000 colonies of *C. perfringens*, Hobb's type 5, per gram.

In preparation for the meal, 8 whole frozen turkeys and 40 frozen turkey breasts had been purchased by a commercial food service company on October 26 and stored at 38°–40° F. On October 30, 4 whole turkeys and 20 breasts were roasted at 375° F for 4 and 2½ hours, respectively. They were then held at room temperature for 2 hours and placed in a walk-in refrigerator. The following day, the turkeys were sliced, placed in steam table pans, and promptly refrigerated. The remaining turkeys and breasts were prepared in the same manner beginning on October 31. On November 2, the day of the buffet, the turkey was warmed in a 250 ° F oven and on surface burners and was subsequently held in insulated hot boxes for 1–3 hours before distribution (*MMWR* 23:19, 1974).

tary personnel wounded during combat has greatly reduced the incidence of gas gangrene associated with battlefield wounds. Antibiotic treatment may help prevent the development of clostridial infection in wounds.

Other Clostridial Diseases

Food poisoning   In addition to producing gangrene, *C. perfringens* is a common cause of food poisoning. Infection is most often associated with consumption of contaminated meat dishes. The spores may survive the normal cooking process then germinate as the meat cools, and within a few hours at warm temperatures massive numbers of bacteria develop. The ingested bacteria grow in the intestines and release toxins as they sporulate. These toxins cause diarrhea, cramps, and abdominal pain. Onset is 8 to 20 hours after ingestion of contaminated meat, and symptoms last about 1 day.

Deaths do not result. In New Guinea, *C. perfringens* (type C) is responsible for a unique type of gastroenteritis referred to as *pigbel*. This condition is often fatal, particularly in children.

Pseudomembranous colitis   A potentially serious form of diarrhea following some antibiotic treatments is caused by *C. difficile*. This bacterium is a normal inhabitant of the intestinal tract but is not able to compete with the normal bacterial flora. When antibiotic treatments reduce the normal bacterial flora, *C. difficile* is able to proliferate rapidly and secrete toxins. These toxins cause fluids to collect in the bowel and damage the cells of the bowel. The first symptoms are abdominal pain with watery diarrhea. Mixtures of fibrin, mucus, and white blood cells accumulate in patches on the mucosa of the colon. These patches are called *pseudomembranes* (false membranes) and are the basis of the name *pseudomembranous colitis*. About one-third of the patients with this disease die, possibly from combined effects of both the primary disease for which they were being treated and the antibiotic-induced **colitis.**

Colitis
inflammation of the colon.

Bacteremia   Several species of *Clostridium* are able to produce bacteremia (bacteria in the bloodstream). This situation is serious not only because of the bacteria that are present, but also because clostridial bacteremia is one of the conditions that frequently accompanies certain types of cancer. When these organisms are found in the bloodstream, the physician usually begins a careful examination for the presence of a tumor.

INFECTIONS CAUSED BY NON-SPORE-FORMING ANAEROBES

Bacteria

In contrast to the clostridia, the non-spore-forming anaerobes are a rather heterogenous group of bacteria comprising a large number of species from several genera. (Figure 20-6) Currently their classification is not complete. But because of the increased interest and research activity involving these microbes, names and classification schemes will undoubtedly undergo frequent revisions. This group of bacteria are not characterized by distinct exotoxins or virulence properties but they are present in as many as 40% of properly collected clinical specimens and are the most common causes of brain, lung, and abdominal abscesses (Table 20-3).

Because the non-spore-forming anaerobes are part of the normal flora of many body tissues, their incrimination as the cause of a given infection can be made only when they are isolated from a tissue that is normally free of these organisms. The source of these

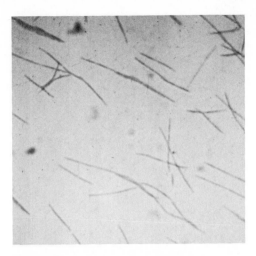

Figure 20-6   A non-sporeforming anaerobe (*Fusobacterium nucleatum*). Note distinctive pointed ends on cells. (Courtesy Centers for Disease Control, Atlanta)

infections is usually **endogenous** and disease results when the integrity of the tissue is altered to allow passage of these bacteria from their normal site of growth to other tissues. Often the anaerobic environment is created by facultative anaerobes that use up the free oxygen and thus act in a synergistic manner to allow the growth of the anaerobe.

A listing of the most common pathogens, their Gram-morphology, and the infections they most often cause is given as Table 20-4.

Endogenous

from inside. Endogenous infections are caused by the normal bacterial flora of the body. The three most likely sources for such bacteria are the mucosa, the skin, and the intestinal tract.

Clinical Diseases

Some general clinical problems attributed to non-spore-forming anaerobes are briefly discussed in the following paragraphs. It should be noted that these infections are often **polymicrobic;** that

Polymicrobic

produced by more than one species of bacteria at the same time. Anaerobic infections are most commonly polymicrobic.

Table 20-3   Commonly Encountered Anaerobes

| | Percent of Organisms Associated with | |
Organism	Pulmonary Infections	Abdominal Sepsis
B. fragilis	17	91
B. melaninogenicus	34	19
Fusobacterium	38	25
Clostridium	10	66
Peptostreptococcus	49	28
Peptococcus	21	12

Table 20-4   Major Anaerobic Bacteria Commonly Associated with Infections

Bacteria	Morphology	Associated Infections
Bacteroides	Gram − bacilli	Peritonitis, liver abscesses, gynecologic, pulmonary, upper respiratory, wounds, bacteremia
Fusobacterium	Gram −bacilli	Liver abscesses, gynecologic, pulmonary, upper respiratory, wounds, bacteremia
Peptostreptococcus	Gram + cocci	Peritonitis, liver abscesses, gynecologic, pulmonary, upper respiratory, wounds, bacteremia
Peptococcus	Gram + cocci	Peritonitis, liver abscesses, gynecologic, pulmonary, upper respiratory, wounds, bacteremia
Propionibacterium	Gram + bacilli	Upper respiratory (pathogenicity uncertain)
Eubacterium	Gram + bacilli	May be isolated from infected tissues, but pathogenic role, if any, is not known
Veillonella	Gram − cocci	May be isolated from infected tissues, but pathogenic role, if any, is not known

is, they are caused by more than one species acting simultaneously.

Infections of the abdominal cavity   Infections may result from passage of fecal material into the abdominal cavity as a result of conditions like injury, surgery, appendicitis, and cancer. Over 90% of abdominal abscesses and infections are caused by anaerobic bacteria. Members of the genus *Bacteroides* (*B. fragilis* in particular) are most frequently involved in these infections.

Infections of the female reproductive tract   About 75% of the infections and abscesses of female reproductive organs are caused by these anaerobes. Such conditions as abortion, surgery, cancer, extensive manipulations, prolonged labor, intrauterine contraceptive devices, and gonorrhea may predispose the tissue to these non-spore-forming anaerobic infections. A serious condition known as *pelvic inflammatory disease* is frequently associated with the presence of these bacteria.

Liver abscesses   Non-spore-forming anaerobic bacteria may reach the liver by direct spread from adjacent tissues or from the blood. One-half or more of the liver abscesses are now known to be caused by these anaerobic bacteria.

Respiratory tract infections   A variety of infections of the respiratory tract are caused by non-spore-forming anaerobes. Between 75% and 95% of such diseases as pneumonitis and lung abscesses are induced by these microbes. More than 90% of patients with aspiration pneumonia (caused by breathing oral secretions down into the lungs) have cultures that are positive for non-spore-forming anaerobes.

Infections of the skin and muscles   Anaerobic infections may develop in skin, muscle, and connective tissue following injury, surgery, or lack of blood supply. Human bites are a common reason for such infections.

Septicemia   Invasion of the blood system may result from any of the preceding anaerobic infections. About 10% of all blood infections detected in hospital patients are caused by non-spore-forming anaerobes.

Brain abscesses   Bacteroides and anaerobic cocci are the most frequent etiologic agents of brain abscesses. Without proper surgical and antimicrobial intervention, these abscesses give the patient an extremely poor prognosis.

Diagnosis

There are a number of clinical clues (e.g., site of infection and foul odor) to infection with non-spore-forming anaerobes, but species identification of the isolated organism can be a difficult task. Recent efforts to provide rapid organism identification have resulted in the development of a variety of colorless enzyme substrates that become brightly colored when they have been changed by their specific enzyme. Use of these *chromogenic substrates* has facilitated rapid (within less than 24 hours) identification of the most common of the anaerobic bacteria. Other, more traditional approaches, such as fermentation reactions and chromatographic analysis may be necessary for the more unusual anaerobic bacteria.

Prevention and Treatment

Because most non-spore-forming anaerobic infections are derived from endogenous (normally present) bacteria, prevention of infection is difficult and largely depends on good medical procedures and nursing care of patients. There are no vaccines and normal human life without these endogenous bacteria is probably not possible.

Treatment of these anaerobic infections is often difficult. Drainage and surgical removal of dead tissue, when possible, are most helpful, and antibiotic therapy is essential. Unfortunately, among these organisms susceptibility to many of the available antibiotics seems to be declining. The *Bacteroides* are largely resistant to penicillins, and susceptibility to the cephalosporins is not uniform. Chloramphenicol, metronidazole, and clindamycin are generally effective across a wide range of these organisms.

CONCEPT SUMMARY

1. Human clostridial infections are serious, life threatening diseases resulting from powerful exotoxins produced by these organisms.

2. Ability to limit disease due to *Clostridium* depends on adequate use of available vaccines, proper food processing and preparation, and effective medical intervention. Such practices have greatly reduced the frequency of these diseases in many countries of the world.

3. Human infections due to anaerobic bacteria are common. Most such infections have an endogenous source of bacteria and are due to non-spore-forming anaerobes. These infections tend to be polymicrobic and serious. Proper medical help, including surgical intervention, is frequently necessary to cure these infections.

4. Anaerobic infections have distinctive characteristics, which facilitate diagnosis. Most anaerobic infections are produced by a relatively small number of different bacterial species.

STUDY SUMMARY

1. Pathogenic anaerobic bacteria can be classified as to their Gram reaction, ability to form spores, and natural habitat. Construct a table that shows the above features for the following anaerobic bacteria: *C. tetani, C. septicum, B. fragilis,* and *F. nucleatum.*

2. What feature of the non-spore-forming anaerobes makes them such a common cause of human infection?

3. What virulence mechanism possessed by most of the clostridia gives them the capacity to produce serious human diseases?

4. DPT vaccine has been used to reduce the incidence of tetanus. At what ages, and how often should this vaccine be given?

5. List the features of infant botulism that are different from those associated with botulism in adults.

6. List the sources of *C. perfringens* that could lead to infection of a wound and possible gas gangrene.

REFERENCES FOR FURTHER STUDY

1. Bacteroides of the Human Lower Intestinal Tract. *Annual Review of Microbiology* 38:161, 1984.

2. *Bacteroides fragilis* Meningitis. *Reviews of Infectious Diseases* 9:783, 1987.

3. *Diagnostic Microbiology,* S. Finegold, 1986. Mosby.

4. Infant Botulism: Clinical Spectrum and Epidemiology. *Pediatrics* 66:939, 1980.

5. Botulism in the United States. *Journal of the American Medical Association* 229:1305, 1974.

chapter 21

GRAM-POSITIVE BACILLI

Ubiquitous
everywhere present.

Etiologic agent
the causative agent; the
microorganism responsible for a
specific infection.

Species from four genera of Gram-positive, facultatively aerobic bacilli—*Corynebacterium, Listeria, Erysipelothrix,* and
Bacillus—are of continuing concern as etiologic agents
of human disease. Although members of each genus are
Gram-positive, this is almost the only characteristic they share in
common. *Bacillus* is a large genus with many endospore-producing,
ubiquitous species, while only a single, nutritionally fastidious
species is found in the genus *Erysipelothrix.* The diseases produced
by these organisms range from classic diphtheria and anthrax to
benign food poisoning due to *B. cereus.* Such variations in pathogenesis is reflective of the physiologic variations that occur
among these four genera. Each genus will be discussed in separate
sections of this chapter.

CORYNEBACTERIUM

Although laboratory isolation of *Corynebacterium* species is a relatively common event, their actual involvement as agents of infection is much less common. Compared to the frequency with which
other microorganisms are recovered as **etiologic agents** of infection, this group of organisms can be considered as uncommon or
even rare.

Diphtheria

The most serious common infection due to bacteria from the genus
Corynebacterium is diphtheria, caused from infection by *C. diphtheriae.* Disease results when the organism produces a powerful exotoxin which is absorbed by various tissues within the body.

   The ability of a given strain of *C. diphtheriae* to produce the
exotoxin is determined by the presence of a lysogenic bacteriophage. As discussed in Chapters 6 and 33, some bacteriophages

have the ability to insert their DNA into the DNA molecule of the host bacterium, a process called *lysogeny*. The gene that directs the production of the diphtheria toxin is carried by the *lysogenic* bacteriophage (known as *beta corynephage*), and the toxin is therefore produced only by those corynebacteria that contain the bacteriophage genes (**phage transformation**). Members of the genus other than *C. diphtheriae* may occasionally be infected with beta corynephage, which enables them to produce diphtheria toxin, but this event seems to be quite rare. Early research on diphtheria, during the last two decades of the 1800s, led to the discovery of the first bacterial exotoxins, and demonstrated that such toxins are the cause of some bacterial disease. This research also led to the development of methods for treating toxic diseases with antitoxins.

Phage transformed cells
cells which produce proteins such as diphtheria toxin under the direction of an integrated bacteriophage genome.

Bacterium   *C. diphtheriae* (Figure 21-1) is a narrow (0.5 to 1 μm), Gram-positive bacillus that may range in length up to 5 μm. When prepared on slides for staining, the cells, which often remain attached on one side during division, are frequently oriented in palisades or in V- and L-shaped arrangements. When mixed together, such cellular arrangements are said to give the appearance of Chinese letters. The cells are *pleomorphic* (multiple shaped), often with bulging at one end that gives a club appearance (Greek *coryne* = club). They may also contain accumulations of phosphates (metachromatic granules) that stain differently from the other cell materials and give the stained cells a beaded appearance. Although

Figure 21-1   Micrograph of *Corynebacterium diphtheriae*. (Courtesy Centers for Disease Control, Atlanta)

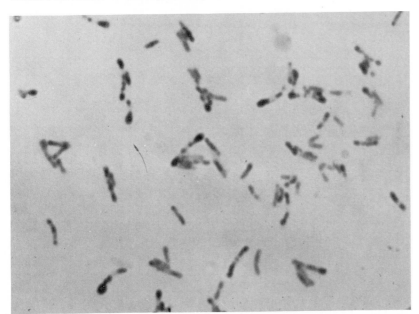

these bacteria can be cultivated on a variety of media, in diagnostic laboratories they are grown on a selective medium containing tellurite salts. Reduction of the tellurite causes these bacteria to produce gray or black colonies. Using this procedure, three different types of *C. diphtheriae*—gravis, mitis, and intermedius—are determined. All three types, however, are capable of producing the same toxin and clinical disease. *C. diphtheriae* is more resistant to drying than many vegetative bacteria and may remain viable for as long as 3 to 4 months in dried respiratory exudates.

Pathogenesis and clinical disease Both toxin-producing and non-toxin-producing strains of *C. diphtheriae* can adhere to and colonize the mucosal tissue of the upper respiratory tract. Humans are the only natural host, and transmission is primarily from person to person by airborne droplets. The disease results entirely from the effects of the exotoxin.

Diphtheria toxin is one of the most frequently studied, and best known of the bacterial exotoxins. This toxin is actually a combination of two peptide molecules (A and B) bound together into a single polypeptide. The B portion of the molecule is not toxic but helps to transport the A portion into the cell. Fragment A then prevents protein synthesis by inhibiting the transfer of the growing protein molecule from the ribosome acceptor site to the donor site (Chapter 6). The toxin specifically adheres to and is initially absorbed into cells around the growing *C. diptheriae.* No structural damage is seen until the lack of newly synthesized proteins causes the death of the cells. As the dead host cells accumulate, the bacteria continue to produce toxin, which causes the lesion to expand. An incubation period of several days to 1 week is required before the patient begins to experience clinical symptoms from diphtheria lesions. These lesions usually appear first in the tonsillar-pharyngeal area, as patches of a thick fibrinous exudate containing many entrapped host cells and bacteria. This layer of exudate, called a *pseudomembrane,* adheres firmly to the epithelial surfaces (Figure 21-2). As the disease progresses, the pseudomembrane may spread upward into nasopharyngeal tissues and/or downward into the larynx and trachea. In severe cases, obstruction of the airway may occur, resulting in suffocation of the patient. The lesions remain superficial and rarely do the bacteria invade deeper tissues, although the toxin may produce necrosis of such internal organs as liver, kidney and adrenal glands.

Besides formation of the pseudomembrane and a sore throat, the patient experiences fever, malaise, and enlarged regional lymph nodes, resulting in the swelling of the neck. The term ''bull-neck'' is sometimes used to refer to this condition. The most frequent and serious damage occurs to the heart and central nervous system (CNS) with death often resulting from damage to the heart. The disease may linger for many weeks and, due to damage

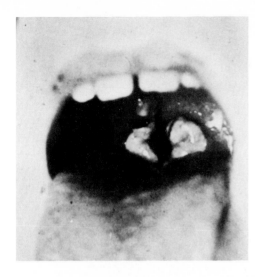

Figure 21-2   Pharyngeal pseudomembrane produced by infection with *Corynebacterium diptheriae.* (Courtesy Centers for Disease Control, Atlanta)

of the CNS, varying levels of paralysis may occur. Aspects of the pathogenesis of diphtheria are shown in Figure 21-3. Before methods of treating or preventing this disease were available, diphtheria was a major killer disease of children. When poor sanitation exists, primary or secondary diphtherial lesions may occur on the skin (Figure 21-4). Because the toxin is also produced in these le-

Figure 21-3   Pathogenesis of diphtheria.

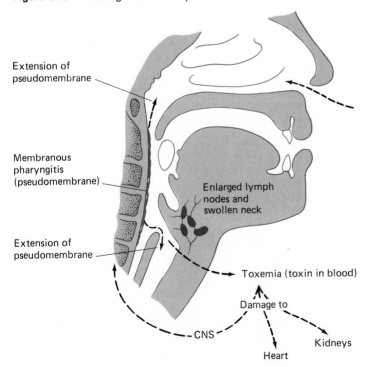

Extension of pseudomembrane

Membranous pharyngitis (pseudomembrane)

Extension of pseudomembrane

Enlarged lymph nodes and swollen neck

Toxemia (toxin in blood)

Damage to

CNS

Heart

Kidneys

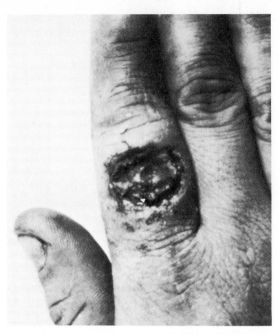

Figure 21-4 Necrotic cutaneous diphtherial lesion about 15 days after onset. (Armed Forces Institute of Pathology, AFIP MIS #44 997-1)

Necrosis
the death and subsequent destruction of cells. Usually appearing as darkened or ulcerated tissue.

sions, patients experience an illness similar to pharyngeal diphtheria.

Transmission and epidemiology Recovery from diphtheria does not necessarily eliminate *C. diphtheriae* from the throat; many patients remain healthy carriers for prolonged periods. The epidemiology of diphtheria was greatly altered during the past several generations in countries where widespread immunization has been practiced. This has also greatly reduced the number of healthy carriers. At present, only a few hundred cases of diphtheria occur each year in the United States (Figure 21-5). Those who develop diphtheria are most often either individuals who have never been immunized or elderly persons who have lost their immune status.

Diagnosis The diagnosis of diphtheria is most frequently made on the basis of clinical or serological evidence. Nevertheless, the isolation of toxin-producing *C. diphtheriae* from the throat or lesion provides a positive diagnosis.

Treatment When diphtheria is suspected, the patient should receive passive immunization with antitoxin. Early antitoxin treatment is necessary in order to be effective because, once the toxin

Fatal Diphtheria: Wisconsin, 1982

A fatal case of diphtheria was reported to the Wisconsin State Department of Health and Social Services. A 9-year-old unimmunized female developed listlessness and a sore throat on June 30, 1982, ten days after arriving at a camp in Colorado operated by a religous group that does not accept immunizations. On July 6, a physician evaluated the patient for her sore throat; a throat culture was taken and oral penicillin prescribed. The patient was hospitalized on July 8 for persistent sore throat, diminished fluid intake, and gingival bleeding. Laboratory tests revealed a white blood cell count of 26,500/mm^3 with 92% polymorphonuclear cells and a platelet count of 10,000/mm^3. The throat culture obtained July 6 was reported to contain normal flora, group A beta-hemolytic streptococci, and large numbers of diphtheroids. The patient was transferred on July 8 to a tertiary care children's hospital.

On admission, she was afebrile and had moderate upper airway obstruction, diffuse ecchymoses (small hemorrhagic spots), bleeding from the nose and gums, prominent swollen cervical lymph nodes, and swelling of the jaw and throat. Initially, the pharynx was poorly visualized due to trismus (spasms with difficulty in opening mouth). On later examination, it revealed severe hemorrhagic and nectrotic tonsillitis; no membrane was observed. Treatment with pencillin G, gentamicin, moxalactam, peritoneal dialysis, and platelet transfusions was instituted. The hospital course was complicated by disseminated intravascular coagulation, cardiac condition abnormalities, and mental confusion. The patient died on July 14. A *Corynebacterium* species isolated from a throat culture obtained July 10 was subsequently confirmed by the Milwaukee Bureau of Laboratories and State Laboratory of Hygiene to be a toxigenic strain of *C. diphtheriae*.

An investigation was undertaken to determine the source of exposure to *C. diphtheriae* and to identify and evaluate the patient's contacts. The camp session had been attended by 108 employees, campers, and counselors from Wisconsin and 12 other states: many were unimmunized. In addition, 119 immediate and extended family members and hospital employees in Wisconsin, who might have had close contact with the patient after onset of illness, were identified. With the aid of state and local health departments and private physicians, 224 of the 227 contacts were evaluated. None reported respiratory illness before or after exposure to the patient, and nasopharyngeal or throat cultures obtained from 218 contacts were negative for *C. diphtheriae* (*MMWR* 31:553, 1982).

has bound to cell receptors, the reaction cannot be reversed. Penicillin or erythromycin should also be given to stop further growth of *C. diphtheriae* in the throat, and to prevent the patient from developing into a carrier. Persons who are asymptomatic carriers can be freed of *C. diphtheriae* by antibiotic treatment.

Prevention and control Diphtheria can be prevented and controlled to a large extent by active immunization with a toxoid vaccine. The vaccine is administered during the second or third month of life in combination with vaccines for tetanus and whoop-

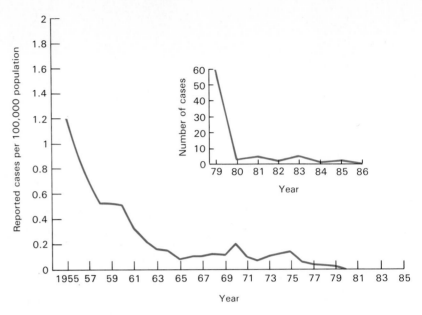

Figure 21-5 Reported case rates of diphtheria in the United States between 1955 and 1987 showing continued decrease in recent years (adapted from CDC reports).

ing cough (DPT vaccine). A booster is given a year later and gain when the child enters school. Revaccination every 10 years thereafter is also recommended.

Unimmunized persons who may have been exposed to diphtheria can be passively immunized with antitoxin. A procedure called the *Schick test* can be used to determine if a person is susceptible to diphtheria. Here a small amount of diphtheria toxin is injected subcutaneously; if the person has no protective antibodies, an inflammatory reaction occurs at the site of toxin injection. Such a person should then be actively or passively immunized, depending on circumstances.

Infections Due to Other Corynebacteria

As already noted, other members of the genus *Corynebacterium* (*C. ulcerans, C. pseudotuberculosis*) can produce diphtheria toxin when they are infected with the beta corynephage. Other members of this genus, which are often referred to as **diphtheroids,** are occasionally the cause of endocarditis and sepsis in immunocompromised patients (Table 21-1). In particular, one of these, known as *JK*, produces serious life-threatening disease with mortality rates as high as 75%. This organism is very resistant to most antibiotics and is found primarily in patients with artificial heart valves or

Diphtheroid

a Gram-positive bacillus of the genus *Corynebacterium*, which is commonly found on body surfaces and is frequently found as contaminating bacteria in clinical specimens.

Table 21-1   Diseases Caused by *Corynebacterium* Species

Corynebacterium	Disease Association
C. diphtheriae	Diphtheria
C. haemolyticum	Pharyngitis
C. xerosis	Endocarditis
C. pseudotuberculosis	Tuberculosis-like illness
C. ulcerans	Pharyngitis
JK	Endocarditis, bacteremia

intravenous catheters. Two species, *C. haemolyticum* and *C. ulcerans* can cause pharyngitis with symptoms similar to those produced by group A streptococci.

LISTERIA

Of the four species in the genus *Listeria,* only *L. monocytogenes* is pathogenic for humans. Human listeriosis is far more common and often as serious as diphtheria. However, it is not so well recognized as a cause of human disease because it doesn't occur in epidemic fashion, and cases are somewhat sporadic. This organism is ubiquitous, occurring in both wild and domestic animals, soils and plants. The organism can be isolated from healthy as well as sick persons, and most human infections can be traced to food or animal contact. It is likely that many persons are regularly exposed to this organism from their environment. It is not clear why such a small percent of individuals develop infections, although it appears that some form of compromise to the immune state may predispose to disease. The organism is a short, motile, non-spore-forming beta-hemolytic bacillus that may be easily confused with group B streptococci on initial isolation (Table 21-2). It is not known to produce a specific toxin.

Table 21-2   Laboratory Tests Used to Identify and Distinguish Between *Listeria* and *Streptococcus* Group B

Test	*Listeria* Reaction	Group B Reaction
Motility	+	−
CAMP test[a]	+	+
Gram morphology	Short bacillus	Coccus
Beta-hemolysis	+	+
Catalase	+	−

[a]The CAMP test is positive if an organism can increase the intensity of beta-hemolysis in the presence of certain staphylococci.

Most infections in the United States are seen as (1) neonatal sepsis or meningitis, (2) spontaneous abortion or stillbirth, (3) sepsis or meningitis in immunocompromised patients, and (4) puerperal sepsis. Of these, meningitis is the most common presentation and patients who are pregnant, newborn, or organ transplant recipients are most likely to be involved. Pencillin is a very effective antibiotic in listeriosis patients.

ERYSIPELOTHRIX

The single species *E. rhusiopathiae* may cause local cutaneous lesions (erysipeloid) or more serious systemic illness. Most infections are associated with animal contact and the disease most frequently occurs in an occupational setting.

BACILLUS

Anthrax

Anthrax is primarily a disease of animals. During the developmental years of medical microbiology anthrax was a frequently encountered disease in sheep and cattle. Because of the relatively large size and definite shape of the bacillus, plus the availability of experimental animals, anthrax served as an excellent model for the study of infectious diseases. Many important discoveries regarding the germ theory of disease and immunity resulted from investigations of anthrax (Chapter 1).

Bacterium *B. anthracis* is a large, aerobic, Gram-positive bacillus 5 to 10 μm long and 1 to 3 μm wide. The spores are highly resistant and may remain viable on animal products or in the soil for years. The bacterium grows readily on laboratory media, where it may be easily confused with other members of the genus (Figure 21-6).

Pathogenesis and clinical disease The spores of *B. anthracis* enter the body either through abrasions of the skin or by inhalation or ingestion. The virulent strains possess an unusual capsule composed of D-glutamic acid around the vegative cell that retards phagocytosis by host cells. A toxin composed of three major components is produced and causes the signs and symptoms of the

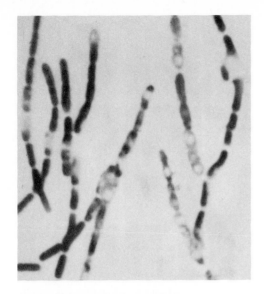

Figure 21-6   Photomicrograph of *Bacillus anthracis* showing both endospores and vegetative cells. (Courtesy Armed Forces Institute of Pathology, Washington, D.C.)

disease. The three main clinical forms of anthrax are shown in Figure 21-7.

CUTANEOUS ANTHRAX   The cutaneous form of anthrax is the most common and results when spores enter the tissues through abrasions or lesions. Infection usually occurs on the exposed skin surface. A local lesion develops that rarely contains pus, but it is swollen, **hemorrhagic,** and forms a black scab called an *eschar* (Figure 21-8). If the infection remains localized, death rates are

Hemorrhagic

lesions or conditions associated with bleeding. Hemorrhagic lesions are usually dark and may be internal or external.

Figure 21-7   Three forms of anthrax that might be contracted by exposure to infected animal products.

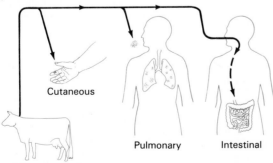

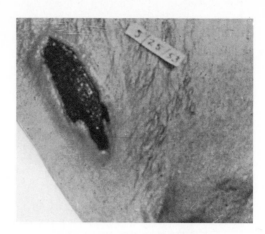

Figure 21-8 Cutaneous anthrax lesion on the neck, fifteenth day of disease. The patient had worked with air-dried goat skins from Africa. (Armed Forces Institute of Pathology, AFIP MIS #75-4203-9)

low. The infection spreads to the blood in about 5% of the cases and this generalized infection is often fatal.

PULMONARY ANTHRAX The pulmonary form of anthrax, which results from inhalation of spores, is seen in persons who handle contaminated animal products and is sometimes referred to as ''woolsorters' disease.'' The onset is sudden, with high fever and respiratory distress. Pneumonia is often followed by sepsis and in untreated cases, death usually results.

INTESTINAL ANTHRAX The intestinal form of anthrax is rare and results from eating contaminated meat. Severe enteritis results and mortality rates are high. This form has not been reported as occurring in the United States.

Transmission and Epidemiology Transmission of anthrax among animals usually occurs from the ingestion of spore-contaminated feed. Anthrax spores may remain viable for 20 to 30 years or longer in a pasture contaminated by the remains of animals dying of anthrax. At present, relatively few cases of anthrax occur in animals in the United States. It is still found in animals in certain countries, however, and this presents a hazard to persons living in those countries who come in contact with contaminated animal products. Since the 1950s, outbreaks in the United States have resulted from contact with contaminated hides covering bongo drums, infected pig bristles used in shaving brushes, goats' hair used in weaving, and similar items, all imported from foreign

Anthrax: California, 1976

The first known anthrax case involving a home craftsman working with yarn occurred in January 1976 in a 32-year-old man who operated a home-weaving business in California. The patient died. *Bacillus anthracis* was isolated from some yarns used by the patient.

The contaminated yarn, obtained from a distributor in Los Angeles, was imported from Pakistan. A second distributor in New York imported materials from the same source. The distributors voluntarily recalled the yarn, according to the Consumer Product Safety Commission.

The patient developed inhalation anthrax on January 17, with fever and symptoms of an upper respiratory infection. He became ill on January 21 and was hospitalized that day with a complaint of fever, chills, pharyngitis, headache, nausea, anorexia, and pleurisy. Admission examination revealed a 38.8° C fever, decreased breath sounds on the left side, spasticity of the left lower and upper extremities, unresponsiveness to simple commands, and a disconjugate gaze. The pleural fluid and a peripheral blood smear contained large Gram-positive bacilli.

Despite intravenous aqueous penicillin (5 million units every 6 hours), intramuscular streptomycin (500 mg every 12 hours), and intensive supportive therapy, the patient died 28 hours after admission. *Bacillus anthracis* was isolated from both clinical and autopsy specimens.

The patient was a self-employed weaver who frequently worked with a variety of imported yarns. He had not traveled outside the local community for at least 2 weeks prior to the onset of his illness and had no probable source of infection other than his work materials.

Yarn from both distributors was obtained and cultured. *Bacillus anthracis* was recovered from various animal-origin yarns obtained from each. The contaminated products, sold in 4-ounch skeins or balls, included camel hair, goat hair, or sheeps' wool in varying combinations. Commonly sold in plastic bags, the yarn was most often used in such handicrafts as wall hangings and macramé objects (*MMWR* 25:33, 1976).

countries. Overall, the risk of contracting anthrax in the United States is slight: an average of only two cases per year have been reported in the past 10 years. Public health personnel should be aware of the threat of anthrax and be able to recognize the possible sources of infection.

Treatment and control Anthrax can be successfuly treated with penicillin or broad-spectrum antibiotics. Vaccines are available to control the disease in animals and humans of high risk. Carcasses of diseased animals should be buried deep in the soil or burned to prevent the spread of spores. Gas sterilization or radiation may be used to decontaminate hides, wool, and related animal products.

CLINICAL NOTE

Bacillus cereus: Maine, 1985

On September 22, 1985, the Maine Bureau of Health was notified of a gastrointestinal illness among patrons of a Japanese restaurant. Because the customers were exhibiting symptoms of illness while still in the restaurant premises, and because uncertainty existed as to the etiology of the problem, the local health department, in concurrence with the restaurant owner, closed the restaurant at 7:30 P.M. that same day.

Eleven (31%) of the approximately 36 patrons reportedly served on the evening of September 22 were contacted in an effort to determine the etiology of the outbreak. Those 11 comprised the last three dining parties served on September 22. Despite extensive publicity, no additional cases were reported.

A case was defined as anyone who had vomiting or diarrhea within 6 hours of dining at the restaurant. All 11 individuals were interviewed for symptoms, time of onset of illness, illness duration, and foods ingested. All 11 reported nausea and vomiting; 9 reported diarrhea; 1 reported headache; and 1 reported abdominal cramps. Onset of illness ranged from 30 minutes to 5 hours (mean 1 hour, 23 minutes) after eating at the restaurant. Duration of illness ranged from 5 hours to several days, except for 2 individuals still symptomatic with diarrhea 2 weeks after dining at the restaurant. Ten persons sought medical treatment at local emergency rooms on September 22; 2 ultimately required hospitalization for rehydration.

Analysis of the association of food consumption with illness was not instructive, since all persons consumed the same food items: chicken soup; fried shrimp; stir-fried rice; fried zucchini, onions, and beans sprouts; cucumber, cabbage, and lettuce salad; ginger salad dressing; hibachi chicken and steak; and tea. Five persons ordered hibachi scallops, and one person ordered hibachi swordfish. However, most individuals sampled each other's entrees.

One vomitus specimen and two stool specimens from three separate individuals yielded an overgrowth of *Bacillus cereus* organisms. The hibachi steak was also culture-positive for *B. cereus*, although an accurate bacterial count could not be made because an inadequate amount of the steak remained for laboratory analysis. No growth of *B. cereus* was reported from the fried rice, mixed fried vegetables, or hibachi chicken.

According to the owner, all meat was delivered two to three times a week from a local meat supplier and refrigerated until ordered by restaurant patrons. Appropriate-sized portions for a dining group were taken from the kitchen to the dining area and diced or sliced, then sauteed at the table directly in front of restaurant patrons. The meat was seasoned with soy sauce, salt, and white pepper, open containers of which had been used for at least 2 months by the restaurant. The hibachi steak was served immediately after cooking.

The fried rice served with the meal was reportedly customarily made from leftover boiled rice. It could not be established whether the boiled rice had been stored refrigerated or at room temperature (*MMWR* 35:25, 1986).

Infections Due to Other *Bacillus* Species

As noted earlier, other members of the genus *Bacillus* are able to produce human disease. Although these diseases are not as severe as those caused by *B. anthracis*, they are more common in the United States, and can be serious. In otherwise compromised patients, *B. subtilus* may produce serious **endophthalmitis,** right-sided endocarditis, and even meningitis. Intravenous drug abuse is frequently an antecedent to such infections. *B. cereus* is not an uncommon cause of gastroenteritis. Eating cooked, improperly stored rice is often the cause of this illness.

Endophthalmitis
inflammation or infection of the inside of the eyeball. This is a serious condition, often requiring removal of the eyeball.

CONCEPT SUMMARY

1. The single, commonly serious infection caused by members of the genus *Corynebacterium* is diphtheria. Diphtheria is caused by lysogenic strains of the bacterium that produce a powerful exotoxin and is generally held under control by appropriate immunization. The organism is frequently found in the human respiratory tract, but superficial wound infections are also known to result in the disease diphtheria.

2. *Bacillus anthracis* is aerobic and only the disease anthrax is of major importance. The disease, though rare in the United States, is a serious, often life-threatening one acquired by associating with infected animals or contaminated animal by-products.

3. Diseases due to Gram-positive bacilli other than diphtheria and anthrax are increasing in frequency and concern. Most of these infections occur as a consequence of some form of host compromise.

STUDY SUMMARY

1. Describe the characteristics of the corynebacteria that are responsible for each of the following observations: (a) toxin production, (b) irregular staining, (c) black colonies on tellurite, (d) palisade formation, and (e) pseudomembrane formation.

2. Draw a diagram that shows the attachment, entry, and inhibitory action of diphtheria toxin.

3. What is the most common disease presentation in individuals infected with *Listeria*?

4. Which of the three clinical forms of anthrax is most unusual in the United States?

5. What activity commonly precedes serious infection due to *B. subtilus*?

REFERENCES FOR FURTHER STUDY

1. The Emerging Role of *Bacillus cereus* Infection. *Reviews of Infectious Diseases* 9:110, 1987.

2. Actinomycosis of the Central Nervous System. *Reviews of Infectious Diseases* 9:855, 1987.

3. Corynebacterium JK. *Reviews of Infectious Diseases* 8:42, 1986.

4. Inhalation Anthrax. *Annals of the New York Academy of Science* 353:83, 1980.

5. *Manual of Clinical Microbiology,* 4th ed., E. Lynnette, 1985. American Society for Microbiology.

chapter 22

MYCOBACTERIA AND RELATED MICROORGANISMS

T uberculosis and leprosy are the major diseases of humans caused by bacteria of the genus *Mycobacterium*. Their impact is difficult to determine, but they would certainly rank among the most devastating of all human diseases. It has been estimated that tuberculosis was the single greatest cause of human disease and death during the past 200 years. During the 1800s as many as 30% of all deaths in the eastern United States were due to this disease.

Although modern medical practices and improved living standards have greatly reduced the **prevalence** of these diseases in developed nations, in some areas of the world up to 40% of the people are infected with *Mycobacterium tuberculosis* and it is estimated that between 10 and 12 million of the world's population suffer from leprosy due to *Mycobacterium leprae*. In the United States, 4.1% of New York City school children are infected with *M. tuberculosis* and 1% of patients admitted to general practice hospitals carry the bacillus. The mycobacteria are distinguished by their acid-fast staining property, which results in part from the high content of lipids in their cell walls. Such lipids also render these bacteria highly resistant to inactivation by dehydration, disinfectants, and other environmental factors.

TUBERCULOSIS

Bacterium

The species *M. tuberculosis*, commonly referred to as the tubercle bacillus, is the major cause of human tuberculosis. The bacterium is a non-spore-forming rod measuring about 0.5×3 μm. It can be grown on simple culture media; in routine laboratory isolation procedures, however, best results are obtained with a medium containing egg yolk and starch, such as the Lowenstein-Jensen

Prevalence
the number of cases of a specific disease existing in a defined population; usually given as a percent of population affected.

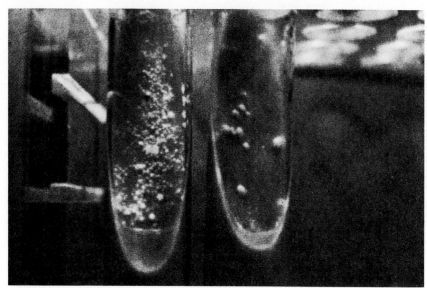

Figure 22-1 Colonies of *Mycobacterium tuberculosis* after several weeks growth on an agar surface. (S. S. Schneierson, *Atlas of Diagnostic Microbiology*, p. 39. Courtesy Abbott Laboratories, Abbott Park, IL.)

medium. This bacterium is an obligate aerobe and grows slowly. Doubling time is from 12 to 20 hours and several weeks may be required for visible colonies to develop (Figure 22-1). Experimental infections can be produced in a variety of laboratory animals.

Pathogenesis and Clinical Diseases

Tuberculosis is a complex disease that may go unrecognized in the human host for many years. Characteristically, it may be seen in different stages. Humans are readily infected with the tubercle bacilli, but progression of the disease depends on many subtle host and environmental factors. In many cases, the bacteria are disposed of with no manifestation of the disease, but in most cases the primary infection develops in the lungs, then becomes dormant and remains in this state for the remainder of the person's life. To provide a better understanding of the complex nature of tuberculosis, the following discussion divides the diseases into various stages. These stages are shown diagrammatically in Figure 22-2.

Primary tuberculosis The primary stage of the disease results when a person becomes infected for the first time. **Aerosolized** bacteria from a person with active tuberculosis are inhaled and the bacilli that reach the **alveoli** are able to cause infection. These bacilli begin to multiply slowly and many are phagocytized by the

Aerosolized

suspended in particles of mucus or saliva that have been released (by sneezing or coughing) into the atmosphere.

Alveoli

small open spaces in the lung where oxygen and carbon dioxide exchange takes place.

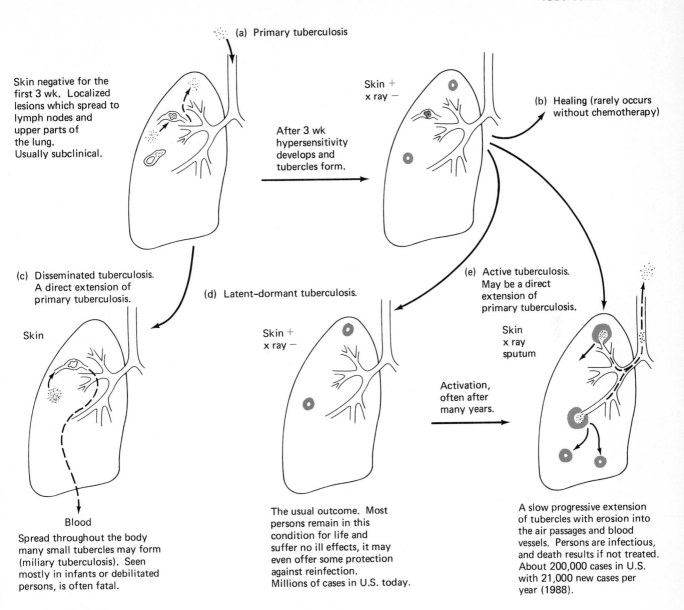

(a) Primary tuberculosis

Skin negative for the first 3 wk. Localized lesions which spread to lymph nodes and upper parts of the lung. Usually subclinical.

After 3 wk hypersensitivity develops and tubercles form.

Skin +
x ray −

(b) Healing (rarely occurs without chemotherapy)

(c) Disseminated tuberculosis. A direct extension of primary tuberculosis.

(d) Latent–dormant tuberculosis.

(e) Active tuberculosis. May be a direct extension of primary tuberculosis.

Skin

Skin +
x ray −

Skin
x ray
sputum

Activation, often after many years.

Blood

Spread throughout the body many small tubercles may form (miliary tuberculosis). Seen mostly in infants or debilitated persons, is often fatal.

The usual outcome. Most persons remain in this condition for life and suffer no ill effects, it may even offer some protection against reinfection. Millions of cases in U.S. today.

A slow progressive extension of tubercles with erosion into the air passages and blood vessels. Persons are infectious, and death results if not treated. About 200,000 cases in U.S. with 21,000 new cases per year (1988).

Figure 22-2   The most common stages in the pathogenesis of tuberculosis.

alveolar macrophages, but these phagocytic cells are generally unable to destroy the bacilli. Consequently, many bacilli are carried by macrophages to regional lymph nodes. Phagocytosis of the bacteria, however, stimulates the development of cell-mediated immunity against the mycobacterial antigens. A brisk reaction then occurs with activated macrophages concentrating around the focus of bacterial growth. The growth of the bacilli inside the macrophages is slowed and a scar tissue barrier forms around the bacilli.

The resulting nodule of scar tissue and cells is called a *tubercle.* A this phase of the disease, the patient develops a positive skin reaction, which is a manifestation of cell-mediated immunity against tuberculosis antigens. This process is commonly called ''converting'' to skin test–positive. The tubercle usually prevents any further spread of the bacilli and the center of the tubercle provides a niche of dead tissue where the bacilli are protected from the host's defense mechanisms. The primary stage of the disease is usually without clinical symptoms. From this point, the disease may enter any one of the following stages.

Healing   The infection may be completely contained and the bacteria destroyed by the primary response. The patient would have experienced no symptoms but would have a positive reaction to the skin test. In persons not receiving adequate chemotherapy it is difficult to determine if this healing does indeed occur.

Disseminated

not localized. Disseminated infections often involve many parts of the body at the same time.

Disseminated tuberculosis   In a small percentage of persons, mostly young children or immunologically impaired individuals, the infection spreads from the primary site of multiplication into the blood and the bacteria may be seeded throughout the body. In some individuals cellular immunity does not readily develop without chemotherapy—the bacilli grow in many body tissues and the patient dies. If dissemination occurs and hypersensitivity develops, numerous small tubercles are formed, a condition called **miliary tuberculosis.** The death rate is high from this type of disease.

Miliary tuberculosis

a condition in which the bacilli are widely disseminated throughout the lung. Each of these bacilli serve as the focus for the development of a tubercle.

Latent-dormant tuberculosis   The latent-dormant stage is the usual outcome of primary pulmonary tuberculosis. During the primary stage, secondary foci usually develop around the initial focus and in adjacent lymph nodes. Tubercles are formed around these foci. The bacilli may remain living inside these tubercles for many years or for the lifetime of the infected person. Before chemotherapy was available, a general saying about tuberculosis was ''Once infected, always infected.''

During this stage the activated host defense mechanisms prevent the bacilli from spreading to other parts of the body and the environment inside the tubercle protects the bacilli from these same defenses. This ''truce'' may last for the lifetime of the person or may be ''broken'' by the influence of various, often not well understood, changes in the physiology of the host. In past years, a vast majority of the world's population had latent-dormant tuberculosis and some estimates place the current number of persons in the United States with latent-dormant tuberculosis at over 20 million. Although these persons have an increased resistance to reinfection due to their activated defenses against the tubercle bacilli, most active cases develop as an extension of this latent infection. So it is not generally considered advantageous to have the latent form of the disease. Persons in the latent–dormant stages remain skin test–positive, but the tubercles may not be large enough to be seen by x ray.

Secondary or active adult-type tuberculosis   The secondary stage of tuberculosis may develop as a direct extension of the primary stage but most cases result from a "reawakening" of the dormant lesion. The exact mechanisms associated with this reawakening or **reactivation,** often after long periods of dormancy, are not understood. It occurs most often in persons who have had their defense mechanisms compromised—for instance, young adults who become run-down, overworked, malnourished, or stressed; elderly persons with general declining health; alcoholics; persons with such diseases as diabetes or silicosis; and those on immunosuppressive therapy.

Reactivation
development of an active, spreading infection in an individual in whom one disease had been latent after an earlier infection.

The previously dormant tubercle begins to expand in size and causes an enlarged central area of dead tissue and debris to form. This material is referred to as *caseous nucrosis* (cheesey, dead tissue). Eventually the expanding tubercle erodes into a bronchial tube and the inner contents are expelled into the airways. At this time, the patient begins to expel large numbers of the bacilli from the respiratory tract. The fibrous and calcified walls of the tubercle then form an air-filled cavity where the tubercle bacilli may continue to grow. At this phase of the disease, healing or treatment is difficult, for the cavity wall forms a barrier not only against the body's defense mechanisms but also against chemotherapeutic agents. Surgical removal of such cavities is sometimes necessary before chemotherapy can be effective. Without treatment, the tubercular lesion may continue to expand and consume the normal tissue until death results. Earlier tuberculosis was called "consumption" because of this progressive destruction or consumption of the tissues. In some cases, the adverse factors that stimulated the "reawakening" of the disease may be removed and the disease may again become stabilized in the dormant stage.

Transmission and Epidemiology

Prior to the studies of tuberculosis by Robert Koch, it was generally agreed that this disease was of genetic origin. This idea probably resulted from the fact that the disease was often observed to occur in families, and among close relatives. However, it wasn't the infection per se that had genetic origins, but rather the response to the infection—that is, the manifestation of disease. Indeed, with the development of skin-testing procedures it was possible to demonstrate that approximately 90% of the population was infected with *M. tuberculosis*, although only a portion of the infected population developed disease symptoms. It has subsequently been shown that host factors (some of which may well be inherited) play a greater role in the outcome of infection by this organism than in possibly any other infectious process (Figure 22-3a, b). Application of Koch's postulates (see Chapter 14) was of considerable significance in demonstrating the role of *M. tuberculosis* in this disease. In fact, because of his monumental work with *M. tuberculosis*, Koch was awarded the Nobel Prize for medicine in 1905.

M. tuberculosis is usually found only in humans and large numbers of bacilli may be disseminated by the airborne route from

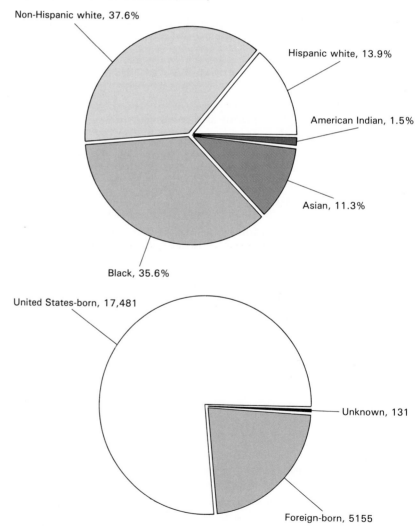

Figure 22-3 (a) Occurrence of tuberculosis by race and ethnic background in the United States in 1986. (b) Occurrence of tuberculosis among American- and foreign-born patients in the United States. (Courtesy Centers for Disease Control, Atlanta)

Non-Hispanic white, 37.6%

Hispanic white, 13.9%

American Indian, 1.5%

Asian, 11.3%

Black, 35.6%

United States-born, 17,481

Unknown, 131

Foreign-born, 5155

Table 22-1   Common Mycobacterial Agents of Disease

Agent	Communicable	Disease
M. tuberculosis	Yes	Human tuberculosis
M. bovis	Yes	Human tuberculosis
M. ulcerans	No	Cutaneous ulceration
M. kansasii	No	Pulmonary tuberculosis
M. avium-intracellulare	No	Pulmonary tuberculosis
M. marinum	No	Cutaneous lesions
M. scrofulaceum	No	Lymph node infection
M. africanum	Yes	Pulmonary tuberculosis
M. fortuitum-chelonei	No	Wound infection
M. szulgai	No	Human tuberculosis
M. leprae	Yes	Human leprosy

persons with active tuberculosis. A person may unknowingly transmit the bacilli for some time before being aware of having the disease. It is generally felt that prolonged close contact with an infectious person is necessary for successful transmission of this disease. Casual contact with an infectious person, such as passing on a street, would normally not result in transmission. Bovine tuberculosis, caused by *M. bovis,* was a problem at one time because transmission was from cow to humans via contaminated milk. But inspection of cows and pasteurization of milk have almost eliminated this source of infection in the United States and many other countries.

There is an increasing concern regarding the occurrence of disease due to **mycobacteria other than** *M. tuberculosis* **(MOTT).** *M. kansasii, M. avium, M. intracellulase, M. chelonei,* and *M. fortuitum* are presently responsible for an increasing number of cases of tuberculosis (Table 22-1). Of considerable epidemiologic interest is the fact that these agents are transmitted to humans from the environment, and human-to-human transmission rarely if ever occurs. Relatively large numbers of persons are infected with these agents but remain healthy unless there is a significant change in their resistance to disease. This fact has been dramatically demonstrated by the occurrence of mycobacterial disease in AIDS patients.

Mycobacteria other than tuberculosis

(MOTT) those mycobacteria of species other than *M. tuberculosis* and *M. leprae* which are capable of producing tuberculosis-like disease in humans.

Diagnosis

Tuberculosis has been the motivating factor in the development of a number of useful clinical diagnostic procedures and tools. The discovery of the stethoscope by René Laennec in the early 1800s was prompted by the clinical necessity of monitoring the progress of tuberculous patients. And the first medical use of the x ray by Wilhelm C. Roentgen was in connection with the diagnosis of tuberculosis (Figure 22-4). Present-day diagnosis of tuberculosis occurs in different stages. The first stage is skin testing, which pro-

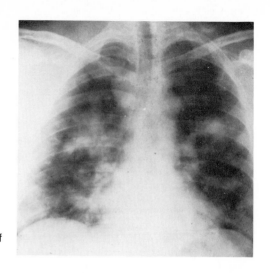

Figure 22-4 Chest x ray of patient with tuberculosis.

vides a rapid, inexpensive procedure for screening large numbers of persons. The second stage involves chest x rays, and the last stage is the isolation of *M. tuberculosis* from the infected individual.

Skin testing
application of an antigen directly to the skin or interdermally to determine the host immune status in relation to the antigen. A positive reaction depends on cell-mediated immunity and is a delayed hypersensitivity response.

Skin testing The highly specific delayed-type hypersensitivity that develops against the tubercle bacilli can be demonstrated by injecting an antigen from the bacillus into the skin (intradermal injection). This antigen is called *tuberculin* and was originally supplied as *old tuberculin* (OT), a crude extract from a broth culture of bacilli. Today a more refined extract called *purified protein derivative* (PPD) is used. The reference skin test—the *Mantoux test*— uses the intradermal injection of standard amounts of tuberculin. More convenient but slightly less reliable tests have been developed for routine screening programs such as the ''Tine'' test, which uses a disposable unit with metal tines that are covered with dried tuberculin and pressed into the skin.

Skin tests are read 48 hours after testing; an area of redness with swelling 10 mm in diameter is considered a strong positive (Figure 22-5). The skin test cannot distinguish clearly between the different stages of tuberculosis, but if someone converts to skin test–positive, it shows that the person has been exposed to the disease and has progressed at least to the primary stage. Further diagnostic tests are then indicated.

Chest x ray Routine chest x rays are discouraged. Such examinations are most appropriately used as a follow-up procedure on those who have converted to skin test–positive or to establish the extent of tissue damage in previously diagnosed cases of active or dormant tuberculosis.

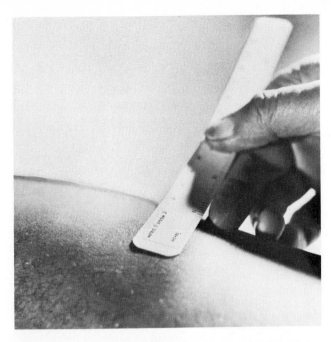

Figure 22-5 A positive Mantoux skin test showing an area of redness and swelling (about 15 mm in diameter) after 48 hours. (Centers for Disease Control, Atlanta)

Bacteriologic tests A definite diagnosis of active tuberculosis requires the isolation of the mycobacterium from the patient. The most effective method for obtaining bacterial specimens is the collection of induced sputum samples. The patient inhales a fine aerosol mist that induces deep coughing. The cough carries sputum and bacilli from the lungs to the mouth. Care should be taken to prevent health care personnel from being exposed to aerosolized bacilli during the collection of induced sputums. Special safety hoods or cubicles are recommended for this procedure (Figure 22-6).

The collected sputum is treated with sodium hydroxide, which kills most microorganisms other than mycobacteria, and an amino acid derivative, *N*-acetylcysteine, which digests the mucus. The bacteria in the sputum are then concentrated by centrifugation, and culture plates as well as slides for microscopic examination are prepared from the sediments. The standard acid-fast stain (Ziehl-Neelsen) provides a specific and reasonably sensitive diagnostic tool. Newer stains, based on the same acid-fast principle, use fluorescent dyes such as auramine-O to ease the microscopic examination of these specimens. The presence of acid-fast bacilli gives a rapid provisional diagnosis. The growth of *M. tuberculosis* on the inoculated culture media confirms the diagnosis.

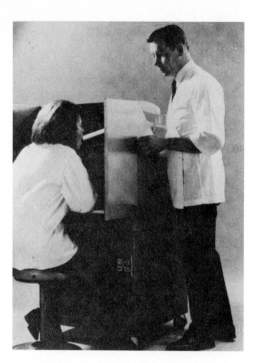

Figure 22-6 A safety hood used during the collection of sputum samples from tuberculosis patients. During the collection process, deep coughing is induced in the patient (seated). All airborne tubercle bacilli expelled by the patient are sucked into this safety hood where they are trapped by filters. The technician (standing) assisting the patient is protected from these airborne bacteria. (Jensen Research Laboratories)

Treatment

Sanitarium

a facility designed to care for persons and help them regain their health. In tuberculosis sanitariums patients were given healthful meals and were kept as free from stress as possible. Surgical and chemotherapeutic treatments were also available at some sanitariums.

Chronic

lasting a long time and tending to progress slowly.

With recognition that tuberculosis is an infectious disease, treatment became a real possibility. Over the years, isolation of patients in **sanitariums,** diet modification, and surgery have all had a significant impact on tuberculosis therapy. However, the ability to treat tuberculosis successfully with chemotherapeutic agents (Table 22-2) has been the most notable advance in controlling this disease and has led to significant changes regarding tuberculosis patients. No longer is it practical to maintain sanatariums specifically for such patients. The majority can be successfully treated in a relatively short time either in a general hospital that has specific facilities to handle tuberculosis or at home. Moreoover, most patients can be rendered noninfectious and then released from the hospital after some weeks. Generally, however, long-term follow-up therapy must be carried out on an outpatient basis. An important phase of the hospitalization program concerns the proper motivation and education of patients so that treatment continues through self-medication and return visits to the clinic. The personnel staffing these clinics must be trained to understand the **chronic** nature of tuberculosis and the need for the patients to return for regular follow-up appointments.

The antibiotic streptomycin was the first highly effective antituberculosis agent to be developed. This agent had such a profound effect on the outcome of disease that its discoverer, Dr. Sel-

Table 22-2   Agents Used to Treat Tuberculosis

Major or Primary Compounds	Minor or Secondary Compounds
Ethambutol (EMB)	Capreomycin
Isoniazid (INH)	Cycloserine
p-aminosalicylic acid (PAS)	Ethionamide
Rifampin	Kanamycin
Streptomycin	Pyrazinamide
	Thiacetazone
	Viomycin

man Waksman, was awarded a Nobel Prize for its discovery. Several years later, in the early 1950s, the synthetic compounds isoniazid (INH) and p-aminosalicyate (PAS), were developed. Later the compound ethambutol (EMB) and the antibiotic rifampin were effectively used to treat tuberculosis.

These chemotherapeutic agents are always given in various combinations. Streptomycin, if used, is given by injection, together with one or more of the less toxic compounds INH, PAS, or EMB given orally. Rifampin, combined with INH, is often administered orally throughout the entire treatment period. The time of treatment may vary, depending on the severity of the infection or the patient's reliability in taking the medication properly. The standard regimen has been daily medication for periods of 6 to 24 months. But it has now been determined that under controlled conditions short-course therapy for about 9 months can be effective. If it is difficult to control daily medication, an intermittently supervised high-dose treatment given twice weekly for the conventional time is effective. Well-regulated programs of administering the antituberculosis drugs are important. Failure to follow prescribed regimens results in the development of resistant strains of the tubercle bacillus. These strains have lead to infections that cannot be readily treated.

Prevention and Control

The prompt diagnosis of active cases is the most important phase in the control of tuberculosis. Once these individuals have been identified, they can be rendered noninfectious by proper chemotherapy. The next major problem is determining who might have become infected from the index cases. All possible contacts should be investigated, starting with those who shared common environmental air at home or work. The investigation should also extend to those who may have had less extensive contact with the patient. Appropriate diagnostic procedures should be carried out on the contacts, beginning with a history of any prior tuberculosis skin tests, vaccinations, or infections. Skin tests should then be done on all contacts and follow-up x rays and sputum specimens

Attenuated
the condition of an organism from which virulence factors have been removed.

used if indicated. Contacts showing conversion to positive skin reactions or having other signs of the disease should be placed on prophylactic chemotherapy. It is sometimes advisable to place the more susceptible close contacts, such as young children, on prophylactic chemotherapy even if they show no signs of the disease.

This program of detection and follow-up has worked quite well in countries with relatively few active cases and with the necessary medical personnel and public health facilities. A vaccine may be advisable in countries where tuberculosis is more prevalent and medical facilities are limited. A live vaccine, containing an **attenuated** M. bovis mutant known as *bacillus Calmette-Guérin*, or BCG, has been available since 1923 and induces an increased resistance to tuberculosis but not complete immunity. BCG vaccination has been used in some countries for many years and appears to offer some protection. But this vaccine induces hypersensitivity against the tubercle bacillus and thus renders the tuberculin skin test useless as a diagnostic aid. It is rarely used in countries where the incidence of tuberculosis is low, for it is considered more valuable to have the diagnostic usefulness of the skin test than the moderate protection provided by the vaccine.

Present-Day Concerns

The study of tuberculosis facilitates the learning of numerous principles and concepts that have application to a broad perspective of infectious disease. However, in spite of remarkable progress in reducing the incidence of this disease from 200 cases per 100,000 population in 1900 to fewer than 2 per 100,000 in 1980, there are significant concerns for the future. During the latter part of the 1980s there has been a small but persistent increase in the number of cases reported in the United States. Perhaps of more significance than the number of new cases has been the number of these cases where the organism is antibiotic-resistant. This primary resistance is not a new phenomenon but occurrence in the United States is relatively recent.

As medical practice and patterns of disease change, new avenues of infection become available to microorganisms, including M. tuberculosis and various MOTT bacteria. M. chelonei and M. fortuitum are somewhat opportunistic in their occurrence, and produce wound infections most often associated with prosthetic surgery. M. avium-intracellulare have taken advantage of the immunologically disabled AIDS patients to produce serious, disseminated mycobacterial disease. M. avium-intracellulare infections are producing an ever-increasing percent of the total mycobacterial disease in the United States. Another significant factor in increasing mycobacterial disease is the number of homeless individuals. These persons often share crowded, hygienically poor conditions, have inadequate diets, and suffer from drug or alcohol abuse; all

Tuberculosis: Maryland, 1974

Ten cases of active tuberculosis were traced to one source, a 30-year-old man, who was diagnosed as having tuberculosis on September 12, 1974. The patient had been ill for about 7 months, with symptoms that included a productive cough, intermittent fever, night sweats, and weight loss of about 60 pounds.

The patient's tuberculosis was classified as: tuberculosis, pulmonary; microscopy-positive (numerous acid-fast bacilli), and culture-positive (50 colonies). He was started on three antituberculous drugs. A report of the case was submitted by the hospital nurse epidemiologist to the county health department and an investigation of the patient's contacts began.

All 24 persons identified as household or close contacts of the patient were examined. Of these individuals, 7 were 21 years of age or older. The other 17 ranged in age from 2 to 12 years. One adult and 9 children had negative initial skin tests and remained negative on retesting.

The remaining 14 contacts (6 adults and 8 children) were found to have tuberculous infection as indicated by skin test reactions of 10 mm or more when tested with purified protein derivative (PPD). Primary active tuberculosis was identified in 7 of these 8 children and in 1 adult; 3 of the children were hospitalized. Daily isoniazid (INH) was given to 13 of these contacts and a 2-year-old child was started on INH and *p*-amino-salicylic acid (PAS). One child (the index patient's daughter) with a 0-mm skin test reaction was started on INH preventive therapy.

It was possible to identify 40 others as casual contacts of the index patient. Of this group, 32 were skin test–negative, 5 were positive reactors, and 3 were known positive. Two of the 5 positive reactors were placed on preventive therapy. One friend, who was a negative reactor on initial testing, refused to be retested. He was subsequently hospitalized and diagnosed as having: tuberculosis, pleural; bacteriology pending. He was treated with multiple antituberculosis drugs.

In addition, another casual contact—not included in the original contact study—was diagnosed as having active tuberculosis in 1975.

Moreover, 6 work contacts were examined; 3 were negative skin test reactors and 3 were previously known positives. Contacts who associated with the index patient's children were skin tested, 13 in all (mostly children); all were negative on initial testing and then on retesting.

Because of concern in the small community where the index patient resided, a tuberculin testing program was offered to community residents. As a result, 66 people were tested; 61 were negative reactors and 5 did not return for a reading (*MMWR* 25:93, 1976).

these circumstances increase the incidence of mycobacterial disease. Present studies show a tuberculosis prevalence as high as 6.8% among homeless persons.

Lastly, there has been a continued drift of the disease into older patient populations. In 1960 tuberculosis was considered as an illness of the middle-aged and young adult patient. By 1985, however, one-third of all cases were seen in patients 65 years of age and older. The incidence of tuberculosis in this group has reached 34.9 cases per 100,000 and the incidence remains less than 14 per 100,000 for persons between 25 and 44 years of age.

LEPROSY

Bacterium

Mycobacterium leprae is the causative agent of leprosy. This bacterium shares many common characteristics with *M. tuberculosis:* it is an acid-fast bacillus containing large amounts of lipid, induces hypersensitivity, and multiples slowly. *M. leprae* is found in enormous numbers of certain lesions of infected persons. This feature allowed Gerhard Hansen in 1874 to make the first reliable causal association between a bacterial agent and a human disease. Leprosy is often referred to as *Hansen's disease,* partly to honor Hansen's discovery and partly to avoid the use of the unpleasant name of leprosy.

Even though this bacterium is found in greater numbers in infected tissues than any other bacterium, it has not been possible to cultivate it on artificial media. Some growth occurs when it is inoculated into the foot pad of a mouse. Today it is known that armadillos are susceptible to this bacillus. Some evidence even suggests that armadillos may be a natural nonhuman host for leprosy. Thus, both mice and armadillos are being used in some limited experimental laboratory studies of leprosy.

Pathogenesis and Clinical Disease

Leprosy is probably transmitted from person to person under conditions of poor sanitation and may gain entry via the respiratory tract or skin lesions. The incubation period averages several years but may extend to 20 years. The major growth of the bacilli occurs in the low-temperature body tissues—that is, nose, ears, and the skin of extremities. The leprosy bacilli are easily phagocytized but not destroyed, and large numbers are found growing inside macrophages. Nerves are uniquely susceptible to infection; early symptoms of leprosy are often associated with anesthesia (lack of feeling) over an area of the body. The exact mechanism of tissue destruction is not understood but probably results from a combination of neurological damage, massive accumulation of bacilli, and immunologic reactions.

Two forms of leprosy are seen, the *lepromatous* and the *tuberculoid* (Figures 22-7 and 22-8). The lepromatous form is the most severe and is characterized by large nodular lesions. In lepromatous leprosy the immune response is impaired, limiting the formation of granulation (scar) tissue. The tuberculoid form is less severe and is associated with a normal immune response that causes

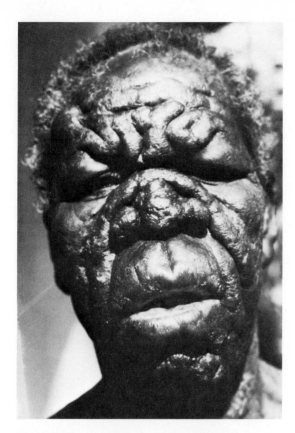

Figure 22-7   A patient with lepromatous leprosy: note the loss of eyebrows and deep furrowing that exaggerates the normal folds of the face. (Courtesy American Leprosy Missions, Bloomfield, N.J. 07003)

granulation-type lesions; bacilli in the lesions are sparse, tissue damage is less, and response to therapy is better. Forms intermediate between lepromatous and tuberculoid are also seen.

Overall, leprosy is a slowly progressing disease that often disfigures and cripples. Death usually results after many years and is commonly associated with **secondary infections.**

Secondary infection
infections which occur as a consequence of other disease processes in the host.

Transmission and Epidemiology

Leprosy is generally found in underdeveloped tropical and subtropical areas. Most cases seen in developed countries were contracted—sometimes years earlier—while the person resided in a tropical or subtropical area. Only about 150 cases occur each year in the United States (Figure 22-9). But the disease is still a major problem worldwide. Estimates are that over 20 million people have leprosy and that only 10% are currently under treatment.

From a historical perspective the epidemiology of leprosy of-

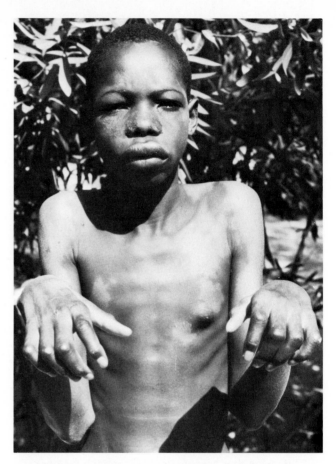

Figure 22-8 A patient with tuberculoid leprosy: note the flat discolored plaques on the shoulder, chest, and hands. Swelling and contraction of the fingers results from inflammation of the nerve fibers. (Courtesy American Leprosy Missions, Bloomfield, N.J. 07003)

fers some unexplainable paradoxes. Early reports suggested that the disease was highly contagious. During the eleventh and fifteenth centuries, for example, leprosy was widespread in Europe. Then a sharp decline in incidence followed in the sixteenth century. The reason for this decline and for the comparative decrease in virulence and communicability of this disease today are not known.

Diagnosis

Bacterial diagnosis is made by direct microscopic demonstration of the presence of acid-fast bacilli in scrapings of fluids from the lesions (Figure 22-10). A skin test using an antigen called *lepromin*, obtained from the heat-inactivated extracts of infected tissues, is

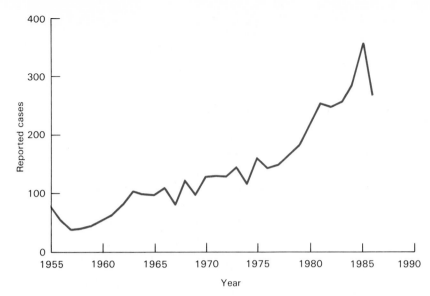

Figure 22-9   Reported cases of leprosy in the United States per year, 1955–1987, The increases in the 1970s and 1980s were due primarily to imported cases among Indochinese refugees (modified from CDC annual summaries).

Figure 22-10   Micrograph of *M. leprae* taken from a lesion and stained by the acid-fast method. (Courtesy American Leprosy Missions, Bloomfield, N.J. 07003)

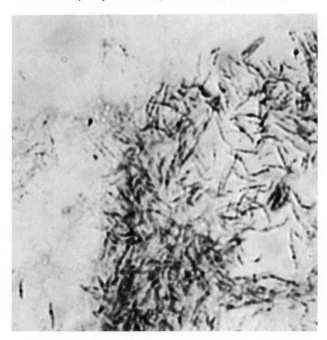

of some value. Clinical findings are often characteristic enough for a tentative diagnosis.

Treatment

Antimicrobial agents called *sulfones,* which are related to the sulfonamides, are fairly effective in arresting progression of the lesions and in allowing them to heal (Figure 22-11). These agents render patients noninfectious and allow them to return to normal daily activities as outpatients. Treatment is prolonged, for months to years, and it is not certain when or if a complete cure is ever obtained. The antibiotic rifampin has been shown to render patients noninfectious in just a few weeks, but the full effect of this promising agent is still under investigation. The other antituberculosis drugs are not effective against leprosy. Unfortunately, there have been reports of increasing bacterial resistance to dapsone, the leading antileprosy drug.

Prevention and Control

Only persons who have prolonged contact with leprosy patients under poor sanitary conditions seem to stand an increased risk of being infected. Young children are more susceptible than adults.

Figure 22-11   (a) A child with leprosy before treatment. (b) The same child after treatment with a sulfone. (Courtesy American Leprosy Missions, Bloomfield, N.J. 07003)

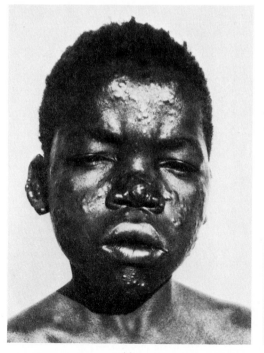
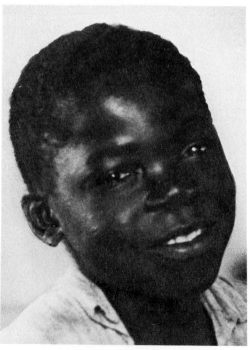

(a)   (b)

Hansen's Disease in Vietnamese Refugees: United States, 1975

Beginning in July 1975 Vietnamese refugees 15 years of age and older living in Camp Pendleton, California, Fort Indiantown Gap, Pennsylvania, and Ford Chaffee, Arkansas, were examined for evidence of Hansen's disease. Among 27,057 adults examined, 39 definite cases were found (1.4 cases per 1000). Only 4 cases (10%) were of the infectious (lepromatous) form. Of the others, 5 were borderline, 3 indeterminate, and 27 tuberculoid. Males numbered 23. The estimated age-specific rates per 1000 (and the numbers of cases) were as follows: 15–19 years, 1.1 (6 cases); 20–29 years, 1.8 (15 cases); 30–39 years, 0.7 (4 cases); 40–49 years, 2.2 (7 cases); 50–59 years, 2.5 (5 cases); and 60+ years, 1.2 (2 cases). Five cases had been recognized in Vietnam, and treatment begun there; 34 cases were newly diagnosed. In addition, 6 suspected but unproved cases were identified. All proved cases were either under therapy or had already completed adequate courses of therapy. Follow-up in each case was coordinated by respective state health departments and public health service hospitals at Carville, San Francisco, and New York.

Several additional cases of Hansen's disease have already been recognized and reported among the refugees who were not screened because they were placed with family or sponsors before July.

Because the prevalence of Hansen's disease in Vietnam has been estimated at 3 to 5 per 1000, it was expected that a number of cases would be found among the 140,000 refugees who entered the country in 1975. In addition, more cases could be expected to develop over the next decade. The risk to U.S. residents, however, is small. The only important risk of untreated lepromatous Hansen's disease patients is to their family contacts. A study in the Philippines showed that the risk of secondary cases of Hansen's disease in such contacts was 6.2 cases per 1000 persons per year. In the years 1949 to 1972 an average of 30 cases of lepromatous Hansen's disease per year were recognized in immigrants to this country. Nevertheless, cases of Hansen's disease in U.S. citizens who have never lived in a leprosy-endemic area are rare. And the few lepromatous cases among the Vietnamese refugees are not thought to be an important additional risk. Early diagnosis and treatment are important, however, to prevent progression of the disease and disability (*MMWR* 24:455, 1976).

Using good sanitary procedures when dealing with patients is recommended. It may also be advisable, in some situations, to remove young children from infectious parents and place them on a course of preventative chemotherapy. Tattooing parlors in endemic areas should be avoided, for contaminated tattooing needles have been shown to transmit leprosy. New cases of leprosy were prevented on a Pacific island by subjecting the entire population of 1500 people to a course of sulfone treatment. Possibly such prophylactic chemotherapy could be used in other endemic areas to block the spread of leprosy.

ACTINOMYCETES AND RELATED MICROBES

Actinomycetes and related microbes are Gram-positive bacteria; some species are acid-fast and related to the mycobacteria. These organisms grow in long filaments (Figure 22-12) with extensive branching and thus resemble the morphology of fungi (Chapter 30). They are procaryotes, however, and possess bacterial-type cellular morphology. Widespread in nature, they are found in soil and are noted for the production of antibiotics and decomposition of organic matter. Some of these organisms are associated with disease in humans and animals. The more prominent human pathogens are briefly discussed here.

Nocardia

The most frequently encountered *Nocardia* species is *N. asteroides*. It is acid-fast and a common inhabitant of soil. Generally it is an opportunistic pathogen-causing disease in patients with other medical problems that have compromised their basic resistance to infections. Lung infection is the most common disease caused by *N. asteroides* and may be misdiagnosed as tuberculosis. The infection may spread from the lungs to the blood and involve various other parts of the body, especially the brain. *Nocardia* species may also cause penetrating lesions of the dermal, subcutaneous, or deeper tissues that are localized and have connecting passages (**sinuses**) to the surface through which the infection drains. Characteristic clumps (granules) made of compact colonies of nocardia are present in the exudate (Figure 22-13). Infections are usually best treated with sulfa drugs.

Actinomyces

Actinomyces are anaerobic Gram-positive, non-acid-fast, filamentous organisms with or without branching. The species *Actinomyces israelii* is the major human pathogen. *A. bovis* is a common

Sinus

an opening or space in a tissue. Infectious processes often produce a non-healing sinus which may connect between tissues or even to the outside.

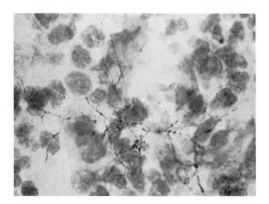

Figure 22-12 A pulmonary specimen containing an actinomycete among many PMNs. Note branching and beading configuration of bacteria. (Courtesy Center for Disease Control, Atlanta)

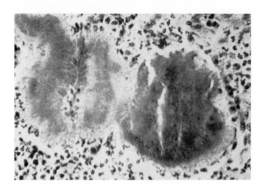

Figure 22-13 Sulfur granule from a patient with actinomycosis. (Courtesy Center for Disease Control, Atlanta)

pathogen of cattle only and causes a disease called "lumpy jaw." *A. israelli* is normally found in the mouth of humans and usually acts as an opportunist by causing infections in damaged tissues. The following types of infection are produced:

1. Head and neck infections following injury to the mouth or jaw, such as tooth extractions or other dental procedures.

2. Pulmonary infections resulting from aspiration of infectious material from the mouth.

3. Abdominal infections, probably resulting from swallowing organisms after abdominal surgery or injury.

4. Human bites that directly introduce the organisms into the tissues or any injury that breaks the skin; foot infections are common in some areas (Figure 22-14).

Figure 22-14 Actinomyces infection of the foot. (Courtesy Centers for Disease Control, Atlanta)

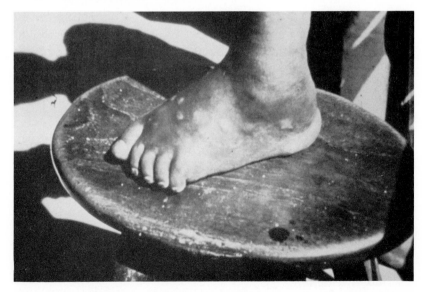

Infections are often characterized by draining abscesses with the actinomyces filaments embedded in yellowish granules in the exudate. Diagnosis is based on clinical appearance and the presence of typical organisms in the granules. Actinomyces are susceptible to various antibiotics, including penicillin, the antibiotic of choice. Surgical removal of the abscess is often necessary before successful treatment is possible.

Streptomyces

Streptomyces form long branching filaments that segment into beadlike structures called *conidia*. Each conidium can develop into a new colony. Most streptomyces are nonpathogens and are found in the soil. Many of the commonly used antibiotics are produced from these organisms. The species *Streptomyces somaliensis*, and perhaps a few other species, causes localized swollen lesions that are distinguishable clinically from lesions caused by *Nocardia* species.

CONCEPT SUMMARY

1. Members of the genus *Mycobacterium* are causative agents of two chronic diseases of great historical interest and significance: tuberculosis and leprosy. The mycobacteria are unique in that their cellullar composition includes a high concentration of lipid. Because of their staining characteristics, they are known as acid-fast bacteria. They are strict aerobes.

2. Tuberculosis is caused by a number of mycobacteria other than *M. tuberculosis* (MOTT). These MOTT are not transferred from person to person but produce a disease that is similar to that caused by *M. tuberculosis*.

3. Tuberculosis therapy has been difficult, requires long periods of antimicrobial use, and has been quite effective. Relatively large numbers of compounds are commonly used in therapy. A vaccine called BCG is available and has produced reliable results in areas where tuberculosis is a major health concern.

4. Leprosy is an age-old human disease. There are millions of cases of this disease throuthout the world, but it is infrequently found in the United States. New approaches to therapy have enabled many leprosy patients to have normal lives.

5. The actinomycetes are very similar in structure and composition to the *Mycobacteria*. They are much less often involved in human infections but the infections are serious and often life-threatening.

STUDY SUMMARY

1. What features of mycobacteria differ from those of other bacteria and may be responsible for the unusual pathogenesis of tuberculosis?

2. What changes in the organism and the host appear to be responsible for adult-type tuberculosis?

3. Describe the use of the skin tests as a means of diagnosing tuberculosis. What are the limitations to the use of this procedure?

4. Explain the advantages and disadvantages of the use of BCG vaccine.

5. Infections due to MOTT are not contagious. What characteristics of lifestyle correlate with tuberculosis due to these organisms?

6. List the two clinical forms of leprosy and the characteristics of this disease that are associated with each type.

7. Discuss the epidemiologic aspects of the transmission of leprosy.

8. What is the major physiologic distinction between the *Nocardia* and the *Actinomyces*?

REFERENCES FOR FURTHER STUDY

1. Opportunistic Pathogens in the Genus *Mycobacterium*. *Annual Review of Microbiology* 39:347, 1985.

2. Leprosy and Leprosy Bacillus. *Annual Review of Microbiology* 41:645, 1987.

3. Mycobacteria Other Than *Mycobacterium tuberculosis:* Review of Microbiologic and Clinical Aspects. *Reviews of Infectious Diseases* 9:275, 1987.

4. Environmental Nonhuman Sources of Leprosy. *Reviews of Infectious Diseases* 9:562, 1987.

5. Tuberculosis in the Native American. *Reviews of Infectious Diseases* 9:1180, 1987.

chapter 23

HAEMOPHILUS AND BORDETELLA

Subtype
a designation used to distinguish among members of a species which have one or more differentiating characteristics.

The two genera, *Haemophilus* and *Bordetella*, discussed in this chapter are composed of small, fastidious, Gram-negative bacilli. Representatives from both genera are capable of producing human respiratory disease. These diseases primarily afflict children and can be serious, even life-threatening. Based on current classification methods, these two genera are not closely related, and so each will be discussed separately in this chapter.

HAEMOPHILUS INFECTIONS

Bacterial species of the genus *Haemophilus* (sometimes spelled *Hemophilus*) require special growth factors that are found only in blood and other body fluids. The name *Haemophilus* means "blood-loving" (Greek *haemo* = blood; *philus* = loving). *Haemophilus influenzae* is the major disease-producing species of this genus. Several other species, such as *H. ducreyi* and *H. aprophilus*, are virulent but are less common agents of serious human infection.

Infections Due to *Haemophilus influenzae*

Bacterium *H. influenzae* is a small (1 × 0.3 μm), Gram-negative coccobacillus (Figure 23-1). It requires blood or blood products—specifically hemin, called *X factor*, and NAD, a coenzyme called *V factor*, for growth in artificial media (Table 23-1).

H. influenzae can be divided into a variety of **subtypes** based on metabolic reactions and antigenic capsular polysaccharides. There are six capsular types (a–f); essentially all serious, systemic disease is due to type b. The type b capsule is a polyribose-ribitol phosphate and is the primary component of the *H. influenzae* type b (Hib) vaccine. The capsule helps retard phagocytosis.

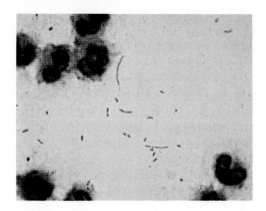

Figure 23-1
Photomicrograph of a spinal fluid containing *Haemophilus influenzae*. Note pleomorphic appearance of bacilli. (Courtesy Centers for Disease Control, Atlanta)

Other virulence factors are less well defined although the bacteria can produce an enzyme that specifically degrades protective IgA molecules that may be produced by the host. These traits may contribute significantly to the virulence of this bacterium. The bacterium does not survive well outside the body and is found only in humans.

Pathogenesis and clinical disease   *H. influenzae* colonizes in the respiratory tract and as many as 50% of young children may be carriers. Only a small number of persons who carry this bacterium develop clinical disease, and disease is most common in young children. Thus, *H. influenzae* generally functions as an opportunist. However, in spite of its opportunistic characteristics, *H. influenzae* is one of the leading causes of serious systemic disease in the United States. Clinical disease often occurs as a nose and throat infection (nasopharyngitis). In some persons, the infection may spread to the sinus and **middle ear** or develop into pneumonia. In a small percentage of cases the bacteria spread to the meninges.

   H. influenzae is the most common cause of bacterial meningitis. An estimated 11,000 to 12,000 cases of this disease occur annually, primarily among children under 5 years of age. Even with treatment, the mortality rate from this infection is about 5%, and

Ear infection
microbial infections of the structures of the ear. These may be external (otitis externa) or internal (otitis media) or both. Otitis media may have serious complications leading to other systemic disease.

Table 23-1   Identification of *Haemophilus* Species

Species	Requirement for		Production of		
	V factor	X factor	Urease	Indole	Beta-hemolysis
H. influenzae	+	+	+/−	+/−	−
H. parainfluenzae	+	−	+/−	−	−
H. hemolyticus	+	+	+	+/−	+
H. aphrophilus	−	−	−	−	−
H. ducreyi	−	+	−	−	−

Epiglottitis
infection of the tissue which normally cover the tracheae during swallowing.

a significant number (25% to 35%) who recover have permanent, residual damage of the central nervous system. In addition to causing bacterial meningitis, *H. influenzae* is responsible for other invasive diseases, including **epiglottitis,** sepsis, cellulitis, pneumonia, and septic arthritis. Patients with altered host defenses such as those patients without spleens or who have sickle cell disease or Hodgkin's disease have a greatly increased risk of serious outcome from Hib infection. Patients with Hib epiglottitis are a true medical emergency because they are in danger of suffocation due to obstruction of the respiratory tract. Other, less serious infections due to *H. influenzae* include otitis media (ear infection), infectious conjunctivitis (pink eye), and nasopharyngitis. Most of these infections are caused by organisms that do not have a capsule and seemingly pose little threat to life.

Transmission and epidemiology The *Haemophilus* bacteria are widespread in humans; most persons develop active antibody immunity against them before reaching adulthood. Newborns receive passive immunity from their mothers and hence valuable protection during the early months of life. Because antibody to the capsular polysaccharide is protective, as long as infants are protected by this transplacental antibody from their mothers they are at little risk of serious *H. influenzae* b infection. However, as this antibody begins to be lost, there is a definite and increasing risk of meningitis until the child develops its own antibody. Children in day-care centers are at increased risk of infection as are **siblings** and other family members of patients. Statistics show that 1 out of every 200 children in the United States will have had a systemic Hib infection by the time they reach 5 years of age. Haemophilus infection also occurs in adults, but at a much reduced rate. Most haemophilus infections occur on a **sporadic** basis, except for conjunctivitis, which is highly contagious, and may occur as an epidemic. *H. influenzae* pneumonia may occur in conjunction with an epidemic viral respiratory disease, such as influenza. The name *H. influenzae* was applied to this bacterium because early studies mistakenly thought it was the primary cause of influenza.

Sibling
a brother or sister.

Sporadic
occurring at irregular intervals. Outbreaks or occurrences of sporadic infections are very difficult to predict.

Diagnosis Diagnosis of *H. influenzae* meningitis can often be made by direct microscopic observation of the bacteria in the spinal fluid. The quellung test on bacteria in spinal fluid, using specific antiserum, will confirm if the observed bacteria are *H. influenzae*. Bacteria can be cultured on chocolate agar and then specifically identified. Some cases are diagnosed through serological procedures that can detect free bacterial capsular antigens in body fluids like urine or spinal fluid.

Treatment Prompt, proper therapy is essential in life-threatening circumstances (e.g., meningitis, sepsis, epiglottitis), and not only reduces mortality but also limits serious sequelae. Delay in treatment greatly reduces the chance for therapeutic success. Ampicillin is considered the drug of choice if the organism is susceptible. However, recent reports indicate that as many as 35% of *H. influenzae* b are now resistant to this antibiotic. Other antibiotics such as chloramphenicol and a cephalosporin called *cefotaxime* may be necessary in cases where ampicillin is not effective. Sensitivity tests to determine the most effective chemotherapeutic agent are generally completed on all strains isolated from serious disease conditions.

Prevention and control Because of the widespread nature of this bacterium, little can be done to prevent exposure. The most effective means of preventing deaths and minimizing neurologic damage are early diagnosis and treatment of meningitis. Most children develop natural immunity during the first six years.

The current use of Hib vaccine has greatly reduced the incidence of serious *H. influenzae* b infection in children over 2 years old. However, the greatest incidence of meningitis is in children between 5 months and 18 months of age. Unfortunately, infants respond poorly to polysaccharide vaccines, and the Hib vaccine does not work well in children under the age of 2 years. Even children less than 18 months of age who have serious Hib disease often fail to develop their own protective antibody. Therefore, it is highly recommended that all children be immunized when they are 2 years of age, regardless of their past history with respect to *H. influenzae*.

Other preventive procedures include the use of chemoprophylaxis for persons who have had close association with a patient. Day-care classmates are at a 20 times greater risk, and siblings are at a 600 times greater risk of developing *H. influenzae* meningitis than is an individual who has no close association with a Hib patient. Therefore, most persons who have close contact with such patients should be given rifampin as a chemoprophylactic antibiotic.

Infections Due to Other *Haemophilus* Species

H. ducreyi is commonly isolated from patients suffering from a sexually transmitted disease known as *chancroid*. This infection is characterized by the development of a small papule or pustule at the point of infection, usually the genitalia. The pustule ruptures and forms an ulcer similar to the chancre observed with syphilis. The ulcer (commonly there are multiple ulcers) is painful and often accompanied by tender, swollen, and suppurative regional

Outbreak of *Haemophilus influenzae* Type b Disease in a Day-Care Center: Kansas, 1976

Four episodes of serious *Haemophilus influenzae* type b infection occurred in three children attending a day-care center in Lawrence, Kansas, during 8 days of October 1976. This outbreak accounted for a third of all *H.influenzae* type b disease reported in Lawrence from January 1, 1974, through October 31, 1976.

The patients were among 13 infants, ages 5 to 14 months, cared for in the same room at the day-care center. There were 59 older children at the center, none of whom became ill. Two children became ill on the same day, one with meningitis and the other with cellulitis of the cheek and bacteremia. Eight days later another child developed meningitis and cellulitis of the cheek. After the child who initially had bacteremia and cellulitis was treated for 6 days with intramuscular ampicillin (100 mg/kg/day), a repeat blood culture was taken; it was negative. However, 7 days after completing this initial therapy, the child developed meningitis. The three children were not related and had no contact with each other except at the day-care center. All *H. influenzae* type b isolates were sensitive to ampicillin.

Children, staff members, and family contacts of patients received ampicillin or rifampin as antibiotic prophylaxis in an attempt to eradicate carriage and prevent transmission of organisms, particularly to young children. Rifampin was prescribed according to recent recommendations for prophylaxis of meningococcal disease and ampicillin was given orally for 5 days. No further cases developed. Although *H. influenzae* is the most common cause of bacterial meningitis in the United States, outbreaks of clusters of the disease are considered unusual (*MMWR* 26:201, 1977).

lymph nodes. Genital ulcers are most frequently seen in male patients. There is often a high correlation between this disease and contact with female prostitutes. Specific diagnosis is made by isolating *H. ducreyi* from the lesion or lymph nodes. Treatment with sulfonamide or tetracycline is generally effective.

WHOOPING COUGH

The clinical term for whooping cough is *pertussis*. Historically it has been one of the prominent childhood diseases and before the advent of an effective vaccine was a frequent cause of death in young children. Vaccination has greatly reduced the number of cases of pertussis in developed countries.

Bacterium

Bordetella pertussis is the causative agent of whooping cough. Morphologically it is similar to *H. influenzae*. It differs from *Haemophilus*, however, in that it is a strict aerobe, does not require specific blood components for growth, and will grow on various types of culture media. Agar containing blood, potato starch, charcoal, and cefalexin is the culture medium of choice. This bacterium survives for only a short time when expelled from the body in respiratory secretions.

Pathogenesis and Clinical Disease

B. pertussis is aerosolized from the throat of a person with whooping cough and is transmitted to others by the airborne route. This bacterium selectively attaches to the epithelial cells of the respiratory tract and growth is limited to the superficial tissues. After an incubation period of 10 days, generalized symptoms of an upper respiratory infection occur, such as sneezing, runny nose, and coughing (the term *catarrhal* refers to such symptoms). This first stage, or **prodrome,** lasts a week or two. The second stage progresses into episodes (paroxysms) of uncontrollable coughs. Each paroxysm may consist of 5 to 20 rapid coughs, with the patient unable to breathe between coughs. At the end of the paroxysm a forced inspiratory breath causes the "whooping" sound. This coughing and whooping form the basis for the common name for this disease. Such prolonged coughing may lead to anoxia (decreased oxygen in the blood), expelling of mucus, and vomiting. The second stage may continue for 1 to 6 weeks. The third stage may include some coughing during convalescence and may last for several more weeks. Various toxins produced by *B. pertussis* are thought to induce the accumulation of mucoid materials and the extensive coughing. The central nervous system is affected and contributes to the morbidity and mortality associated with whooping cough. Respiratory distress and secondary bacterial pneumonia also contribute to the seriousness of many cases of whooping cough, particularly in young children. About 25% of the cases are mild or subclinical and are passed off as a nonspecific respiratory infection.

Prodrome
an early phase of infection leading to disease. The prodromal phase of disease is usually not associated with specific diagnostic symptoms, but may include a variety of nonspecific host changes.

Transmission and Epidemiology

B. pertussis is found only in humans and is transmitted, in most cases, only by persons with an active infection. Up to 90% of the unimmunized household contacts of a clinical case may develop whooping cough. Pertussis is found worldwide and has no seasonal distribution. Widespread immunization in the United States has caused a steady decline in the number of cases. In 1950, for instance, 120,000 cases with 1100 deaths occurred compared to

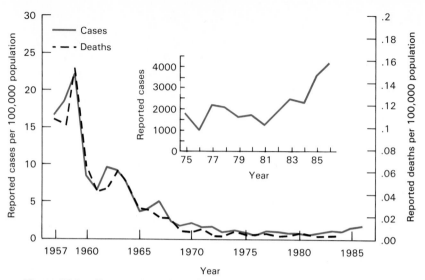

Figure 23-2 Reported yearly cases and deaths from pertussis (whooping cough) in the United States, 1957–1987. (*CDC Annual Summary*)

about 4500 cases in 1985 with just a few deaths. Similar decreases are seen in other countries where wide-scale immunization is used. Reported cases in the United States are shown in Figure 23-2.

Diagnosis

Fluorescent-tagged antibodies can be used for a rapid and specific identification of *B. pertussis* obtained directly from nasopharyngeal swabs (swabs passed through one nostril into the nasopharynx). Culture can be obtained by having the patient cough directly onto the open plate or by streaking the plate with the nasopharyngeal swab.

Treatment

Although no antibiotic is always successful against *B. pertussis*, the antibiotic erythromycin is the most effective chemotherapeutic agent. Tetracyclines and chloramphenicol have also been used but are somewhat less effective. Removal of respiratory secretions, oxygen therapy to aid breathing, and general supportive measures are of value in treating patients with severe symptoms.

Prevention and Control

A killed pertussis vaccine has been widely used for many years and is associated with a steady decline in the number of cases of whooping cough. The vaccine is usually given in combination

Pertussis: Maine and Georgia, 1977

Two outbreaks of pertussis, one in Maine, the other in Georgia, have been reported to the Centers for Disease Control in Atlanta. Details of these outbreaks are as follows.

Maine. Pertussis was diagnosed in a 2-year-old girl from Bridgeton, Maine, in April 1977 after a 6-week history of cough. The child had been seen several times both as an outpatient and in the hospital, where diagnoses of asthma, bronchitis, and cystic fibrosis were considered before the diagnosis of pertussis. Direct fluorescent antibody (FA) stain of a nasopharyngeal smear from the patient and from an ill sibling confirmed pertussis in both. Two other siblings, the parents, and a neighbor's child also had had a clinical illness compatible with pertussis. All the children had received the recommended number of immunizations for diphtheria and tetanus toxoids and pertussis vaccine (DPT) for their age. The cases were treated with erythromycin and an immunization clinic was set up in the community.

Georgia. An outbreak of pertussis occurred among students of a Decatur, Georgia, elementary school over a 5-week period in May and June 1977. Of the school's 580 students, 26 had a clinical syndrome of fever and catarrhal symptoms, followed by prolonged cough, as did 4 preschool siblings of sick children. None developed clinical pneumonia or required hospitalization and most had a relatively mild cough. Of the 30 cases, 26 were students in the third grade or their contacts.

Nasopharyngeal swabs were obtained for culture and FA staining from 28 ill schoolchildren and their siblings. *Bordetella pertussis* was isolated from 6 children; it was identified by FA staining in 1 culture-positive child and 3 other children.

Immunization histories of the ill children were compared with those of the well children. Of 75 children who gave a history of complete DPT immunization for their age, 18 were ill. Of 19 children who had a history of incomplete immunization, 12 became ill. No child had a certain history of no prior pertussis immunization. The majority of children with incomplete immunization lacked a preschool booster of DPT. Thus complete immunization provided 62% more protection than partial immunization.

Editorial note: Pertussis occurs more frequently than is generally recognized. It is often not considered in the differential diagnosis of cough (as weith the index case in the first outbreak) or in older children because the disease may be mild and manifested simply as a persistent cough (as in the second outbreak). Diagnosis is further complicated by the various capabilities of laboratories in identifying the organism by culture or FA staining (*MMWR* 26:250, 1977).

with tetanus and diphtheria toxoids as the DPT vaccine. Little passive immunity to this disease is transferred to newborn infants; therefore vaccination should be initiated as soon as possible (Figure 23-3). The first immunization of a series of three should be given at about 6 weeks of age and the other two at monthly intervals. Booster immunizations should be given at about 1 year of age and again just before starting school. When a person under 4 years of age who has been immunized is exposed to someone with whooping cough, a booster injection should be given. When

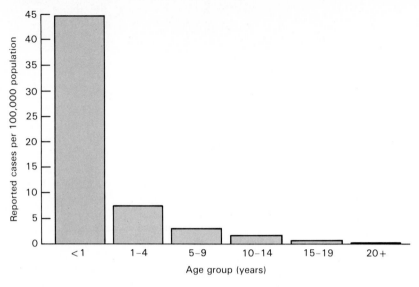

Figure 23-3 Distribution of pertussis by patient age in the United States in 1986. (Courtesy Centers for Disease Control, Atlanta)

exposed, unimmunized children should be given prophylactic treatments with erythromycin for about 10 days.

Brain damage following administration of the vaccine has been reported in about 1 in 100,000 vaccinated infants; consequently, some countries with low rates of whooping cough have begun limiting the use of the vaccine in young infants. Still, young infants are the ones who need the protection most; the balance between benefits and hazards in the use of this vaccine is sometimes difficult to determine. When use of this vaccine was discontinued in England for a period of time, a dramatic rise in the number both of cases and fatalities due to whooping cough occurred. There is current interest in developing an improved whooping cough vaccine.

CONCEPT SUMMARY

1. *Haemophilus* is a genus of fastidious Gram-negative bacilli that are responsible for a wide variety of clinical diseases. These organisms are particularly serious pathogens of children.

2. Because of some problems associated with use of pertussis vaccine, there has been a worldwide decrease in the use of DPT. Reduction in immunization use has been accompanied

by a corresponding increase in the reported number of cases of whooping cough.

STUDY SUMMARY

1. What virulence feature is almost always associated with serious *Haemophilus* infection?
2. Discuss the observation that serious *Haemophilus* infection usually occurs between the ages of 6 months and 6 years.
3. What determines the age at which the Hib vaccine should be administered?
4. What explanation can you provide to account for the observation that antibiotic therapy has only limited effect on the course of pertussis?
5. How do you justify the use of DPT in view of the toxic response that occurs in some persons?

REFERENCES FOR FURTHER STUDY

1. Virulence Factors of *Bordetella pertussis*. *Annual Review of Microbiology* 40:661, 1986.
2. Lipooligosaccharide and Virulence of *Haemophilus influenzae* Type b. *Microbiology—1986*, p. 49. American Society for Microbiology.
3. Pertussis Toxin: Mechanism of Action, Biological Effects and Roles in Clinical Pertussis. *Microbiology—1986*, p. 75. American Society for Microbiology.
4. Nontypable *Haemophilus influenzae:* A Review of Clinical Aspects. *Reviews of Infectious Diseases* 9:1, 1986.
5. *Haemophilus influenzae* Type b Infectious in Day Care Attendees. *Review of Infectious Diseases* 8:558, 1986.

chapter 24

ENTEROBACTERIACEAE

Nitrate test

a test to determine whether an organism is able to convert nitrate to nitrite or nitrogen gas. This is a relatively simple biochemical test.

Oxidase test

a test to determine the presence of specific enzymes associated with the electron transport pathway.

Enterobacteriaceae is a family of commonly isolated Gram-negative bacilli. It is a large family containing more than 100 species of bacteria. These organisms are related biochemically; they all ferment glucose, they are **nitrate** positive and **oxidase** negative, and they are not benefited by increased concentrations of sodium chloride.

Because of the close relationship of many of these microbes, it is sometimes difficult to determine the exact classification categories. Over the years, various classification arrangements have been used and the names of some species were periodically changed. For example, as of 1972 there were only 12 genera and 26 species in this family; by 1988 there were more than 30 genera, 17 of which contain organisms of clinical significance (Table 24-1). The number of species presently exceeds 100 with additions being made regularly. In the following discussion, references are chiefly to the genus or species names and less emphasis is given to larger taxonomic categories. In the clinical setting these microorganisms are referred to as the Gram-negative or the enteric bacilli.

The Enterobacteriaceae primarily inhabit the large intestines of humans and animals. Some are also found in soil, water, and decaying matter. Some of these bacteria are of moderate to high virulence and are able to cause disease when they infest susceptible hosts. Members of this group are referred to as primary pathogens and include species of the genera *Salmonella*, *Shigella*, and *Yersinia*—the causative agents of typhoid fever, dysentery, and bubonic plague, respectively. Most other enteric bacilli are of lower virulence and function as opportunistic pathogens; these organisms are regular inhabitants of the intestinal tract of humans or are routinely found in the general environment. The opportunistic species cause disease only when they gain access to normally sterile body compartments or tissues or when the host defenses become compromised.

TABLE 24-1   Genera of Clinically Significant Enterobacteriaceae

Cedecia	*Hafnia*	*Salmonella*
Citrobacter	*Klebsiella*	*Serratia*
Edwardsiella	*Kluyvera*	*Shigella*
Enterobacter	*Morganella*	*Tatumella*
Escherichia	*Proteus*	*Yersinia*
Ewingella	*Providencia*	

The endotoxins contained in the cell wall of these enteric bacteria may play an important role in the pathogenesis of the diseases they cause. Some pathogenic strains also produce exotoxins. A number of species produce an exotoxin called **enterotoxin** that specifically affects the intestinal tract, causing diarrhea and fluid loss from the body. Various species of the Enterobacteriaceae are able to cause pneumonia and are also the most common cause of urinary tract infections. These microorganisms are now recognized as a major cause of wound infections and other **nosocomial** infections acquired by hospital patients. They may also cause severe systemic infections such as bacteremia and occasionally meningitis. It has been estimated that infections by these enteric bacilli may be contributing factors in about 100,000 deaths per year in the United States. Infections caused by these bacteria are often difficult to treat with routinely used chemotherapeutic agents.

Enterotoxins
microbial toxins which have intestinal tissues as their primary site of action.

Nosocomial
acquired in the hospital. Nosocomial infections are a major concern in today's highly immunocompromised hospital patient population. Although any organism may be obtained in a hospital setting, most nosocomial infections are due to endogenous bacteria.

GENERAL CHARACTERISTICS OF THE ENTERIC BACILLI

The members of the family Enterobacteriaceae are relatively small (0.5 × 2 μm), non-spore-forming bacilli (Figure 24-1). Some are motile, others are not. Some have capsules, but others do not. They ferment a variety of different carbohydrates and the patterns of carbohydrate fermentation are used to help differentiate and classify these bacteria. The bacterial colonies appear similar on nondifferential media. Various differential and selective media, however, are used to help in the preliminary classification of the Enterobacteriaceae. Once these microorganisms have been classified by biochemical tests to the genus or species level, further differentiation is made by serologic tests.

People in a clinical bacteriology laboratory spend much time identifying and differentiating the species of these Gram-negative bacilli. Being widespread, normal inhabitants of the body, they are often found in clinical specimens and it is a rather laborious

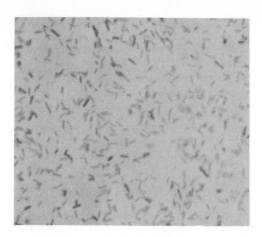

Figure 24-1
Photomicrograph of
Salmonella.

task to determine if pathogenic strains are present among the non-pathogens. When dealing with an infected patient, particularly a compromised host, it is also necessary to determine if the disease is caused by a low-virulence strain. Trying to find the involvement, if any, of these bacteria in a given clinical disease is a challenge to physicians and laboratory workers.

Because these bacteria are found in large numbers in the intestinal tract, they are often transmitted by the fecal-oral route and are frequent contaminants of food and water. The enteric bacilli are able to survive for extended periods when adequate moisture is present. They can be carried in water supplies over long distances and may be found on foods or in other environmental niches where moisture is present. Freezing does not destroy these bacteria and frozen foods or ice can remain contaminated for extended periods. They are responsive to relatively low concentrations of common disinfectants and are effectively reduced in water supplies treated with small amounts of chlorine. However, their antibiotic susceptibility is unpredictable, and they are frequently resistant to common antimicrobials.

SALMONELLA

Enteric fever
bacteremia due to organisms from the genus *Salmonella.*

Members of the genus *Salmonella* are so closely related that they could easily be considered a single species. However, for epidemiologic and clinical purposes it is useful to characterize at least three species, *S. typhi*, *S. cholerasuis*, and *S. paratyphi A*. Other species are divided among more than 1500 serotypes. The major diseases caused by *Salmonella* bacteria are **enteric fever** and gastroenteritis. The classic example of enteric fever is known as typhoid fever.

Typhoid Fever

Pathogenesis and clinical disease Typhoid fever is caused by *S. typhi* which attaches to and penetrates the epithelial lining of the small intestines. Following penetration, the bacteria are phagocytized by macrophages; unfortunately, they are not destroyed but are actually able to multiply within the macrophages. The macrophages carry the *S. typhi* throughout the RES. These events occur during the first week of infection and may be accompanied by fever, malaise, lethargy, and aches and pains. During the second week, extended bacteremia is present and the foci of infection may occur in various tissues; often the gallbladder becomes infected. Bacteria may be shed from the gallbladder back into the intestinal lumen. During this time ulcerative lesions of Peyer's patches may develop and the patient is often severely ill with a constant fever as high as 40° C (104° F), abdominal tenderness, diarrhea or constipation, and vomiting. By the third week, in uncomplicated cases, the patient is exhausted, may still be febrile, but shows improvement. Death may result in up to 10% of the untreated patients. After people recover from the clinical disease, *S. typhi* may continue to multiply in the gallbladder of about 3% of the patients. These persons may become chronic carriers and serve as a source of future outbreaks. The pathogenesis of typhoid fever is shown in Figure 24-2.

Transmission and epidemiology The primary mode of transmission of the typhoid bacillus is the fecal-oral route through contaminated food or water. In developed countries, typhoid fever cases have declined significantly because of adequate water and sewage systems. Most outbreaks of typhoid fever in the United States today are associated either with persons living in undeveloped areas or with **point-source** outbreaks due to contamination of a food or beverage by a carrier. The threat of typhoid is always present when normal water and sewage systems are disrupted by disasters like floods and earthquakes. Normally between 400 and 500 cases of typhoid fever occur each year in the United States. The typhoid fever rate in the United States is seen in Figure 24-3.

Point source
a single source from which dissemination of an infectious agent occurs. Sometimes referred to as *common source* (e.g., contaminated milk).

Diagnosis Typhoid fever, particularly in early stages, is easily confused with other diseases. A positive diagnosis depends on the isolation of *S. typhi* from the blood, feces, or other parts of the body. Agglutination tests showing a rise in specific antibodies are also used.

Treatment Treatment is with ampicillin or chloramphenicol. It must be continued for several weeks to ensure killing bacteria that became sequestered in the phagocytic cells. Carriers are best cured by daily treatment with ampicillin for three months. If this treatment fails, surgical removal of the gallbladder may be necessary.

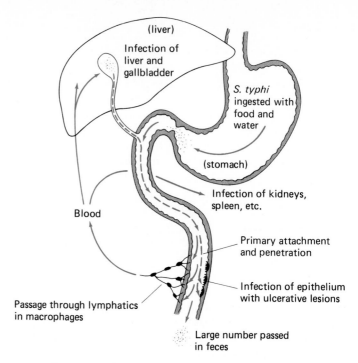

Figure 24-2 The pathogenesis of typhoid fever.

Prevention and control Proper water treatment and sewage disposal are the most important factors in controlling typhoid fever. Pasteurization of milk and exclusion of chronic carriers as food handlers are also helpful. Killed vaccines have been used for many

Figure 24-3 Occurrence of typhoid fever in the United States, 1955–1987. (Courtesy Centers for Disease Control, Atlanta)

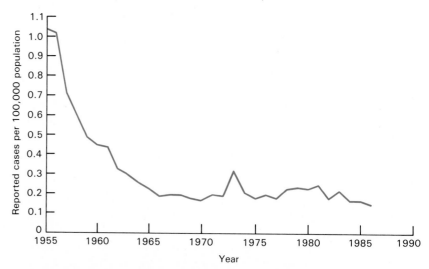

Typhoid Fever: Michigan, 1981

During October and November 1981, 18 cases of typhoid fever were diagnosed in Jackson, Michigan, among 310 United Way volunteers who consumed a luncheon served at a community banquet hall on October 8, 1981. Although no specific food could be incriminated, a probably chronic carrier of *Salmonella typhi* was identified among the food handlers who prepared the luncheon.

Dates of onset ranged from October 12 to November 11, 1981, for an incubation period of 4 to 33 days (mean = 13.5). Older individuals tended to have shorter incubation periods. The attack rate was 5.8%. Sixteen of the 18 cases were confirmed by blood and/or stool culture. All isolates of *S. typhi* were phage type E_1 and were sensitive to chloramphenicol, ampicillin, and trimethoprim-sulfamethoxazole.

All patients experienced fever (mean temperature 103.3° F [39.6° C]), fatigue, and headache, and most had chills, sweats, and anorexia; 39% reported diarrhea, and 33% had constipation. No instances of gastrointestinal hemorrhage or perforation were reported. There were no deaths and no evidence of secondary transmission.

Self-administered questionnaires asking about foods eaten at the luncheon and subsequent illness were distributed to all attendees; 289 (93%) returned completed questionnaires. Food histories of the 16 culture-confirmed cases were compared with those of asymptomatic controls and failed to incriminate any food item.

A probably chronic carrier of *S. typhi* was identified among the food handlers. This individual, an asymptomatic 68-year-old female with previously undiagnosed cholelithiasis (gallstones), had participated in the preparation of all or most of the foods served. *S. typhi* of the same phage type and antimicrobial-sensitivity pattern as that obtained from cases was isolated from her rectal swab and all her stool specimens; her serum antibody titer was 20. She subsequently underwent cholecystectomy (removal of gallbladder) in combination with high-dose amoxicilin therapy. Culture of the gallstone after antimicrobial therapy and all follow-up stool cultures have been negative (*MMWR* 31:544, 1982).

---

years but are of limited value. A recently developed oral (living attentuated) vaccine has been used in highly endemic countries. Unfortunately, results from this vaccine are not always as good as was originally predicted.

Gastroenteritis

Pathogenesis and clinical diseases   Many serotypes of *Salmonella* are found as normal flora in the intestinal tract of animals and birds. However, when ingested by humans, salmonella proliferate in the intestines and symptoms of **gastroenteritis** may begin within 18 to 36 hours. These symptoms include fever, nausea, abdominal pain, and diarrhea. This condition is usually self-limiting and complete recovery occurs within several days. In serious or

Gastroenteritis
an infection or intoxication of the intestinal tract. Gastroenteritis is commonly characterized by nausea, diarrhea, and malaise.

Lumen

opening. Often used to refer to the hollow space in a tubelike structure.

prolonged cases, extensive dehydration may occur; this is particularly true in very young or elderly persons. Fluid imbalance resulting from dehydration may be life-threatening. Human infection by these organisms is usually limited to the **lumen** of the intestine, but on occasions may progress to enteric fever. Such infections constitute a form of infectious food poisoning.

Transmission and epidemiology   Salmonellosis is one of the most common infectious diseases in the United States. It is estimated that more than 2 million cases occur annually. Infections results from ingesting salmonella-contaminated foods. Poultry products, including eggs, are the most common source of salmonella infections, but meat and meat products, in general, are frequently contaminated. Any food that comes in contact with rodents or animal products may become contaminated. Pets or other animals may harbor salmonellae and transmit the infection directly to humans. Pet turtles are often infected; consequently, their sale is regulated throughout the United States. Outbreaks of *Salmonella* gastroenteritis often occur after such holidays as Thanksgiving and Christmas. The increased use of widely distributed mass-produced foods may result in an increase in the rate of salmonellosis in the United States. The numbers of reported cases of salmonellosis occurring in this country are shown in Figure 24-4.

Diagnosis   Isolation of *Salmonella* from the intestinal tract is required for a positive diagnosis.

Figure 24-4   Cases of salmonellosis reported in the United States, 1955–1987. (Courtesy Centers for Disease Control, Atlanta)

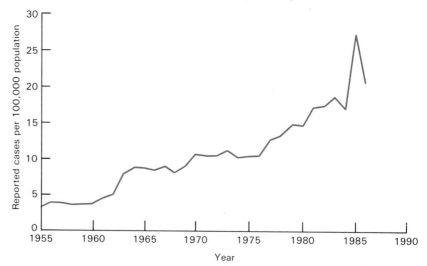

Multistate Outbreak of Salmonellosis Caused by Precooked Roast Beef: Northeastern United States, 1981

In the first week of August 1981, three outbreaks of salmonellosis that affected more than 100 people in three northeastern states were reported to CDC. The first two outbreaks were traced to precooked roast beef from a Philadelphia meat-processing plant, and the third to delicatessen-style sliced sandwich meat served at a hospital cafeteria. Some of these meat slices were of the precooked roast beef processed in the Pennsylvania plant.

The first outbreak followed a wedding reception held on July 25 at Claymont, Delaware, attended by approximately 150 people, mostly residents of Delaware County, Pennsylvania. Of the 58 persons contacted for interview, 37 had had diarrhea. *Salmonella* group B was isolated from the stools of 13 patients (11 *S. chester*, 2 *S. typhimurium*). Illness was significantly associated with eating precooked roast beef at the reception. None of the meat served at the reception was available for culture.

The second outbreak followed a wedding reception held on July 25 in southern New Jersey; 47 of 92 persons who attended became ill, and illness was again associated with eating precooked roast beef. *Salmonella* was isolated from 18 of 20 stool cultures (17 *S. typhimurium*, 1 *S. newport*). *S. typhimurium* and *S. johannesburg* were isolated from an opened package of precooked roast beef provided by the caterer of the reception. Another unopened package of the same brand from the same caterer contained *S. typhimurium*, *S. newport*, and *S. anatum*.

The third outbreak, which occurred in a hospital in Philadelphia, Pennsylvania, was first recognized on July 24 after two patients had severe diarrhea. Subsequent investigation revealed 42 cases of diarrheal illness between July 20 and August 11. Six of the persons involved were inpatients, and 36 were hospital employees. *Salmonella* group B was isolated from stools from 18 persons (including 4 patients); *Salmonella* group C_2 was isolated from 1 employee. *Salmonella* group B was isolated from 5 of 71 asymptomatic

dietary and nursing staff in a stool-culture survey. Preliminary analysis of a case-control study demonstrated an association between illness and eating sandwich-meat slices served at the hospital cafeteria. The meat slices included the same brand of precooked roast beef involved in the other outbreaks. Some of the infected persons had not eaten the beef; the other meats may have been contaminated by it. The suspected beef samples were not available for culture, but *Salmonella* group B was recovered from meat drippings in a tray containing remnants of meat from the cafeteria delicatessen.

On August 5, the U.S. Department of Agriculture (USDA) asked the Philadelphia producer to temporarily halt further distribution of the implicated beef. *S. typhimurium* was isolated from 1 of 64 specimens tested by the USDA. Assessment of the internal temperature of these products by the protein coagulase test showed that the core temperature ranged from 130° to 152° F, ± 5° (54.4° to 66.7° C ± 2.8°). On August 10, the USDA issued a recall order of all precooked roast beef that had been processed by the Philadelphia company before August 6, 1981.

Editorial note: This is the first reported multistate outbreak of salmonellosis attributable to commercially produced precooked roast beef in 4 years. Until 1977, when multiple outbreaks of the disease involving several meat-processing companies were reported from Connecticut, Georgia, New York, New Jersey, Pennsylvania, and Virginia, the USDA instituted regulations requiring that raw beef be cooked until heated throughout to at least 145° F (62.8° C).

The outbreaks reported here may have resulted from failure to achieve the required minimum temperature, as indicated by the USDA study. Also, recent evidence shows that under certain conditions even heating raw meat to 145° F (62.8° C) may not produce a completely *Salmonella*-free product. Further studies on the survival of *Salmonella* in raw beef may be indicated (*MMWR* 30:391, 1981).

Treatment Supportive therapy is the recommended treatment for salmonellosis. Antibiotics are not recommended except in extreme cases of disseminated disease or cases involving infants or elderly persons.

Prevention and control Proper cooking and refrigeration of meats eliminate or prevent the growth of salmonellae. Sanitary procedures in slaughterhouses help reduce the level of contamination. Some foods are routinely monitored for the presence of salmonellae.

SHIGELLA

Shigella neurotoxin
a powerful toxin produced by *S. dysenteriae* which acts on tissues of the central nervous system.

Dysentery
serious diarrhea, accompanied by mucus and blood in the stool along with severe abdominal cramping.

The *Shigella* are primarily pathogens of humans and are not naturally found in other environments. The four species of the genus *Shigella*—*S. dysenteriae*, *S. flexneri*, *S. boydii*, and *S. sonnei*—can all cause **dysentery** in humans. *S. sonnei* is by far the most commonly involved species, and *S. dysenteriae* causes the most severe type (Table 24-2).

Bacillary Dysentery

Pathogenesis and clinical disease Following ingestion, the shigellae are usually unable to penetrate the intestine into the deeper body tissues or into the blood, but multiply in the small intestines. The bacteria are mechanically carried to the large intestines; here they specifically attach to, and penetrate into, the epithelial cells, where further multiplication occurs. Generally, penetration is not deeper than the submucosal cells. Inflammation, together with sloughing of the epithelial cells, results in ulcerative lesions. After 1 to 3 days of incubation the patient experiences a sudden onset of symptoms—abdominal cramps, fever, and diarrhea. The diarrheal stool frequently contains mucus and blood. Significant loss of water and salts may occur and in young and/or debilitated patients this dehydration and electrolyte imbalance may cause death. In

Table 24-2   Distribution of Shigella Species Recovered from Diarrhea in the United States

Species	Group	Percent of Total
S. dysenteriae	A	<1
S. flexneri	B	28
S. boydii	C	<1
S. sonnei	D	70

otherwise healthy persons the disease is usually self-limiting and recovery occurs in 3 to 7 days. The death rate from dysentery in young children is significant in countries with poor sanitation and nutrition.

Infections due to *S. dysenteriae* are always potentially more serious than those due to other species. This organism produces a very powerful exotoxin (neurotoxin) that greatly increases its virulence. Although not endemic in the United States, this species has recently been introduced by tourists returning from Central America and Mexico. Most residents in areas where dysentery is endemic develop immunity to the disease either through clinical or subclinical cases. Many such persons, however, remain carriers of the organism and serve as a source of infection for new susceptibles, such as visitors or newborns entering the population.

Transmission and epidemiology Transmission is from human to human via the fecal-oral route by "fingers, foods, feces, or flies." Infection by *Shigella* is commonly associated with poor or crowded living conditions. Most of the approximately 20,000 causes occurring annually in the United States are associated with institutionalized individuals, where hygienic conditions may be difficult to maintain because of crowding and lack of individual capabilities. This relationship between an ability to maintain personal hygiene and the frequency of shigella infection is reflected in the age distribution of the disease in the United States (Figure 24-5).

This disease is endemic in underdeveloped countries. Historically, dysentery has been a problem in military populations and entire armies have become temporarily disabled when living un-

Figure 24-5 Occurrence of shigellosis in the United States, 1955–1987. (Courtesy Centers for Disease Control, Atlanta)

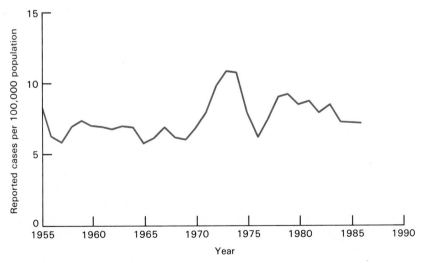

Outbreak of Shigellosis: Fort Bliss, Texas, 1976

An outbreak of food-borne shigellosis occurred on November 5, 1976, in a tactical unit conducting field-training exercises at Fort Bliss, Texas. Of 850 soldiers at risk, 176 became ill with diarrheal disease; 53 were hospitalized.

The onset of the majority of the cases (92) was between 1 A.M. and noon on November 5; an additional 34 cases occurred during the second half of the day. Excluding the suspected index case, the range of onset was from November 4 to 9.

The disease was characterized by rapid onset with fever up to 41° C (105° F), abdominal cramps, profuse diarrhea (bloody in several cases), and frequent vomiting. Many of the more serious cases with high fevers complained of severe myalgia with backache. The mean duration of the disease was 4 days, with a range from 1 to 8 days. The longest period of hospitalization was 5 days; however, most hospitalized cases were discharged within 48 hours. All cases recovered without sequelae. Stool cultures were positive for *Shigella boydii,* serotype 2, in 29 individuals.

The distribution of times of onset and the nature of the illness typified a food-borne infection originating from a common source. Although the unit was operating under field conditions, most of the personnel ate their meals in a common mess hall. A limited number of meals were prepared separately and delivered to troops at various outlying areas; most of these meals were distributed at noon.

Interviews with a large sampling of soldiers concerning food ingestion on November 3 and 4 revealed a statistically significant association between eating spaghetti at the evening meal on November 3 and subsequent diarrheal disease.

The mean incubation period calculated from the time of ingestion of the spaghetti at the evening meal of November 3 was 50.5 hours. The spaghetti was not available for culturing. However, water, milk, and several other foods that were available failed to demonstrate any contamination with enteric pathogens.

Of the 26 food handlers working in the mess hall at the time of the outbreak, 12 were sympto-

---

der unsanitary conditions existing during combat. Often people from countries like the United States contract bacillary dysentery within a short period after entering a country where dysentery is endemic.

Diagnosis Diagnosis is made by isolating *Shigella* from the feces or intestinal tract.

Treatment In contrast with *Salmonella* gastroenteritis, most cases of shigellosis are improved by chemotherapy. The recent development of **multiresistant** strains of *S. sonnei* (resistant to ampicillin, tetracycline, and trimethoprim-sulfamethoxazole) has complicated the approach to therapy, but several available antibiotics remain effective.

Multiresistant
bacteria which are resistant to a variety of antibiotics with different mechanisms of antimicrobial action.

matic with diarrheal disease. Positive stool cultures for *S. boydii*, serotype 2, were reported for 9 of the symptomatic and 1 of the asymptomatic food handlers. One food handler responsible for preparing the spaghetti reported having had diarrheal disease at the time he did so. This food handler had spent the preceding weekend (October 30–31) in Juarez, Mexico; 2 days later he had onset of illness.

The meat sauce was prepared on the morning of the outbreak whereas the spaghetti was prepared in the afternoon, several hours before being served. The spaghetti and sauce were reportedly reheated before serving. Field mess facilities, including those for hand washing, were limited, however, and there is some question whether the reheating was performed as prescribed.

The following control measures were taken:

1. All food handlers associated with the outbreak were removed from the mess line and rectal swabs were taken. The food handlers were not allowed to work at that job until they had consecutive negative cultures taken at least 24 hours apart. Cultures were not taken until at least 48 hours after discontinuance of antimicrobials. (Symptomatic food handlers were placed on 2 g ampicillin daily for 7 days.)

2. Meticulous attention to food preparation procedures, especially handwashing for mess personnel, which included brushing of fingers and nails, was instituted. All food service personnel were continuously monitored for signs or symptoms of disease and proper food handling techniques were emphasized.

3. All persons who were ill or had a positive culture were instructed in proper sanitary practices by a community health nurse. Special attention was given to soldiers with families to ensure that secondary cases did not occur in family units. All family contacts were instructed to report any occurrence of diarrheal disease (*MMWR* 26:107, 1977).

Prevention and control   Prevention of person-to-person transmission by following good sanitary practices is the most effective means of avoiding shigellosis. Patients with the disease should be isolated.

YERSINIA

The other genus in addition to *Salmonella* and *Shigella* that has primary pathogenic species is *Yersinia*. This genus contains *zoonotic* species (organisms that cause disease in animals that are transmissible to humans). In fact, the most widely known disease from this genus, bubonic plague, is primarily a disease of rats and other rodents, not humans.

Plague

The bacterial species, *Yersinia pestis,* was the cause of epidemic plague also known as the "black death" during the Middle Ages. Due to improved living conditions, and perhaps changes in other factors influencing host-parasite relationships, plague is no longer the devastating disease it once was. Sporadic cases still occur in the western United States and it remains endemic in Asia.

Bipolar stain

bacteria which stain more intensely at the poles (ends) of the cell than in the center. This often gives cells a "safety pin" shaped appearance.

Bacterium   *Y. pestis* (Figure 24-6), a Gram-negative coccobacillus, shows **bipolar staining** that produces a "safety pin" appearance when viewed with an optical microscope. It can easily be grown on common laboratory media, and grows best at 30° C. It is non-motile.

Pathogenesis and clinical disease   A variety of toxins are associated with *Y. pestis.* The most significant of these toxins are the V

Figure 24-6   Scanning electron micrograph of *Y. pestis* magnified 40,000×. (T. H. Chen and S. S. Elberg, *Inf. Imm. 15:*972–977, Figure 4, with permission from ASM.)

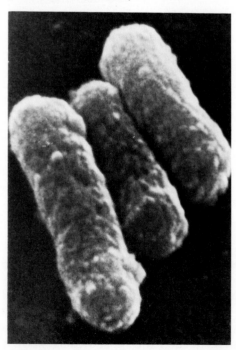

and W toxins, which are transferred among these organisms by a plasmid. Organisms without the plasmid are avirulent and have been used as vaccine strains.

Y. pestis is able to multiple in a variety of different mammalian and insect hosts and exists in three cycles. The first, or natural cycle, is found in wild rodents and is called *sylvatic plague.* Sylvatic plague is transmitted among rodents by fleas. The most frequent carriers of plague are squirrels, mice, prairie dogs, and chipmunks; over 200 different animals have been shown to be susceptible. Some animal species die of the disease whereas others experience subclinical infections.

The second cycle occurs when plague is spread to urban rodents, mainly rats, that live in close proximity to humans. This cycle is called *urban* or *domestic plague.* Urban rats frequently die of plague, which causes their fleas to seek new hosts and results in an increased chance of spread to other animals as well as humans.

The third cycle, called *human plague,* starts when humans are bitten by an infected flea from either the sylvatic or urban cycles. Generally the fleabite occurs on the legs and the bacteria spread to regional lymph nodes in the groin, where extensive multiplication and swelling occur. The swollen lymph nodes are called *buboes,* especially in older medical writings, and this form of the disease is called *bubonic plague* (Figure 24-7). The buboes usually appear less than a week after the fleabite. Fever, chills, nausea, malaise, and pains may precede and accompany the buboes. The spread of the bacteria is not stopped by the lymph nodes and so bacteremia results. The presence of the *Y. pestis* in the blood is called *septicemic plague.* Massive involvement of blood vessels occurs, resulting in purpuric (purple) lesions in the skin. This manifestation was responsible for the ''black death'' title earlier applied to this disease. Bacterial **emboli** may become trapped in the lungs, where the lesions erode into the air sacs and cause *pneumonic plague.* Pneumonic plague gives an added dimension to this disease, for the bacteria can be readily transmitted from the patient to other persons by the airborne route. Those contracting pneumonic plague in this way rapidly develop severe signs of the disease and die within 2 or 3 days. The epidemiology and pathogenesis of plague are shown in Figure 24-8. The death rate from untreated bubonic and septicemic plague is 50% to 75% whereas that from pneumonic plague is close to 100%. Some persons do develop mild nonfatal cases of plague.

Transmission and epidemiology   Plague has occurred in **pandemics** in earlier periods and throughout history was one of the most devastating diseases of humankind. The first well-documented pandemic occurred in A.D. 550 and resulted in an estimated 100 million deaths over a 60-year period. The next major pandemic

Embolus
an abnormal particle that blocks a blood vessel. Emboli are usually small blood clots, but may be composed of gases (such as air), fat, or other material.

Pandemic
an epidemic that involves the population of more than one country. Often thought of as worldwide occurrence.

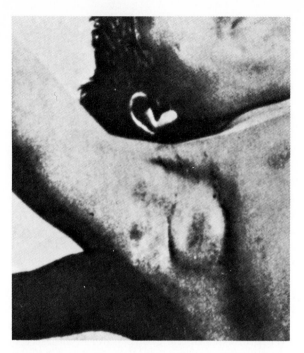

Figure 24-7 Swollen axillary lymph nodes (bubo) in a patient with plague. (Armed Forces Institute of Pathology, AFIP MIS #219900(7-B))

took place in the fourteenth century when 25% of the population of Europe died. Smaller epidemics continued until about 1800; then a general decline set in. The last major epidemic happened in China at the end of the 1800s. During the nineteenth century, plague was carried to most parts of the world, including to the West Coast of the United States, by rat-infested ships. Today, most cases of plague are reported in southeast Asia. Virtually all plague seen today results from fleabites and not from airborne transmission from person to person. Sylvatic plague still exists in the western United States in over 50 species of rodents and their fleas. Most cases seen in the United States occur among persons who live in rural areas or who camp in the West. At present, 10 to 20 cases of plague per year have been diagnosed in humans in the United States (Figure 24-9). Urban plague from domestic rats in seaport cities is a possible threat; however, no such outbreaks have occurred for many years.

Diagnosis Preliminary laboratory diagnosis of plague may be made by direct microscopic examination of smears of fluids from lymph nodes or lesions. The appearance of Gram-negative, bipolar-staining coccobacilli is suggestive of *Y. pestis*. A confirmed diagnosis can be made by culturing the bacteria and by serologic tests.

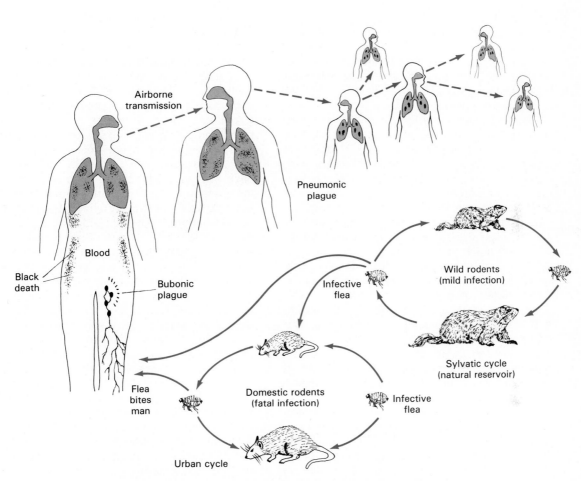

Figure 24-8 The epidemiology and pathogenesis of plague.

CLINICAL NOTE

Plague: South Carolina, 1983

On August 5, 1983, plague was diagnosed in a 13-year-old girl in South Carolina. She became ill while en route to Maryland from her previous residence in Santa Fe, New Mexico, and subsequently died. The area in which she had lived had been recognized as a locality where sylvatic plague was enzootic.

On July 25, the girl, a horsewoman who spent considerable time outdoors, handled and then released a wild chipmunk. On July 27, she flew to Atlanta, Georgia, and spent the night with friends; the following day she was driven to Seneca, South Carolina. That evening, she complained of a sore throat and tenderness in her right groin and reportedly had a temperature of 40.0° C (104° F). On July 29, she saw a physician, who noted an oral temperature of 38.3° C (101° F), pharyngeal erythema, tender cervical lymph nodes, and 1- × -2-cm tender right inguinal lymph node. Laboratory tests, including complete blood count, urinalysis, and throat culture, and tests for mononucleosis, were done, and oral penicillin was prescribed. Three days later she was seen again, still febrile and with expanding right inguinal nodes. Her white blood cell count was 20,500, and a chest x ray was normal. Because of her history of residence in a plague-enzootic state, a diagnosis of plague was considered. She was hospitalized and given parenteral therapy, including streptomycin. By the following morning, she was tachypneic (rapid, shallow respiration), with productive bloody sputum, and appeared moribund. She was transferred to a large, regional medical center where, despite intensive supportive care and therapy with intravenous chloramphenicol, she developed overwhelming sepsis and died on August 2. A chest radiograph taken before death revealed extensive pulmonary infiltrates.

Antemortem aspiration of the right inguinal lymph node demonstrated Gram-negative bipolar staining bacilli on Giemsa stain. Both this aspirate and multiple cultures of blood yielded *Yersinia pestis*. In addition, fluorescent antibody (FA) stains for *Y. pestis* were positive for specimens consisting of blood smears, culture material, and pulmonary secretions.

Editorial note: This is the fifth documented case of plague east of the hundredth meridian (south-central Texas to north-central North Dakota), exluding laboratory accidents, since 1920. All five patients were exposed in enzootic areas (four in the western United States, one in Vietnam). Considering this patient's outdoor activities and area of residence, exposure possibilities are numerous; her exact exposure will probably never be known, since the chipmunk was not captured. That she was able to handle the animal suggests that it was not healthy.

Because the patient had no evidence of pneumonia before hospitalization, no chemoprophylaxis was recommended for the friends with whom she stayed in Georgia; there were no secondary cases. Based on the clinical picture and the positive FA results from sputum, it appears that pneumonic plague and the potential for human-to-human transmission existed terminally. Local health care providers had placed her in complete isolation before this development. Hospital staff directly in contact with her at this point were placed on prophylactic tetracycline and followed up for evidence of illness. No secondary cases appeared during the expected incubation period (*MMWR* 32:417, 1983).

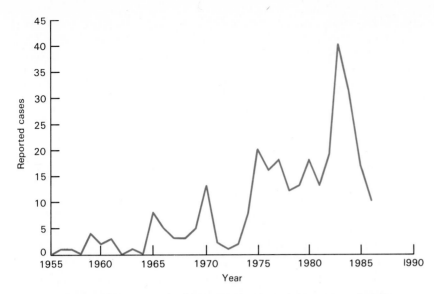

Figure 24-9   Occurrence of human plague in the United States, 1955–1987. (Courtesy Centers for Disease Control, Atlanta)

Extreme care is needed to prevent laboratory-acquired infections when working with *Y. pestis.*

Treatment   *Y. pestis* is highly susceptible to streptomycin, tetracyclines, and chloramphenicol. Early treatment is extremely important, especially for pneumonic plague because treatment after the first day may not be successful. Proper early treatment of bubonic plague reduces the mortality to less than 5%.

Prevention and control   Both living and killed plague vaccines are available. Three doses of the killed vaccine are used in the United States and this dosage is recommended for persons going to southeast Asia. Plague vaccinations were effective in protecting U.S. military personnel during the Vietnam War. In general, plague can be controlled by improved living conditions that reduce close contact between humans and rodents. Efforts to prevent the importation of rats by ship or airplane have been quite effective and are a necessary phase of plague control.

Yersinia Enterocolitica Infection

By far the most common disease in humans caused by *Yersinia* is that caused by *Y. enterocolitica.* This bacterium is associated primarily with domestic animals but may be transmitted to humans through contaminated foodstuffs or directly from such animals as poultry and swine. The organism is frequently associated with large outbreaks of disease. This is typical of point-source food-borne infections, and *Y. enterocolitica* has often been transmitted to relatively large groups of individuals in milk. An interesting feature of this organism is that it is motile when grown at room temperature, but not when grown at 37° C.

The infection is characterized by acute abdominal pain, profuse (sometimes bloody) diarrhea, and headache. Vomiting may occur in some patients. These symptoms are characteristic of many cases of appendicitis and so have led to the removal of normal appendixes in patients with this infection. Patients may also have an inflammation of the abdominal lymphatic structures, a condition referred to as *mesenteric adenitis.* Recovery is usually uneventful and complete.

Y. enterocolitica is most often isolated by plating a stool specimen on a selective medium. However, when present in low numbers, it can be cultured by a cold-enrichment procedure in which the culture specimen is held in saline at 4° C for up to 3 weeks. Periodic cultures are made from the cold enrichment to regular media and incubated at 35° C to recover the organism.

OPPORTUNISTIC ENTERIC BACILLI

The bacteria discussed in this section are generally of low virulence and are often present as normal or transient inhabitants of the intestinal tract of humans and animals. Some are also found in water, sewage, and soil. Members of the genera *Escherichia, Klebsiella, Enterobacter, Serratia,* and *Citrobacter* usually ferment the sugar lactose and share a number of other properties; they are sometimes called **coliforms.**

Coliform
enterobacteriaceae that are commonly normal flora of the intestinal tract.

All these opportunistic bacilli are capable of producing similar infections. When they gain access to such tissues as the urethra, bladder, lungs, wounds, or internal organs, they may be capable of causing disease, particularly in a compromised host. The most frequent problems are urinary tract and wound infections. Pneumonia, gastroenteritis, septicemia, and meningitis may also result from these microbes. The more commonly encountered genera or species are discussed briefly in this section, with emphasis on some unique characteristics of each. The short Gram-negative morphology and physiologic characteristics generally associated with the enteric bacilli are typical for this group of bacteria.

Klebsiella

Primary pneumonia
pneumonia which occurs as a result of infection without previous compromise to host defenses.

The major *Klebsiella* species is *K. pneumoniae.* It is a cause of **primary pneumonia** in older persons with such predisposing medical problems as chronic bronchitis, diabetes, or alcoholism. It is also a common cause of septicemia as well as urinary tract and wound infections. Many antibiotic-resistant strains are found in hospitals; treatment is often difficult.

Enterobacter

The *Enterobacter* are closely related to the *Klebsiella* and cause similar infections. The most commonly encountered species is *E. cloacae*. These bacteria are frequently resistant to antimicrobial therapy and therefore cause serious infections.

Serratia

The most frequently encountered *Serratia* is *S. marcescens*. This bacterium may produce red-pigmented colonies when grown at room temperatures. For many years it was considered a nonpathogen and, because of the pigmented colonies, it was used in various experiments to follow the movement of airborne particles in hospitals and other environments. It is now recognized that *S. marcescens* may cause pneumonia, cystitis (inflammation of the urinary bladder), and other infections in compromised hosts. Treatment is difficult because of its resistance to many commonly used antimicrobials.

Proteus, Providencia, and Morganella

Proteus, Providencia, and *Morganella* are closely related. Bacteria of these genera are found in waters, soil, sewage, and the intestinal tracts of humans and animals. Most clinical infections are of the urinary tract or burns. These bacteria are responsible for 10% of hospital-acquired (nosocomial) infections. Treatment with antibiotics is often difficult.

Citrobacter

The genus *Citobacter* is closely related to *Salmonella*. *Citrobacter* bacilli have occasionally been incriminated as the cause of infections in humans, particularly urinary tract infections.

Escherichia

The most commonly occurring *Escherichia* species is *E. coli*. Like many other enteric bacilli, *E. coli* was considered a nonpathogen for many years. It is one of the predominant facultative anaerobic bacteria of the intestinal tract and so is used as an indicator organism in determining the amount of fecal contamination in water and food. Many strains are used in experimental work in cell research. Much of the current work in molecular biology and recombinant DNA uses *E. coli.* More is probably known about this organism than any other bacterium.

It became increasingly apparent over the past several decades that *E. coli* of varying degrees of pathogenicity exist and that these bacteria are responsible for numerous human infections. Certain strains of *E. coli*, called *enterotoxigenic E. colli* (ETEC), produce enterotoxins that function like those produced by the cholera bacillus *V. cholerae.* These strains are the most frequent cause of infectious diarrhea throughout the world. Often referred to as ''traveler's diarrhea,'' it is considered by many to be one of the nuisances of international travel. In adults it is usually self-limited, after a few days of nausea and profuse watery diarrhea. In global terms, it is not so benign, and is the leading cause of child mortality throughout the world. The extent of such intestinal diseases is not known because most cases are self-limiting and a specific laboratory diagnosis is difficult. Epidemics in hospital nurseries have been reported and infections are probably widespread in infants living under impoverished conditions. Where infants are malnourished and supportive therapy is not given, a significant number of deaths result from dehydration and electrolyte imbalance due to *E. coli* enteritis. The use of oral rehydration therapy has produced remarkable results in reducing mortality due to ETEC.

Other infections that are commonly due to *E. coli* include urinary tract infections, (where *E. coli* is the most common cause); bacteremia (where *E. coli* is among the leading causes), and neonatal meningitis (where *E. coli* is associated both with regular occurrence and a high mortality rate). Of recent concern has been the isolation of a specific *E. coli* serotype, 0157:H7, from cases of bloody, sometimes fatal diarrhea. These organisms, referred to as *verotoxin-producing E. coli* (VETC) because the toxin they produce will kill vero tissue culture cells, have also been shown to produce a rare but frequently fatal disease known as *hemolytic-uremic syndrome.*

CONCEPT SUMMARY

1. The enteric bacilli consist of a large group of Gram-negative bacilli that are normally found in the intestinal tract of humans and animals. They are transmitted by the fecal-oral route and usually are commensals with only a few primary pathogens, such as *Salmonella* and *Shigella.*

2. Typhoid fever, a disease caused by *Salmonella typhi,* is of a considerable significance worldwide. Most frequently transmitted in contaminated water, this organism causes a serious

life-threatening illness. Proper sewage and water treatment, as well as adequate food-handling laws, are necessary to prevent the spread of this organism. Other *Salmonella* species cause disease in humans but these infections are nearly always transmitted through contamination of our environment by animal feces.

3. Shigellosis or bacillary dysentery is a human disease and is transmitted through human fecal contamination of food, water, or inanimate objects. The disease is severe but usually self-limiting.

4. The plague bacillus is endemic in the United States. A small number of cases occur in humans each year. These cases are usually associated with outdoor activities in endemic areas and can be effectively treated with early antibiotic therapy.

5. The opportunistic enteric bacilli are common environmental inhabitants that are responsible for a high percentage of hospital-associated infections, and are the leading cause of urinary tract infection.

STUDY SUMMARY

1. How would you respond to a statement that the Enterobacteriaceae are low-level pathogens of minimal medical significance?

2. What feature of the Enterobacteriaceae makes antibiotic therapy of their infections difficult?

3. Contrast the following terms: (a) diarrhea and dysentery; (b) food poisoning and gastroenteritis.

4. Describe the normal route of infection for each of the following organisms: (a) *Salmonella*, (b) *Shigella*, (c) *Y. enterocolitica*, (d) *Y. pestis*, and (e) *E. coli*.

5. Describe the following three cycles: (a) domestic plague, (b) human plague, and (c) sylvatic plague.

6. List the cultural, morphologic, and virulence features that are common to the genera of the opportunistic enteric bacilli.

REFERENCES FOR FURTHER STUDY

1. *Microbiology—1985*, L. Leive, 1985. American Society for Microbiology.

2. Urinary Tract Infections. *Infectious Disease Clinics of North America* 1:4, 1987.

3. Genetics of Bacterial Enterotoxins. *Annual Review of Microbiology* 40:577, 1986.

4. Traditional Enteropathogenic *Escherichia coli* of Infantile Diarrhea. *Reviews of Infectious Diseases* 9:28, 1987.

5. *Yersina enterocolitica:* A Primary Model for Bacterial Invasiveness. *Reviews of Infectious Diseases* 9:64, 1987.

6. Travelers' Diarrhea. *Review of Infectious Diseases* 8:5109, 1986.

chapter 25

NONFERMENTATIVE GRAM-NEGATIVE BACILLI

A significant number of genera of bacteria are of relatively low virulence and produce disease only as a consequence of host immunocompromise. Although these organisms produce primary infection in such hosts, their natural habitat is almost always the environment and in that sense, they are true opportunists. These organisms are all non-spore-forming, Gram-negative bacilli, motile or nonmotile. The most characteristically distinguishing feature of the group is that they are not fermentative. And while they utilize carbohydrates, they do so oxidatively without producing the acid or alcohol end products of fermentation.

A common feature of this group of genera is that they produce similar infections, and they are not known for a particular type of disease. It is also characteristic of these bacteria that they are commonly responsible for *nosocomial* (hospital-acquired) infections. About 15% of all clinical bacterial isolates are from these genera. Therefore, they are most likely to be found in cases of urinary tract infections (as a consequence of catheterization) or burn infections (as a consequence of a reduction in the immune status of the patient), and bacteremia or pneumonia (in patients with reduced phagocyte function). Microbiologists frequently refer to these bacteria as ''water bugs'' because they can often be found in any amount of standing moisture, and they pose a particular patient care problem due to this association. Therapy is often difficult because of high levels of antibiotic resistance.

Of the many genera (Table 25-1) of bacteria that fit the above description, only those most frequently involved in clinical disease will be presented in this chapter.

OUTLINE

PSEUDOMONAS
ACINETOBACTER
ALCALIGENES
MORAXELLA
EIKINELLA
CONCEPT SUMMARY
STUDY SUMMARY
REFERENCES FOR FURTHER STUDY

Table 25-1   Nonfermentative Gram-Negative Bacilli of Clinical Significance

Achromobacter	Alcaligenes	Moraxella
Acinetobacter	Eikinella	Pseudomonas
Agrobacterium	Flavobacterium	

PSEUDOMONAS

There are more than 300 species within the genus *Pseudomonas*, but of these only a few are commonly associated with human disease (Table 25-2). *P. pseudomallei* and *P. mallei* differ from others of this genus in that they are primary pathogens and are extremely virulent. *P. pseudomallei* is endemic in Southeast Asia, but infections outside of this area are uncommon. The three pseudomonads most frequently seen in human disease are *P. cepacia, P. maltophelia,* and *P. aeruginosa*. About two-thirds of all the clinically significant isolates of nonfermentative Gram-negative bacilli are *P. aeruginosa*.

P. aeruginosa is a motile bacillus that is usually about 2 μm long. It is an obligate aerobe and grows well on most culture media. More than 90% of *P. aeruginosa* isolates produce a blue-green water-soluble pigment (pyocyanin) that diffuses into the culture medium. The growing colonies give off a sweat odor variously described as grapelike or corn tortilla–like. It grows well at 42° C and is oxidase positive.

Table 25-2   *Pseudomonas* Species Associated with Human Disease

Species	Disease
P. areuginosa	Opportunistic
P. cepacia	Opportunistic
P. mallei	Glanders
P. pseudomallei	Melioidosis
P. maltophelia	Opportunistic
P. fluorescens	Opportunistic
P. stutzeri	Opportunistic
P. putrifaciens	Opportunistic
P. acidovorans	Opportunistic
P. paucimobilis	Opportunistic
P. diminuta	Opportunistic

Otitis due to *Pseudomonas aeruginosa* Serotype 0:10 Associated with a Mobile Redwood Hot Tub System: North Carolina, 1982

From March 19 to April 2, 1982, six cases of *Pseudomonas aeruginosa,* serotype 0:10, infection occurred following common exposure to a hot tub in Orange County, North Carolina. Clinical illness included severe hemorrhagic external otitis (inflammation of the external ear), which, although commonly associated with swimming pools, has not been previously reported in the literature for whirlpool/spa settings.

Among 24 members of a university coeducational fraternity who used the implicated tub from March 26 to 29, 2 had simple dermatitis, and 4 developed severe external otitis, 1 of whom, a 19-year-old male, had concurrent cellulitis of the chest wall and thigh. He was hospitalized and treated with intravenous tobramycin for 4 days. His infection began as an area of erythema approximately 1½ inches in diameter below the left nipple, accompanied by tender, swollen left axillary lymph nodes and a pustule below the right nipple. The patient also noted severe pain and drainage from his left ear. Cultures from the chest pustule and the draining left ear were positive for *P. aeruginosa* serotype 0:10 (resistant to cephalothin, ampicillin, tetracycline, and trimethoprim-sulfamethoxazole and sensitive to gentamicin and carbenicillin). His symptoms began 48 hours after last exposure to the tub. The 3 persons with severe external otitis that began within 48 hours of last exposure to the tub had visited the student health service for treatment. In 2 of those, disease was bilateral and was associated with profound erythema or bloody discharge. The first had onset on March 27; the other, with onset on March 29, had a positive culture of ear drainage for *P. aeruginosa* of the same resistance pattern as the 19-year-old male. Neither responded to topical antibiotics, but both were treated successfully with intramuscular gentamicin.

A survey of fraternity members showed an association of illness with exposure to the tub, which was rented and used from March 26 to March 29. Of 15 students who responded to a questionnaire, 5 (described above) met the case definition of ear infection or skin rash developing within 7 days after exposure to this tub. Total duration of exposure to the tub over the 4-day period was significantly associated with illness. Patients had a mean duration of 10.2 hours exposure; nonpatients had a mean duration of 5.1 hours exposure.

Inspection and culturing of the tub on April 15, after a previous night's usage at another fraternity, showed a pH 7.6 and free bromine level of <0.5 parts per million (ppm). Of 12 environmental swabs of the tub, 4 were positive for *P. aeruginosa* serotype 0:10. No other serotypes were identified in the specimens. The positive sites included a recirculation port, two areas of the dual filter, and filter intake line.

Procedures involved in maintaining and using the tub were reviewed. Usage peaked during the four evenings, when 15 or more persons at a time were in the tub. Despite written instructions to check the free-bromine level every 4 hours, water sampling was performed only once before use each day. The tub was emptied and rinsed with water from a garden hose daily, and filters were sprayed with water on March 27 and 28. No hyperbromination or scrubbing of internal surfaces was performed (*MMWR* 31:541, 1982).

Infection of compromised patients
many bacteria which are unable to produce a primary infection have little difficulty in causing disease in host compromised patients.

Leukopenic
having a reduced number of circulating white blood cells (PMNs). When the number of white blood cells is less than 500/cc, there is serious concern for infection.

Several exotoxins produced by *P. aeruginosa* have been identified. These along with its endotoxic cell wall and occasionally a mucoid capsule probably account for the virulence associated with this organism. The organism is commonly found on plants, in areas where there is any collected water, and occasionally as transient flora in the human intestine. This organism is so ubiquitous in the environment that no open wound, burn, or **immunocompromised patient** is free from exposure.

As is characteristic for the Gram-negative nonfermenters, *P. aeruginosa* infection most often occurs in a hospital setting. Several clinical conditions are highly correlated with *Pseudomonas* infection including cystic fibrosis, burns, urinary catheterization, cancer chemotherapy, or any condition that renders the patient severely **leukopenic**. From any such infection the patient may develop *Pseudomonas* pneumonia or bacteremia. These conditions are serious and have mortality rates in the order of 60% to 70%. *P. aeruginosa* is a regular cause of eternal *otitis* (ear infection) sometimes referred to as "swimmer's ear." *Pseudomonas* infection of the eye is a serious condition often leading to perforation of the cornea and subsequent loss of the eye.

P. aeruginosa infections are often malignant and very resistant to therapy. The remarkable metabolic capabilities and diverse plasmids associated with these organisms have resulted in the development of a high level of resistance to a broad range of antimicrobials. A number of new antibiotics have been specifically designed for treatment of *Pseudomonas* infections. As yet, the ideal antipseudomonal compound has not been discovered.

Control and prevention rely on proper aseptic techniques when dealing with burns and open wounds. *Pseudomonas* species are able to grow in water with minimal nutrients and are found in such places as water baths used for heating baby bottles, vases for fresh-cut flowers, and water sumps in humidifiers. Certain precautions, such as not allowing fresh-cut flowers in critical areas of a hospital and routine monitoring of water held in baths and air systems, help reduce the hazard of these infections. *Pseudomonas* species are among the most resistant vegetative bacterial cells to chemical disinfectants.

ACINETOBACTER

Acinetobacter is an interesting genus with but one species. *A. calcoaceticus*, that has two variants or subspecies, *anitratus* and *lwoffi*. These organisms, while fitting the description for Gram-negative nonfermenting bacilli, are not closely related to the pseudomonads, but are part of the family Neisseriaceae, which also includes the *Neisseria* species presented in Chapter 18 (Figure 25-1).

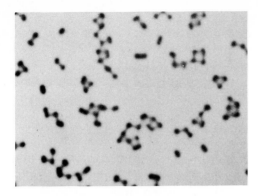

Figure 25-1
Photomicrograph of
Acinetobacter. Note the
paired coccobacillary
structure of the cells.
(Courtesy J. M. Matsen,
University of Utah)

Acinetobacter is an oxidase-negative, nonmotile, non-spore-forming coccobacillus (1.0 × 0.7 μm) that is normally found in soil, water, and on moist skin areas (axilla, groin, etc.) of humans. Although it is capable of producing primary infection, most of the infections are nosocomial, and infection of any kind is somewhat unusual, accounting for only about 1% of nosocomial infections.

Infections by *A. calcoaceticus* var. *anitratus* are far more common than those due to *A. calcoaceticus* var. *lwoffi*. Most infections are of the lower respiratory tract, but urinary tract infections, and bacteremia following intravenous catheterization also occur. Most unusually, there is a marked seasonal occurrence associated with infections due to these organisms (Figure 25-2). Control of these infections depends largely upon good patient care procedures.

Figure 25-2   Seasonal variation in the occurrence of *Acinetobacter* infections. (Courtesy Centers for Disease Control, Atlanta)

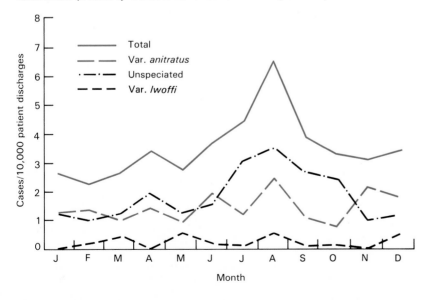

ALCALIGENES

Alcaligenes are similar in morphology and biochemical characteristics to bacteria of the other genera listed in Table 25-1. They are, however, unable to break down any of the sugars commonly used for bacterial identification. They are obligately aerobic and motile. The natural habitat of the most commonly isolated species, *A. faecalis*, is similar to that of pseudomonads. Not frequently isolated, *A. faecalis* is occasionally found in wounds, ear infection, blood, and urine of infected patients. Patients suffering from these infections are somewhat more easily treated than those infected with the organisms previously discussed in this chapter.

MORAXELLA

Moraxella species are Gram-negative coccobacilli that are nonmotile and oxidase-popsitive. As with the other genera in this chapter, they are unable to ferment glucose. These organisms grow well on supplemented laboratory medium.

There has been, and continue to be, some disagreement regarding the proper classification of these species (Table 25-3). The clinical status of this group is also under question, although these bacteria have been isolated from a variety of clinical conditions such as conjunctivitis, septic arthritis, bacteremia, and urethritis. Reports of such isolations have not always correlated with patient status, and there are many who feel that these organisms are commensals, or at best, low-grade opportunists. They complicate the laboratory responsibility because they are difficult to classify. They are somewhat unusual among this group of nonfermenters because they are susceptible to penicillin.

Table 25-3   Characteristics of *Moraxella* Species

Species	Biochemical Reactions					
	Litmus Milk	Urease	Citrate	Nitrate	Growth on MacConkey	Catalase
M. osloensis	−	−	+	+/−	+/−	−
M. lacunata	+	−	−	+	−	+
M. phenylpyruvica	−	+	−	+/−	+/−	+
M. urethralis	+	−	+	−	+	+
M. nonliquificiens	−	−	−	+	−	−

EIKINELLA

The genus *Eikinella* has only a single species, *E. corrodens*. This organism is of interest here because it fits the description of the organisms under discussion, and also because of the rather unusual infections with which it is associated. *E. corrodens* is somewhat difficult to grow in the laboratory, and does best on blood supplemented medium in a 10% CO_2 atmosphere. It is part of the normal flora of the mucous membranes of the human respiratory tract. Most infections are wounds that have become contaminated with human saliva. They are the most likely cause of human bite wound infections, and a wound appropriately described as a "clenched fist" injury. The latter is often the result of a hasty decision to enter the pugilistic arena and may be serious, with extensive cellulitis, osteomyelitis, or even bacteremia resulting in some instances. The organism is very susceptible to penicillin, which is used as the treatment of choice.

CONCEPT SUMMARY

1. The nonfermentative Gram-negative bacilli are environmental organisms of low virulence that are not uncommonly found in agents of human disease in compromised hosts. Antibiotic therapy cannot be empirically applied to disease caused by this group of bacteria and is often difficult because of resistance among these bacteria.

2. These organisms are frequently nonreactive with a variety of sugars and other metabolic substrates. This nonreactivity often makes identification and phenotypic classification of these bacteria very difficult.

STUDY SUMMARY

1. Describe the most common types of infections due to the nonfermentative bacteria.

2. What host-parasite relationship is demonstrated by infection and pathogenesis by the nonfermentative bacteria?

3. What feature of *Acinetobacter* species may lead to their being confused with *Neisseria* species.

4. Which of the genera presented in this chapter are aerobic?

REFERENCES FOR FURTHER STUDY

1. Genome Organization in *Pseudomonas. Annual Review of Microbiology* 40:79, 1986.

2. Infections with *Eikinella corrodens* in a General Hospital. *Reviews of Infectious Diseases* 8:50, 1986.

3. *Medical Microbiology,* J. Sherris, 1984. Elsevier.

chapter 26

VIBRIO AND CAMPYLOBACTER

*V*ibrio and *Campylobacter,* at one time considered to be but one genus, are closely related in morphology and biochemistry. Both genera are comprised of slightly curved Gram-negative bacilli, and there are many similarities in the diseases they produce. *Vibrio* species are **free-living** and have marine water as their most common natural habitat, while *Campylobacter* species are natural animal parasites.

VIBRIO INFECTIONS

The genus *Vibrio* belongs to the family Vibrionaceae, which includes Gram-negative, motile, oxidase-positive, facultative anaerobes that use glucose as a source of energy. Of the more than 20 species of *Vibrio,* 11 have been responsible for human infection. These infections have generally produced one of two types of disease: localized infection, such as the gastroenteritis of classical cholera, and a severe disseminated bacteremic disease only recently recognized.

Cholera

Bacterium *Vibrio cholerae,* the causative agent of human cholera, is similar to the enteric bacilli in many respects. This bacterium can be grown on simple media and differentiated from the enteric bacilli by using selective and differential media. The bacilli are slightly curved on initial isolation, giving comma-shaped cells (Figure 26-1; the first name given to this bacterium was *Kommabacillus*). Based on the outer lipopolysaccharides, *V. cholerae* can be divided into more than 100 serotypes. Of these, sero group O1 is responsible for classical cholera, although some organisms from the non-O1 groups are also capable of producing a choleralike illness. *V. cholerae* has also been subclassified into various biotypes.

Free-living
organisms which are capable of living outside of the parasite relationship.

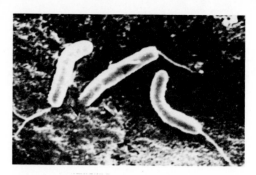

Figure 26-1 Electron micrograph of *Vibrio cholerae* on intestinal epithelial cells. Note the polar flagellum and the curved bacilli. (Courtesy J. S. Teppema et al., *Inf. Imm. 55:*2093)

The biotypes *classical* and *El Tor* (hemolytic) are responsible for the more serious epidemics of cholera.

Pathogenesis and clinical disease *V. cholerae* produces a powerful heat-labile enterotoxin. This toxin, composed of two proteins (A and B), is bound to intestinal cell receptors by part B. Part A then enters the cell and activates an enzyme known as *adenyl cyclase.* This enzyme acts as an internal messenger within the cell and the cell responds by secreting large volumes of water and dissolved salts, or **electrolytes,** into the lumen of the intestine. As much as 20 liters per day of fluid is withdrawn from the body with resultant acidosis, shock, and often death.

The disease of human cholera, often referred to as *Asiatic cholera,* can be devastating, especially in crowded populations with poor sanitary and medical facilities. The term *cholera* itself refers to any condition characterized by violent diarrhea. The bacterium is transmitted via contaminated food or water. The organisms attach to and proliferate in the small intestines but do not invade the tissues. The incubation time averages 2 to 3 days and the onset is abrupt. The initial signs are vomiting and diarrhea. The solids in the intestinal tract are purged early in the disease and the subsequently voided fluid is watery, without odor, and contains such electrolytes as sodium chloride, potassium, and bicarbonate. The patient develops sunken eyes and cheeks and the skin becomes wrinkled. Death results from rapid dehydration and resulting electrolyte imbalance.

No direct tissue damage occurs. *V. cholerae* may remain in the intestinal tract for a period after recovery and the patient may act as a carrier and continue to shed the bacteria up to a year. Persons over 50 years of age may become chronic carriers and intermittently shed the organism for many years. The pathogenesis of cholera is outlined in Figure 26-2. Without treatment, death rates

Electrolytes
sodium, potassium, chloride, and bicarbonate ions present in the bloodsteam. These ions are normally carefully regulated within the body. An electrolyte imbalance can rapidly produce severe morbidity or even mortality.

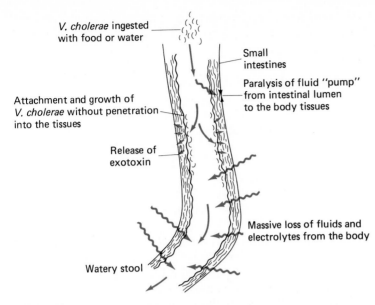

V. cholerae ingested with food or water

Small intestines

Paralysis of fluid "pump" from intestinal lumen to the body tissues

Attachment and growth of V. cholerae without penetration into the tissues

Release of exotoxin

Massive loss of fluids and electrolytes from the body

Watery stool

Figure 26-2   The pathogenesis of cholera showing the toxin-mediated effects of the *V. cholerae* on the intestinal mucosa.

are known to exceed 60%. With treatment, death rates may be reduced to less than 1%.

Transmission and epidemiology   In epidemic cholera, transmission follows the typical fecal-oral routes with carriers and clinical cases serving as sources of infection.

Cholera is endemic in regions of India and Bangladesh and periodic epidemics erupt throughout Asia and Africa. Occasional outbreaks occur in other parts of the world. Because of today's rapid international travel, cholera could break out in any part of the world.

During the mid-1800s major outbreaks of cholera occurred along the Mississippi and Missouri river valleys. No cases were reported between 1911 and 1973. In 1973 a single case occurred in Texas. Then in 1977 a case developed in Alabama, and 11 cases were reported in Louisiana in 1978. Subsequently cases have continued to occur along the Gulf coast (see clinical note). Their sources were shown to be due to improperly cooked shellfish. The source of infection of these shellfish is not known, but evidence now indicates that *V. cholerae* is widespread along the Gulf Coast and provides the source of a number of sporadic cases of cholera each year in the United States.

Diagnosis   Cholera is generally diagnosed by clinical observation, although isolation of *V. cholerae* from the patient is needed to confirm diagnosis. A serologic test of acute and convalescent serum may be helpful in confirming the diagnosis. Direct fluorescent antibody tests on stools from patients have been successfully used in making a rapid diagnosis.

Treatment   Effective treatment of cholera, if initiated soon enough, is amazingly simple. Inasmuch as death results from loss of fluids and not tissue damage, the patient can be maintained by replacing the lost fluids and electrolytes. For severe cases, intravenous **isotonic electrolyte** solutions are given until the patient recovers, often within hours. The fluid balance can then be maintained by oral administration of electrolyte solutions containing glucose. Fluid therapy is continued until antibodies are produced to neutralize the enterotoxin. Oral therapy alone can be highly effective, especially if the initial fluid loss is not excessive. Such a procedure is appropriate for clinics in rural areas that are staffed with paramedical personnel. Under proper treatment death rates may be reduced to less than 1%. Such oral rehydration therapy (ORT) has been used in treatment of enterotoxic diarrheas throughout the developing world. The results of its use have been remarkable, and literally tens of thousands of lives are saved each year by its use. Some medical observers have suggested that use of this simple ORT solution may represent the greatest single medical advance in history. Tetracyclines are effective and help eliminate the organism from the intestinal tract but are not used routinely in endemic areas.

Prevention and control   Proper sewage treatment and water purification systems are the most important preventative measures. Countries with adequate systems have few, if any, outbreaks of cholera. Rapid detection, isolation, and treatment of patients and carriers are also important.

Persons traveling in countries where cholera exists should avoid consuming uncooked fruits or vegetables, raw seafood, and nonsterilized beverages. Considering the outbreaks along the Gulf Coast in the United States, care should be taken to properly cook shellfish taken from these waters.

A killed vaccine has been used for many years and numerous countries require an international certificate of vaccination against cholera from travelers arriving from cholera-infected areas. The killed vaccine is not highly effective and work is currently underway to develop more effective vaccines.

Other Vibrio Infections

Recent recognition that the non-O1 vibrios (Table 26-1) are responsible for a variety of clinical illness has prompted considerable interest in this group of bacteria. These organisms are all from ma-

Isotonic electrolytes
concentrations of common metabolic ions (Na$^+$, K$^+$, CL$^-$) in the same concentration as found inside the cell.

Table 26-1 *Vibrio* Species Pathogenic for Humans

Species	Growth in NaCl			Fermentation of		Human Disease
	0%	3%	8%	Sucrose	Salacin	
V. cholerae	+	+	−	+	−	Cholera
V. parahemolyticus	−	+	+	−	−	Gastroenteritis
V. valnificus	−	+	−	−	+	Bacteremia, cellulitis
V. fluvialis	−	+	+/−	+	+	Gastroenteritis
V. mimicus	+	+	−	+	−	Gastroenteritis
V. alginolyticus	−	+	+	+	−	Cellulitis
V. damsela	−	+	−	−	−	Cellulitis

rine habitats and some are true **halophiles,** requiring increased sodium chloride concentrations for growth.

The most common illness produced by the non-O1 serotypes of *V. cholerae* is gastroenteritis. Cases range from mild to severe, and are nearly always associated with the ingestion of seafood. A recent study showed that more than 80% of such victims had recently consumed oysters or crabs and that only 10% of these patients could not associate their illness with seafood. Most of the patients (96%) had diarrhea, 82% had cramping, and 70% suffered headaches; more than 50% were hospitalized. The illness appears to result from the production of an enterotoxin similar to cholera toxin and the heat-labile (LT) toxin of *E. coli.*

Vibrio species other than *V. cholerae* are also implicated in human disease. *V. parahemolyticus* infection is acquired by eating improperly cooked or stored seafood. The illness is accompanied by a watery diarrhea that lasts for a number of days. It is now recognized that about half the cases of diarrhea during the summer in Japan are caused by *V. parahemolyticus.*

V. vulnificus is a halophilic vibrio found in warm sea waters. It has long been known that persons with liver disease occasionally became infected with this organism. It is now recognized that persons who have open wounds, or who injure themselves in a marine setting, run the risk of developing severe *V. vulnificus* cellulitis, which may lead to bacteremia (infection of the blood). The usual source of bacteremia due to this organism is from ingestion of contaminated seafood such as raw oysters. In approximately 50% of patients with bacteremia due to this organism, the disease is fatal.

Other species of *Vibrio* listed in Table 26-1 are occasionally involved in human diseases. As more and more attention is given to this group of bacteria, it becomes apparent that they are increasingly involved in human infections.

Halophile
a microorganism which prefers high concentrations of salt in its growth medium.

Follow-up on *Vibrio cholerae* Infection: Louisiana, 1978

According to the record, 4 more cases of cholera and 2 asymptomatic infections were identified in Louisiana, bringing the total number of persons known to be infected in August and September 1978 to 11. The 6 most recent infections were discovered after a 58-year-old woman from Lafayette had onset of a diarrheal illness on September 24, was hospitalized, and had *Vibrio cholerae* isolated from her stool. On September 22 she ate crabs that were caught in White Lake, boiled, and then held without refrigeration for approximately 6 hours. Investigation found that 5 of 9 other persons who ate the crabs at the same time also developed diarrheal illnesses; *V. cholerae* organisms were isolated from the stools of 3 of these ill persons. Some of the boiled crabs left over after the meal had been refrigerated and *V. cholerae* organisms were isolated from one of them. Other crabs, caught in White Lake at the same time by the same man, were bioled separately on September 22 and eaten at once by 6 persons; none became ill, but *V. cholerae* organisms were isolated from the stools of 2 of the 6 persons. All previously reported isolates of *V. cholerae* from Louisiana in August and September were also of the same serotype.

The eight infected persons with symptoms had eaten boiled or steamed crab within 5 days before onset of illness. A case-control study of foods eaten by the first five symptomatic patients and ten age- and sex-matched neighbor controls found that none of the controls had eaten crabs during comparable periods. The three asymptomatic infected persons had eaten crabs within 9 days before culture. As noted, *V. cholerae* was isolated from a boiled crab. The organism was also isolated from raw shrimp caught south of Pecan Island. These epidemiologic and laboratory data indicate that crabs collected in Louisiana in the area between Mud Lake, west of Cameron, and Vermilion Bay, south of Abbeville, have been the vehicles of infection for the cases of cholera. Crabs prepared in large lots by commercial establishments have not been implicated.

Preliminary results of studies on the effect that boiling has on crabs artificially infected with *V. cholerae* from one of the Louisiana cases showed that the organism can be isolated from iced crabs individually boiled after 2, 4, 6, and 8 minutes of boiling but not after 10 minutes. At 8 minutes the crab shell was red and the meat was firm; so these criteria are not adequate to determine when crabs are safe to eat. In practice, crabs are cooked in varying numbers and via a variety of methods and containers. The crabs eaten by the persons with cholera were reportedly steamed for up to 35 minutes or boiled for 10 to 20 minutes (*MMWR* 27:388, 1978).

CAMPYLOBACTER INFECTIONS

Bacteria

Bacterial species now belonging to the genus *Campylobacter* were classified as vibrios for many years. The term *campylobacter* means "curved rod" in Greek and describes the shape of these bacteria.

They are Gram-negative, motile, **microaerophilic** microorganisms and are best isolated on a selective agar medium in an atmosphere of reduced oxygen concentration and 10% CO_2. Microscopically, they are often seen in pairs or short chains giving them a typical "gull wing" appearance (Figure 26-3). Although they grow well on most laboratory media, they grow slowly, and are easily missed if other bacteria are present. Laboratories often use highly selective media incubated at 42° C in order to isolate *Campylobacter* from clinical material.

Pathogenesis and Clinical Diseases

Long recognized as part of the intestinal microbial flora of many mammals and birds, campylobacter have been incriminated as a cause of abortions in domestic animals. Today it is recognized that these bacteria cause enteritis and are occasionally disseminated in humans. The most common human infection due to campylobacter is acute gastroenteritis. Of the species shown in Table 26-2, *C. jejuni* is most often the etiologic agent involved. This organism is usually acquired from food, milk, or contact with infected animals. The disease is accompanied by fever, bloody diarrhea, headache and abdominal pain. It is usually self-limited, lasting 6–10 days, although chronic cases are known. Systemic infection, usually due to *C. fetus* subspecies *fetus* is known to occur, particularly among immunocompromised persons.

Two recent observations have extended our appreciation of the pathogenesis of this group of bacteria. Evidence is increasing that *C. fetus* subsp. *fetus* infection may induce spontaneous abor-

Microaerophile
a microorganism which prefers a limited supply of oxygen in its growth environment.

Figure 26-3 *Campylobacter jejuni* on the intestinal epithelium of a colonized mouse. Scanning electron micrograph; bar represents two micrometers. (Courtesy A. Lee et al., *Inf. Imm. 51:*536)

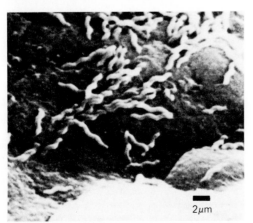

2µm

Outbreak of *Campylobacter* Enteritis Associated with Raw Milk: Kansas, 1981

During the week of March 23, 1981, the Wichita–Sedgwick County Department of Community Health was notified that a patient admitted to a local hospital with gastrointestinal illness had *Campylobacter jejuni* isolated from his stool. The hospital's clinical laboratory, which routinely reports isolations from communicable agents, noted that the patient regularly drank raw milk from a commercial dairy. *C. jejuni* was isolated from rectal swabs from two of three other members of the patient's family, all of whom also drank raw milk from the same dairy. The dairy voluntarily stopped selling raw milk on April 1 and cooperated in an investigation of the problem.

News coverage of the preliminary investigation prompted telephone calls from persons in 104 families (representing 264 individuals), who reported that members of their families had recently had a gastrointestinal illness and that the families purchased raw milk from the same dairy. *C. jejuni* was isolated from the stools of 60 of 116 (52%) persons in households that had one or more ill family members.

A cohort study was conducted of families who belonged to a local food cooperative that purchased raw milk from the dairy in question the week of April 6. Then 17 of 24 member families completed a questionnaire about exposure to pets, live poultry or cattle, and persons outside the household who had diarrhea. Questions also concerned recent travel and food-intake patterns, including consumption of chicken, rare meat, uncooked eggs, cheese, raw milk, and water.

No significant association was found between illness and any risk factor except raw milk. Gastrointestinal illness had affected members in all 11 families that purchased raw milk from the dairy but did not affect 6 families that did not purchase the milk. Of those who drank raw milk, 39 out of 55 (71%) were ill, as were 4 of 36 (11%) persons who did not drink raw milk ($p < .01$, t test). These 43 persons all became ill in the period of March 1–April 4. Predominant symptoms included diarrhea, abdominal cramps, and headache. Duration of illness ranged from 1 to 9 days; few people sought medical advice. *C. jejuni* was isolated from 17 of 29 (59%) ill and 4 of 8 (50%) well persons; all 21 isolates were from persons who drank raw milk.

Rectal swabs collected on April 8 from well cows and those with mastitis at the implicated dairy and from well cows (none with mastitis was seen) from two other local dairies that also sell raw milk were positive for *C. jejuni*. Cultures of milk samples obtained at all three dairies were negative for *C. jejuni*. In the period March 31 to April 7 bulk-tank milk samples from the implicated dairy, but not samples from the other two dairies, exceeded the generally recommended standard plate count level of 100,000 organisms/ml. The count fell below this level on April 8 and 9.

The dairy implemented hygienic measures during the investigation, such as not using milk from cows suspected of having mastitis, using a disinfectant solution to wash teats, and immersing milking claws in a disinfectant solution before putting them on each cow. The dairy began selling milk again on April 10. No new cases of raw milk–associated gastrointestinal illness had been reported as of May 6 (*MMWR* 30:565, 1981).

Premature Labor and Neonatal Sepsis Caused by *Campylobacter fetus,* subsp. *fetus:* Ontario, 1984

A 900-g male infant was delivered vaginally in a Toronto, Ontario, Canada, hospital, 5 hours after the spontaneous onset of labor at 26 weeks gestation. Apgar scores were 1 and 5 at 1 and 5 minutes, respectively. The infant was intubated, given penicillin G (25,000 U), and transferred to the neonatal intensive care unit. On arrival, his temperature was 34.8° C (95° F) rectally; systolic blood pressure, 78; heart rate, 164 beats per minute; and respiratory rate, 48 per minute. The infant was lethargic, with moderate respiratory distress. A chest radiograph showed a normal cardiac silhouette, with a bilateral reticular pattern and air bronchograms in both lung fields. The infant was felt to be premature, with neonatal respiratory distress syndrome and sepsis. Ampicillin (100 mg/kg/day) and gentamicin (5 mg/kg/day) were given. A Gram stain of a gastric aspirate revealed numerous curved Gram-negative bacilli with an appearance typical of *Campylobacter;* erythromycin (40 mg/kg/day) was also started. *C. fetus,* subsp. *fetus,* was isolated from this aspirate, as well as from blood and stool. Cerebrospinal fluid (CSF) obtained after antibiotics were started was clear, had six red blood cells, 106 white blood cells (55% polymorphonuclear cells), and a glucose of 2.6 mmol/L. No organisms were seen on Gram stain.

The infant steadily improved over the next few days and was extubated after 6 days. He received ampicillin and gentamicin for 3 weeks; erythromycin was discontinued after 1 week.

The infant's mother was a 28-year-old office worker. Her first pregnancy 4 years earlier had been uneventful, and she had carried her infant to term. She had felt well during the current pregnancy until 2 weeks before her premature delivery, when she had fever and chills for 1 day and watery diarrhea for 3 days. No other family members had been ill, and there was no history of contact with family pets or other animals. She had not consumed unpasteurized milk or milk products.

C. fetus, subsp. *fetus,* was isolated from the mother's vagina and stool 2 days postpartum. The organism was identified by its unique morphology and motility when viewed by phase-contrast microscopy and its bioehcmical characteristics. Disk diffusion antibiotic susceptibility testing showed that all isolates from both mother and infant were susceptible to ampicillin (10 μg), erythromycin (15 μg), gentamicin (10 μg), and chloramphenicol (30 μg) but resistant to tetracycline (5 μm). CSF culture was negative (*MMWR* 33:483, 1984).

Table 26-2 *Campylobacter* Species and Associated Human Diseases

Species	Growth at 42°C	Clinical Significance in Humans
C. fetus	−	Systemic infection/bacteremia
C. jejuni	+	Acute gastroenteritis
C. coli	+	Proctitis/gastroenteritis
C. hyointestinalis	−	None
C. laridis	+	Rare in humans
C. pylori	+	Gastritis
C. sputorum	−	None

tion in humans. This organism has long been known to cause fetal loss in lower animals but has recently been associated with similar pathology in pregnant humans. Recent isolation of *Campylobacter pylori* from the stomachs of individuals with stomach ulcers or gastritis has raised questions as to the nature of the relationship. Some researchers feel strongly that this organism may be one of the causes of these diseases.

Epidemiology

Although the *Campylobacter* group of bacteria is less commonly known by the general public than are *Salmonella* and *Shigella,* it appears to be responsible for as many cases of infectious enteritis as the other two groups combined. Intestinal infection occurs in patients of all ages; it is common in young children and may account for up to 30% of all acute diarrhea in children under 8 months of age living in underdeveloped countries. The presence of the organism in the normal gut flora of domestic animals (particularly poultry) widely disseminates these organisms in our environment. Most reported cases (60%) are associated with consumption of contaminated milk, and sporadic cases occur in individuals who are infected from their house pets.

Diagnosis

Diagnosis of *Campylobacter* infections is made by observing the bacteria among blood cells in fecal specimens, or by culture of the organism. Systemic cases are nearly always diagnosed by culture.

Treatment and Control

Even though most cases of *Campylobacter* infection are self-limiting, therapy is usually recommended to reduce the length and severity of the disease. A number of antibiotics, including the quinolones are effective agents when given properly. Control is best achieved by good hygiene, with special emphasis on avoiding transmission of microorganisms from animals to food and water consumed by humans.

CONCEPT SUMMARY

1. The genus *Vibrio* is represented by several highly virulent species that cause a variety of human diseases. Most of the organisms in the genus are halophilic, curved, Gram-negative, motile bacilli.

2. Asiatic cholera is a disease known for its great human plagues. This fecally transmitted disease can cause death in its victims within hours of infection. Infections have resulted from eating improperly cooked shellfish or drinking contaminated water.

3. *Campylobacter* produces a painful, sometimes serious gastrointestinal disease. Usually transmitted from domestic animals, the disease is generally self-limiting.

STUDY SUMMARY

1. Describe the mechanism of action of cholera toxin.

2. Why is cultural diagnosis of cholera a questionable approach in highly endemic areas?

3. List four reasons why oral rehydration therapy is such a valuable therapeutic procedure.

4. What is the difference between O1 and non-O1 vibrios?

5. Compared to the more classic *Shigella* and *Salmonella* gastroenteritis, how common is *Campylobacter* gastroenteritis?

REFERENCES FOR FURTHER STUDY

1. Epitopes in the Cholera Family of Enterotoxins. *Reviews of Infectious Disease* 9:544, 1987.

2. *Medical Microbiology*, J. Sherris, 1984. Elsevier.

3. Food Poisoning due to *Vibrio parahemolyticus*. *Annual Review of Medicine* 25:75, 1974.

4. Diseases of Humans (Other than Cholera) Caused by Vibrios. *Annual Review of Microbiology* 34:341, 1980.

5. Campylobacter Enteritis in the United States. *Annals of Internal Medicine* 98:360, 1983.

chapter 27

MYCOPLASMA AND LEGIONELLA

There are few similarities between *Mycoplasma* and *Legionella*. They both cause human pneumonia and are commonly treated with the same antibiotic, but they are vastly different in their epidemiologic, morphologic, and clinical properties. *Mycoplasma* infection is common in young adults. This primary pneumonia, while serious, is rarely life-threatening, and the organism is a true parasite which must be transmitted from person to person. *Legionella* is a much more rare cause of pneumonia, occurs most often in compromised elderly patients, is frequently life-threatening, and is not communicated among patients.

Scientists seeking to resolve the role of these two organisms in disease have been puzzled by both. For many years *Mycoplasma* were thought to be viruses, while the etiologic role of *Legionella* defied characterization because it could not be grown on the usual bacteriologic media nor stained with the usual analine dyes. In some ways, both organisms were an enigma to researchers seeking to determine their roles in human health. They have been included in a common chapter primarily for convenience, but provide the student with an interesting study in contrasting biological properties.

MYCOPLASMA INFECTIONS

The mycoplasmas are a group of free-living and parasitic microorganisms that are unique in that they possess no cell wall. They are widespread and are found as natural flora in the mouth, throat, and genitourinary tract of mammals and birds. There are three genera of mycoplasmas: *Acholeplasma*, which includes the free-living forms, and *Ureaplasma* and *Mycoplasma*, which contain only parasitic agents.

Bacteria

Mycoplasma cells, except for the lack of a cell wall, have the same intracellular components and metabolic activities as other bacteria. The cell membrane differs from that of other bacteria and their shapes are variable due to the flexibility of this membrane (Figure 27-1). Smallest cell sizes are about 300 nm in diameter for the spherical-shaped cells. Other forms may be filament- or branch-shaped. Multiplication is by binary fission, which sometimes takes the form of fragmentation into groups of **daughter cells**. Mycoplasmas can be grown in enriched agar media and produce small colonies about 0.5 mm in diameter that have the appearance of a fried egg (Figure 27-2).

Daughter cell
a cell which is produced by binary fission or budding directly from another cell.

Pathogenesis and Clinical Disease

Various diseases caused by the mycoplasmas have been diagnosed in mammals and birds. The first mycoplasma to be discovered was isolated from cattle suffering from a disease called *pleuro-*

Figure 27-1   Scanning electron micrograph of a small colony of *Mycoplasma pneumoniae* showing a filamentous shape around the periphery and pleomorphic shapes in the center. Bulbous swellings (arrows) are seen in some individual cells. (K. E. Muse, D. A. Powell, and A. M. Collier, *Inf. Imm. 13*:229–237, Figure 1b, with permission from ASM)

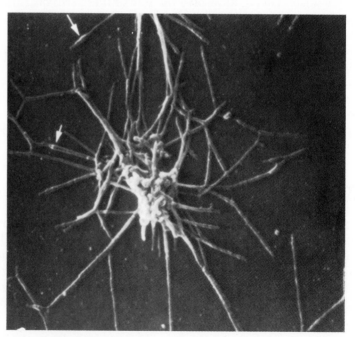

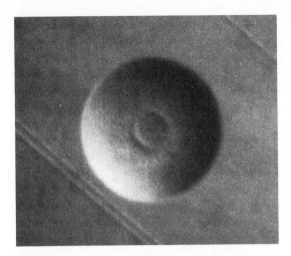

Figure 27-2 Figure of *Mycoplasma hominis* colony showing the "fried egg" colony appearance. This unusual colony form is produced by the colony growing down into the medium as well as across the surface of the agar.

pneumonia; consequently, other mycoplasmas have often been referred to as pleuropneumonialike organisms or PPLOs. The best-known disease of humans caused by mycoplasmas is called *primary atypical pneumonia;* the causative microbe is *Mycoplasma pneumoniae.* This form of pneumonia is called *atypical* because it does not have the characteristics of the typical bacterial pneumonias but resembles pneumonias caused by viruses. The species *Ureaplasma urealyticum* appears to be the cause of a form of nonspecific (nongonococcal) urethritis that is transmitted by sexual contact. Mycoplasmas are also incriminated as the possible agents of such diseases of humans as lupus erythematous and rheumatoid arthritis, for which other specific microorganisms have not yet been shown to be responsible. Nevertheless, there is not yet enough evidence to prove that mycoplasmas cause these diseases.

Transmission and Epidemiology

Primary atypical pneumonia is widespread and may account for 20% of pneumonia in urban populations. It is chiefly responsible for pneumonia in persons between 5 and 30 years of age. Outbreaks are often associated with schools, families, summer camps, or military barracks. The organisms seem to be transmitted efficiently by aerosol from person to person during the acute stages of the disease, which lasts for 1 to 2 weeks.

Diagnosis

Pneumonia caused by mycoplasmas can be differentiated from viral or rickettsial pneumonias by clinical and laboratory tests. Both specific and nonspecific serologic tests can be used. The most common test is for **cold agglutinins**—substances that agglutinate red blood cells when held at about 4° C and occur in about 80% of the patients with mycoplasma pneumonia. *M. pneumoniae* can be cultured from the respiratory tract by using enriched media.

Cold agglutinins

proteins produced in response to some infectious diseases which are able to agglutinate red blood cells at low (refrigerator) temperatures.

Treatment

Antibiotics of the tetracycline and erythromycin groups are effective in reducing the severity and duration of mycoplasma pneumonia. Such antibiotics as penicillin that affect only bacterial cell walls are obviously of no value against microorganisms that have none.

Prevention and Control

The best prevention is to avoid contact with persons suspected of having the disease. Antibiotics can be taken prophylactically to prevent the spread of infection to members of a group or family where a known index case has been diagnosed. Research is being conducted to develop a vaccine, but as yet no effective vaccine is available.

LEGIONELLOSIS

The disease now called the *Legionnaires' disease* or legionellosis is a pneumonialike illness that went unrecognized as a specific disease until the late 1970s. Attention was dramatically focused on it in the summer of 1976 when some 5000 members of the American Legion attended a convention in Philadelphia. Within 2 weeks of the convention's close, many of these legionnaires complained of chills, fever, and muscle aches. Over the next week 12 of the legionnaires died of a pneumonialike illness. During the ensuing weeks, 170 of those attending the convention were hospitalized with pneumonia; 29 deaths occurred.

An extensive investigation was immediately launched to find the cause of this newly recognized disease. Tests were run with all known pathogenic microorganisms or toxins that might be responsible and all tests were negative. After several months of continued research a previously unidentified bacterium was found to be the culprit.

Bacterium

The causative bacterium grows in guinea pigs, in the yolk sac of embryonated eggs, and on special nutrient media containing extra amounts of the amino acid cysteine and iron. The bacterium seems to have the shape of a bacillus (Figure 27-3). It does not stain well with the Gram stain; therefore special stains, such as

Figure 27-3 Electron micrographs of *Legionella pneumophila.* (Courtesy Centers for Disease Control, Atlanta).

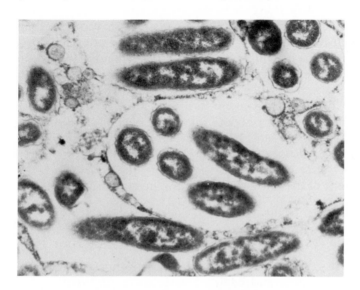

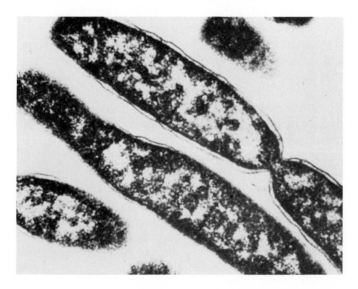

Table 27-1   *Legionella* Species Isolated from Human Disease

L. bozemanii	L. maceachernii
L. feeleii	L. micdadei
L. gormanii	L. pneumophila
L. hackeliae	L. wadsworthii
L. longbeachae	

Pleomorphic

having many morphological shapes. Pleomorphic bacilli often appear as long drawn-out cells or as short coccobacilli. These figures are often found in the same microscopic field.

Malaise

a general feeling of uneasiness or discomfort usually associated with the earliest indication of impending illness.

Subclinical

occurrence of infection with such mild symptoms that no diagnostic signs are evident. Antibody responses are usually as strong as with clinical infections.

the Gimenez silver-impregnation stain, are used to demonstrate the presence of these cells. When grown in yolk sacs, the cells have both coccoid and bacillary forms. The shape is **pleomorphic** when grown on culture media but is predominantly bacillary. These bacteria are quite stable and may remain viable for up to 1 year in water. Evidence indicates that they may be free-living in soil or streams and possibly in water held in air-conditioning systems. No close relationship has been found between this bacterium and any of the previously characterized bacteria. Thus a new family, Legionellaceae, has been established that contains but one genus *Legionella* and at present 22 species (Table 27-1). There are a variety of serogroups associated with some of the species, and only some of the known species have been associated with human disease.

Pathogenesis and Clinical Disease

The pathogenesis of Legionnaires' disease most closely resembles lobar pneumonia and begins 2 to 10 days after exposure. Some early symptoms are diarrhea, weakness, headache, muscle aches, **malaise**, anorexia, and a dry cough. An increasing temperature to 40° C (104° F) may be seen after several days, along with prostration and pulmonary consolidation. Some patients experience stupor and show signs of involvement of the kidneys and liver. The primary involvement, however, appears to be in the lungs. The duration of the disease is from 5 to 16 days. Most cases are seen in older or immunosuppressed persons, although all ages may be afflicted. Risk factors inlcude alcoholism, advanced age, smoking, and immunosuppressive therapy. Most sporadic cases occur in renal transplant or cancer patients.

Humoral immunity plays only a limited role in resistance to Legionnaires' disease. Some patients who have expired from this infection have been found to have high antibody titers. It appears that the development of cellular immunity is important in predicting a good outcome following infection. Unless treated, 20% of those patients requiring hospitalization die. Evidence now indicates that many mild or **subclinical** cases may occur.

Transmission and Epidemiology

Person-to-person transmission does not seem involved. When clusters of cases occur, it appears that exposure was from a common environmental source. The organisms are ubiquitous in fresh water and are readily isolated from streams, water found in air-conditioning systems, or in domestic water supplies. Airborne dissemination via dust or water sprayed in air-conditioning systems or from showers has been suggested.

Once the causative bacterium was isolated, thus providing a known antigen, it was possible to study serum samples that had been collected from patients who had suffered from unknown types of pneumonia before 1976. Many of these samples contained specific antibodies against *L. pneumophila*, indicating that this disease has been around for many years. Since the initial recognition of this disease in 1976, numerous outbreaks have been recognized in all parts of the United States and in many foreign countries. Many isolated cases occur as well as some clusters of infection. Several hundred severe cases are diagnosed each year in this country. An estimated 20,000 to 30,000 additional mild or subclinical cases are thought to also occur yearly. It is presently determined that between 3% and 6% of all hospital-associated pneumonias are due to *L. pneumophila*.

Diagnosis

A tentative diagnosis is based on symptoms when no other causative agent can be demonstrated. Cultivation of *L. pneumophila* from the lung tissues or blood is possible but is often difficult. Specific laboratory tests rely mostly on serologic procedures that show specific increases in, or high levels of, antibodies against the *L. pneumophila*. The presence of *L. pneumophila* in sputum or lung tissues can sometimes be demonstrated by direct microscopic examination, using special stains or specific fluorescent-labeled antibodies.

One of the benefits of the techniques of molecular biology has been evidenced in the development of a DNA probe for *Legionella*. Use of this probe has been approved by the Federal Food and Drug Administration. The radiolabeled DNA probe is mixed with disrupted bacterial cells and is designed to form a recombinant duplex, not with DNA (of which there may be but one copy per cell) but with a portion of bacterial RNA— which may be present as hundreds of copies in the cell. Thus, using a DNA probe for specific bacterial RNA greatly increases the sensitivity of the test procedure. It is estimated that the probe technique has about the same sensitivity as does culture, but it is much more rapid (test results are available on the day of testing) and it is 100% specific.

Isolates of Organisms Resembling Legionnaires' Disease Bacterium from Environmental Sources: Indiana, 1978

Organisms identical to *Legionella pneumophila* were isolated from two environmental specimens collected in the investigation of the outbreak of Legionnaires' disease in Bloomington, Indiana. The positive specimens included water from an air-conditioning cooling tower atop the Indiana Memorial Union, a hotel student union complex in which 19 of 21 confirmed cases had stayed overnight in the 2 weeks before onset of illness, and water from a creek approximately 50 m from the Union.

The water specimens were initially examined for *L. pneumophila* by direct fluorescent antibody (FA) methods and were positive. Aliquots were inoculated into guinea pigs. Guinea pigs were sacrificed when fever was noted, or if no fever was noted, 7 days after inoculation. Splenic tissue was negative by direct FA, but FA-positive organisms were recovered from yolk sacs of embryonated hens' eggs inoculated with suspensions of guinea pig splenic tissue. The organisms were isolated directly on charcoal yeast extract agar from the splenic tissue of a guinea pig inoculated with the creek water. The isolates from the cooling tower were strongly FA positive, but the creek water isolates gave weak FA staining. Organisms from both sources had colonies on special agar typical of pneumophila. Subcultures did not grow on trypticase soy agar or trypticase soy blood agar. Isolates from each water specimen showed a pattern of cellular fatty acids on gas-liquid chromatography typical of the *L. pneumophila*. Studies of the DNA relatedness of these isolates showed them to the same as *L. pneumophila*.

The cooling tower is located on the roof of the Union, adjacent to and higher than the wing with guest rooms. Studies are underway to determine whether water droplets released from the cooling tower in the process of evaporative cooling could be drawn into air intakes serving hotel rooms and meeting areas. Procedures were undertaken to decontaminate the cooling tower water (*MMWR* 27:191, 1978).

Treatment

Erythromycin has been the most effective antibiotic in treating this disease. Often recovery is prompt and dramatic following the use of this agent. Therapy usually lasts for about 2 weeks. Prompt treatment greatly decreases the death rate. Rifampin may also be effective.

Prevention and Control

No vaccines are available. Elimination of possible contamination of water used in some air-conditioning systems may reduce the number of cases. Avoiding exposure to high concentrations of dust from such activities as soil excavation could be helpful. Pro-

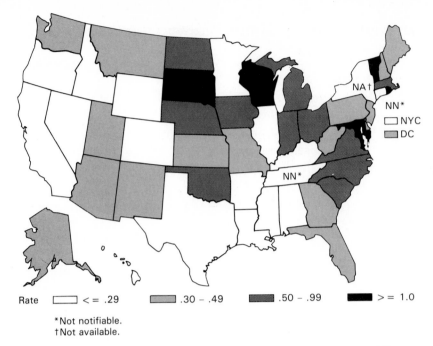

Rate　☐ < = .29　▨ .30 – .49　▨ .50 – .99　■ > = 1.0

*Not notifiable.
†Not available.

Figure 27-4　Occurrence of legionellosis in the United States in 1986.
(Courtesy Centers for Disease Control, Atlanta)

tecting compromised patients from excessive dust is recommended. As more is learned about the epidemiology of this disease, additional preventive measures can be developed (Figure 27-4).

CONCEPT SUMMARY

1. Mycoplasmas are unique bacteria without cell walls. They produce a number of diseases in animals but only one in humans. This primary pneumonia is common among children and young adults. Older individuals seem somewhat refractory, probably due to antibodies from earlier infection.

2. Legionnaires' disease is due to a bacillus normally present in water environments. Individuals with pulmonary compromise are usually the victims of this organism. Frequently nosocomial, the infection represents upward of 5% to 6% of all pneumonias in hospitalized individuals. Diagnosis is difficult because the organism is characteristically refractile to the analine stains used in early diagnosis.

STUDY SUMMARY

1. How important is *M. pneumoniae* as a cause of human pneumonia?
2. What feature of *Legionella* would make it very difficult to prevent exposure to these bacteria?
3. Why did Legionnaires disease "suddenly" appear as a cause of human disease in the 1970s?
4. What is the primary clinical symptom associated with Legionnaires' disease?
5. What risk is there to family members and friends of a patient with Legionnaires' disease?

REFERENCES FOR FURTHER STUDY

1. *The Biologic and Clinical Basis of Infectious Diseases,* 3rd ed., G. Youmans, 1986. Saunders.
2. *Manual of Clinical Microbiology,* 4th ed., E. Lennette, 1985. American Society for Microbiology.
3. *Diagnostic Microbiology,* S. Finegold, 1986. Mosby.
4. *International Perspectives on Neglected Sexually Transmitted Diseases,* K. Holms, 1983. McGraw-Hill.

chapter 28

CHLAMYDIA AND RICKETTSIA

T he two groups of bacteria presented in this chapter are not closely related, but they share a number of character-istics. Both contain **zoonotic** species, with animals act-ing as both reservoir and **vector** in some instances. Both of these groups of bacteria are obligate intracellular parasites and lack the metabolic ability to grow outside of host cells. Both are very small, have Gram-negative type cell walls, and contain both RNA and DNA. Disease due to *Rickettsia* is generally much more severe than that due to *Chlamydia,* although the latter is by far the most com-mon and contributes extensively to human misery and suffering.

CHLAMYDIA INFECTIONS

Bacteria

Chlamydiae are obligate intracellular parasites that depend com-pletely on the host cell for energy, for they have no ability to pro-duce their own ATP molecules. They go through a unique devel-opmental cycle inside intracytoplasmic vacuoles of the host cell (Figure 28-1). The basic structure, called an *elementary body,* is 0.2 to 0.4 μm in diameter. It is infectious, metabolically inert, and en-ters the host cell by phagocytosis. The replication occurs in the **phagosome,** which becomes enlarged and is called a *vacuole.* Be-fore replication can occur, the elementary body changes into a large structure, 0.7 to 1.0 μm in diameter, that is called an *initial body.* The initial body is not infectious, is metabolically active, sur-vives only intracellularly, and is the replicating form of chlamyd-iae. It divides by binary fission to fill the vacuole with new parti-cles. The initial bodies next change into the smaller, infectious elementary bodies that are not able to multiply. The growth of chlamydiae may cause the death and breaking up of the host cell that result in the release of the elementary bodies. The released elementary bodies enter new host cells and the cycle is repeated.

Zoonotic
pertaining to an infectious disease of lower animals that can be transmitted to humans.

Vector
a living animal, usually an insect, capable of transmitting an infectious agent from one host to another.

Phagosome
the phagocytic vesicle that contains the ingested bacterial particle.

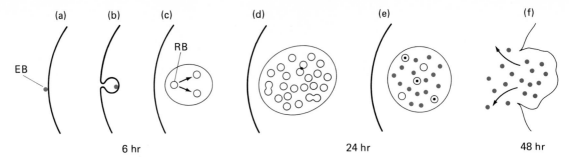

Figure 28-1 Stages in the replication of chlamydiae. (a) attachment of elementary body (EB) to cell membrane; (b) phagocytosis of EB; (c) EB changes into a reticulate body (RB) that divides by binary fission; (d) continued replication of RBs inside of vacuole; (e) RBs change into EBs, and (f) lysis of cell membrane and vacuole with release of EBs.

Two species of the genus *Chlamydia*—*C. trachomatis* and *C. psittaci*—cause diseases in humans.

Diseases Caused by *C. trachomatis*

Disease categories Three categories of diseases of humans caused by *C. trachomatis* are listed in Table 28-1 and include (1) trachoma, (2) a complex of diseases transmitted by direct (primarily sexual) and indirect routes, and (3) lymphogranuloma venereum. The ability of a single species to cause such varied clinical diseases probably stems from slightly different variations in virulence or host tissue affinity for different serotypes of this microbe. Specific serotypes of the chlamydiae are characteristically associated with the different disease manifestations. This diversity is also a function of the different routes of transmission and the degree of natural resistance of the persons being infected. In many cases, the chlamydiae are apparently able to persist in the cells of the host for prolonged periods without causing disease.

Table 28-1   Diseases for Which Chlamydiae Have Been Implicated as Etiologic Agents

Chlamydia	Normal Host	Disease in Humans
C. psittaci	Birds	Psittacosis, ornithosis
C. trachomatis serogroups A, B, C	Humans	Trachoma
Serogroups D–K	Humans	Nongonococcal urethritis (NGU), inclusion conjunctivitis, infant pneumonia
Serogroups L_1–L_3	Humans	Lymphogranuloma venereum

TRACHOMA Trachoma (Figure 28-2) is an infection of the eyelid (conjunctivitis) and, in some cases, of the cornea (keratitis). Cases of varying degrees of severity appear and range from asymptomatic infections to those showing extensive scarring of the cornea with resultant blinding. This disease is widespread in areas where poverty, overcrowding, and unsanitary conditions exist. Humans are the only hosts; infection is spread by direct and indirect contact. Trachoma is most prevalent in Asia and Africa, but also occurs in the United States. An estimated 400 million people worldwide suffer from this disease and of them, about 6 million are blind. The number of persons with severely impaired vision or blindness in countries where trachoma is prevalent definitely impairs socioeconomic progress. Trachoma ranks among the major infectious disease problems of humankind. Most trachoma seen in the United States appears on Indian reservations in the Southwest or in Appalachia. This disease is rarely seen in persons living under modern sanitary conditions. If treated early, cure is obtained. However, in many circumstances treated individuals readily become reinfected.

INCLUSION CONJUNCTIVITIS, URETHRITIS, AND ASSOCIATED DISEASES The clinical conditions discussed in this section are caused by serotypes of *C. trachomatis* that are passed by sexual contact or vaginal delivery. In many cases, these infections are asymptomatic or involve only mild symptoms that go undiagnosed. This form of urethritis is commonly called *nongonococcal* (NGU) or *nonspecific urethritis* (NSU) and is now recognized as a common sexually transmitted disease. *C. trachomatis* can be isolated from approximately 60% of males suffering from NGU. This infection seems to be widespread but is often without symptoms. As many

Figure 28-2 Trachoma with infection of the eye lid (conjunctivitis). (Centers for Disease Control, Atlanta)

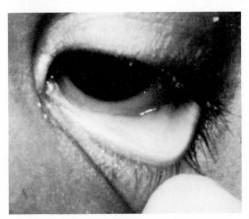

Cervicitis
inflammation of the cervix.

Ectopic pregnancy
a pregnancy in which the embryo develops and grows in the fallopian tube or peritoneal cavity instead of implanting in the uterus. Such pregnancies pose serious health threats to the female.

as 10% of cervical specimens taken from females without symptoms who were undergoing routine medical examinations contained chlamydiae.

The organism is found most often in sexually active female adolescents and can be found in as many as 27% of pregnant adolescents. It is the most common sexually transmitted pathogen. Although as many as 50% of infected females are asymptomatic, others commonly develop **cervicitis,** pelvic inflammatory disease, urethritis, or inflammation of the fallopian tubes (salpingitis). Salpingitis is often followed by infertility and a marked increase in tubal (**ectopic**) **pregnancies.** Ten percent of women with a single occurrence of salpingitis become infertile. There is some evidence of ascending infection in pregnant women. Studies have shown that chlamydia-infected women deliver a stillborn child or a child that suffers a neonatal death ten times as often as uninfected women. As many as 33% of chlamydia-infected women deliver prematurely or have stillborn children.

It is now recognized that *C. trachomatis* infection of neonates occurs at birth during vaginal delivery through an infected cervix. Infants who are exposed to *C. trachomatis* at birth may manifest their infections as conjunctivitis or pneumonitis. Infants born to untreated culture-positive mothers have an overall chlamydial infection rate varying from 23% to 70%, including conjunctivitis in 17% to 50%, and pneumonia in 11% to 20%. Other infants may exhibit isolated nasopharyngeal carriage or positive serology as their only evidence of infection. Multiple sites have yielded positive culture, including conjunctiva, nasopharynx, rectum, and vagina. Positive nasopharyngeal cultures have been found in up to 78% of infected infants (including those with conjunctivitis or pneumonia, and those who were asymptomatic). Sporadic cases may occur in adults whose eyes become infected through contact with contaminated towels, fingers, and similar items. Transmission can also occur in unchlorinated swimming pools. This form of conjunctivitis, known as *inclusion conjunctivitis,* is much less severe than trachoma and is readily treated with erythromycin or tetracycline.

LYMPHOGRANULOMA VENEREUM (LGV) Lymphogranuloma venereum is transmitted by sexual contact and is caused by distinct chlamydial serotypes (Table 28-1). A variety of nonspecific symptoms may be experienced in the early stages of illness, with lesions on the skin and mucous tissues of the genital organs. This condition is followed by the characteristic signs of enlarged and painful lymph nodes in the inguinal area (buboes). The enlarged lymph nodes may break (suppurate) and drain. Patients often have fever, nausea, headache, and conjunctivitis or skin rash. If untreated, the disease can lead to permanent obstruction of the lymphatic or rectal stricture (blockage).

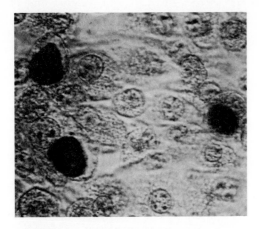

Figure 28-3   Chlamydia infected cells in cell culture. Dark inclusions are aggregates of chlamydia. (Courtesy Centers for Disease Control, Atlanta)

Diagnosis   *C. trachomatis* infections are diagnosed by observing **inclusion bodies** (cell vacuoles filled with the chlamydiae) (Figure 28-3) in cells scraped from infected tissues, by culturing the chlamydiae in cell cultures or embryonated eggs, and by showing a rise in specific antibodies. A recently developed antigen detection system has given good specificity and sensitivity with very rapid results.

Treatment   Sulfonamides, tetracyclines, and rifampin are effective agents in treating these chlamydial infections.

Prevention and control   Vaccines against chlamydia infections have been tried but generally do not induce a high enough level of protection to warrant their use. Proper hygiene and sanitation are the most effective means to preventing eye infections. Some persons may remain chronic carriers and serve as a reservoir of infections, a factor that makes control difficult.

Diseases Caused by *C. psittaci*

Psittacosis is a zoonotic disease, and *C. psittaci* is able to infect a wide range of birds and animals. This microbe was first recognized as an infection of psittacine birds, such as parrots and parakeets; hence the name *psittacosis*. Today the disease is also known as **ornithosis** because it infects many species of birds besides those of the Psittacine family. Recent studies have also demonstrated the organism in a variety of domestic animals from which human infection is possible.

   Many tissues of the bird are infected and a wide variety of

Inclusion bodies
intracellular inclusion often found in the cell cytoplasm as a consequence of infection. These inclusions are usually masses of developing microorganism being formed within the parasitical cell.

Ornithosis
a disease associated with birds from the Ornithine family.

Psittacosis Associated with Turkey Processing: Ohio, 1981

An outbreak of psittacosis occurred among employees of an Ohio turkey-processing plant in July 1981. Approximately 27 of the plant's some 80 employees were ill; 3 were hospitalized. Turkeys being slaughtered at the plant were the probable source of infection, but no specific group of birds could be implicated.

Most patients had an illness characterized by weakness, headache, fever, chills, and cough. To a lesser extent, patients had photophobia, conjunctivitis, generalized joint pains, stomach cramps, and diarrhea. Eight patients who had chest x rays showed evidence of pneumonia consistent with psittacosis.

Paired serum specimens from 27 workers were tested for complement-fixing antibodies to chlamydial group antigen. Of 15 workers who had recently had an illness compatible with psittacosis, 7 had a $\geq$ fourfold titer rise, and 5 had a titer of $\geq$ 16 in at least 1 specimen. Of 12 workers who had not recently had a compatible illness, none had a significant titer change. Single serum specimens were obtained from 29 other workers 1 to 3 days after onset of the last-recognized case in the employee group. Eight of 11 workers in this group who had recently had illness compatible with psittacosis had a titer of $\geq$ 16; 2 of 18 who had not had such an illness had a titer $\geq$ 16.

The plant, which operates approximately 40 hours per week, 10 months a year, processes turkeys only, which are delivered by truck from various locations, and slaughtered and defeathered on the day of arrival in the "kill-pick" area. Then they are conveyed on a continuously moving line into the evisceration area, where deep tissues are exposed, the birds are inspected and trimmed, edible organs are removed, and the remaining inedible internal and external parts are discarded.

Because most employees worked in various job stations in several departments on a given day, it was difficult to assess the relative importance of respiratory, skin, and conjunctival exposure. However, the attack rate by work department was significantly higher for workers in the kill-pick and evisceration areas than in other departments of the plant. Furthermore, there was no apparent correlation between degree of skin exposure and clinical psittacosis, suggesting that infections were the result of aerosol transmission or that multiple routes of exposure may have been involved (*MMWR* 30:638, 1981).

clinical signs may be seen. Diarrhea is a common finding in infected birds and chlamydiae are shed in the feces. The organism remains viable in dried avian feces for several months. Many birds have latent infections that may develop into acute diseases when such stresses as crowding and shipping occur. Ornithosis can be a major problem in the shipping and holding of pet birds and in the poultry industry.

Persons who work or live closely with birds stand the greatest risk of being infected. Exposure is usually by the airborne route via contaminated dust. Symptoms in humans are varied and may be subclinical or mild and simply passed off as a common minor

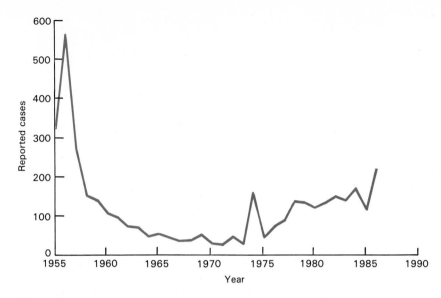

Figure 28-4 Cases of human psittacosis reported in the United States between 1955 and 1987. (Courtesy Centers for Disease Control, Atlanta)

respiratory disease. Occasionally (in about 50 to 100 cases per year in the United States) severe respiratory infections develop. Some deaths result, but early treatment with antibiotics usually reduces the mortality rate (Figure 28-4).

Very recently a new strain of *C. psittaci,* the TWAR strain, has been identified. This strain has been isolated from human pneumonia and pharyngitis patients, but not from animals. It is suggested that this may be a ''human'' strain that can be spread from person to person without animal contact.

RICKETTSIA INFECTIONS IN GENERAL

Bacteria

Rickettsiae are a group of small bacteria that traditionally have been considered separately from the typical bacteria. In fact, the rickettsiae have many characteristics, such as methods of laboratory cultivation and modes of transmission, that suggest a close relationship to the viruses. For many years the rickettsiae were considered a separate group of microorganisms positioned between the bacteria and viruses and the study of rickettsial diseases was usually included in the general subject area of virology. It is now well established, however, that rickettsiae are small **obligate parasitic** bacteria.

Obligate parasite
organisms that depend on a living host for their nutrition, growth, and development.

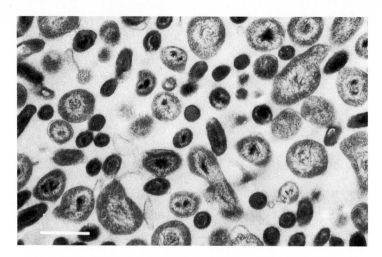

Figure 28-5 Transmission electron micrograph of the rickettsia *Coxiella burnettii* showing the pleomorphic nature of this microorganism (bar = 0.6 μg). (T. F. McCaul and J. C. Williams, *J. Bact. 147:*1063–1076, Figure 1b, with permission of ASM)

Rickettsiae are about 0.3 μm in diameter and up to 1.0 μ in length (Figure 28-5). Their shape ranges from pleomorphic to coccobacillary to bacillary and they are procaryotic cells. Their metabolic activities are highly dependent on energy received from living host cells and all but one (*Rochalimea quintana*) are able to multiply only inside the living host cells and are thus called *obligate intracellular parasites.* They are grown in the laboratory in cell cultures, embryonated eggs, or in animals, much like viruses (see Chapter 32). These bacteria are very specific in their intracellular growth: those causing spotted fevers grow in the nucleus of infected cells, while the typhus fever organisms are found only in the cytoplasm. Most rickettsiae are readily inactivated once they leave the host. Therefore their transmission depends on direct contact or vector transmission and all rickettsial diseases except

Table 28-2   Diseases Caused by Rickettsiae

Disease	Reservoir	Vector	Rickettsial Species
Trench fever	Human	Human louse	*Rochalimaea quintana*
Q fever	Lower animals	Tick	*Coxiella burnetii*
Rocky Mountain spotted fever	Tick	Tick	*Rickettsia rickettsii*
Epidemic typhus	Human	Human louse	*Rickettsia prowazekii*
Endemic typhus	Rodent	Flea	*Rickettsia typhi*
North Asia tick typhus	Rodent	Tick	*Rickettsia sibirica*
Boutoneuse fever	Rodent	Tick	*Rickettsia conorii*
Rickettsial pox	Mouse	Mite	*Rickettsia akari*
Scrub typhus	Rodent	Mite	*Rickettsia tsutsugamashi*

Q fever require an arthropod vector for successful transmission between hosts. Three genera of rickettsiae are described: the genus *Coxiella* contains only the Q fever agent, *Rochalimea* contains the agent of trench fever, and *Richettsia* contains the other species (Table 28-2).

Most rickettsiae and rickettsial diseases share some common features. These features are discussed first and are then followed by several of the more important rickettsial diseases of humans.

Pathogenesis

Except for *Rickettsia prowazekii* and the agent of trench fever, *Rickettsia* are zoonotic disease agents for which humans are only accidental hosts. The rickettsiae are usually introduced into the tissues by the bite of an arthropod and have a predilection for the cells that line the small blood vessels (endothelial cells). These bacteria multiply and spread along the blood vessels of the body. The signs and symptoms result from inflammation and swelling of the small blood vessels. This condition may cause blockage or a reduced blood flow to some tissues and some leakage of blood into the surrounding tissues. The leakage of blood in the skin produces the spots and rashes seen with most rickettsial diseases (Figure 28-6). Headache, chills, and fever are due to the generalized inflammation; and stupor, delirium, and shock may occur due to alterations in blood flow to the brain and other vital organs. Symptoms may last for several weeks. Death rates may be as high as 70% with epidemic typhus or less than 1% with rickettsial pox. Lifelong immunity usually results after recovery.

Figure 28-6   Rash of Rocky Mountain spotted fever consists of generally distributed, sharply defined purpuric macules involving the palms and soles which are usually unaffected in typhus fever. The rash may be gangrenous in regions such as the scrotum. (Armed Forces Institute of Pathology, AFIP 67987-3)

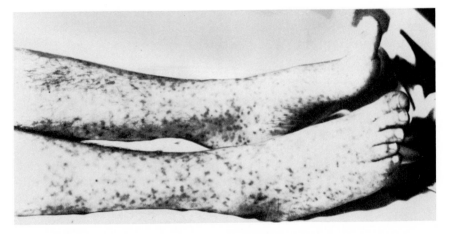

Diagnosis

Most rickettsial diseases are diagnosed by patient history and clinical signs or in the laboratory by an increase in specific antibodies between the acute and convalescent sera. Two general types of serologic tests exist. The first type uses specific rickettsial antigens prepared by growing the rickettsiae in embryonated eggs. Methods of measuring antigen-antibody reactions like complement fixation, agglutination, or immunofluorescence may be used. The second type, called the *Weil-Felix test,* is an agglutination test that uses certain strains of *Proteus* bacteria as the antigens. Some antigens present in these strains of *Proteus* cross-react with antibodies against certain rickettsiae. This procedure used to be widely used because it is relatively simple to run and is less expensive than using rickettsial antigens. Unfortunately, neither the sensitivity nor the specificity of the Weil-Felix test makes it a reliable procedure and currently it is seldom used.

Treatment

Rickettsial diseases respond well to treatment with tetracyclines. Chloramphenicol is also effective, but its use is restricted due to its greater toxicity to humans. Death rates are greatly reduced when chemotherapy is applied.

Prevention and Control

Two general methods are used to prevent rickettsial diseases. First, vaccines developed to fight some rickettsial diseases may be used on persons who have a high risk of being exposed to a specific rickettsial disease. The second method is to eliminate or reduce the animal reservoir and/or the arthropod vector of a given rickettsia.

SPECIFIC RICKETTSIAL DISEASES

Epidemic Typhus

Epidemic typhus is caused by the species *Rickettsia prowazekii,* named after Howard Ricketts and S. von Prowazek, two early investigators of this disease. Both scientists died following accidentally acquired laboratory infections of typhus. Without treatment, death rates from epidemic typhus may be as high as 70%.

The typhus rickettsia infects humans and the body louse of humans. The louse becomes infected when it feeds on infected humans and it leaves when the human body temperature significantly increases or decreases from normal. The louse can move only a short distance when searching for a new host. The louse will die of typhus in 1 to 3 weeks, but during this period the rickettsiae proliferate in its digestive tract and are excreted in the feces. When the infected louse infests and bites a new human host, louse feces are deposited on the skin. The louse bite causes itching, which is scratched, and the scratching forces the contaminated feces into the bite wound, thus initiating a new infection. Because of the short distance the louse can travel from human to human, epidemic typhus is associated with conditions of poor hygiene where humans are crowded together. These conditions are found in times of war, flooding, or other major disruptions of normal human activities. These conditions have existed often enough over the years to have allowed epidemic typhus to be a major killer of humankind. Armies of the past were frequently stricken with typhus fever and the outcome of many military campaigns was determined not so much by the strategies of the generals as by the epidemics of typhus fever. In 1489 during the Spanish siege of Granada, for example, 3000 Moorish troops died in battle and 17,000 died of typhus; in 1528, as the French army was on the verge of victory at Naples, typhus struck down 30,000 French troops and the tide of battle changed, resulting in a French defeat. During his campaign to conquer Moscow, Napoleon's army of 500,000 troops was reduced to fewer than 200,000 by disease. About 180,000 died of typhus. The last major epidemic typhus outbreaks occurred in southeastern Europe during World War I and in Russia just afterward. In the Russian epidemic an estimated 30 million people contracted the disease and over 3 million deaths resulted. The mode of transmission of epidemic typhus is shown in Figure 28-7.

Epidemic typhus has greatly decreased over the past 60 years. A few limited outbreaks occurred during World War II, but effective use of DDT as a delousing agent and vaccination of military personnel have generally controlled this disease.

Some humans who have recovereed from typhus can appar-

Figure 28-7   The transmission of epidemic typhus from human to human by the body louse.

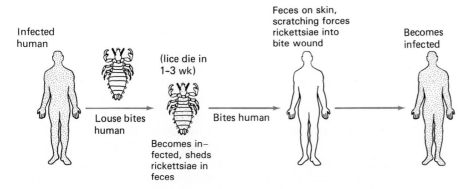

Infected human

Louse bites human

(lice die in 1-3 wk)

Becomes in- fected, sheds rickettsiae in feces

Bites human

Feces on skin, scratching forces rickettsiae into bite wound

Becomes infected

Epidemic Typhus: Georgia, 1984

On January 3, 1984, a 12-year-old male resident of middle Georgia became ill with a fever of 40° C (104° F) and a mild sore throat. No other symptoms or signs, including rash, were noted. Treatment with erythromycin for 4 days provided no clinical improvement, and the patient was hospitalized for further evaluation. Physical examination remained unchanged. No antibiotics were administered during the 8-day hospitalization, and the patient was discharged with the diagnosis of fever of undetermined origin. During the next 2 weeks, he gradually recovered.

Acute- and convalescent-phase serum specimens obtained from the patient were submitted to the Georgia Department of Human Resources, where testing indicated infection with either spotted fever group or typhus group rickettsiae. Additional testing at CDC revealed a fourfold increase in antibody titer against *Rickettsia prowazekii*, the causative agent of epidemic typhus. In February, state and CDC investigators visited the patient's residence and found a colony of eastern flying squirrels (*Glaucomys volans*) in the attic near the patient's bedroom. Four flying squirrels were trapped and returned to the CDC laboratories. Three of the four captured squirrels had antibodies against *R. prowazekii*.

Blood specimens obtained from the patient's parents showed no antibodies against *R. prowazekii*. Specimens were also obtained from 30 residents of 13 neighboring homes, including two residents of a house known to have been infested with flying squirrels. None of these persons had antibodies against *R. prowazekii*; no additional flying squirrels were captured in their homes (*MMWR* 33:618, 1984).

ently carry the rickettsiae in their tissues for the remainder of their life. Some of these carriers may experience a mild case of clinical typhus, called *Brill-Zinsser disease.* These persons could serve as a focus of a new epidemic if they were part of a crowded, deprived environment where body lice are present.

Endemic or Murine Typhus

Endemic or murine typhus, which is cased by *Rickettsia typhi*, is milder then epidemic typhus. Only sporadic cases are seen in humans; the death rate is less than 5% among untreated cases. The natural infection is found in rats, mice, and other rodents and is sporadically transmitted to humans by fleas. The disease in rodents and fleas is mild or subclinical and *R. typhi* may be carried in these hosts as a latent infection. The infection is occasionally transmitted to humans when they are bitten by an infected flea. Persons who live, work, or play around rodent-infested areas stand the greatest risk of infection. No human-to-human transfer occurs. Endemic typhus is found worldwide. In the United States

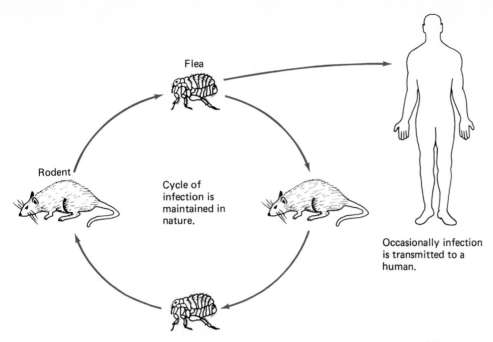

Figure 28-8   The transmission cycle of endemic typhus involves rodents and fleas.

it appears most in the southeastern states. Generally fewer than 75 cases per year are reported in this country. Deaths are rare when chemotherapy is applied. The transmission of endemic typhus is seen in Figure 28-8 and Figure 28-9 shows cases reported in the United States.

Figure 28-9   Cases of endemic typhus reported between 1955 and 1987 in the United States. (Courtesy Centers for Disease Control, Atlanta)

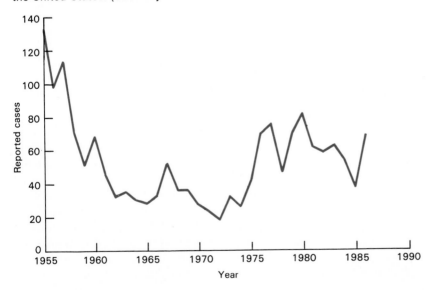

Outbreak of Murine Typhus: Texas, 1982

A cluster of cases of murine (endemic) typhus has been reported from Texas. From October 25 to November 11, 1982, five persons became ill with fever (temperature $\geq$ 40° C [$\geq$104° F]), headache (three patients), and myalgia (two patients). On the fourth or fifth day of illness, three patients developed a macular rash that began on the trunk and spread to the extremities. Blood specimens obtained on December 16, 1982, from three patients demonstrated indirect fluorescent antibody titers of 1:512 or greater to typhus-group rickettsiae; cross-absorption studies performed at CDC using antigens to *Rickettsia typhi* (the causative organism of endemic typhus) and *R. prowazekii* (the causative organism of epidemic typhus) indicated the former as the cause of the elevated titers. No serum specimens were obtained from the other two patients. Four patients received appropriate antimicrobial therapy with tetracycline; all five recovered without sequelae.

Three patients—a 27-year-old male, a 25-year-old female, and a 6-year-old female—lived in a house that had been unoccupied for 5 years before being moved in July 1982 to its present site on a peanut farm in Comanche County in north-central Texas. The other two cases occurred in a 24-year-old female who visited this family at their home every week or two, and a 48-year-old female, the grandmother of the 6-year-old, who lived ¼ mile away and visited the house at least once a month. Inspection of the house revealed holes in the roof, walls, and floors, and a large space beneath the house. Family members had heard rodents in the attic before the outbreak, and a mouse had recently been killed in the bathroom. Two or 3 weeks before the outbreak, rat poison had been placed inside the house. Five cats, present in the home before the outbreak, died during the outbreak period, four of unexplained causes, one in an accident. The cats slept indoors and had fleas. The family also owned three dogs, which usually slept underneath the house; they remained healthy during the outbreak period. None of the patients recalled being bitten by fleas.

An exterminator visited the house on November 19, 1982, and applied insecticide and rat poison. No further illnesses among family members or visitors to the house have been reported (*MMWR* 32:131, 1983).

Rocky Mountain Spotted Fever

Rocky Mountain spotted fever was first recognized around the year 1900 in the Rocky Mountains—hence the name. Yet it is found throughout North and South America and in Russia. Currently the greatest number of cases in the United States occur in the southeastern regions (Figure 28-10). The causative agent, called *Rickettsia rickettsii*, is primarily a parasite of ticks. This rickettsia infects many tissues of the tick without apparent ill effects. The eggs of the female tick may be infected and so the infection is passed directly to her progeny. This process is called **transovarian passage.** The rickettsiae are in the saliva of the tick and are transmitted to humans or animals by a tick bite. Ticks may become

Transovarian passage
a process whereby eggs are infected by an etiologic agent present in the female. When the eggs hatch, the insect is infected and capable of transmitting the agent to a new host or, if female, to her own eggs.

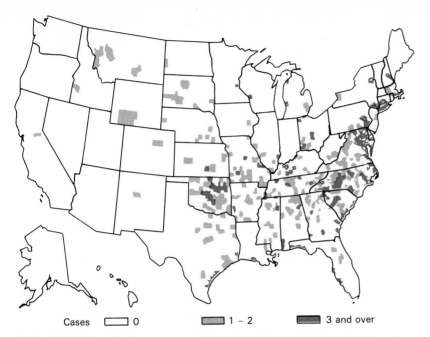

Cases ☐ 0   ▨ 1 – 2   ▧ 3 and over

Figure 28-10   Distribution of tick-borne Rocky Mountain spotted fever in the United States, by county, in 1986. (Courtesy Centers for Disease Control, Atlanta)

infected by feeding on infected animals or by transovarian passage from tick to tick without the involvement of an animal reservoir. No human-to-human transfer occurs. The transmission of Rocky Mountain spotted fever is shown in Figure 28-11. Death rates vary in different areas, suggesting that strains of varying degrees of virulence exist. Overall the death rates are generally from 3% to 10%.

Symptoms of the disease are similar to those for other rickettsial diseases; headache, fever, myalgia, and rash. Opposite to the typhus fevers, rashes of the rickettsial spotted fevers usually appear first on the arms and legs and later involve the body. These rashes also involve the palms and soles of the feet. There are presently about 700 reported cases of Rocky Mountain spotted fever in the United States each year. During the late 1970s and into the mid-1980s there was a marked increase in the number of reported cases (Figure 28-12). However, this unexplained increase in cases seems to have subsided to a present incidence rate of less than 0.32 cases per 100,000.

Q Fever

A rickettsia called *Coxiella burnetii* is the cause of Q fever. The name *Q fever* comes from "Query" fever, for the cause of this disease was not known for some time. *C. burnetii* is more stable than

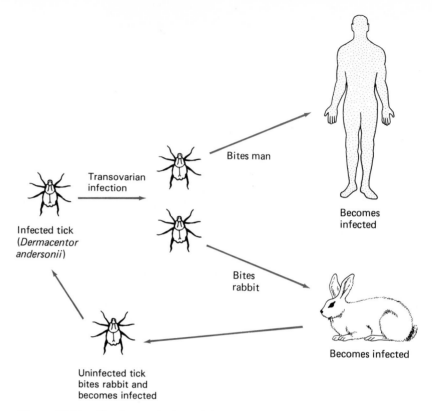

Figure 28-11   The transmission of Rocky Mountain spotted fever.

other rickettsiae and is able to survive for long periods outside the host, allowing transmission by indirect means. Current research indicates that this rickettsia forms a resistant endospore (Figure 28-13). Natural infections are found in many species of ticks and apparently can be spread by tick bites to birds and mammals in which asymptomatic infections develop. Rickettsiae are shed in saliva, urine, and milk. High concentrations are present in the placenta and amniotic fluids of infected animals. These rickettsiae remain viable on drying and may be carried on dust particles by the airborne route. Humans may be infected by the bite of ticks, ingesting contaminated milk, direct contact with infected tissues, or by the airborne route. The airborne infection results in pneumonitis whereas other routes may produce a nondescript disease with chills, malaise, and fever similar to influenza. A rash is not seen with Q fever. Asymptomatic infections seem widespread in cattle, and rickettsiae may be found in unpasteurized milk. Q fever is found throughout the world and occurs most frequently in persons working in the livestock or meat-producing industries.

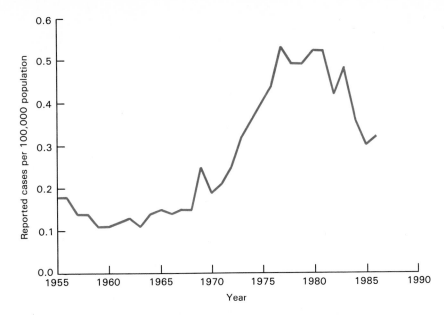

Figure 28-12   Cases of Rocky Mountain spotted fever reported in the United States, by year, between 1955 and 1987. Reasons for the sharp increase in cases between 1973 and 1983 are unknown. (Courtesy Centers for Disease Control, Atlanta)

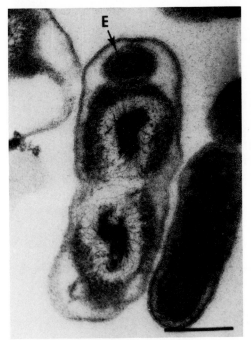

Figure 28-13   Transmission electron micrograph showing the presence of an endospore (E) in the rickettsia *Coxiella burnettii.* This cell is undergoing division (bar = 0.2 μm). (T. F. McCaul and J. C. Williams, *J. Bact. 147:*1063–1076, Figure 3c, with permission of ASM)

Q Fever Among Slaughterhouse Workers: California, 1985

During May 1985, five cases of hepatitis were reported to the Solano County (California) Health Department among workers at a local meat-packing plant that processes sheep. Illnesses were characterized by fever, malaise, myalgias, severe headache, and abdominal pain, but no jaundice. Symptoms lasted at least 1 week, then gradually resolved. Hepatitis was suspected because all cases had moderately elevated SGOT values. However, none had serologic evidence of acute infection with either hepatitis A or B (i.e., negative immunoglobulin M [IgM] antibody to hepatitis A and hepatitis B surface antigen). Since all five patients were exposed to domestic animals in the course of their work, the differential diagnoses included Q fever, brucellosis, and leptospirosis. Sera from four of the patients who were originally thought to have had hepatitis from other causes were positive for IgM antibody to Q fever by the immunofluorescent antibody test (IFA), indicating recent infection.

A serosurvey was conducted to identify the extent of the outbreak. Forty-two of approximately 100 employees agreed to be surveyed, including the 5 employees described above. Twelve (29%) had complement-fixation (CF) titers to Q fever rickettsiae; 8 (67%) of the 12 had recently experienced a clinical illness compatible with Q fever. Nineteen (45%) of the surveyed employees were positive by IFA test (but negative by CF test) for IgG antibody. Eleven of the 42 employees were negative both by CF and IFA. The 31 persons with serologic evidence of infection worked in a variety of jobs in areas throughout the plant, but no further investigation was performed to determine areas of highest risk.

Employees were educated about the illness through printed material and a question-and-answer session. A letter was mailed to physicians in the vicinity of the meat-packing plant informing them about Q fever. An investigation conducted by the California Occupational Health and Safety Administration resulted in the implementation of a surveillance program that included screening for Q fever by serology and for valvular heart disease among new employees. No feasible environmental control measures were identified (*MMWR* 35:223, 1986).

Other Rickettsial Diseases

In addition to the preceding varieties, other rickettsial diseases are found in different geographic areas throughout the world. Scrub typhus, which occurs over a wide area of southeast Asia, is the most important. The most common rickettsial diseases of humans are listed in Table 28-2.

CONCEPT SUMMARY

1. The chlamydiae are obligate intracellular parasites and are parasites of humans or animals. Numerous diseases occur from these organisms, including trachoma, LGV (a sexually

transmitted disease) and a serious but usually not fatal form of pneumonia. These diseases respond well to therapy.

2. The rickettsiae are obligate energy parasites of animal cells, are not found as free-living forms, and are accidental parasites of humans. They are transmitted to humans by vectors and produce serious generalized infections characterized by high fever and a rash. Members of the genus *Coxiella* may be found in domestic animals and can be transmitted to humans by the airborne route. These infections respond well to antibiotic therapy and vaccines are available for some diseases.

STUDY SUMMARY

1. How does trachoma differ clinically from inclusion conjunctivitis?
2. What is the most common chlamydial disease in the United States?
3. Define the nature of the risk to a newborn infant who is born to a woman infected with *C. trachomatis*.
4. What is the host range for *C. psittaci*?
5. Construct a table listing the rickettsial agents of infection that shows the common features of clinical presentation, transmission, and culture of these organisms.
6. Briefly outline the effect epidemic typhus has had on military operations.
7. Describe the relationship between Brill-Zinsser disease and epidemic typhus.
8. List the ways that members of the genus *Coxiella* differ from the organisms of the genus *Rickettsia*.

REFERENCES FOR FURTHER STUDY

1. Natural History of *Rickettsia rickettsi. Annual Review of Microbiology.* 40:287, 1986.
2. Early Phases in the Interaction between *Chlamydia trachomatis* and Eucaryotic Cells. *Microbiology—1986,* p. 82. American Society for Microbiology.
3. Epidemiology and Ecology of Rickettsial Diseases in the People's Republic of China. *Reviews of Infectious Diseases* 9:823, 1987.

4. *Manual of Clinical Microbiology,* 4th ed., E. Lennette, 1985. American Society for Microbiology.

5. *International Perspectives on Neglected Sexually Transmitted Diseases,* K. Holmes, 1983. McGraw-Hill.

chapter 29

INFREQUENTLY OCCURRING PATHOGENS

O rganisms presented in this chapter are a mixture of families, genera, and species that may be related only in that they produce human disease. The sporadic occurrence of disease due to these organisms should not suggest that they are not serious. Many of the infections discussed have a serious morbidity and significant mortality.

BRUCELLOSIS

Four of the six species of *Brucella* (Table 29-1) produce disease in humans. These organisms have their normal habitat in lower animals, and human infections are zoonotic. Humans become infected by contact with contaminated animal products or ingestion of contaminated unpasteurized milk or milk products.

Of the three most common *Brucella* species, *B. abortus* normally causes infections of cattle, *B. melitensis* is usually found in sheep or goats, and *B. suis* commonly infects swine. Humans are susceptible to all three species. Brucellae are small, Gram-negative, pleomorphic, coccobacillary-shaped bacteria (Figure 29-1). Because they grow slowly on artificial culture media, incubation for several days to several weeks is sometimes necessary before colonies develop. These microorganisms may survive from several days to several weeks when shed in the body fluids of an animal.

Pathogenesis and Clinical Disease

The *Brucella* organisms enter the body via lesions or cuts, ingestion, or inhalation. The bacteria are readily phagocytized by white blood cells; however, they are able to survive inside both PMNs and macrophages and much of the pathogenesis of brucellosis is associated with this intracellular survival.

Table 29-1   Common Reservoir Host and Human Infections of *Brucella* Species

Species	Reservoir Host	Human Disease
B. abortus	Cattle	Brucellosis (undulant fever)
B. canis	Dogs	Brucellosis
B. melitensis	Goats	Brucellosis (Malta fever)
B. neotomae	Rodents	None
B. ovis	Sheep	None
B. suis	Swine	Brucellosis (Bang's disease)

Bacteria are carried with the phagocytic cells through the lymphatic system to the blood and into such organs of the RES as the liver and spleen, which may, in turn, become enlarged. Circulating antibodies are produced but are unable to neutralize the bacteria sequestered inside the white blood cells.

The onset of clinical symptoms of brucellosis is usually gradual and often occurs weeks or months after exposure. Clinical symptoms are quite generalized and include fever, weakness, malaise, body ache, headache, and sweating. The fever may occur in cycles with febrile periods alternating with afebrile periods. The fever pattern has prompted the use of the name **undulant fever** for this disease. When cell-mediated immunity develops, the body is better able to contain or eliminate *Brucella* infections. Recovery from the disease is gradual and partial disability is often prolonged. Some infections are not apparent or go unrecognized. Brucellosis induces abortions in animals, an important factor in the economics of the cattle and swine industries. This is not, however, a feature of the human disease.

Undulant fever

one of several common names applied to the disease *brucellosis*. *Bang's disease* is also commonly used to refer to infection by the *Brucella*.

Figure 29-1   Photomicrograph of *Brucella suis*.

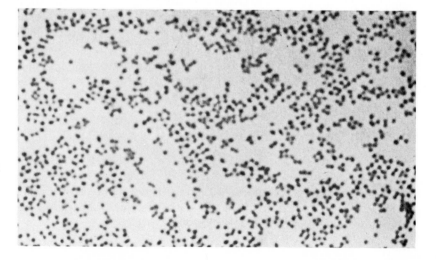

Transmission and Epidemiology

Large numbers of *Brucella* organisms are shed in urine, placental fluids, milk, and other secretions of infected animals. Transmission among animals occurs by direct contact with contaminated materials. Similarly, transmission to humans is by contact with contaminated animal products. Thus infections are most often seen in persons who work with animals or in meat-processing plants. Between 1980 and 1987, 1187 cases of brucellosis were reported in the United States. More than half were in persons working in meat-processing jobs. But the number of cases of brucellosis has decreased significantly in the past three decades (Figure 29-2) due to intensive control programs with domestic animals. Currently many states are certified as being free of brucellosis. Still, a slight increase in the number of cases has occurred in the past few years among persons working with cattle. Drinking of unpasteurized milk is a major transmission route of brucellosis in some parts of the world.

Diagnosis

Various clinical findings in persons most likely to be exposed are suggestive of the disease in humans. Diagnosis is confirmed by cultivation of the *Brucella* organism from the blood or tissues of the patient. However, culture is difficult and positive in only about 20% of cases. Most clinicians rely on the development of

Figure 29-2   The reported occurrence of brucellosis in the United States, 1945–1986 (modified from CDC annual summaries).

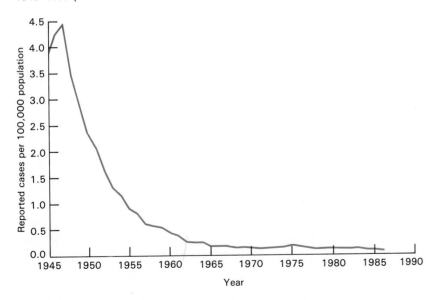

Brucellosis: Texas, 1983

On April 7, 1983, a case of possible brucellosis was reported to the city of Houston, Texas, Health Department's Bureau of Epidemiology. Three weeks later, 12 suspected cases had been reported, and by July 19, 29 cases were identified. Six of the cases were reported by physicians and nurses, and the remainder were discovered during epidemiologic investigation in the community.

The patients ranged in age from 2 to 81 years. All were Mexican emigrants living in northeast Houston. Twenty-eight of the 29 patients reported eating goat cheese ("queso blanco") before the onset of symptoms. Twenty-three patients reported purchasing cheese from neighborhood weekend vendors selling the product from their motor vehicles.

None of the patients interviewed had any leftover cheese, but one was able to purchase additional cheese for analysis from a vendor in his neighborhood. The cheese was reportedly produced in Linares, Mexico, and laboratory analysis determined that it was unpasteurized; all attempts to isolate *Brucella* sp. from the cheese were unsuccessful. On May 6, a news release was circulated to the media, and the public was made aware of the potential dangers of purchasing cheese from unlicensed food vendors. Since that time, neighborhood contacts reportedly have not seen the street vendors.

As of this report, 19 of the 29 patients have had blood cultures positive for *B. melitensis,* and one had *B. melitensis* isolated from blood and bone marrow. Three additional cases were confirmed by a fourfold rise or fall in agglutinating titer. Seven patients with presumptive diagnoses displayed clinical symptoms compatible with brucellosis in addition to agglutinating titers of > 1:160. (MMWR 32:616, 1983).

humoral antibody to confirm their diagnosis. The serologic test is not specific for brucellosis and in veterinarians and meat industry workers, antibody titers may be high because of repeated exposure to the organisms.

Treatment

Tetracyclines are the most effective antibiotics against brucellosis and generally cure the clinical disease within a few days. Prolonged therapy for 3 to 4 weeks is recommended, however, to ensure killing of the bacteria sequestered in the white blood cells and to prevent relapses. Streptomycin is sometimes used in conjunction with tetracyclines to help prevent recurrences of this disease.

Prevention and Control

Pasteurization of milk is effective in preventing transmission of brucellosis. Most control efforts are directed against the animal reservoir and extensive serologic and skin testing of domestic animals is required by law in most states. Infected animals are destroyed. An effective living vaccine is available for animals. Serologic tests or certification of vaccination is required to transport cattle into brucellosis-free areas or across state lines. These measures have resulted in a general decline in the number of brucellosis infections in both humans and animals.

TULAREMIA

Tularemia, like brucellosis, is a zoonotic disease. However, in this instance, the animal reservoir is wild animals, and transmission is extended beyond direct contact and ingestion of contaminated foods to vector transmission which may also occur.

Bacterium

Francisella tularensis is the cause of the disease tularemia. It is a small (0.5 × 0.3 µm) Gram-negative coccobacillus. **Cysteine** and blood or serum must be present in culture media before this bacterium will grow and even then growth is slow.

Cysteine
one of the sulfur containing amino acids.

Pathogenesis and Clinical Disease

Tularemia is a widespread disease in many species of animal and insects. Humans become infected by being bitten by an infected insect, by handling blood or tissues from infected animals, or by drinking contaminated water. An **ulcer**-type lesion usually develops at the site of inoculation or bite (Figure 29-3) and regional lymph nodes become swollen and painful. Systemic signs, such as dizziness, headache, chills and fever, sweating, and prostration, develop. Gastrointestinal symptoms may result from ingesting contaminated water or meats. Pneumonia may also be part of the clinical picture, either as a result of airborne exposure or as an extension of the systemic disease. The lesion heals in 4 to 7 weeks without treatment and complete recovery may require 3 to 6 months. Some relapses may occur, for *F. tularensis* is able to remain sequestered inside certain host cells and not be removed by normal host defense mechanisms. Unless treated, a death rate of 10% is possible, but death rates are less than 1% with antibiotic therapy.

Ulcer
an area of tissue erosion. Skin ulcers are typical of a variety of diseases such as syphilis and tularemia.

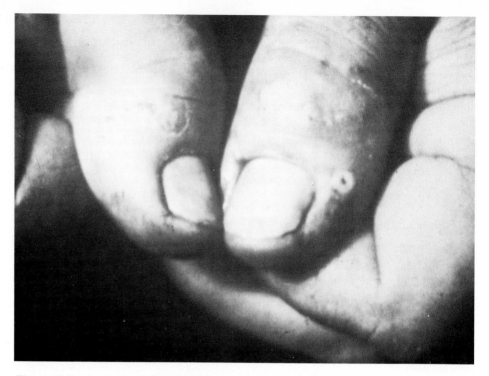

Figure 29-3   Lesions at the site of exposure to *Francisella tularensis.* (Courtesy Centers for Disease Control, Atlanta)

Transmission and Epidemiology

Most cases occur in rural areas and among persons who came in contact with wild animals or who are routinely exposed to ticks, deerflies, or other biting arthropods. Rabbits and rodents are the most common animal sources of human infection and transmission occurs during handling or dressing of an infected animal. Tularemia is sometimes referred to as ''rabbit fever'' or ''deerfly fever.'' Open streams of water may become contaminated from infected beavers or muskrats. Infections can be maintained in ticks by the passage of *F. tularensis* from the female to her offspring (transovarian passage). No human-to-human transmission happens under natural conditions and the occurrence of diseases in humans is sporadic. From 100 to 200 cases are reported each year in the United States (Figure 29-4).

Diagnosis

Growth of *F. tularensis* occurs slowly, even on some specialized culture media, and isolation of the microbe from clinical specimens is difficult. Diagnosis is usually made on the basis of clinical

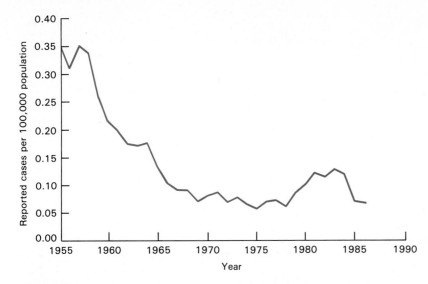

Figure 29-4 Occurrence of tularemia in the United States. (Courtesy Centers for Disease Control, Atlanta)

symptoms and a history of possible exposure. Serologic agglutination tests are available; a sharp rise in antibodies against *F. tularensis* is needed to confirm the diagnosis.

Treatment

Streptomycin, the treatment of choice, is highly effective against *F. tularensis*. It is more effective than some other broad-spectrum antibiotics in preventing recurrent diseases. Penicillin is ineffective.

Prevention and Control

The best methods of preventing tularemia are to avoid possible infected animals, especially sick rabbits, and to take precautions to reduce the chance of being bitten by anthropods. When working with *F. tularensis*, care should be taken to prevent laboratory-acquired infections. Because of the widespread nature of this disease in wild animals and arthropods, it cannot be controlled by the eradication of these natural hosts.

A live attenuated vaccine is available to persons who have a high risk of exposure, including laboratory personnel working with this microorganism, sheepherders, and those who work with wild animals or process hides or other produces from these animals.

Tularemia: Colorado, Alaska, and Georgia, 1979

Through October 13 of 1979, CDC received reports of 166 cases of tularemia. Three reports exemplify several clinical and epidemiologic characteristics commonly observed with this disease.

Colorado. A sheep-shearing crew was working west of Rangely during the week of April 23 when four of nine members became ill with fever and headache. Three persons developed left axillary lymphadenopathy (enlarged lymph nodes) with lesions on the dorsum of the left hand. The other patient, who did not have adenopathy or a skin lesion, suffered a more severe illness associated with a pulmonary infiltrate. All patients consulted a physician approximately 10 days after the onset of illness and recovered with tetracycline therapy. One patient had a fourfold rise in antibody to *F. tularensis* whereas the other three had single titers of > 1:160. Before becoming ill, these men had sheared sheep that seemed ill and that were covered with wood ticks (*D. andersoni*). The presence of lesions on only the left hand is explained by the procedure that the workers use in shearing sheep. The men part fleece with their bare left hand while shearing with the right hand—often rupturing ticks in the process and spilling blood onto the left hand.

In late June a 31-year-old laboatory technician was hospitalized in Grand Junction, with an illness of 2 weeks duration that began several days after working with an isolate of *F. tularensis.* Symptoms included fever to 105.8° F (41° C), headache, and pleuritic chest pain; pneumonitis and pleural effusion were confirmed by x ray. A diagnosis of tularemia was made, based on a 16-fold rise in titer. The patient recovered with streptomycin therapy.

Alaska. On August 31 a 49-year-old man in Fairbanks became ill 3 days after dressing a rabbit killed by his dog. Initial symptoms were a fever of 105° F (40.5° C) and vomiting; within 2 days he developed bilateral axillary adenopathy, with two ulcerations just proximal to a cut on his left hand. Culture of a lymph node aspirate grew *F. tularensis* and the patient made an uneventful recovery with tetracycline therapy. A number of dead rabbits were recently observed in the area.

PASTEURELLA INFECTIONS

The genus *Pasteurella* formerly included both the etiologic agents of plague, *Yersinea pestis* and of tularemia *Francisella tularensis.* There are presently four species in the genus, and, as with brucellosis and tularemia, the diseases are zoonotic. The bacteria are small Gram-negative coccobacillary forms that stain with difficulty, but give safety pin–type staining when Wright's or Giemsa methods are used. They all grow on normal laboratory media at 37° C and all are oxidase-positive.

Pasteurella multocida is the most frequently recovered species of the genus, and gets the name *multicida* as a consequence of both

Georgia. In mid-September two boys aged 10 and 11 from Calhoun became ill after handling a dead rabbit they had found. Both boys developed fever, swollen axillary lymph nodes, and ulcerative lesions on their hands. When seen in October 1, both patients were still ill and cultures of both hand lesions and one lymph node aspirate grew *F. tularensis.* Both patients recovered following streptomycin therapy (*MMWR* 28:529, 1979).

Tularemia: New Mexico, 1981

On May 13, 1981, a 31-year-old man living in Taos County who had been bitten by his pet cat 4 days earlier had onset of fever, rigors, myalgia, non-productive cough, pleuritic pain, and vomiting. When examined by a physician on May 17, the patient appeared acutely ill and had a temperature of 102.9° F (39.4° C). Skin lesions resembling insect bites were noted on several areas of his body.

Tularemia was suspected, and streptomycin, 1 g intramuscularly every 12 hours, was given as outpatient therapy and was continued for 9 days. The patient was clinically improved after 48 hours of treatment, but his fever persisted for 3 more days. Tests of acute- and convalescent-phase serum specimens, using the microaggluti-nation technique for detection of *F. tularensis* antibody, revealed a rise in titer from < 20 on May 19 to ≥ 640 on June 2.

On May 9, the patient had found his cat eating a dead rabbit under the bed. While removing the cat and rabbit from the house, the patient was bitten on the hand. On May 12, the cat became anorectic and listless; when examined that day by a veterinarian, it had a temperature of 105.1° F (40.6° C; normal temperature 100.5°–102.5° F) but appeared normal otherwise. No therapy was given. The cat appeared healthy when examined again on May 19, and a serum specimen obtained at that time had an *F. tularensis* antibody titer of 160 (*MMWR* 31:39, 1981).

its broad host range (many animals can be infected) and the serious consequence of infection. In poultry *P. multocida* causes a serious disease known as *fowl cholera,* and in other domestic animals it is responsible for a frequently fatal hemorrhagic septicemia. The organism can be found in the upper respiratory tract of normal dogs and cats. Human infection often (40%) follows a bite or scratch by one of these animals. The onset of disease is rapid with marked swelling and pain at the site of the injury. Fever usually occurs and is accompanied by swollen regional lymph nodes. If treated, the infection can be fairly easily terminated, or it may go on to produce **septicemia** with systemic and life-threatening consequences.

Septicemia
a condition in which an infecting microorganism is found in the bloodstream of the patient. This is a negative prognostic sign, and suggests that the host may be losing its battle with the infecting agent.

AEROMONAS AND PLESIOMONAS INFECTIONS

Saccharolytic
able to break down and metabolize sugars.

Organisms from the genera *Aeromonas* and *Plesiomonas* have increasingly been implicated as causes of diarrhea. Both are normally found in aqueous habitats, both fresh and marine. Both are Gram-negative, **saccharolytic,** facultative bacilli that grow readily on common laboratory media.

Although the taxonomy of *Aeromonas* is not completely worked out, there appear to be four species in the genus of which three, *A. hydrophilia, A. sobria,* and *A. caviae* have been isolated from stool specimens from persons with diarrhea. Although *Aeromonas* organisms can be isolated from up to 25% of normal individuals, the frequency of their occurrence in persons with diarrhea is statistically greater than in healthy individuals. Such data, repeatedly obtained from a variety of countries throughout the world, has given strength to the argument for the pathogenic nature of this genus. Diarrhea due to *Aeromonas* may be watery and last for up to two weeks. More severe forms of the disease such as bloody dysentery also occur, and in some patients the illness has been prolonged. The most likely source of infection is contaminated drinking water. It appears that this genus will take its place among the other enteric disease agents.

The case for *P. shigelloides* as an enteric pathogen is less clear. In an attempt to demonstrate the pathogenicity of this organism by fulfilling Koch's postulates, volunteers who intentionally drank water containing *P. shigelloides* remained well. However, implication of this bacterium as an etiologic agent persists due to its repeated isolation from cases of self-limited gastroenteritis. It is not considered as part of the normal human intestinal flora, and has been isolated from both sporadic and epidemic outbreaks of diarrhea.

GARDNERELLA AND MOBILUNCUS INFECTIONS

The organisms from the genera *Gardnerella* and *Mobiluncus* are, like those from *Aeromonas* and *Plesiomonas*, possible emerging pathogens. However, the disease they produce is not diarrhea but vaginitis. Many cases of vaginitis do not have a definite known etiologic cause and are referred to as *nonspecific vaginitis*. As is the case with diarrhea, there are a variety of known vaginosis agents, including *N. gonorrheae, Chlamydia, Candida,* and several viruses, but even when all of these are added together they account for much less than 100% of the cases.

Gardnerella vaginalis is the only species of the genus and is a nonmotile, relatively biochemically inert Gram-negative bacillus. It has a propensity for staining as a Gram-positive organism and was at one time classified among the corynebacteria. However, it has a cell wall composition consistent with Gram-negative bacilli and uses an anaerobic metabolism. This organism is part of the normal vaginal flora in about 10% of females. However, in females with vaginosis the number of patients with the organism rises to about 40%. Whether or not this is cause or effect of the disease is not entirely clear. The presence of these organisms in the vagina is associated with the development of "clue cells." These are *epithelial* (surface) cells to which *G. vaginalis* attach in large numbers, and can be readily detected by microscopic observation. Treatment of this condition leads to both a reduction in the presence of *G. vaginalis* and recovery from this disease.

Mobiluncus is a genus of highly fastidious, oxygen-sensitive, curved, Gram-negative, anaerobic bacilli. Like *Gardnerella* organisms, these bacteria are present in the normal female vagina, but increase significantly during the course of vaginosis. The organism is so oxygen-sensitive that culture is extremely difficult and most cases are diagnosed by Gram stain of vaginal secretions.

CONCEPT SUMMARY

1. Zoonotic disease agents are able to produce infection in both animals and humans. They are characterized by a wide range of bacteria of which *Brucella*, *Francisella*, and *Pasteurella* are typical.

2. A classic zoonotic disease, brucellosis is usually transmitted to humans through contact with contaminated animals or animal products. Individuals in the animal industry, particularly males, have an increased risk of getting the disease. Meat, milk, and meat products have been implicated in the spread of infection. Several species exist. In the United States the most common cause of human disease is due to *Brucella abortus*.

3. Tularemia, resulting from infection by *F. tularensis*, is a not uncommon infection of humans, particularly in some areas of the world. Because its normal habitat is rodents, it is most often found or contracted in a rural setting. Antibiotics have been successful in treating the infection.

STUDY SUMMARY

1. What is the method by which *Brucella* infect humans?

2. What aspect of *Brucella* infection promotes chronic disease?

3. What features characterize the epidemiology of zoonotic diseases?

4. What aspects of infection are common to both *Gardnerella* and *Mobiluncus*?

5. What is the source of most human infections due to *P. multocida*?

REFERENCES FOR FURTHER STUDY

1. Brucella Meningitis. *Reviews of Infectious Diseases* 9:810, 1987.

2. *Manual of Clinical Microbiology,* 4th ed., E. Lennette, 1985. American Society for Microbiology.

3. Human Brucellosis. *Reviews of Infectious Diseases* 5:821, 1983.

4. *Diagnostic Microbiology,* S. Finegold, 1986. Mosby.

5. *International Perspectives on Neglected Sexually Transmitted Diseases,* K. Holmes, 1983. McGraw-Hill.

chapter 30

FUNGI

F ungi are eucaryotic organisms existing both as single cells, as in the case of yeast, or as muticellular filaments, as seen in the molds and mushrooms. The multicellular fungi are plantlike in their structure, but they carry out no photosynthetic activities and depend on preformed organic matter for their nourishment (i.e., they are heterotrophic).

The term *mycology* refers to the study of fungi and is derived from the Greek term *mykes*, which means ''mushroom.'' Fungi are widespread, with approximately 100,000 species having been identified. Fungi are involved in the decomposition of organic matter and play an important role in recycling organic compounds in nature. Many plant diseases are caused by fungi; however, these diseases will not be covered in this book. Only about 100 species of fungi are associated with diseases in humans or animals. Most fungal diseases of humans are caused by only 10 to 15 different fungi (Table 30-1). This chapter summarizes the major fungal (mycotic) infections of humans.

MORPHOLOGY AND REPRODUCTION

Yeasts

Yeasts are single oval or spherical fungal cells ranging from 3 to 20 μm in diameter. As a rule, they reproduce by budding, which first entails dividing the nucleus, followed by passage of one nucleus to a bud that forms from the wall of the mother cell (Figure 30-1). A wall forms between the bud and the mother cell. The bud separates from the mother cell and becomes a daughter cell. Many daughter cells form from a single mother cell. Initially the daughter cell is smaller than the mother cell, but it gradually increases in size and, in turn, produces its own buds (Figure 30-2).

Table 30-1   Most Common Clinically Significant Fungi

Classification	Body Site	Fungi
Superficial	Skin	*Malassezia fur fur*
		Exophiala werneckii
Dermatophyte	Hair	*Piedraia hortae*
		Trichosporon beigelii
	Skin, hair	*Microsporum* sp.
	Skin, nails	*Epidermophyton* sp.
	Skin, hair, nails	*Trichophyton* sp.
Subcutaneous	Subcutaneous/ lymphatic (chromoblastomycosis)	*Sporothrix schenckii*
		Cladosporium sp.
		Phialophora sp.
		Fonsecaea sp.
Systemic	Respiratory	*Histoplasma capsulatum*
		Coccidioides immitis
		Fusarium sp.
		Penicillium sp.
	Respiratory/ subcutaneous	*Blastomyces dermatitides*
	Respiratory/CNS	*Cryptococcus neofurmans*
Opportunistic	Various	*Aspergillus* sp.
		Mucor sp.
		Candida sp.
		Rhizopus sp.

Figure 30-1   Replication of yeast cells by budding.

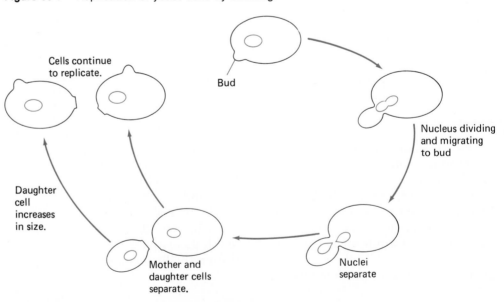

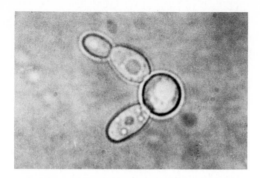

Figure 30-2   Phase microscope picture of budding yeast cells. (Courtesy Abbott Laboratories, Chicago)

Molds

The growth of a mold usually starts with the germination of a spore (also called *conidium*), which sends out a filament that grows by elongation at its tip. This filament is the basic structure of growing molds and is called a *hypha*. Many branches of hyphae are formed and masses of hyphae are called *mycelium*. Some hyphae grow above the surface of the substrate, resembling branches of a plant, and are called *aerial hyphae* or *aerial mycelia* (Figure 30-3). Other hyphae grow into the surface to absorb nutrients, similar to roots of plants, and are called the *vegetative hyphae*. The hyphae vary from about 2 to 10 μm in diameter, depending on the species of mold. Many nuclei are contained within the hyphae; in many

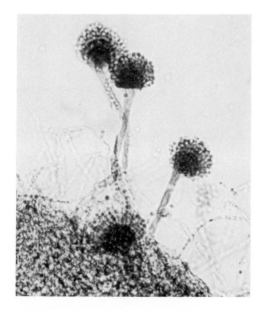

Figure 30-3
Photomicrograph of *Aspergillus* species showing aerial hyphae and sporangia. (Courtesy Centers for Disease Control, Atlanta)

Septum

a crosswall or membrane between compartments. Molds are classified into two groups by the presence or absence of septa; when present, septa divide fungal hyphae into complete cellular units.

Dimorphism

the property of having two morphologic shapes. Some fungi are dimorphic and exist as either yeasts or molds depending on their growth environment.

species crosswalls called **septa** are located at frequent intervals along the hyphae.

Molds reproduce by developing spores (conidia) on the aerial hyphae. Spores act as "seeds" for new colonies of molds. A reproductive cycle of one type of mold is shown in Figure 30-4. Many variations are seen in the morphology of the mycelium, spores, and reproductive structures of molds. These features are useful in identifying the different species. Some general structural variations of common molds are shown in Figure 30-5.

A typical mold colony is able to produce many reproductive structures and each structure may produce hundreds of spores. These spores are easily disseminated through the air and so mold spores are carried to virtually every unprotected environmental habitat on the earth. This type of reproduction is called *asexual*. Some fungi carry out a form of sexual reproduction in which two different reproductive bodies connect and haploid cells from each body fuse to form diploid cells.

Certain species of fungi are able to grow as either the yeast or the filamentous form—a trait called **dimorphism** (Figure 30-6). Under certain growth conditions the yeast form will develop, whereas under other conditions the filamentous form is produced. This phenomenon is important in the diagnosis of some fungal infections because certain pathogenic fungi exist in the yeast phase when growing in body tissues but change to the filamentous form when growing on an artificial laboratory medium. Most fungi can be cultivated on artifical media in the laboratory,

Figure 30-4　An asexual reproduction cycle of a conidial-type fungus.

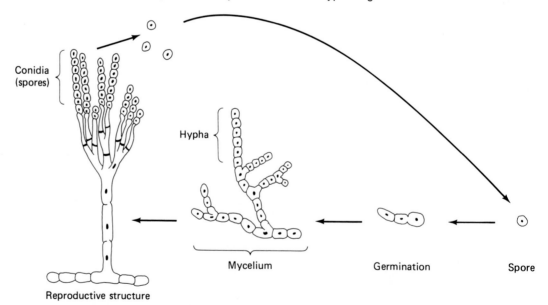

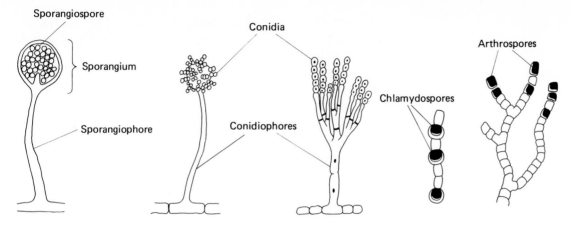

Figure 30-5 Some of the different types and arrangements of fungal spores.

through variations of the same basic methods used to cultivate bacteria.

CLASSIFICATION OF FUNGAL DISEASES

Fungal diseases are called *mycoses*. When found in humans, these diseases can be divided into four groups, based on the level of penetration of the infection into the body tissues, as follows:

1. Superficial mycoses, diseases caused by fungi that grow only on the surface of skin and hair

Figure 30-6 Dimorphism of the fungus *Sporothrix schenckii.*

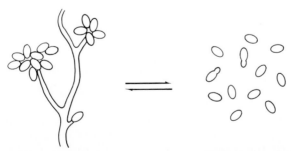

Filamentous form with conidia when grown on Sabouraud's agar at room temperature

Yeast form when grown on blood agar or in animal tissues at 37°

2. *Cutaneous mycoses or dermatomycoses,* including are such infections as athlete's foot and ringworm in which fungal growth occurs only in outer layers of skin, in nails, or in hair shafts

3. *Subcutaneous mycoses,* fungal infections that are able to penetrate below the skin and involve the subcutaneous, connective, and bone tissues

4. *Systemic or deep mycoses,* fungal infections that are able to infect internal organs and become widely disseminated throughout the body

Superficial Mycoses

The superficial mycoses are of minor importance because the infections are limited to hair surface or to the surface of the skin. The resulting tissue damage is minimal. These diseases are seen most often in warm climates. The lesions appear as scaly or pigmented areas on the skin or as nodules on the shafts of hair. Treatment involves removing the skin scales with a cleansing agent and removing the infected hair. Good hygiene generally prevents these infections.

Dermatomycoses

Tinea
wormlike. Cutaneous mycotic infections are often called "ringworm." This name derives from the concentric circles formed in the skin of some infected patients.

The fungi that cause dermatomycoses are able to infect only the epidermis, hair, or nails. About 30 different species of the genera *Epidermophyton, Microsporum,* and *Trichophyton,* collectively referred to as *dermatophytes,* cause these infections. Dermatomycoses are known by such lay terms as "athlete's foot," "jock itch," and "ringworm." The term **tinea,** along with the area of the body involved, is also used when referring to these infections. For example, *tinea capitis* is an infection of the scalp (Figure 30-7), *tinea corporis* is an infection on the body (Figure 30-8), *tinea cruris* (jock itch) is in the groin area, and *tinea pedis* (athlete's foot) is on the foot.

Because many dermatophytes may cause similar types ot infections, specific diagnosis can only be made by laboratory tests. Although these diseases do not cause death and are rarely serious, they may produce uncomfortable symptoms and sometimes unsightly lesions. The hyphae of the dermatophytes grow into the tissues of the epidermis, into the hair shaft, or into finger- or toenails. In young children, growth of these fungi in the epidermis of the scalp moves outward in concentric circles. The term "ringworm" was applied to this type of lesion years ago when it was thought that the lesion was caused by worms coiled under the skin. The lesions on the feet that characterize *tinea pedis* (athlete's foot) often start between the toes as small fluid-filled vesicles. The vesicles rupture, leaving shallow lesions that itch and may become

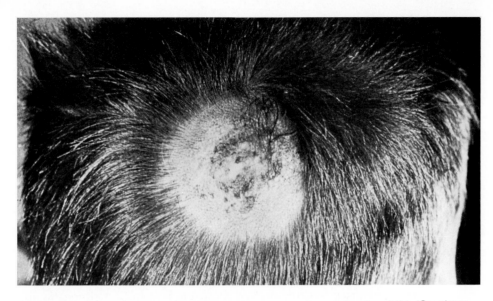

Figure 30-7 *Tinea capitis,* or ringworm infection, on the scalp of a child. (Courtesy Centers for Disease Control, Atlanta)

secondarily infected with bacteria. Infections of the nails cause puffy-chalky lesions (Figure 30-9). Infections may persist for years in some persons if not treated whereas in others the cure is spontaneous. Reinfection may occur because typical antibody-type immunity does not seem to develop.

Figure 30-8 Dermatomycosis of the foot (Athlete's foot). (Courtesy Centers for Disease Control, Atlanta)

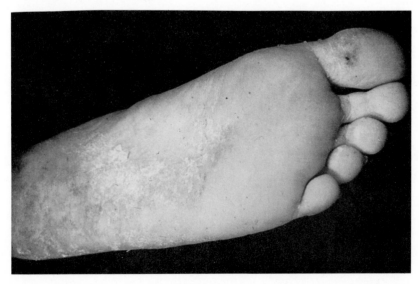

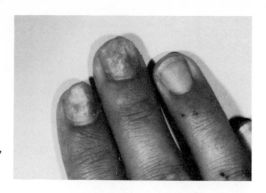

Figure 30-9 *Tinea unguim,* infection of the fingernails by dermatophyte.

Transmission and epidemiology Dermatophytes are usually parasites of humans and animals. Transmission is apparently from person to person by direct or indirect contact with bits of sloughed-off tissues that contain the fungus. *Tinea capitis* is seen mostly in children, *tinea pedis* in adolescents and adults. Some dermatomycoses are transmitted from pets and other domestic animals to humans. Infections are found worldwide and a significant number of people have been or are currently infected. Clusters of ringworm infection may occur in elementary school–age children.

Diagnosis Dermatomycoses are usually diagnosed by clinical signs and symptoms. Microscopic examination of tissue scrapings shows the presence of hyphae (Figure 30-10). Tissue scrapings can

Figure 30-10 Microscopic appearance of fungal hyphae in infected tissue. (S. S. Schneierson, *Atlas of Diagnostic Microbiology,* p. 45. Courtesy Abbott Laboratories, Abbott Park, IL.)

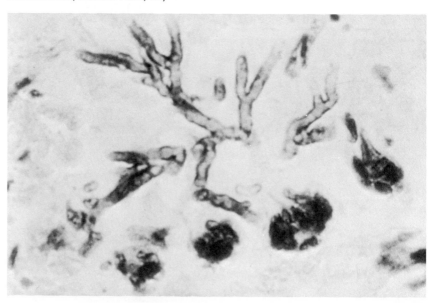

be inoculated onto an agar medium and after incubation at room temperature for a week or two, fungal colonies develop. Specific species can be identified by the gross appearance of the colony and by microscopic examination of the structure of the fungus. This procedure uses Sabouraud's agar medium, which contains antibiotics and a low pH to inhibit bacterial growth.

Treatment Numerous ointments, powders, and solutions are available as nonprescription treatments. Many are effective in providing symptomatic relief; when combined with good hygiene, they may help to produce a cure in some persons. The most effective systemic treatment is the antibiotic griseofulvin. When taken orally, it accumulates in the **keratin** tissues and exhibits a fungistatic effect. Treatment must be continued long enough to allow the infected tissues to be sloughed off. For infections of the scalp and skin, treatment for 2 to 3 weeks is required. Longer periods are needed for infections of nails. Infected nails may be removed surgically if prolonged treatment with griseofulvin is not practical.

Keratin
an insoluble protein found in skin epithelium, hair, and nails; sometimes used to refer to skin.

Subcutaneous Mycoses

Some fungi that are normal inhabitants of the soil or organic matter are able to cause infections when introduced into the skin. These infections tend to remain in the adjacent subcutaneous tissues but on occasion may spread to deeper tissues. The most common type of subcutaneous mycoses is caused by the fungus *Sporothrix schenckii* and the disease is called *sporotrichosis* (Figure 30-11). This infection is seen in all parts of the world and occurs most often in gardeners, farmers, or other workers who come in contact

Figure 30-11   Sporotrichosis on the arm. (Courtesy Centers for Disease Control, Atlanta)

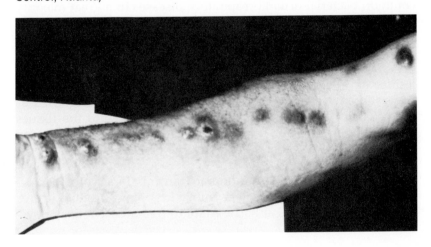

with soil. An ulcerative lesion develops at the site of inoculation; then infection may spread to regional lymph nodes, where swelling occurs. Diagnosis is made by culturing the fungus from lesion exudate. This fungus is dimorphic with a yeast phase at 36° C and a mycelial phase at room temperature. Treatment is often difficult, but doses of potassium iodide over a 4- to 6-week period are fairly effective.

Other forms of subcutaneous mycoses occur primarily in the tropics and subtropics. The two major forms, *chromomycosis* and *maduromycosis,* are caused by several different fungal species. Lesions are usually on the feet or lower extremities where the fungi have the most likely chance of entering traumatized tissues. The lesions of chromomycosis appear as ulcerative, warty, cauliflower-like growths. The lesions of maduromycosis are deeper and purulent, with openings draining to the outside. Treatment is often difficult but usually includes surgical removal of diseased tissues in the case of maduromycosis, with chemotherapy being used to control secondary bacterial infections. The lesions of maduromycosis appear similar to the subcutaneous lesions caused by *Nocardia, Actinomyces,* or *Streptomyces* (Chapter 22); it is important to determine which agents are causing the disease, for it can be treated with antibiotics if bacterial agents are responsible.

Systemic Mycoses

General pathogenesis   The systemic mycoses occur in two basic forms. The most prevalent is a subclinical or mild respiratory infection whereas the other is a severe disseminated infection involving many tissues. Unless treated, the disseminated form is usually fatal. The fungi that cause systemic mycoses live in the environment as saprophytes. The spores are inhaled into the respiratory tract, where an acute, self-limiting pneumonitis may result. This initial infection is generally mild and passed off as a common bacterial or viral respiratory disease. In a great majority of cases, the infection terminates after this mild pulmonary phase. In a relatively small number of persons, often those with compromised defense mechanisms, a chronic form of the disease develops. Slowly progressing, purulent, or granulomatous pulmonary lesions develop and resemble the lesions of tuberculosis in many ways. Often systemic mycoses of the lungs are misdiagnosed as tuberculosis. These lesions may extend directly into the tissues around the lungs or the fungi may be carried via the blood to any organ of the body, where secondary lesions will develop.

Transmission   No human-to-human transmission is known to occur. The fungi growing in soil or animal droppings produce spores that are carried by the airborne route to humans. The major systemic mycoses are discussed below; some have worldwide distribution whereas others are limited to specific geographic areas.

Diagnosis   Most fungi that induce systemic mycoses are dimorphic and diagnosis is aided by observing the yeast form of the fungus in tissue specimens. The fungi may be cultivated on various nutrient agars, in which either the yeast or filamentous forms may be produced; serologic tests are available for some infections. Delayed hypersensitivity is induced and antigens prepared from the fungi can be used in skin tests for some.

Treatment   The chemotherapeutic agents amphotericin B and 5-fluorocytosine are the treatments of choice for most systemic mycoses. Surgical removal of large pulmonary lesions may be useful in some cases.

Prevention and control   No vaccines against mycotic infections are routinely available. Avoiding areas like bird roosts and caves where spores are most likely to be found may be wise.

SELECTED SYSTEMIC MYCOSES

Coccidioidomycosis

Coccidioidomycosis is caused by fungus *Coccidioides immitis*. The fungus is found in some desert areas and is prevalent in the southwestern United States and in some areas of Central and South America. *C. immitis* grows as a mold on the soil and produces **arthrospores** that are carried with air currents into the pulmonary spaces, where they cause infection. As many as 50% to 80% of the people living in some areas of the central valleys of California have a positive skin test to this agent, which indicates that they have at least had the mild respiratory form of this disease. Coccidioidomycosis is called ''valley fever'' by residents of California's San Joaquin Valley. A small percentage of those persons infected develop the disseminated disease. *C. immitis* grows in spherical forms in tissues (Figure 30-12).

Arthrospore
a fungal spore formed as the cell walls increase in thickness. Each of the cells in the hyphae may become an arthrospore. These spores are very resistant to drying.

Histoplasmosis

The fungus *Histoplasma capsulatum* (Figure 30-13) causes the disease of histoplasmosis. This fungus grows well in soil enriched by bird or bat droppings and produces infectious spores. It is most

Coccidioidomycosis: California, 1978

A violent windstorm in the San Joaquin Valley on December 20 and 21, 1977, created extensive dust clouds that spread to many areas of California. State and local health officials became concerned that dust bearing the arthrospores of *Coccidioides immitis* would expose people outside the regions endemic for coccidioidomycosis to the disease. During the first 24 days of January 1978, 11% of 656 sera obtained from persons with suspected coccidioidomycosis and submitted to the Kern County (California) Health Department for tube precipitin tests were positive for *C. immitis;* in comparison, 2% of 300 sera submitted in January 1977, 9% of 400 sera submitted in January 1976, and 6% of 250 sera submitted in January 1975 were positive. During the same period (January 1978) the University of California at Davis reported that 18% of 356 sera submitted were positive compared with 4% of 206 sera tested in January 1977. Several of these patients lived outside endemic regions of the state.

Editorial note: Persons who traveled through the San Joaquin Valley during the storm and those who were subsequently exposed to dust clouds from the area may have been exposed to *C. immitis.* Because the incubation period is 1 to 3 weeks, physicians should suspect the diagnosis in exposed persons who developed flulike symptoms in January. The diagnosis can be confirmed by the early appearance of *C. immitis* precipitins or by the later appearance of antibodies detected by complement-fixation or immunodiffusion tests or skin-test conversion (*MMWR* 27:55, 1978).

prevalent in the Ohio and Mississippi river valleys. Skin testing shows that upward to 80% of the population in some areas give evidence of having been infected. Infection results from inhaling the spores. Mild lung infections usually result and go unnoticed, but on healing they leave small, thin-walled calcified nodules that are easily mistaken for tuberculosis lesions on chest x rays. This

Figure 30-12 Spherules of *Coccidioides immitis* in sputum from patient. (Courtesy Centers for Disease Control, Atlanta)

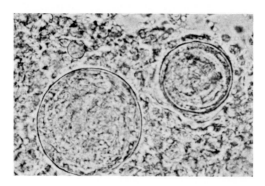

Histoplasmosis Outbreak: Tennessee, 1977

During the first weekend in May 1977 several families gathered at a friend's home in a suburb of Nashville, Tennessee, to cut and remove a large oak tree that had fallen during a thunderstorm the previous day. The tree was not noted as a prominent bird roost. There were 42 people (ages 2½ to 52 years) who either observed or helped clear debris with chain saws, hand saws, rakes, or their bare hands. Then 12 to 25 days later, 18 persons (average age, 23) developed symptoms of fever, malaise, chest pain, cough, myalgia, weight loss, and difficult breathing. Pulmonary infiltrates and/or enlarged lymph nodes were observed on chest x rays of 13 of the 14 patients examined. Three patients were hospitalized; all recovered.

Although *Histoplasma capsulatum* could not be isolated from cultures inoculated with induced sputum from 14 patients, a majority of these patients had a titer rise in yeast phase or mycelial-phase complement-fixation (CF) antibodies in the month following illness. Two dogs present at the activities also became ill and showed a titer rise in *Histoplasma* CF tests.

Numerous soil and tree samples have been cultured; so far all have been negative. The tree was burned at the suggestion of the country health department and topsoil 2 inches deep was laid over the area.

Editorial note: This outbreak demonstrates the continued endemicity of histoplasmosis in an area that has been known since the mid-1940s to have a high prevalence of this infection. The high attack rate (43%) in this outbreak could be partially explained by the young age of the patients or by the dosage of spores to which these patients were exposed, which was sufficiently high to overcome any residual immunity they might have had.

H. capsulatum is difficult to isolate from sputum cultures; the diagnosis is often established only by serologic changes in CF antibodies or histoplasmosis immunodiffusion tests. Although spraying a 3% formalin solution on soil contaminated with *Histoplasma* spores has often been the preventive measure of choice in large outbreaks of histoplasmosis, covering the area with topsoil and burning the tree in this instance were probably adequate measures, for the soil area was small and only one tree, not notable as a bird site, was involved (*MMWR* 26:322, 1977).

fungus is dimorphic and grows in the form of yeast in tissues. Disseminated infections are rare.

Blastomycosis

Blastomycosis is caused by the fungus *Blastomycoses dermatidis*. It probably grows in the soil as a mold and produces connidia that infect humans by the airborne route. This fungus is found worldwide, but most reported diseases occur in the central river valleys of the United States. Along with common mild respiratory infection and the less common disseminated infection, skin lesions

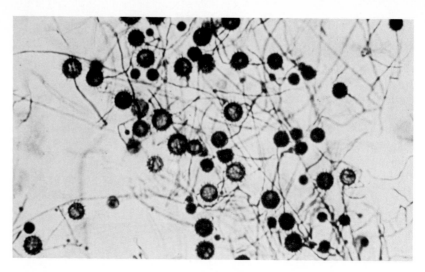

Figure 30-13 Photomicrograph of *Histoplasma capsulatum*, mycelial phase. (Courtesy Centers for Disease Control, Atlanta)

may also be produced. *B. dermatitidis* grows as a budding yeast in human tissues (Figure 30-14).

Cryptococcosis

Cryptococcosis occurs throughout the world and is caused by the yeast *Cryptococcus neoformans*. This yeast has been isolated from soil and habitats of pigeons and exists only in the yeast form. Most infections are associated with mild respiratory tract involvement. In compromised persons, however, the infection may spread through the body with a characteristic involvement of the central nervous system (Figure 30-15).

Figure 30-14 Budding yeast phase cells of *Blastomyces dermatitadis.* (Courtesy Centers for Disease Control, Atlanta)

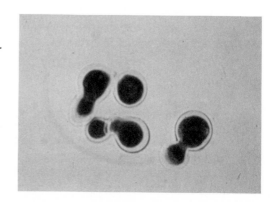

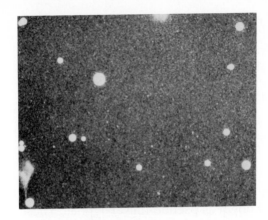

Figure 30-15 *Cryptococcus neoformans.* India ink preparation of spinal fluid from patient with cryptococcal meningitis.

OPPORTUNISTIC FUNGAL INFECTIONS

The number of individuals kept alive in immunocompromised conditions continues to increase. These persons are at considerably increased risk of infection, and the variety of caustive agents responsible for opportunistic disease in them continues to expand. With no group of microorganisms is this more apparent than with the fungi. Many organisms, traditionally considered as saprophitic or comensalistic, manage to obtain a foothold in the promising soil of the immunocompromised host. By far the majority of mycotic diseases are the result of this relationship.

The nature of the immunocompromise determines to some extent the genus of those fungal agents most likely to be responsible for infection (Table 30-2). Thus, patients with bone marrow

Table 30-2 Fungi Most Commonly Associated with Specific Immunocompromise

Immune Compromise	Opportunistic Fungi
Leucopenia (bone marrow failure)	*Candida* sp.
	Aspergillus sp.
	Phycomyces sp.
Cellular immunity (tissue transplants)	*Candida*
	Cryptococcus
	Coccidioides
	Histoplasma
Diabetes	*Zygomyces*
	Rhizopus
	Mucor
	Absidia
Steroid therapy	*Zygomyces*
Malignancy (leukemia, lymphoma, Hodgkin's disease)	*Candida*
	Cryptococcus
	Histoplasma

transplants seem uniquely susceptible to *Fusarium* infection; children on long-term steriod therapy often develop infections due to *Rhodotorula;* the *Trichsporon* species often infect those patients with tumors of the blood, and patients with leukemia are frequently victims of *Mucor* or *Rhizopus.* However, the most frequent cause of mycotic infection regardless of the kind of immunocompromise is *Candida.*

Candidiasis

Candida is a genus of true yeasts that are not dimorphic, although chains of yeast cells, each measuring 4–6 μm, sometimes link together forming structures known as pseudo-(false) hyphae. These yeast are Gram-positive, budding cells that ferment a variety of sugars. They produce reproductive spores (chlamydospores) and the species *C. albicans* produces **germ tubes** (Figure 30-16) when placed in a nutrient environment. The yeast-like fungus *C. albicans* is often part of the normal microbial flora of the mucous membranes of the mouth, vaginal canal, and intestinal tract. Inflammation of the mouth, called *thrush,* may occur in newborn infants, who become infected during birth, or in immunocompromised persons (Figure 30-17). Vaginal tissues may show signs of candidiasis during pregnancy or in diabetics. Candidiasis of the skin may occur where the skin is damp or irritated, such as between the upper leg or under the arms. Candidiasis seems to be more prevalent in persons on broad-spectrum antibiotic therapy, because many normal indigenous bacteria are destroyed, leaving niches into which *C. albicans* can grow. Members of this genus produce serious disease such as endocarditis, septicemia, protracted urinary tract infection including kidney and lung infection, esophagitis, and other soft tissue infection. Even with proper treatment,

Germ tube

the hyphaelike growth of yeast cells that occurs when the cells are placed in an appropriate growth medium.

Figure 30-16   Typical germ tube formation by *Candida albicans.* (Courtesy W. H. Flemming III, *J. Clin. Microbiol.* 5:236)

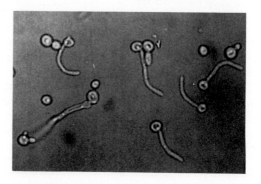

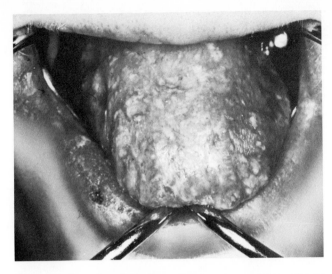

Figure 30-17   Candidiasis on the tongue and lips. (From: Council on Dental Therapeutics, American Dental Association)

which may be difficult, a high mortality rate is associated with these infections.

An increasing incidence of systemic candidiasis (canidia in the blood) is being recognized in various compromised patients. Candidiasis can be treated with imidazoles, various ointments, or with antifungal antibiotics, such as nystatin and amphotericin B.

Aspergillosis

Species of the genus *Aspergillus* (Figure 30-3) are widespread in nature and several species are known to cause infections in humans. When persons with compromised immune defense mechanisms encounter large concentrations of aspergillus spores, infections may result. Respiratory infections are the most common and lesions containing masses of mycelia may develop in the lungs or bronchi. Lesions may also develop in the ear canal, sinuses, and subcutaneous tissues. Systemic aspergillosis may occur in severely immunosuppressed patients, such as those with leukemia or Hodgkin's disease. Treatment is not always successful, but amphotericin B seems to be the most effective chemotherapeutic agent.

Mucormycosis

Mucormycosis refers to fairly rare diseases produced by a variety of common fungi of the order *Mucorales* (Figure 30-18). These infections are seen in severely immunocompromised patients. The

Eye Infections after Plastic Lens Implantation: California, Florida, Montana, and Ohio, 1975

During October and November 1975 physicians in California, Florida, Montana, and Ohio noted 11 cases of unusual ocular infection in patients who had had a prosthetic plastic lens implanted in the eye after cataract extraction. The infections were suspected 2 to 6 weeks after lens implantation, when the usual short-term postoperative inflammatory changes persisted despite the topical corticosteroid therapy frequently used in these patients. Ocular cultures from 8 of the patients grew *Paecilomyces libaeinus,* a penicilliumlike organism, resistant in vitro to amphotericin B. In most cases, the plastic lens was removed after infection was suspected and local antifungal therapy was instituted. Vision was seriously impaired in all patients (*MMWR* 24:437, 1975).

fungi may penetrate the respiratory or intestinal mucosa or enter through breaks in the skin. Localized lesions may develop, followed by spread to the blood and dissemination to all organs. Death often results from a combination of the predisposing illness and the fungal infection.

Figure 30-18 Photomicrograph of *Mucor* sp. (Courtesy Centers for Disease Control, Atlanta)

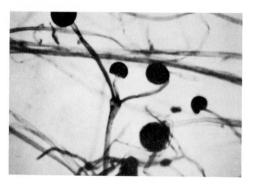

CONCEPT SUMMARY

1. Fungi are eucaryotic, nonphotosynthetic, often multicellular organisms, some of which cause disease in humans and animals. Forms causing disease in humans include the yeasts and simple multiple-celled forms called *molds*. Because fungi do not have bacterial-type cell walls, infections are often difficult to treat. Fungi are ubiquitous in the environment and cause much economic loss through their destructive growth processes.

2. Mycotic infections range from the benign "athlete's foot" to serious systemic disease that is frequently fatal. These diseases are far more common in compromimsed hosts than in normal individuals.

STUDY SUMMARY

1. List the reproductive structures found in fungi.

2. Make a table listing the systemic fungi and showing the diseases produced, cultural characteristics (dimorphism, etc.), unique morphologic features, and recommended treatments.

3. What ecological feature of *Coccidioides imitis* is responsible for its restricted geographic occurrence?

4. Characterize the role of *Candida* as etiologic agents of disease.

5. List four normally saprophytic fungi that can cause disease in humans.

REFERENCES FOR FURTHER STUDY

1. *Candida ablicans:* Biology, Genetics and Pathogenicity. *Annual Review of Microbiology* 39:579, 1985.

2. Specific and Rapid Identification of Medically Important Fungi by Exoantigen Detection. *Annual Review of Microbiology* 41:209, 1987.

3. Rapid Diagnosis of Candidiasis and Aspergillosis. *Reviews of Infectious Diseases* 9:398, 1987.

4. *Manual of Clinical Microbiology,* 4th ed., E. Lennette, 1985. American Society for Microbiology.

5. *Fungal Infection in the Compromised Host,* D. Warnock, 1982. Wiley.

chapter 31

PROTOZOA

The microorganisms presented in this chapter are animal-like in their structure and function. They are the smallest of the animal parasites and are normally included in the discipline of medical parasitology. Medical parasitology includes study of parasites from four large phyla in the animal kingdom. These phyla are Protozoa (of the kingdom Protista), Platyhelminthes (flatworms), Nematodes (roundworms), and Arthropoda. The worms and arthropods are multicellular organisms, usually macroscopic in size; in fact, some, like tapeworms, may attain lengths of several meters. It is not within the scope of this book to cover the diseases caused by these multicellular types of parasites. However, a table listing some of these diseases is included in Appendix B. The protozoa are briefly reviewed in this chapter because of their small size and because their pathogenesis parallels that of the bacteria and fungi.

GENERAL CHARACTERISTICS

Protozoa are eucaryotic cells and have many of the intracellular components characteristics of higher forms of life. They range in size from 5 μm to more than 100 μm in diameter, and most protozoa have some form of active locomotion. Locomotion is an important feature used to group them into major subdivisions. Protozoa are found in soil, in most bodies of water, and in many higher forms of life, either as commensals or parasites. Of approximately 30,000 species, relatively few are able to cause diseases in humans and most protozoa are beneficial contributors to the various biological cycles in nature.

Protozoa and other parasitic diseases are common in underdeveloped, tropical, and subtropical areas. In many such areas most of the population is infected with a variety of parasites. The overall effects of these diseases on the general well-being of the inhabitants of these areas are of major importance. In industrialized nations, particularly in temperate-climate regions, parasitic diseases are of relatively minor importance. There are, however, several protozoal diseases of significance in the United States. These include diarrhea due to *Giardia* or *Coccidia*, congenital disease due to *Toxoplasma*, pneumonia due to *Pneumocystis*, and vaginitis due to *Trichomonas*.

The diagnosis, treatment, and control of protozoal diseases differ in some ways from those used for other microbial diseases. The protozoa are not easily cultured on artificial media or inoculated into experimental animals or cell culture systems for isolation. Serologic tests are not as useful, because high levels of antibody do not readily form against many protozoa that infect the intestinal tract or other superficial tissues. Some infections, however, do stimulate an antibody response, and serologic tests are now available to aid in the diagnosis of these protozoal diseases. The diagnosis of most protozoal diseases depends mainly on demonstrating the presence of the parasite by microscopic methods. The feces are examined to determine intestinal infections, and the blood and/or other tissues are examined for systemic infections. Scrapings of mucosal tissues or biopsies of infected organs may also be examined. Because of the large size and distinct shapes of the protozoa, directed microscopic identification is the routine method of diagnosis. The symptoms of many protozoal diseases are quite general and often are not used solely as a basis for a specific diagnosis.

No vaccines are available against protozoal diseases and chemotherapy is not as specific nor readily available as it is against procaryotic microbes; however, a few compounds are fairly effective against certain protozoal diseases. Toxic side effects are common with antiprotozoal drugs.

Some disease-producing protozoa go through a life cycle that involves more than one kind of animal host. In many of these situations such as with malaria, humans are **intermediate hosts** and not *definitive hosts* (the host in which the parasite goes through sexual reproduction, sometimes refered to as primary host); and with some infections such as toxoplasmosis, humans are terminal (sometimes called *blind*) hosts because there is no way that the parasite can be transmitted from them.

Many protozoa exist in two basic forms: the active, growing form, called the *trophozoite*, and the dormant, resistant form, called the **cyst** (Figure 31-1). The trophozoite form proliferates in the tissue and causes the damage that results in the clinical disease. The cyst is able to survive in the external environment and is the form of the protozoa that is usually transmitted from host to host by indirect routes. Some protozoa go through intermediate development stages in bloodsucking insects and the infected insect may serve as the vector in transmitting the disease.

Intermediate host
a parasitic host in which the parasite goes through asexual reproduction. The intermediate host is often an essential step in the life cycle of the parasite.

Cyst
a closed, walled sac or pouch, usually filled with fluid or solid tissue.

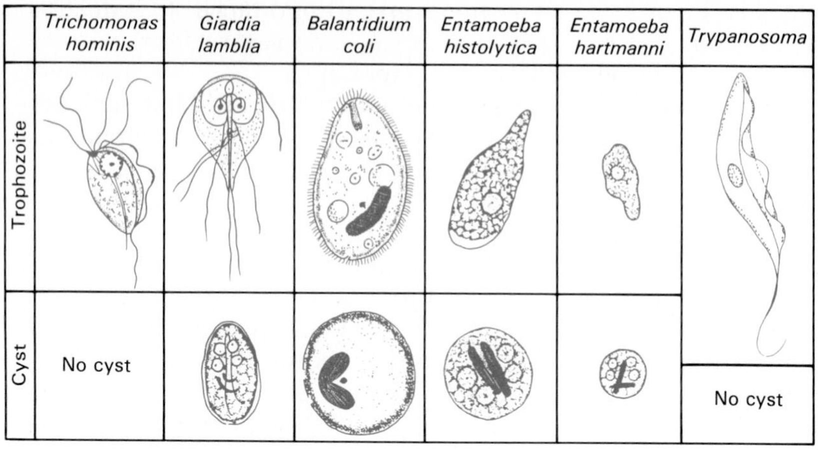

	Trichomonas hominis	Giardia lamblia	Balantidium coli	Entamoeba histolytica	Entamoeba hartmanni	Trypanosoma
Trophozoite						
Cyst	No cyst					No cyst

Figure 31-1
Trophozoite and cyst stages of some protozoa. All except *Entamoeba hartmanni* are human pathogens.

PROTOZOAL DISEASES

Amebiasis

The class Sarcodina (which includes the subclass Rhizopoda) contains protozoa that move by ameboid action—that is, by extending a section of their cytoplasm in one direction and then causing the remainder of the cytoplasm to flow in the extension. This extension is called a *pseudopodium* (false foot). The amebae are members of the Sarcodina and six species from three genera are parasites of humans. Only one species, *Entamoeba histolytica*, however, causes widespread or major diseases in humans. The disease is called *amebiasis*.

Amebiasis The pathogenesis of amebiasis is outlined in Figure 31-2. Only the cyst stage of *E. histolytica* is infectious. The trophozoite stage readily dies once out of the body; if it survives long enough to be swallowed, it will be destroyed by stomach acids. Once the cyst, which contains four nuclei, passes into the small intestine, excystment occurs; that is, the cyst changes into four small trophozoite forms of the ameba. Each continues to grow and divides by binary fission, thereby producing large numbers of offspring. These trophozoites release an enzyme that lyses tissues. This trait is the basis for the species with the name *histolytica* (Greek *histos* = tissue; *lysis* = dissolving). The histolytic enzyme allows the amebae to penetrate into the intestinal mucosa, where subsurface lesions develop. These lesions may coalesce into extensive ulcerative areas, thus leading to severe dysentery with stools containing bloody mucus. In a small percentage of the cases, the amebae may penetrate into the mesenteric venules and lymphat-

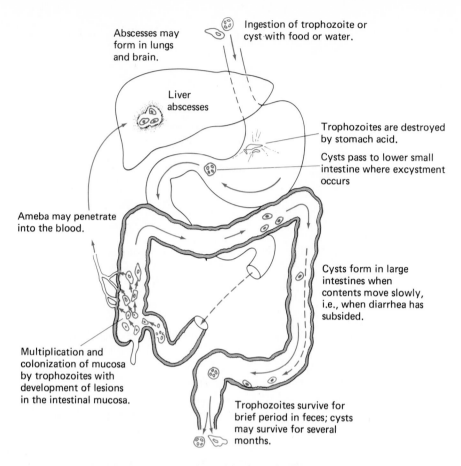

Ingestion of trophozoite or cyst with food or water.

Abscesses may form in lungs and brain.

Liver abscesses

Trophozoites are destroyed by stomach acid.

Cysts pass to lower small intestine where excystment occurs

Ameba may penetrate into the blood.

Cysts form in large intestines when contents move slowly, i.e., when diarrhea has subsided.

Multiplication and colonization of mucosa by trophozoites with development of lesions in the intestinal mucosa.

Trophozoites survive for brief period in feces; cysts may survive for several months.

Figure 31-2   The pathogenesis of amebic dysentery.

ics and be disseminated to various internal organs. With disseminated amebiasis, abscesses usually develop in the liver (4% to 5% of cases) but may also develop in the brain, lungs, heart, or other tissues. Death may result from the disseminated disease.

When a person is experiencing the acute symptoms of intestinal amebiasis, called *amebic dysentery*, the contents of the intestinal tract pass rapidly through the system. Under such conditions the amebae do not have time to develop into the cyst stage and normally only the trophozoites are released. As the body begins to establish an equilibrium with the ameba, possible by developing neutralizing antibodies against the lytic enzymes, the lesions heal and the contents of the intestinal tract move more slowly, allowing time for the development of cysts. Thus persons showing no signs of the disease may be infectious. A large segment of the adult population in developing countries where amebiasis is prevalent lives in semibalance with this ameba; yet this group serves as a source of infection to susceptible persons. Some amebiasis is

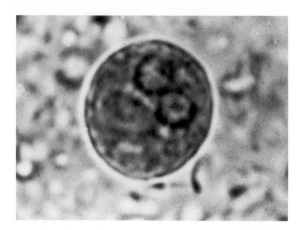

Figure 31-3 Microscopic appearance of cyst of *Entamoeba histolytica* in fecal material. (Courtesy Centers for Disease Control, Atlanta)

found in the United States, with most cases occurring in the South.

Specific diagnosis is made by observing the trophozoite or cyst stage of the ameba in the feces (Figure 31-3). Serologic tests are helpful in diagnosing disseminated amebiasis.

Several chemotherapeutic agents are available for the treatment of amebiasis. Tetracyclines, in combination with diloxanide furoate, is effective. A compound called metronidazole can be used with good results and chloroquine is often used in combination with the preceding drugs.

Control of amebic dysentery is best achieved by following good sanitary practices, particularly in the handling and treatment of human fecal wastes.

Infections due to Free-Living Amebae

Two amebae that are normally found in water or moist organic matter have been responsible for serious human infection. *Naegleria fowleri* live in freshwater lakes or streams and can produce serious encephalitis in swimmers. Though rare, the disease is usually fatal. *Acanthamoeba* species live in soil and fresh or even brackish water. There has been a significant increase in infections due to these organisms during recent years. These infections most frequently occur in individuals who wear contact lenses, but who do not properly care for these lenses. Because *Acanthamoeba* are ubiquitous, they can easily contaminate homemade lens-cleaning solutions. The wearing of contaminated lenses may lead to infection of the cornea resulting in reduced vision or even **enucleation** of the eye.

Enucleation
removal of the entire eyeball from its socket.

Ciliophora Infections

Protozoa of the subphylum Ciliophora are surrounded by many fine cilia that beat in rhythmic patterns to propel the organism. Only one species, *Balantidium coli*, causes disease in humans. This organism is a large (50 to 100 μm in length), ovoid-shaped cell. Its normal habitat is the intestinal tract of hogs. Transmission is by the fecal-oral route. Diseases in humans are rare and symptoms range from mild intestinal discomfort to severe diarrhea.

Mastigophora Infections

Protozoa of the class Mastigophora, also called *flagellates*, have whiplike flagella that serve as their organs of locomotion (Figure 31-4). Some mastigophora inhabit the superficial tissues of the intestinal or genital tract of mammalian hosts. Others require a bloodsucking arthropod for part of their life cycle with the other part of their life cycle in the blood and internal tissues of the mammalian host. Two relatively minor diseases, *trichomoniasis* and *giardiasis,* found in the United States, and the serious diseases of *trypanosomiasis,* found in Africa and South America, are typical flagellate diseases.

Trichomoniasis   Trichomoniasis is caused by the protozoan *Trichomonas vaginalis. T. vaginalis* is a globular-shaped cell about 25 μm in length with four anterior flagella and a short **undulating membrane**. It exists only in the trophozoite stage and inhabits the vagina and urethra. Transmission is usually by sexual contact. A large number of cases are asymptomatic. Males having the clinical infection may experience some irritation of the urethra, with a slight discharge and pain during urination. In the female, *T. vaginalis* may cause the pH of the vagina to become slightly alkaline.

Undulating membrane

an external membrane found on the surface of some protozoa. This membrane may be of various sizes and appears to be capable of wavelike movement.

Figure 31-4 *Leishmania tropica* in artificial culture. Note prominent flagella. (R. Barlow and T. Minnick, *ASM News*, vol. 51, 1985, with permission of ASM)

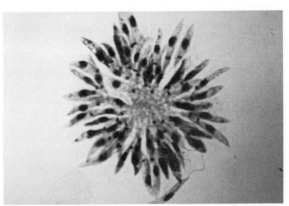

Giardiasis: Colorado, 1978

A multistate outbreak of giardiasis in visitors to and residents of Vail, Colorado, occurred from March 14 to April 20, 1978. At least 38 confirmed cases were reported.

On April 13 a gastroenterologist in Petoskey, Michigan, reported the occurrence of giardiasis in 6 members of the family who had vacationed in Vail, Colorado, from March 23 to 25. All had epigastric pain, nausea, and weight loss. *Giardia lamblia* was confirmed in the stool specimen of 1 of the 6 patients. Additional information obtained from the Colorado State Health Department revealed that 13 cases of confirmed giardiasis had been reported from Colorado (7 from Colorado Springs, 6 from Denver) and 12 more confirmed cases from the state of New York—all in individuals who had visited Vail during the last week in March.

An epidemiologic investigation was begun by the Colorado Department of Health and CDC. Information was obtained on 777 long-term Vail residents by means of a questionnaire and stool survey. Of those surveyed, 465 (60%) gave a history of diarrheal illness within the past 3 months. A rise in the number of acute diarrheal illnesses began March 14 to 16 and reached a peak April 1 to 12.

Preliminary analysis demonstrated no differences in attack rate by age or sex. Long-term (>7 days) and short-term (<7 days) diarrheal illness peaked at similar periods of time. The local hospital's routine examinations of stools for bacterial pathogens were negative.

Because contaminated water is a frequent cause of giardiasis outbreaks, the Environmental Protection Agency (EPA) and CDC reviewed the city's recent records of weekly sewage output. During the week of March 28 to April 3 the number of gallons of sewage produced dropped approximately 50%. This drop coincided with a sewer-line obstruction and leak into the creek supplying water to the city.

Editorial note: The fact that many cases occurred after discovery of the sewer-line obstruction is probably a reflection of the long incubation period of giardiasis (variable, but approximately 7 days) and the continued use of water from contaminated storage tanks. Illness disappeared with dilution of freshwater (MMWR 27:155, 1978).

This condition may be accompanied by a foul odor, a slight discharge, itching, and burning sensations. These symptoms may be caused in part by secondary bacterial infections resulting from the altered pH.

Diagnosis is made by direct microscopic examination of smears from the vagina or urethral discharge. Treatment of individuals and their sex partners by oral administration of the drug metronidazole effectively cures this infection.

Giardiasis Giardiasis is caused by the flagellate *Giardia lamblia*. Giardia has a distinctive appearance (that resembles a human face) because of its teardrop-shaped cell, with four pairs of flagella, and two nuclei (Figure 31-1). The cell is 9 to 16 μm in length and exists in both the trophozoite and cyst stages. The cyst is able to persist for prolonged periods outside the body and transmission is by the typical fecal-oral route. Infection is in the upper small intestines; many infections are asymptomatic or go undiagnosed and are passed off as minor intestinal disturbances. Following ingestion of the cyst, gastroenteritis and diarrhea may result, along with dark, greasy, foul-smelling feces, considerable abdominal discomfort, and flatulence. Symptoms may continue for 2 to 3 weeks with gradual improvement. The infection may become chronic in some patients, with continued intermittent bouts of diarrhea. Infection is often accompanied by anorexia, weight loss, and nausea. Giardia is the most common intestinal pathogenic protozoan of humans in the United States. Infections have occurred among campers and hikers who drank untreated water. Even water from numerous municipal sources has been implicated as a source of infection.

Giardiasis is a recognized problem among children attending day-care centers. It is commonly associated with individuals who are deficient in IgA, and is frequently diagnosed in homosexual men. Diagnosis is made by demonstrating the parasite in feces or **duodenal** aspirates. Treatment with furazolidone or metronidazole is frequently effective. This disease may not respond to treatment, however, and may be difficult to eliminate.

Duodenal
pertaining to the portion of the small intestine that attaches directly to the stomach. In adults the duodenum is about 25 cm in length.

Trypanosomiasis   Three species of the genus *Trypanosoma* cause serious diseases in humans. *T. brucei gambiense* and *T. brucei rhodesiense* cause African sleeping sickness and *T. cruzi* causes South American sleeping sickness or Chagas' disease. The morphology of these protozoa is shown in Figure 31-5.

African sleeping sickness is found only in geographic areas of Africa where the *tsetse* (glossina) fly lives. The tsetse fly is a necessary link in the life cycle of *T. brucei gambiense* and *T. brucei*

Figure 31-5   Photomicrograph of *Trypanosoma brucei*, cause of sleeping sickness.

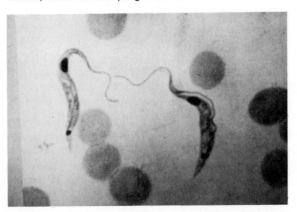

Reduviid bug
a small biting bug.

rhodesiense and functions as the vector for transmission to humans and animals. Cattle, swine, and various wild animals are the major hosts and serve as a reservoir for these protozoa. When a person is bitten by an infected tsetse fly, the trypanosomes cause a local lesion at the site of the bite. The protozoa then spread and become lodged in the lymph nodes and produce a chronic infection. In some cases, the trypanosomes spread to the CNS and result in the well-recognized symptoms of African sleeping sickness. During this stage, the patient becomes somnolent and eventually goes into a coma and dies. African sleeping sickness has a significant impact on the economy of the African continent, for large areas of otherwise productive land cannot be inhabited by humans due to the presence of infected animals and tsetse flies.

T. cruzi is found in South and Central America and is transmitted by **reduviid bugs**. Dogs, cats, and various wild animals serve as the reservoir of infection. The reduviid bugs bite humans at night and defecate when they feed. *T. cruzi* are in the feces, which contaminate the bite wound or other skin abrasions or are carried by fingers to the mucosa of the mouth or nose or to the conjunctiva of the eyes to cause the infection. Persons living in huts with dirt floors or walls are most likely to become infected, especially if they sleep on the floor or ground. Lesions are produced by the parasite at the site of the bite. The protozoa then spread through the body. Many infections are nondescript and may remain latent for years. Acute diseases occur in some persons, especially children, involving the heart and CNS, and result in a 10% death rate.

Diagnosis of trypanosomal diseases is generally made by demonstrating the presence of the protozoa in the blood, lymph node aspirates, or spinal fluid. There is no effective treatment for South American trypanosomiasis. Two drugs, suramin sodium and pentamidine, however, are used with some success in treating the African diseases.

Sporozoa Infections

Malaria Of all the infectious diseases of humans, malaria is probably the most important as far as total number of cases, deaths, and debilitation are concerned. Possibly hundreds of millions of people worldwide are infected with malarial parasites resulting in more than 1 million deaths each year. The family Sporozoa includes four species of the genus *Plasmodium* that cause most infections in humans. They are *P. vivax, P. malaria, P. falciparum,* and *P. ovale.* Most malaria is found in the subtropics or tropics. Malaria cases seen in the United States currently involve persons who were infected while visiting or residing in endemic areas outside the country. During military operations like the Vietnam War a marked increase in malaria was seen in the United States. (Figure 31-6).

The female anopheles mosquito is the primary host for the malarial parasite; humans serve as an intermediate host. The life cycle of the plasmodia is quite involved, with different stages of development occurring in the human and the mosquito. A simplified general outline of this life cycle is shown in Figure 31-7.

The mosquito becomes infected by taking a blood meal from an infected person. Within the mosquito, the plasmodia go through a sexual reproduction cycle. This results in the accumulation of large numbers of infectious *sporozoites* in the salivary glands of the mosquito. The sporozoites are then inoculated into a susceptible host as the mosquito feeds. The sporozoites are rapidly filtered from the blood and specifically infect liver cells. The parasite matures through a series of stages in the liver cells and after a week or so parasitic forms called **merozoites** are released into the blood. The merozoites infect red blood cells and go through another series of developmental stages that end with the bursting of the red blood cells, thus releasing new merozoites (Figure 31-8). These merozoites infect more red blood cells and the cycle is repeated. The cycles of infection in the red blood cells become synchronized and with each cycle more and more cells become infected and then burst. When the red blood cells burst and release cellular debris, parasites, and by-products, the onset of a malarial *paroxysm* is triggered. A paroxysm is a periodic sudden recurrence of symptoms. The paroxysms of malaria start with

Merozoite

the asexually reproducing form of the malarial parasite. The merozoite is infective for human red blood cells and the mosquito.

Figure 31-6   Reported cases of malaria in the United States, 1933–1986. Of all the reported cases in 1980, 81% were among foreign civilians (modified from CDC annual summaries).

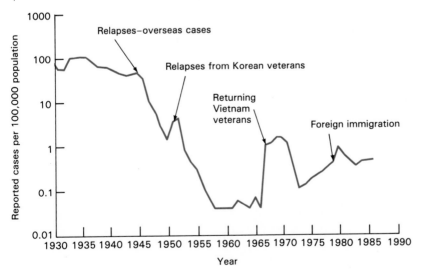

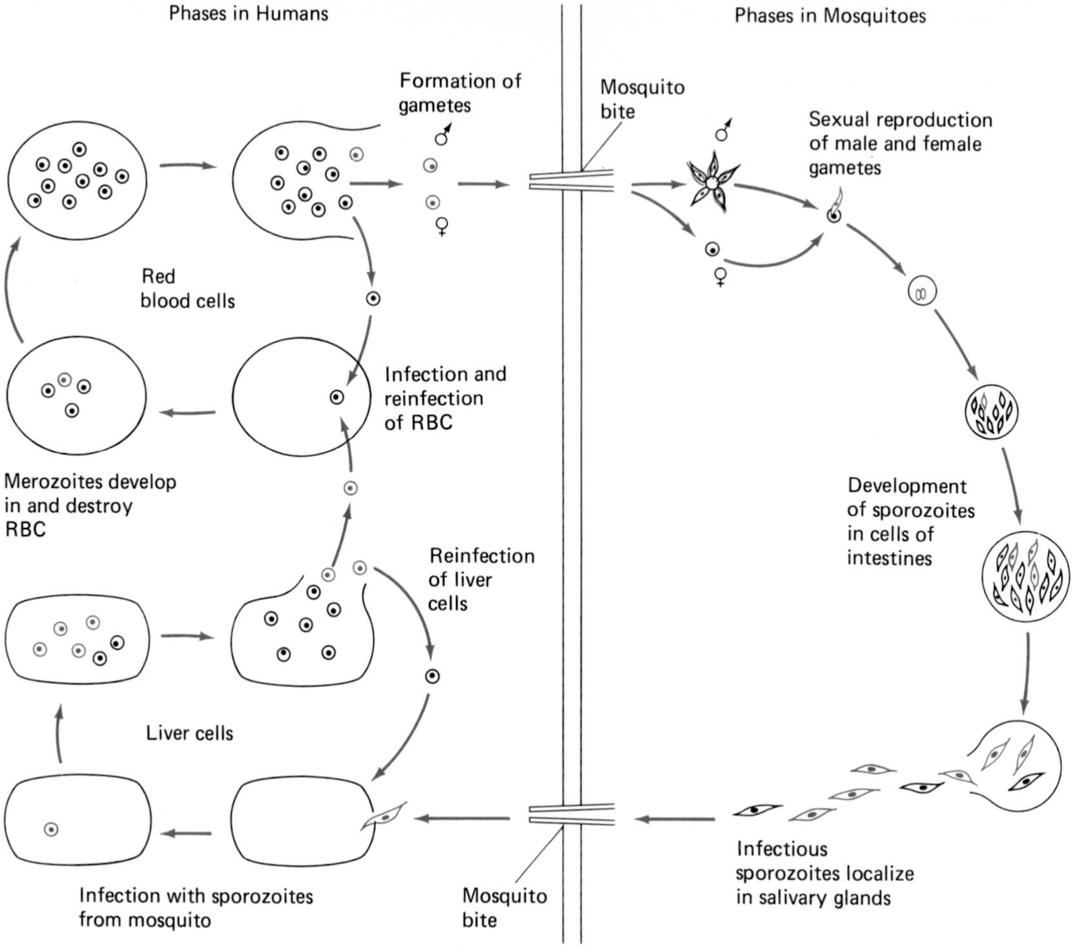

Figure 31-7 A simplified outline of the phases of the life cycle of a plasmodium parasite in humans and mosquitoes.

Figure 31-8 Malaria infected human red blood cells. (Courtesy Abbott Laboratories, Chicago)

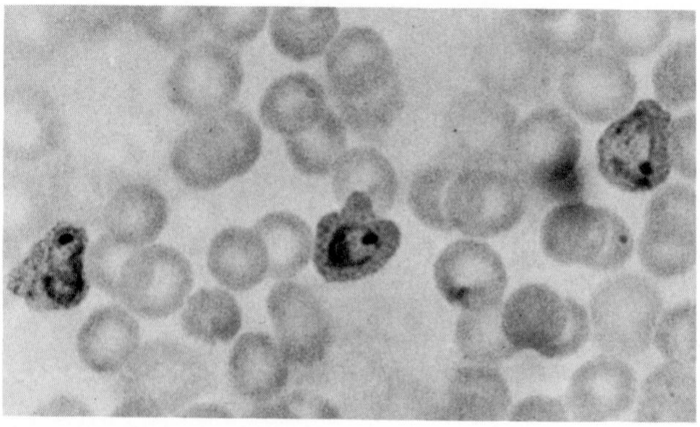

chills that last for 15 to 60 minutes. During this time the patient may have a headache, vomit, and generally feels nauseated. As the sensation of chilling stops, a high fever develops and lasts for several hours. It may be accompanied by a severe headache, increased nausea and vomiting, profuse sweating, and often mild delirium. The paroxysm lasts 8 to 12 hours and terminates as the exhausted patient goes to sleep. On awakening, the patient usually feels relatively well. The growth of the parasite inside the red blood cells occurs at fixed intervals and this factor determines the frequency of paroxysms. The interval is 48 hours for *P. falciparum*; and paroxysms occur every 72 hours for *P. malariae*.

The severity of clinical symptoms produced varies among the different species. Generally infections with *P. falciparum* are the most severe. The continued destruction of red blood cells, with concurrent damage to the capillaries, RES, and various internal organs, may lead to the death of the patient. In many patients, the infection is somewhat suppressed and develops into a chronic disease. In others, the infection is suppressed and remains asymptomatic for many years. Occasionally symptomatic diseases may reoccur in these chronically infected persons.

The major mode of transmission of malaria is by the bite of the anopheles mosquito. A few cases may be transmitted by other means. Occasionally a chronically infected female may congenitally transmit malaria to her offspring. Blood transfusions or unsterilized paraphernalia used in the injection of illicit narcotics may also transmit malaria. Persons who have had malaria or who have, within the past three years, visited areas where malaria is endemic, are requested not to give blood for transfusions.

Laboratory diagnosis is made by observing the malarial parasites in stained slides of blood examined with a microscope.

Perhaps more effort has been made to develop methods for the treatment and control of malaria than for any other infectious disease. Although significant progress has been made, as yet no ''magic bullet'' or ''wonder drug'' is available as an easy cure of this disease. Control of the anopheline mosquito has been one of the major methods used to control or reduce the number of cases. Malaria has been significantly reduced in countries where wide-scale mosquito control programs were carried out. DDT was a highly effective insecticide in these programs and there is concern that the reduction in the use of DDT (for other environmental reasons) may result in an increase in malaria in some countries. Mosquito nets and insect repellents are of some value.

Chloroquine, primaquine, and pyrimethamine have been used with some success against malaria. These drugs can terminate a clinical disease, prevent recurrent attacks, and, if given long enough, result in a cure. These chemotherapeutic agents can also be used prophylactically to prevent the parasite from growing once it has infected the tissue. This type of prophylaxis is widely

Chloroquine—Resistant *Plasmodium falciparum* Malaria in West Africa: Nigeria, 1986

On May 27, 1986, a 50-year-old American helicopter mechanic traveled to Enugu, a city in the eastern state of Anambra, Nigeria. While in Nigeria, he took chloroquine 300 mg base weekly for malaria chemoprophylaxis and continued this regimen after returning to the United States via Lagos on December 6. He traveled only in eastern Nigeria and did not travel to other malarious countries. On December 9, he developed fever, chills, and headache, and was hospitalized in California on December 18.

On December 20, a peripheral blood smear revealed that 0.5% of red blood cells were infected with asexual *Plasmodium falciparum* parasites, and treatment with chloroquine 1500 mg base was administered over a 3-day period. He became afebrile on December 22, and a peripheral blood smear on December 23 showed rare trophozoites. On December 27, he again became febrile, and a blood smear on December 31 revealed a parasitemia of 1.0%. A whole-blood specimen collected on December 31 was analyzed by high performance liquid chromatography and contained 151 ng of chloroquine/ml, indicating that the treatment dosage of chloroquine had been adequately absorbed.

A parasite isolate collected on December 31 was assayed by the 48-hour in vitro test of Nguyen-Dinh and Trager and found to be resistant to chloroquine: parasite multiplication was inhibited only at 0.3 μmol of chloroquine/per liter of medium, a concentration higher than the accepted limit of in vitro chloroquine resistance (0.06 μmol/L). The patient responded promptly to treatment with quinine (650 mg three times daily for 3 days) and tetracycline (250 mg four times daily for 7 days) and has remained well. (*MMWR* 36:13, 1987).

used when large numbers of military personnel must enter malaria-infested areas, as they did during World War II and the Vietnam War. Malaria constituted one of the major problems in these military operations. Medications taken orally on a rigid daily or biweekly regimen can be quite effective. Military personnel in the field, however, often ignored the prescribed regimen because nausea and intestinal disturbances sometimes result from the medication. Furthermore, some military personnel, particularly in an unpopular war like Vietnam, preferred to contract malaria and be sent home for a cure rather than to remain at their combat positions with the possibility of an even less desirable fate. Research is currently in progress on a vaccine against malaria.

Toxoplasmosis In contrast to many protozoal diseases found mainly in tropical regions and under unsanitary conditions, toxoplasmosis occurs in all parts of the world and can be transmitted in cosmopolitan populations. Research has shown that from 25% to 50% of the world's population have been, or are now, infected with the toxoplasmosis parasite. Yet this disease in humans went virtually unrecognized until the 1940s and only a handful of cases had been specifically diagnosed during the 1950s.

The causative agent is a sporozoan called *Toxoplasma gondii*, which is a small, crescent-shaped organism (Figure 31-9), 4 to 8 μm long, with no appendages or prominent internal structures other than a nucleus. *T. gondii* is able to infect many animals and birds where it may set up an ideal parasitic relationship. Only in the past two decaces has the life cycle of *T. gondii* begun to be understood. It is now apparent that the primary hosts are various felines, with domestic cats the chief transmitters to humans (Figure 31-10). Cats become infected by eating mice, birds, or raw meat; they can also be infected by the feces of other cats. The *T. gondii* goes through a sexual phase of reproduction in the intestinal tract of cats. Reproductive structures called *oocysts* are shed in the feces and in 3 to 4 days, if warm and damp, eight infectious sporozoites develop within each oocyst. This mature oocyst may remain viable for up to 1 year and infect humans and animals when ingested. No sexual reproduction of the parasite occurs in nonfeline animals or humans. However, it is able to proliferate by bineary fission and circulate throughout the body. The parasite penetrates into cells and continues to proliferate until the cell bursts. As this process continues, clinical disease may result with such symptoms as fever, weakness, respiratory illness, myocarditis, or an infectious mononucleosislike illness with swollen lymph

Figure 31-9   Micrograph of the crescent-shaped *Toxoplasma gondii*. (S. S. Schneierson, *Atlas of Diagnostic Microbiology*, p. 69. Courtesy Abbott Laboratories, Abbott Park, IL.)

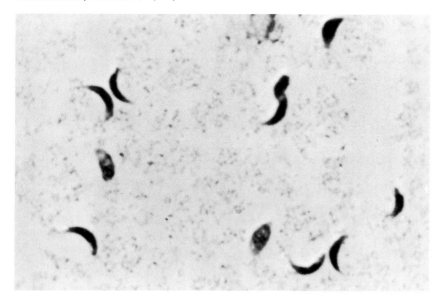

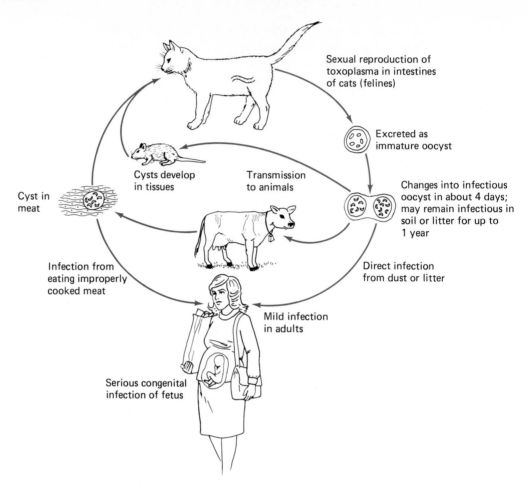

Figure 31-10   Transmission of toxoplasma in nature and to humans.

nodes. The disease is often asymptomatic or is passed off as some other disease. Only lately has a diagnosis of toxoplasmosis even been considered when dealing with such nondescript illnesses. As the immune mechanisms of the host respond and antibodies are produced, *T. gondii* remains inside the infected cells and forms aggregates of several thousand parasitic cells that become enclosed in a fine membrane to form a cyst. The cyst evokes no further response from the host. It does not cause any tissue damage and the enclosed parasites are protected from the host's defense mechanisms. Thus a near ideal parasitic relationship is established and may persist for the lifetime of the host. These cysts, however, may serve as a source of infection to a new host that may ingest the tissue. Undoubtably this is a major means of transmission to various carnivorous birds or animals in nature. It has also been well established that humans may become infected by eating raw or rare meat.

Toxoplasmosis: Pennsylvania, 1974

On September 2, 1974, two male members of a wedding party became ill with low-grade fever, chills, generalized aches, fatigue, and swollen cervical lymph nodes. On September 4 another male member similarly became ill. On September 30 a female member also became ill with identical symptoms but did not have swollen cervical lymph nodes. The fever, chills, and generalized aches in these four persons subsided unevenly over a period of weeks; the fatigue and swollen lymph nodes persisted for months.

The patients were at first treated symptomatically and with antibiotics by their respective physicians. When the illness persisted, however, toxoplasmosis was suspected, and sera were drawn in November and December from three of the four ill persons. Results by indirect fluorescent antibody (IFA) test were positive in all three persons for toxoplasmosis.

These results indicated a possible common source outbreak and epidemiologic investigation revealed that on August 23, 1974, the 4 ill persons were among a group of 19 people attending a wedding rehearsal supper at a Syrian restaurant. Food histories were obtained from 15 of the 19 guests and all 15 reported having eaten Kibee Nayee, a meat dish made from raw beef. Sera obtained 2 to 5 months after the common meal were then collected from 12 more of the guests. Of the total of 15 persons from whom sera were obtained, 8 had titers of $> 1:64$, compatible with a recent exposure to *Toxoplasma gondii* organisms. In all cases, however, serology was performed too long after the implicated meal to demonstrate a rise in titer and to confirm the meal's possible role in transmission. Moreover, 6 of the 9 individuals with antitoxoplasma antibody titers $> 1:16$ had a history of habititual ingestion of rare or raw meat. Of the 8 individuals with titers 1:64, 4 were clinically ill, but no statistically positive correlation was found between presence of symptoms and seropositivity. In cases of acquired toxoplasmosis, however, it is often impossible to obtain a history of symptomatic illness.

Editorial note: Although this investigation did not study serologic data from a control group of nonill persons, it appears likely that the illness resulted from eating raw meat at this restaurant. The high prevalence of antibodies (56%) among the 14 guests of Middle East origin may reflect their habit of eating undercooked meat. In Paris, France, where eating undercooked meat is perhaps the most important means of exposure to toxoplasma organisms, the prevalence of antibodies was 84% among 378 pregnant women studied.

Only one documented outbreak of food-borne toxoplasmosis has occurred in the United States, when five persons associated with the Cornell University Medical College acquired acute lymphadenopathic toxoplasmosis after eating inadequately cooked hamburger.

Because toxoplasma cysts have been found in samples of mutton, pork, and beef intended for human consumption, such meat should be heated to 56°C for 10 to 15 minutes to protect against toxoplasmosis infection. Freezing is considered a probable means of killing the tissue cysts, although viable toxoplasma organisms have been isolated from the carcass of a monkey frozen for 16 days at −20°C (*MMWR* 24:285, 1975).

In a great majority of cases, toxoplasmosis is mild and self-limiting. The major concern is congenital toxoplasmosis. This condition occurs when a pregnant female develops a primary case of toxoplasmosis by being in contact with cats or by eating raw or rare meat. During the systemic phase of the infection *T. gondii* is able to pass the placental barrier and infect the developing fetus. Congenital infection is most serious if it occurs after the first trimester of pregnancy. In such cases, there is a 50% chance that serious congenital defects will develop. Generally the tissue of the brain or eyes are involved. Some infants die in utero; others are born with serious CNS defects and die shortly after birth. In some cases, infected infants show no signs of disease but carry the toxoplasma parasite as a latent infection. Later in life the parasite may begin to proliferate, causing tissue damage. Other congenitally infected infants may remain symptomless throughout life. About 1 of every 1000 children born in the United States has congenital toxoplasmosis, which makes this disease one of the major congenital diseases.

If a female has acquired toxoplasmosis with the resultant antibody immunity before becoming pregnant, the developing fetus is protected against congenital infection. About 30% of the women of childbearing age in the United States have antibodies against this parasite. Some health officials are recommending serologic tests for toxoplasmosis during early pregnancy and suggest that those who are negative should avoid contact with cats or their feces, and also avoid rare or raw meat during their pregnancy. Such procedures should be followed by all pregnant females who have not had a serologic test for toxoplasmosis.

Diagnosis is made by examining tissues or fluids for the cysts of *T. gondii* and using serologic tests. Treatment is only effective during the systemic phase of the disease. A mixture of three different sulfa drugs in combination with the antimalarial drug pyrimethamine is used. There is no vaccine.

Other sporozoa infections Two ubiquitous sporozoa *Pneumocystis carinii* and *Cryptosporidium* have increasingly been recognized as causes of serious morbidity in immunocompromised patients. Pneumonia due to *P. carinii* has been recognized for many years as a complication of organ transplantation or cancer chemotherapy. However, as the epidemic of AIDS developed, this disease became the most common serious complication in these patients. The source of the organism is not clear. It is widely distributed in nature and probably occurs in otherwise healthy humans without producing disease. Diagnosis of this infection is difficult and frequently requires removal of fluids or tissues directly from the infected lung. Trimethoprim-sulfa or pentamidine are effective therapeutic agents. However, even with therapy as many as 30% of

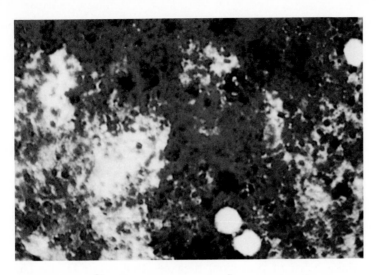

Figure 31-11 Photomicrograph of cryptosporidium parasites found in human intestinal specimen.

patients die, and the disease is the leading direct cause of death among AIDS patients.

Cryptosporidium (Figure 31-11) is also a sporozoan with a very broad host range. Many domestic animals harbor this organism in their intestinal tract, and it appears that most humans have had one or more infections due to this organism. Cryptosporidia cause a profuse watery diarrhea that appears to be self-limiting in the otherwise healthy host. However, in individuals with immune deficiencies such as AIDS, the diarrhea is severe and often prolonged. In AIDS patients the infection may be associated with malnutrition, malabsorption, and significant weight loss and may last for many months. No effective therapeutic agents are available.

CONCEPT SUMMARY

1. The protozoa are a diverse group that includes both free-living forms and animals parasites. A number of protozoa require a second animal host in addition to humans in order to complete their development. Such life cycles provide a variety of alternatives for exercising control measures against these organisms.

2. Protozoal diseases range in seriousness from the relatively benign giardiasis and trichomoniasis to the very common and severe diseases of malaria and amebic dysentery. Proto-zoan diseases are not only among the most common world-wide but are also among the most serious. Therapy of such infections remains limited and is often ineffective.

STUDY SUMMARY

1. List the morphologic and physiologic features of the proto-zoa that separate these organisms from the bacteria.
2. What features of pathogenesis associated with *E. histolytica* are responsible for the severity of disease due to this or-ganism?
3. Make a list of protozoal diseases that occur in the United States.
4. What features of protozoa limit possible antimicrobial ther-apy in humans?
5. Diagram and label the life cycle of *Plasmodium.*
6. Describe the sporozoa-host relationship.

REFERENCES FOR FURTHER STUDY

1. *Atlas of Human Parasitology,* L. Ash, 1980. American Society of Clinical Pathologists.
2. *Manual of Clinical Microbiology,* 4th ed., E. Lennette, 1985. American So-ciety for Clinical Microbiology.
3. Evaluation of Commercial Serodiagnostic Kits for Toxoplasmosis. *Jour-nal of Clinical Microbiology* 25:2262, 1987.
4. Infection and Diarrhea Caused by Cryptosporidium sp. among Guate-malan Infants. *Journal of Clinical Microbiology* 26:88, 1988.
5. *The Biologic and Clinical Basis of Infectious Diseases,* G. Youmans, 1985. Saunders.
6. Cryptosporidium and Cryptosporidiosis. *Reviews of Infectious Diseases* 8:1012, 1986.

chapter 32

VIRUSES

B efore the germ theory of disease was established, people believed that many diseases were caused by poisons. The Latin term for poison is *virus*. Then as discoveries during the nineteenth century showed that microorganisms were the cause of infectious diseases, the various pathogenic microbes were identified as bacteria, fungi, or protozoa and were removed from the category of poisons or viruses. Due to the inability to propagate viruses on artificial culture media or to observe them with standard optical microscopes, the virus particles went undiscovered during the so-called Golden Age of Microbiology in the late 1800s. Yet during this time it was recognized that many diseases were caused by agents that had not been identified and such unidentified agents were still referred to as virus. Around the turn of the century it was shown that the causative agents of some diseases could pass through filters that would hold back bacterial-sized cells and by the 1930s it was possible to crystallize these agents. This latter procedure showed that they were particulate agents and not chemical poisons. By this time, however, the term virus had become permanently associated with these agents and the original meaning was, to a large extent, lost.

All forms of life seem to have specific viruses that parasitize their cells. There are viruses of animals, plants, insects, bacteria, algae, fungi, and so on. The viruses that attack bacteria are called *bacteriophages* or just *phages* and are much easier to work with in laboratory experiments than animal or plant viruses. Thus many significant discoveries on the nature of viruses were made using phages. Fortunately, most viruses, regardless of the types of hosts they attack, function by many similar mechanisms and the information obtained through studies with phage has aided in studies of animal viruses. A great deal of information regarding the structure and function of viruses has been obtained in the past several

OUTLINE

decades. This chapter presents a brief summarization of the major characteristics and functions of viruses that infect animals.

STRUCTURE OF VIRUSES

Viruses range in size from about 20 nm to 300 nm in diameter. A virus possesses no independent metabolic capabilities and is thus totally dependent on a living host cell to supply all the needed energy and building blocks for its replication. A given virus contains only one molecule of one type of nucleic acid, which can be either DNA or RNA. Furthermore, the nucleic acid molecule may be either single-stranded or double-stranded. Some simple viruses consist only of the single molecule of nucleic acid and a protein coat. Other viruses may possess an envelope over the protein coat; in addition, some may have internal proteins and/or small projections called *peplomers* (Figure 32-1). The complete virus particle, regardless of its structure, is called a *virion*. Five basic morphological shapes (spherical, cylindrical, brick, bullet, and tailed) are seen among the viruses and are shown in Figure 32-2.

Most animal viruses contain fairly small amounts of genetic information, which means that they are limited in the number of different types of protein molecules that can be synthesized under their direction. Many viruses that cause disease in humans contain from 5 to 15 cistrons (genes) in their nucleic acid. Many viruses must construct their protein coat, called a **capsid**, out of just one or a few different types of polypeptides. The individual protein molecules that make up the building blocks of the capsid are called *structure units*. Viral capsids are symmetrical. Many capsids are constructed as regular icosahedrons—that is, an enclosed shell of 20 triangular faces, 12 vertices, and 30 edges (Figures 32-3 and 32-4). To form the icosahedral capsid, the structure units must first

Capsid

the external protein structure of a virus. The capsid is the "virus" observable by electron microscopy and is composed of external capsomers and internal nucleic acid.

Figure 32-1   A schematic outline of a virus. The protein coat is called the capsid. An envelope is present on some viruses and not on others. Peplomers are present on some viruses. One molecule of nucleic acid is contained inside the capsid. Some viruses may have additional internal proteins. The entire virus is called a virion.

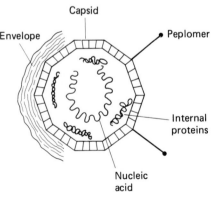

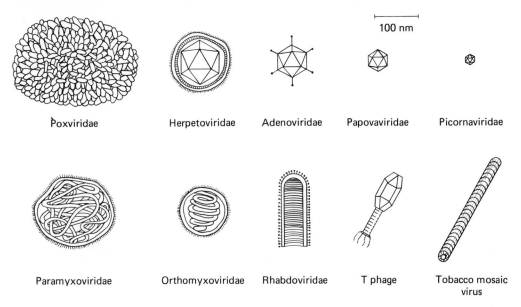

Poxviridae   Herpetoviridae   Adenoviridae   Papovaviridae   Picornaviridae

100 nm

Paramyxoviridae   Orthomyxoviridae   Rhabdoviridae   T phage   Tobacco mosaic virus

Figure 32-2   The basic shapes and relative sizes of some representative groups of viruses.

form into clusters of five, called *pentamers*, and clusters of six, called *hexamers*. These clusters are called *capsomers*. The number and arrangement of the capsomers in an icosahedron are restricted geometrically. The 12 vertices must be pentamers and one of the smallest possible icosahedrons is composed of only the 12 pentamers. As the icosahedron increases in size, hexamers are

Figure 32-3   Models of viruses made from repeated copies of identical interconnecting structure units (plastic triangles) to form capsids with either cubical or helical symmetry. (Jensen Research Laboratories)

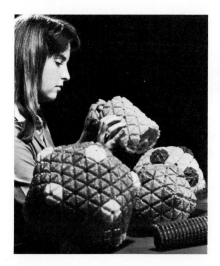

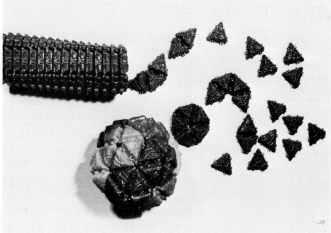

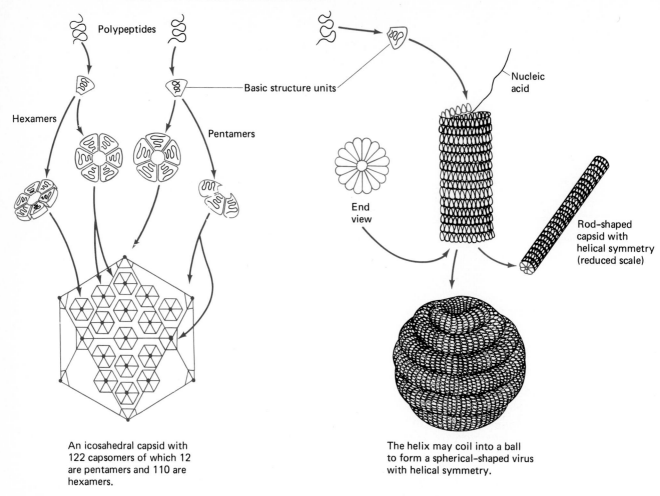

An icosahedral capsid with 122 capsomers of which 12 are pentamers and 110 are hexamers.

The helix may coil into a ball to form a spherical-shaped virus with helical symmetry.

Figure 32-4 The formation of viral capsids with cubical and helical symmetry from polypeptides that form the basic structure units.

added between the pentamers in regular increments. The number of pentamers remains constant at 12, however. The smallest number of hexamers that will fit is 20—that is, one for each triangular face of the icosahedron. The result is a virus with a total of 32 capsomers (12 pentamers and 20 hexamers). Other increments of capsomers that can form into icosahedrons are 42, 72, 92, 122, 162, 252, and so on. The number of capsomers of a given virus is constant and serves as a useful characteristic in classifying and identifying viruses. Icosahedral viruses are said to have *cubical symmetry*. The nucleic acid is packaged inside the icosahedral capsid.

Other viruses have *helical symmetry*, which refers to an arrangement of structure units connected side by side in a continuous ribbon that spirals into a tubular helix. The nucleic acid is connected to each structure unit much like a string that is connected along a row of beads. The tubular helix may remain extended to form a cylindrical-shaped virus or it may coil into a ball to form a spherical-shaped virus (Figures 32-3 and 32-4). A few larger viruses have more complex structures.

CULTIVATION OF VIRUSES

Viruses can only be propagated in living host cells, and a major activity in a viral laboratory is to provide a suitable supply of such cells. The main sources of cells for the propagation of animal viruses are intact animals, **embryonated eggs**, and organ, tissue, or cell cultures. The injection of viruses into susceptible living animals gives useful information on the pathogenesis of viral diseases but is usually not a useful method of producing large amounts of viruses for vaccines or experimental studies. When dealing with human viruses, an attempt is made to find an experimental animal that will support the multiplication of the virus and produce a disease similar to that seen in humans. Such attempts are not always successful, however, for many viruses are host-specific; that is, human viruses will only multiply in human cells, cat viruses in cat cells, and so forth. Yet it is possible to get some specific human viruses to multiply in such primates as monkeys or chimpanzees, an experimental procedure that is expensive and cumbersome. If there is no chance that the virus will cause death, permanent damage, or undue discomfort, human volunteers may be used in virus research. For example, human volunteers have been used in research on the common cold for many years. Even though research using intact hosts has many limitations, it is often the only means available to study some diseases.

Embryonated eggs
fertilized eggs in which the embryo has been permitted to grow to a recognizable stage of development.

Embryonated eggs provide an inexpensive, easy-to-handle, sterile container full of a variety of living cells (Figure 32-5). Some animal viruses will multiply in embryonated eggs; others will not. Often, embryonated eggs are used to produce large amounts of viruses for vaccines. A small hole can be drilled through the egg shell and virus can be injected into the appropriate embryonic tissue. Generally embryos between 7 to 10 days of age are used.

The development of methods to grow living animal cells routinely in test tubes (in vitro) greatly accelerated research work with animal viruses by making it possible to discover many new viruses, grow large amounts of viruses, and develop sensitive quantitative assays for many viruses. The impact of cell-culturing procedures is dramatized by the fact that in the late 1940s, when these procedures first came into wide use, only about 35 viruses associated with human diseases had been discovered. During the fol-

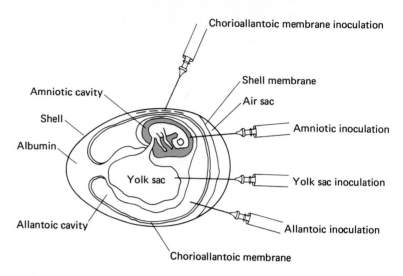

Figure 32-5   An embryonated egg showing the routes of inoculation.

lowing 15 to 20 years, 500 additional viruses associated with humans were identified and tremendous advances were made in our understanding of the nature of viruses. *Organ culture* is a procedure in which a section of an organ is taken from an intact host and the cells of that organ are kept alive by immersing them in a nutrient fluid in a test tube. This procedure is difficult to carry out and has limited use. The terms *tissue culture* and *cell culture* are often used interchangeably. In the technical sense, however, tissue culture means implanting tissue fragments into test tubes and allowing cells to grow out from these fragments. Cell culture is the most widely used method of growing cells in vitro. A wide variety of tissues can be used, but tissues from embryos generally work best. To produce cell cultures, the tissue is cut into small pieces and treated with an enzyme that splits proteins (i.e., is proteolytic); this process causes the cells to separate into a suspension of single cells or small clumps of several cells. These cells are then washed, suspended in a nutrient medium, and placed in specially cleaned glass or plastic containers. The cells settle onto and adhere to the surface and begin to divide. Usually after several days a continuous monolayer (a layer that is one cell deep) will form over the surface. These cells can again be treated with a proteolytic enzyme and the cells of the monolayer will disassociate into a suspension of single cells. The cells can then be passed to new containers where they will continue to multiply. Enough cells can be obtained from one container to seed two or three new containers. Some cells can be passed only 5 or 6 times, others up to 100 times, and yet other cells adapt so well to cell cultures that they can be passed indefinitely. One particular cell culture line, called *Hela cells*, was started from human cancer tissue in 1952 and is still being passed at the present time. A procedure for setting up a cell culture is shown in Figure 32-6. It is now possible to grow some cell cultures in fluid suspensions without forming a monolayer and to grow monolayers of cells on large numbers of small beads in a container. Both of these procedures greatly increase the density of cells that can be grown in a given container.

Much current work in virology uses cell cultures for the detection, propagation, and measurement of viruses. When viruses are placed on a monolayer, the cells become infected and are usually destroyed. Different patterns of cell destruction, referred to

Figure 32-6 A procedure for setting up a cell culture and the production of viral plaques in the cell monolayer.

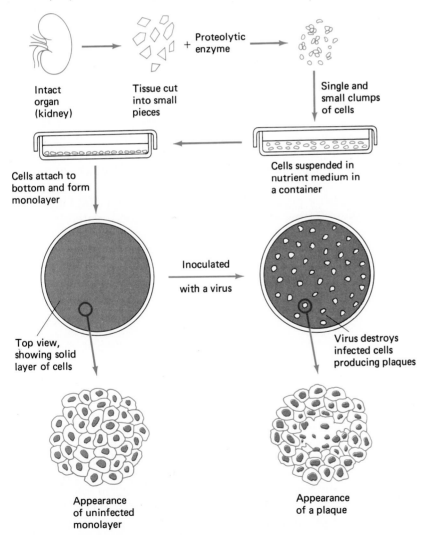

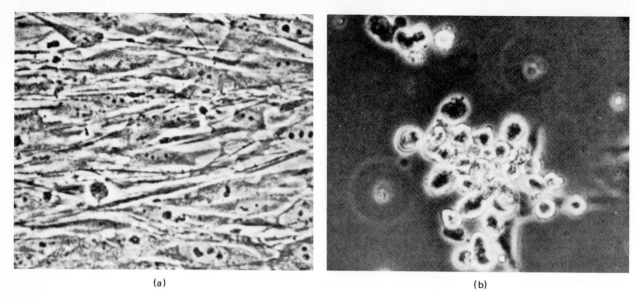

Figure 32-7 Cytopathic effect of toxic materials or viruses on tissue culture cells; (a) Normal tissue culture; (b) cells in the presence of cytotoxic materials. (vero cells ×200) (Courtesy M. R. Popoff, *Inf. Imm. 55:35*)

Plaque

an area of cell destruction caused by the propagation of a single virus in a monolayer of cells.

as the *cytopathic effect*, are produced by different viruses and can be observed with an optical microscope (Figure 32-7). If the viruses are sufficiently dilute, an isolated area of cells in the otherwise continuous monolayer is destroyed. This area of destroyed cells is called a **plaque** and is a useful method of counting the number of viruses in a given sample.

Cell culture procedures are useful in areas of biology other than virology. Using this technique cells can be isolated from the complex interactions of an intact animal and studied under controlled conditions in a test tube. The process of isolation and subsequent propagation of a single cell taken from a multicellular organism is called *cloning* and has many useful applications in various areas of biology.

MULTIPLICATION OF VIRUSES

When studying the subject of viral multiplication, the virus should be viewed as a segment of genetic information that becomes inserted into the "genetic pool" of the host cell. The only contribution of the virus to its host cell is a single molecule of nucleic acid (the *viral genome*) and, in some cases, an enzyme for the transcription of this nucleic acid. All other components involved in the multiplication of the virus are supplied by the host cell. Some viruses have a profound effect on the host cell, for they redirect most of the cellular metabolic processes to the production of new viral components. Such a redirection usually results in the destruction of the infected cell. Other viruses may set up a less dramatic relationship in which they do not seriously interfere with the cell's metabolic processes and redirect only a small percentage of the cellular components into the production of new virus particles. Some viruses are able to insert their nucleic acid into the DNA of the host cell, where no influence is manifested and the viral genome replicates and rides along with the DNA of the host cell. In some cases, the viral genome that becomes inserted into the host cell DNA is partially transcribed and imparts specific traits to the host cell.

Throughout all other biological processes in nature, protein synthesis is directed by the same reliable mechanism of information contained in double-stranded (ds) DNA molecules being transcribed into single-stranded (ss) mRNA molecules, which, in turn, direct the synthesis of polypeptides through the process of translation. These reactions are summarized as ds-DNA→mRNA→ protein. When dealing with viruses, however, not only is the conventional ds-DNA→mRNA→protein pathway used but so are a variety of other modified pathways. Viruses can be divided into at least the following six classes, based on the type of nucleic acid they contain and on the pathways used to express their genetic information.

Class 1: Viruses with ds-DNA   The flow of information is ds-DNA→mRNA→protein. This is the classical pathway seen in all higher forms of life. An example of this class of viral multiplication is outlined in Figure 32-8.

Class 2: Viruses with ss-DNA   The flow of information is ss-DNA→ds- DNA→mRNA→protein. The ss-DNA must first be changed into ds-DNA, which is done by cellular enzymes after the viral nucleic acid enters the cell. Afterward the flow of information is the same as in Class 1.

Class 3: Viruses with ds-RNA   The flow of information is ds-RNA→mRNA→protein. This class of viruses presents a unique problem because ds-RNA is not found in normal cells. Thus no enzyme is present in a cell to direct the transcripton of ds-RNA molecules. To solve this problem, these viruses direct the synthesis of a special enzyme that will transcibe mRNA from the ds-RNA molecule. This enzyme is packaged inside the viral capsid along with the ds-RNA.

Class 4: Viruses with ss-RNA of the same polarity as mRNA (called ss-RNA⁺)   The information flow is simply mRNA→protein. The viral nucleic acid acts directly as mRNA once inside the cell and completely bypasses the regular step of transcription.

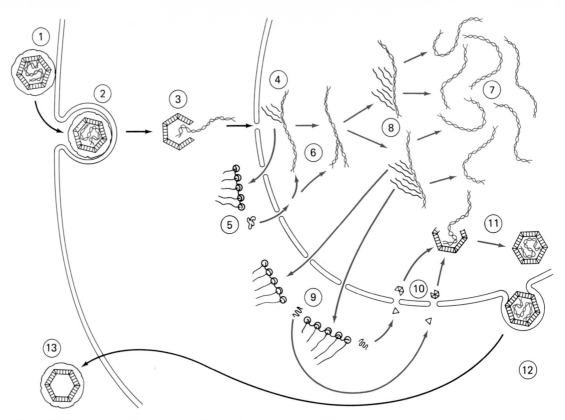

Figure 32-8 Some of the steps in the replication of a ds-DNA virus (i.e., a herpesvirus). (1) Specific attachment. (2) Penetration. (3) Release of viral nucleic acid and its migration to the cell nucleus. (4) Early transcription of viral DNA, directed by cellular enzymes. (5) Translation of viral *m*RNA and synthesis of an enzyme needed to replicate viral DNA. (6) Replication of viral DNA. (7) Synthesis of many viral DNA molecules. (8) Late transcription of viral DNA. (9) Translation of late viral *m*RNA with the synthesis of basic structure units. (10) Formation of capsomers. (11) Assembly of capsid around viral DNA. (12) Budding of virus from the nuclear membrane and picking up of an envelope. (13) Release of virus from the cell. The herpesviruses are able to produce about 500 new viruses in 10 hours from each infected cell.

Class 5: Viruses with ss-RNA of the opposite polarity from mRNA (called ss-RNA⁻) The information flow is ss-RNA⁻→mRNA protein. As in Class 3, this is a unique situation in which a function not found in a normal cell must be carried out—that is, the transcription of mRNA from a ss-RNA molecule. It is therefore necessary to provide a specific enzyme to accomplish this task. These viruses carry this special enzyme and also direct its formation as part of their replication process. An example of this class is outlined in Figure 32-9.

Class 6: Viruses with ss-RNA⁺ and a special enzyme called reverse transcriptase or RNA-dependent DNA polymerase Some viruses of Class 6 are associated with the induction of cancer in animals

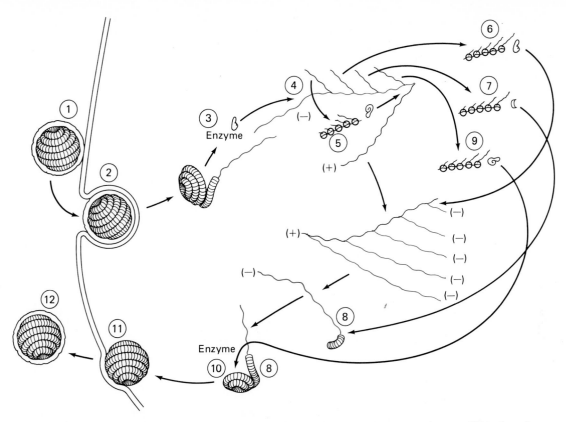

Figure 32-9   An interpretation of some of the major steps in the replication of an ss-RNA virus (i.e., a virus with a ss-RNA molecule of opposite polarity from the *m*RNA and thus it must carry its own enzyme for transcribing *m*RNA). All steps occur in the cytoplasm. (1) Attachment. (2) Penetration. (3) Uncoating with release of viral RNA and enzyme. (4) Transcription of viral RNA to *m*RNAs by the enzyme carried by the virus. (5) Translation of a viral *m*RNA with the formation of an enzyme that will direct the synthesis of complimentary copy of the viral RNA. (6) Synthesis of an enzyme that directs the synthesis of negative ss-RNA copies off the positive copies synthesized in step 5; these negative copies are identical to the original viral RNA. (7) Synthesis of structure units. (8) Formation of helical capsid around the viral RNA. (9) Synthesis of the enzyme to be packaged in the virus. (10) Packaging of enzyme in the virus. (11) Budding capsid and picking up of an envelope. (12) Release of complete virion. Hundreds of viruses are made in each infected cell.

and others cause the immunodeficiency syndrome (AIDS). These viruses change the genetic information on their ss-RNA molecule into a ds-DNA molecule or, in other words, move backward from the normal flow of genetic information. The information flow is ss-RNA→ss-DNA→ds-DNA→mRNA→protein. The enzyme reverse transcriptase is needed for the step from ss-RNA to ss-DNA. Normal cellular enzymes are able to direct the other functions. When the ds-DNA is formed, it may insert into the DNA of the host cell. Under certain conditions that are not well understood some of the information in this inserted DNA may be transcribed and direct changes in the cell that may cause cancer. Under other conditions the inserted DNA may be transcribed and direct the formation of new virus particles.

Steps in Viral Replication

The replication of animal viruses can be divided into the following general steps:

Viral attachment
the attachment of virus particles to specific receptor sites on a cell. These receptor sites and attachment sites define the host-range of viruses.

Pinocytosis
a process analogous to phagocytosis where the ingested material is a liquid or very small particle.

1. *Attachment to the cell surface.* **Viral attachment** is a specific reaction and only cells that have the correct receptor site can be infected by a specific virus. This phenomenon accounts for the ability of a virus to infect only a certain animal species or only a given tissue within the infected animal.

2. *Penetration into the cytoplasm.* After attachment has occurred, the plasma membrane invaginates into the cytoplasm and forms a vacuole around the virus. This process is called **pinocytosis**.

3. *Release of viral nucleic acid.* The viral capsid is broken down by cellular enzymes and the nucleic acid is released. This procedure may occur in either the nucleur or the cytoplasm, depending on the type of virus.

4. *Transciption of viral nucleic acid.* This process occurs in the cytoplasm for some viruses and in the nucleus for others. The various modes of transcription were discussed earlier.

5. *Translation of viral-directed mRNA.* Cellular ribosomes, tRNA, amino acids, energy, and other inputs are used in this step to bring about the synthesis of the proteins needed for the synthesis of new viral particles.

6. *Replication of viral nucleic acid.* One or more proteins produced under the direction of the viral genome function as enzymes for directing the synthesis of new viral nucleic acid molecules. The original viral nucleic acid molecule must serve as a template.

7. *Assembly of virus particles.* Viruses do not replicate by dividing as cells do but are assembled from pools of the viral nucleic acid and protein structure units. Many copies of a virus may be forming simultaneously within a single cell. Assembly may occur in the nucleus or cytoplasm, or partly in one and partly in the other area, depending on the type of virus. Assembly of the protein structure units into capsomers and then into capsids was described earlier. As the capsid forms, it encloses the viral nucleic acid. This process is not efficient, however, and often the capsid forms without enclosing the nucleic acid. It is called an *empty virus particle*. Often enough viral building blocks are produced to make 10,000 to 20,000 new virus particles per infected cell. Because of the inefficient assembly, however, only 200 to 300 particles will be properly

Rapid Laboratory Virus Diagnosis

Recent advances in rapid diagnostic techniques: Existing rapid diagnostic techniques and recent relevant advances pertaining to a number of viral infections were reviewed. The major advances in viral respiratory disease diagnosis include the successful extension of immunofluorescence techniques to more laboratories, use of large-scale production of antibodies in eggs, and development of sensitive solid-phase immunoassays for detection of virus antigens in nasopharyngeal secretions. For diarrheal diseases, immunoassays for both rotaviruses and adenoviruses have been further refined and standardized, and monoclonal antibodies have been used in ELISA tests for rotavirus. In the hepatitis area, advances include growth of hepatitis. A virus in tissue-culture systems, use of antigens for IgM immunoassays, the recent production of hepatitis B core antigen from bacteria through genetic engineering, and development of immunoassays for both antigen and antibody associated with the "delta" antigen. The diagnosis of dengue has been facilitated by development of monoclonal antibodies to all four dengue types. Detection of IgM antibodies during the acute phase of both dengue and Japanese encephalitis is of value in rapid diagnosis. Development of microscopic slides containing stable, inactivated, formalin-fixed antigens for Lassa and Ebola viruses has facilitated the detection of antibodies by immunofluorescence.

General recommendations: The Group recommended that a coordinated program be developed to ensure the availability of reagents within the network of WHO Collaborating Centres and National Laboratories for the diagnosis of the following diseases: viral hepatitis; respiratory viral diseases, including measles; viral gastroenteritis; anthropod- and rodent-borne viral diseases; rubella; and herpes-virus-group diseases.

To implement a program in each of these areas, it was agreed that coordinators within the WHO Collaborating Centers, together with their associates, be appointed and assume responsibility for (1) identifying specific tests recommended for rapid diagnosis, taking into account considerations of cost, simplicity, and accuarcy; (2) defining reagents and test material required and identifying specific suppliers of reagents; (3) defining minimum standards of quality and performance of reagents and other material; (4) developing a strategy for distributing reagents within the network of WHO Collaborating Centres for Reference and Research and cooperating national laboratories; (5) assisting WHO in developing and implementing training courses and selecting suitable candidates for training; (6) evaluating rapid virus diagnostic tests performed in field situations; and (7) soliciting and reviewing informations on new tests and new reagents, including monoclonal antibodies that might have application in rapid virus diagnosis (*MMWR* 31:568, 1982).

assembled. Even so, the fact that the entire process may only take an hour or two to produce several hundred offspring makes it an effective means of reproduction.

8. *Release of viruses.* Some viruses are released when the cell disintegrates as a result of the damage produced by the replication process. These viruses would have no envelopes. Other

viruses migrate to a cell membrane and bud out through the membrane. The membrane pinches off and remains attached to the virus, thus forming the envelope. With some viruses, viral-directed proteins are formed and become embedded in the cell membrane and thus incorporated into the envelope.

CONCEPT SUMMARY

1. Viruses are submicroscopic structures containing both nucleic acid and protein. These structures are not capable of self-replication but require living host cells for synthesis and development. Hundreds of viruses have been identified, but it is possible that thousands exist. They are known to be responsible for many human, plant, and animal diseases and yet also appear to exist as commensals without harming their host cells.

2. Viruses have specific host cells that they infect. This specificity is determined by viral protein surface structure and corresponding host cell receptors. For convenience in studying viruses, they are frequently cultivated in vitro in organ or cell culture systems.

3. A variety of viral replication methods have evolved. The exact nature of these replicative processes depends upon the type of nucleic acid in the virus genome. There are at least six variations of virus replication although the procedures involved in attachment, penetration, release of nucleic acid, and other activities are similiar among all viruses.

STUDY SUMMARY

1. Write a short paragraph that describes the general properties of viruses.

2. What are the two most common forms of symmetry of viral capsids?

3. Define each of the following terms: (a) capsid, (b) organ culture, (c) cytopathic effect, (d) cell culture, (e) tissue culture, (f) plaque, and (g) clone.

4. Diagram the process of nucleic acid replications for each of the six classes of viruses illustrated in the chapter.

5. What feature of possible host cells and virus accounts for host specificity?

6. Describe the process of viral maturation (virus assembly).

REFERENCES FOR FURTHER STUDY

1. *The Microbial World*, 5th ed., R. Stanier, 1986. Prentice-Hall.

2. How an Animal Virus Gets into and out of Its Host Cell. *Scientific American* 246:58, 1982.

3. *Fundamental Virology*, B. Fields, 1986. Raven.

4. *Molecular Virology*, Y. Becker, 1983. Martinus Nijhoff.

5. The First Human Retrovirus. *Scientific American* 255:88, 1986.

6. Progress and Problems in Creating RNA Virus Vaccines. *Microbiology—1985*, p. 282. American Society for Microbiology.

INTRODUCTION TO VIRAL DISEASES

The outcome of the multiplication of viruses in an animal host may vary from rapidly progressing destruction of tissues with resulting disease and death to a completely inconsequential relationship in which the viruses multiply at a low level or are dormant and cause no damage or disease. Some general effects of viruses on individual cells and the general characteristics of viral infections are discussed in this chapter.

EFFECTS OF VIRUSES ON CELLS

Cellular Destruction

Many viruses enter the host cell and promptly rearrange the cellular components into those needed for the assembly of viruses. These viruses are often able to turn off the metabolic pathways of the cell. The result is a rapid degradation of the cellular components with the resultant disintegration of the cell. This process may require 15 minutes for some viruses to several hours for many others. During this process, changes may be observed in the infected cells. Aggregates of viral materials or cell debris may collect in areas of the cell and are called *inclusion bodies*. Characteristic inclusion bodies occur with some viral infections and serve as useful diagnostic aids (Figure 33-1). Usually within a few days these cell-destroying viruses have caused enough damage that symptoms of the clinical diseases begin to appear in the host. The common acute viral diseases are caused by these cell-destroying viruses.

Cellular Alterations

Some viruses enter the host cells and replicate without significantly interfering with normal cellular functions. Only about 1% of the cellular components is "pirated" for the production of new

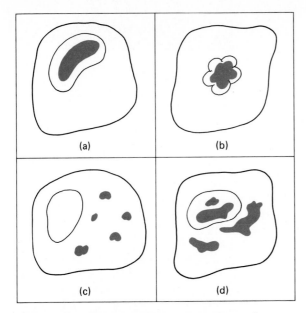

Figure 33-1 Some examples of the types of inclusion bodies formed when different viruses infect cells. (a) Intranuclear inclusions from a herpes-virus infection. (b) A rosette-type intranuclear inclusion from an adenovirus infection. (c) Intracytoplasmic inclusions (Negri bodies) from rabies virus infection. (d) Both intranuclear and intracytoplasmic inclusions in the same cell from a measles virus infection.

viruses. These viruses are gradually released from the cell by budding through the cell membrane without causing apparent damage. With such infections a balance may be maintained for years between the host cell and the infecting virus, a situation known as **viral latency**. Because of the lack of observable changes, this type of virus-cell relationship has been difficult to study. There is evidence, however, that after many years the host's immune mechanisms may react against these latently infected cells. The immune reaction or other effects of the virus may lead to the slow degeneration of the infected tissue. It has now been determined that several chronic degenerative diseases of humans may be caused by such infections, which are called *slow virus infections*. Only two such diseases of humans have been shown to be caused by slow viruses: *Creutzfeldt-Jakob disease* and *kuru*. Both are rare; kuru is found only in one tribe of natives living under primitive cannibalistic conditions in New Guinea. There is some indirect evidence that such diseases as multiple sclerosis and muscular dystrophy may also be caused by yet-unidentified slow viruses.

Viral latency
viral infection of a cell where there is no apparent effect of the infection, or where new virus develops so slowly that the infected cell survives for a long time.

Update: Creutzfeldt-Jakob Disease in a Patient Receiving a Cadaveric Dura Mater Graft: United States, 1987

CDC and the Food and Drug Administration (FDA) have investigated a case of Creutzfeldt-Jakob disease (CJD) in a 28-year-old woman who died 22 months after receiving a lyophilized, irradiated human cadaveric dura mater graft. They found that the most likely source of the disease was the graft, LYODURA (Lot 2105), produced by B. Braun Melsungen AG, Federal Republic of Germany. The CDC/FDA investigators were unable to obtain the identity of the donor of the implicated graft or to trace the disposition of other tissues from this donor. A representative of the producer of LYODURA reported that the company does not maintain records identifying donors and mixes dura from multiple donors during processing of a single lot. As a result of this investigation, FDA issued a Safety Alert on April 28, 1987, recommending disposal of all LYODURA from packages bearing a four-digit lot number beginning with the digit "2" (the code for material packaged in 1982) as well as all unmarked LYODURA.

CDC conducted a telephone survey of ten other known producers of dura mater used in the United States. All reported maintaining records that allow identification and tracing of each donor of a particular lot of product and of the recipient institution. In addition, it was found that these producers process dura from each donor individually so that there is no contact with or co-mingling of dura from different donors.

Editorial note: Because of the differences between the processing of LYODURA and of other products, LYODURA may carry a higher risk of transmitting CJD than other dura mater products used in the United States. As indicated in the FDA Safety Alert, current procedures used to sterilize human dura mater are not adequate to inactivate the CJD agent, and even the most stringent donor screening cannot exclude asymptomatic prepatent carriers of CJD. Thus, the use of any human dura mater product carries some risk of transmission of CJD, and procedures that minimize the risk are important. Alternatives to these products, such as autologous fascia or synthetic materials, are available.

The potential for human tissue products to transmit infectious agents has been documented for several procedures other than this single case in a recipient of a dura mater graft. There have been reports of presumed transmission of rabies and CJD by corneal transplantation, of human immunodeficiency virus (HIV) by organ transplantation, and of hepatitis B and HIV by artificial insemination.

The methods of production and distribution of human tissue products are not routinely subjected to FDA inspection and approval. Health care providers are urged to use human tissue products that have been handled according to strict guidelines such as those established by the American Association of Tissue Banks. In addition, hospitals should maintain records so that infections associated with human tissue products can be linked with specific lot numbers of these products *MMWR* 36:325, 1987).

Certain DNA viruses are able to enter a cell and their DNA becomes integrated into the DNA of the host cell. This integrated DNA may impart new characteristics to the cell but will not direct the formation of new viruses. This phenomenon has been well studied in bacteriophages and is called *lysogeny*. In some cases, the bacteriophage carries a gene for an important cellular product. The ability to produce diphtheria toxin in the bacterium *C. diphtheriae* is made possible by the presence of a genome from a bacteriophage. The phenomenon of lysogeny is not well documented with animal viruses; however, such DNA viruses as herpesvirus (Chapter 35) and adenovirus (Chapter 34) seem able to insert their DNA into that of the host cells, where the viral genome may be carried in a latent form for many years. At a later time, when the viral genome is released from the cellular DNA, it may then direct the formation of new viruses with the resultant cell destruction and disease.

Cellular Transformation

A special type of alteration, called *transformation*, may occur following the insertion of viral nuclei acid into host cell DNA. Transformed cells are cancer cells that multiply rapidly and do not respond to the normal mechanisms that control cellular proliferation. The causes of many types of cancer are not known, but animal experiments have shown that certain types are caused by viruses. Well-documented studies have demonstrated that a number of ds-DNA viruses are able to produce **tumors** in animals. The papovaviruses (Table 33-1) are primarily tumor-producing viruses and certain strains are able to produce tumors in mice, rabbits, and other experimental animals. These tumors are most effectively produced when the papovaviruses are injected into newborn animals. The only tumors known to be induced in humans by a papovavirus are common warts. Some human adenoviruses (Chapter 34) have been shown to produce tumors when injected into baby rodents, but there is no evidence of adenovirus-induced cancer in humans. Herpesvirus (Chapter 35) are able to produce cancer in their specific animal hosts. Some herpesviruses of humans are suspected of causing cancer.

At present, there is much interest in the cancer-producing capabilities of the RNA-containing retroviruses (Table 33-1). Retroviruses are the members of replication Class 6 described in Chapter 32. They contain ss-RNA and the reverse transcriptase enzyme. The ability to carry out reverse or *retro* transcription from RNA to DNA is the basis for the current name of this group of viruses. As early as 1910 it was shown that a retrovirus, called *Rous sarcoma* virus, could produce cancer in chickens. In the past few decades retroviruses that cause cancer in mice, cats, baboons, and other experimental animals have been found. At first the induction of cancer by these ss-RNA viruses presented a dilemma, for it is impossible for the ss-RNA molecule to become inserted into the ds-DNA molecules of the host cells. This dilemma was resolved when the phenomenon of reverse transcription was discovered in the 1960s and showed how it is possible to change the

Tumor
abnormal cell growth.

Table 33-1   The Classification into Families of Viruses that Infect Animals

Type of Nucleic Acid	Symmetry of Capsid	Envelope	(Size (nm)	Number of Capsomers	Family
RNA	Cubical	−	24–30	32	Picornaviridae
	"	−	35–39	32	Caliciviridae
	"	−	60–80	32	Reoviridae
	"	+	60–70	32	Togaviridae
	"	+	40–50	32	Flaviviridae
	Helical	+	80–120	—	Orthomyxoviridae
	"	+	150–300	—	Paramyxoviridae
	"	+	60 × 180[a]	—	Rhabdoviridae
	"	+	80 × 800[b]	—	Filoviridae[c]
	"	+	60–220	—	Coronaviridae
	"	+	80–110	—	Bunyaviridae
	Uncertain	+	80–100	—	Retroviridae
	"	+	50–300	—	Arenaviridae
DNA	Cubical	−	18–26	32	Parvoviridae
	"	−	45–55	72	Papovaviridae
	"	−	70–90	252	Adenoviridae
	"	+	40–50	?	Hepadnaviridae
	"	+	120–200	162	Herpesviridae
	"	+	130–300	1500	Iridoviridae
	Complex	−	230–300	—	Poxviridae

[a]Bullet-shaped.
[b]Filamentous.
[c]Proposed new family.

genetic information in a ss-RNA molecule into genetic information in a ds-DNA molecule. The ds-DNA molecule is able to insert into the host cell DNA to induce the cellular transformation. Evidence suggest that certain forms of cancer in humans, primarily leukemia and breast cancer, may be caused by retroviruses.

Not all retroviral infections result in cell transformation. The human immunodeficiency virus (HIV), which causes AIDS, is a retrovirus but is able to produce lytic (destructive) infections in some cells. Other cells infected with HIV may permit long-term chronic infection with a rather gradual release of the virus. Integration of the viral DNA into host DNA is possible with this virus, but direct tumor formation is not a usual consequence of these infections.

INTERFERON PRODUCTION

Considering the rapid multiplication of cell-destroying viruses, it would seem that massive numbers of cells of the infected host could be destroyed in a relatively short time. Along with host defense mechanisms, such as phagocytosis and antibody formation, cells have a special built-in defense mechanism that produces a group of substances called *interferons* that limit the proliferation of viruses. Interferons are a group of different proteins produced by cells of vertebrates following infections by viruses and following stimulation by some antigens. Three distinct types of interferons have been identified and are called *alpha, beta,* and *gamma.* About 12 different varieties of alpha and one or two varieties of beta interferon have been found. Alpha and beta interferons are induced by any virus in most infected cells. Only one variety of gamma interferon has been identified and it is produced only by lymphocytes following antigenic stimulation. Gamma interferon seems to function much like some of the lymphokines discussed in Chapter 12. In fact, as our knowledge of interferons increases, it appears that interferons and lymphokines represent a large group of **immunomodulating** proteins and the full actions and interactions of these proteins are as yet not fully understood.

Immunomodulation
regulation of the immune system.

Interferons induce protection against all viruses, not only the type of virus that stimulated their production, and are thus nonspecific in their antiviral action. It has been hoped that interferons might prove to be effective antiviral chemotherapeutic agents; in fact, much effort has been made to use interferons in treating viral infections. A major limitation has been the species specificity of interferons; that is, interferons produced by human cells will induce protection only in other human cells. Therefore it was not possible to produce interferon in such hosts as experimental animals or embryonated eggs for use in treating humans. In the 1970s methods were developed for producing some interferon in human white blood cells and fibroblasts grown in cell culture systems. This interferon was effective in treating some human viral infections, but only small amounts could be produced, which made treatments very expensive. Most applications were limited to research trials. Another limitation is the short duration of protection offered by interferon, which is about 2 weeks.

In the 1980s, the genes for human interferons were cloned into bacteria and yeast cells using genetic engineering technology. This made large amounts of human interferons available for research and clinical trials. There has been much optimism that interferons would function as the long-sought-after effective antiviral therapeutic agents. While these genetically engineered interferons have shown some effects in treating certain viral infections, the hoped for dramatic effect on treating many viral diseases has as yet not been realized. Much research work is still going on with various forms and combinations of interferons which may yet yield effective ways of using these proteins for antiviral treatments. Some interferons have also shown promise in treating certain forms of cancer.

Most evidence indicates that interferons function in intact animal hosts as important rapidly mobilized natural defense mechanisms against viral infections. Interferons probably play a vital role in slowing down the destructive effects of rapidly multiplying viruses during the early stages of the infection and thus allow the host to survive long enough for the humoral and cell-mediated immune responses to be mobilized to react specifically against the invading virus.

The mode of interferon production and action is outlined in Figure 33-2. Interferons are proteins that are stable and readily diffuse out of the cells in which they are produced. When they reach adjacent cells, they attach to specific receptors on the cell membrane and induce a series of cascading reactions that eventually result in blocking the replication of viruses in these cells. In these reactions, at least three new enzymes are induced that catalyze the synthesis of short segments of nucleotides; these in turn activate endonuclease enzymes that then destroy mRNAs, which prevents the synthesis of proteins that are needed to produce the infecting virus. Some of these intermediate proteins have now been produced through genetic engineering and may also prove to be effective agents for treating viral infections.

Figure 33-2   A simplified outline of the production and action of interferon. (1) Viral or chemical inducer of interferon enters the cell. (2) The virus induces derepression of the interferon-producing gene. (3) New viruses produced and released from cell. (4) *m*RNA for interferon synthesized. (5) Interferon produced and secreted from cell. (6) Interferon binds to wall of adjacent cells. (7) The binding triggers secondary reactions that induce mechanisms that interfere with the replication of any viruses that might enter this cell.

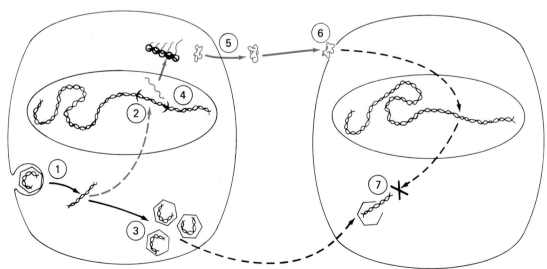

SIGNIFICANCE OF VIRAL DISEASES

Many of the infectious diseases of humans are caused by viruses. Fortunately, today, most are not serious; that is, they are not life-threatening and they do not require hospitalization. Still, they cause discomfort and incapacitation and are disruptive overall to normal human activities. Many serious problems still result from viral infections and, as patterns of human behavior change, a new environment may be created that allows a new virus to enter the human population and be transmitted to large numbers of persons with devastating results; an example is the acquired immunodeficiency syndrome (AIDS), which reached epidemic levels in the 1980s. On the other hand, several serious viral diseases have been either eradicated or greatly reduced through active immunization programs. Smallpox, once the greatest killer of all viral diseases, has been completely eradicated. Such diseases as poliomyelitis, measles, and rubella, which up until the past few decades caused many deaths and left thousands crippled or impaired, have been greatly reduced in number.

Most viral diseases are unresponsive to antibiotics or other "wonder drugs" that are so effective in treating bacterial infections. And most treatments are symptomatic—that is, use procedures that reduce the discomfort and maintain the proper physiological functions of the body. Recovery results primarily from the patient's own natural defense mechanisms. Procedures or activities that would weaken the host, such as malnourishment, lack of sleep, and immunosuppressive drugs, should be avoided. Vaccines are very effective in preventing some viral infections and a new generation of vaccines against additional viral disease is being developed using genetic engineering technology. Viral infections may cause sufficient tissue damage to predispose a patient to secondary bacterial infections. In such cases, chemotherapy to combat the bacterial complications would be appropriate.

The impact of viral diseases on humans is most apparent with infections of the respiratory tract. It is estimated that about 75% of all infectious diseases are of the respiratory tract and about 80% of them are caused by viruses. A great majority of these viral infections are of the upper respiratory tract and cause such clinical diseases as common colds (rhinitis) and sore throats (pharyngitis). A fair number of infections, however, involve the lower respiratory tract and may cause serious problems, particularly in infants and small children. Approximately 150 different viruses are associated with respiratory infections and it is estimated that, on the average, each person will experience about six such infections per year. Because of these infections, approximately 100 million work days are lost per year in the United States. In addition, they are

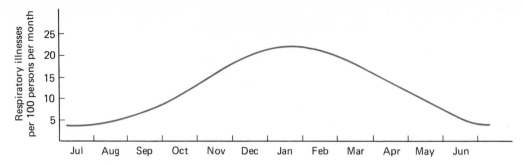

Figure 33-3 An approximate representation of the number of respiratory illnesses during each month of the year in persons living in the United States.

responsible for 50% of the absences from school and a third of all patient visits to general practitioners or clinics. Most of these common respiratory infections occur during the cooler months with peak incidences in the winter, although some are seen year-round (Figure 33-3). The second most prevalent type of viral disease involves the gastrointestinal tract. Well over 50% of the cases of gastroenteritis in humans are caused by viruses, and viral gastroenteritis is a major cause of death of undernourished infants. Should the interferons produced by recombinant DNA procedures prove effective in treating these common viral diseases, it would constitute a major medical advance.

CLASSIFICATION OF VIRUSES

It is possible to classify viruses into groups of families or related members according to chemical and morphological characteristics. Table 33-1 shows the major families of animal viruses based on the following characteristics: type of nucleic acid, symmetry of capsid, presence or absence of an envelope, size of virion, and number of capsomers if the symmetry is cubical. The use of binomial Latin names for species is not well established in virology and attempts to introduce Latinized names have met with varying degrees of success. The Latinized suffix-*viridae* is now used to designate the families of viruses, for example, Poxviridae. At the genus level, the name of the virus or an acronym followed by the suffix- *virus* is used, for example, poliovirus and echovirus. The species or sub-species level is usually designated by a letter or number after the genus level name. Thus viruses might be referred to as adenovirus 4 or 7, and influenza A or B, and so on.

Some species of each group listed in Table 33-1 cause diseases in animals. The papovaviruses and retroviruses are primarily associated with cancer and their possible role as causative agents of cancer in humans is still under investigation.

The viruses causing important diseases of humans will be discussed in the following chapters.

CONCEPT SUMMARY

1. Intracellular multiplication of viruses may result in one or more of several effects on the host cell. These responses vary from rapid and complete destruction of the host cell to long-term coexistence within the cell with no apparent adverse effect.

2. Cell transformation is a unique response to viral infection in which the host cell is not injured but is changed from its normal function. Virus-induced tumors are the result of this type of host-parasite interaction.

3. Response of the host cell to viral infection includes the production of interferons, which increase the protection of other cells to viral replication.

STUDY SUMMARY

1. List the possible outcomes of viral infection of a host cell.

2. What aspect of host cell–virus interaction is essential if cellular transformation is to be the result of virus infection?

3. List four characteristics of viruses that can be used to identify and classify these particles.

4. Why haven't scientists been able to produce interferon in experimental animals for use in treatment of human disease?

5. Write a paragraph on your own experience with viral infections.

REFERENCES FOR FURTHER STUDY

1. Genetic and Molecular Mechanisms of Viral Pathogenesis: Implications for Prevention and Treatment. *Nature* 300:19, 1982.

2. Classification and Nomenclature of Viruses: Fourth Report of the International Committee on Taxonomy of Viruses. *Intervirology* 17:1, 1982.

3. Interferon: The First Quarter Century. *Journal of the American Medical Association* 248:2513, 1982.

4. *Viral Infections of Humans*, A. Evans, 1982. Plenum Medical Books.

5. *Mechanisms of Interferon Actions*, vols. 1 and 2, L. Pfeffer, 1987. CRC Press.

6. Antiviral Therapy. *Scientific American* 256:76, 1987.

chapter 34

ADENOVIRUSES AND POXVIRUSES

I n terms of clinical significance the adenoviruses and poxviruses provide an interesting contrast. The major human
disease caused by poxvirus is smallpox, a disease of great
historical significance that has been responsible for almost
untold human misery and suffering. Among the first known viral
diseases, smallpox was the first for which immunization was available. It has now been completely eradicated as a result of extensive world-wide disease preventive efforts. On the other hand, adenoviruses are a large group of viruses whose clinical significance
is still being described, and for which only limited immunization is
possible. These viruses cause some of the most common respiratory diseases of humans, but have also recently been implicated as
a source of human disease ranging from conjunctivitis to
gastroenteritis. The properties and clinical role of these two groups
of DNA viruses are presented in this chapter.

ADENOVIRUSES

Adenoviruses are widespread in nature and currently 41 distinct
serotypes have been isolated from humans. They are designated
types 1, 2, and so forth up to type 41. Additional adenoviruses
are also found in various avian and nonhuman mammalian species. The adenoviruses were so named because they were first isolated from tonsils and adenoids. Many adenoviruses have been
shown as the cause of some common upper respiratory infections
of humans and some are associated with diarrheal diseases in infants. Less frequently, they may cause infections in other tissues.
The adenoviruses have the ability to remain sequestered in lymphatic tissues and tissues of the intestinal tract long after the primary exposure. About 50% of surgically removed tonsils and adenoids are found to contain some of these latent adenoviruses.

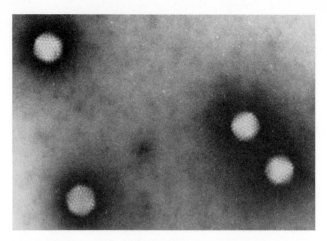

Figure 34-1 Transmission electron micrograph of adenoviruses magnified 150,000 × . (Courtesy Robley C. Williams, University of California, Berkeley)

General Properties of the Viruses

Adenoviruses have a distinct appearance and can often be identified by direct observation with an electron microscope (Figure 34-1). The capsid is 60 to 90 nm in diameter, has cubical symmetry with 252 capsomers, and has no envelope. These viruses contain ds-DNA and can be cultivated in various types of cell cultures. Adenoviruses are quite stable and are able to survive for long periods once expelled from a host.

Pathogenesis and Clinical Diseases

Acute respiratory diseases Close to 100% of the children living under crowded conditions become infected with adenoviruses early in life. The infectivity rates are less, but still 50% or more, in children living in less crowded conditions. About half the infected children develop definite clinical symptoms. The most common clinical disease is an acute respiratory infection with such common symptoms as sore throat, cough, runny nose (coryza), and headache. Tonsillitis and pneumonia may be seen occasionally. Adenovirus infections are also seen in adults but generally are less frequent and less severe.

A unique form of acute respiratory disease caused by adenoviruses is seen in training centers for military recruits. Quite typically, military recruits begin to develop adenovirus infections after several weeks of training and during the next month or so more than 80% of the recruits may experience this respiratory disease syndrome. Symptoms may last up to 10 days; overall this disease may be quite disruptive to the recruit-training program. Typically outbreaks among the recruits are caused by type 4, 7, and 21 adenoviruses. The reason for this unique epidemiologic pattern among military recruits is not known but may be associated with assembling large numbers of young persons from diverse backgrounds and subjecting them to the crowding and "stresses" of military life.

Pharyngoconjunctival fever and keratoconjunctivitis Adenovirus-induced pharyngoconjunctival fever is a disease characterized by fever, conjunctivitis (inflammation of the eyelids), and sore throat. This disease occurs in sporadic outbreaks associated with swimming pools, summer camps, and small lakes. It usually involves children and young adults. All evidence indicates that transmission is by direct contact with contaminated water. Several outbreaks have occurred in swimming pools that were not properly chlorinated. The incubation period is 6 to 9 days.

Keratoconjunctivitis is an infection transmitted by adenovirus-contaminated instruments or medications in ophthalmological (eye) clinics. The adenoviruses are quite stable and often survive disinfection procedures that use alcohol and many other common chemical disinfectants. This syndrome starts with inflammation of the eyelid and spreads to the cornea. Damage to the cornea may lead to impaired vision. The incubation period is 8 to 10 days.

Keratoconjunctivitis
an infection of the eye surfaces that leads to inflammation of the conjunctiva as well as the cornea of the eye.

Gastroenteritis Besides their extensive multiplication in the respiratory tract, adenoviruses are also able to grow in and are shed from the intestinal tract. It is becoming increasingly apparent that some of the adenoviruses, e.g. adenovirus 40 and adenovirus 41 are major causes of diarrhea in children. Although the full extent of these diseases is not known, in the United States it appears that about 15% of the cases of viral gastroenteritis of children that require hospitalization are caused by adenoviruses. Some scientists have suggested that adenoviral gastroenteritis is second only to enterotoxigenic *E. coli* as a cause of mortality among the world's children.

Transmission

Adenoviruses are spread from person to person by direct and indirect contact. The fecal-oral route is probably a major means of spread in children and the airborne route in all age groups. Contact with contaminated materials is the major route of transmission for eye infections.

Diagnosis

Adenoviruses can be isolated on a variety of cell cultures. Isolation should be correlated with a specific rise in antibody titer before an adenovirus can be considered the cause of a specific disease, for

Adenovirus Type 7 Outbreak in a Pediatric Chronic Care Facility: Pennsylvania, 1982

In July 1982, an outbreak of respiratory disease caused by adenovirus type 7 (Ad 7) occurred in a chronic care facility in a pediatric hospital in Pennsylvania. On June 6, a physician, the presumed index case, developed infected conjunctiva; 2 days later, conjunctivitis; and on June 12, an acute upper respiratory tract illness (URI, coryza and/or pharyngitis). Between June 15 and July 9, 4 of the 14 children in the facility became ill with an acute respiratory illness characterized by either URI or lower respiratory tract illness (LRI; fever and respiratory distress). These 4, and 3 other asymptomatic children, were culture-positive for Ad 7. Three of the 4 ill children had LRI and required mechanical ventilation; 1 with congenital heart disease and 1 with bronchopulmonary dysplasia died. In addition, 3 of the other 35 staff members (physicians, nurses, and play therapists) developed acute URI, and Ad 7 was isolated from cultures from 2 of them.

The chronic care facility has a nurses' station, treatment room, playroom, and three patient rooms—with four, six, and seven beds, respectively. All 14 children remained in the facility throughout the outbreak. Culture-positive children resided in two of the three rooms.

The index case had contact with all 14 children on June 6 and 7 and from June 14 on. Both culture-positive staff members had contact with the first ill child as early as June 15. Ultimately, one of these staff members had contact with all seven culture-positive and three of seven culture-negative children. The other had contact with three culture-positive children and one culture-negative child. When these staff members became ill, they were excluded from patient contact. When the extent of the outbreak was recognized on June 22, children culture-positive for Ad 7 were moved into one room, and staff members with acute respiratory illness were excluded from contact with the children (*MMWR* 32:258, 1983).

---

adenoviruses are frequently isolated from healthy persons. Adenovirus respiratory infections in the general population cannot be distinguished on clinical grounds from the many respiratory infections caused by a variety of other infectious agents. The specific laboratory tests required to identify an adenovirus infection are generally not done.

Treatment

No treatment is available other than measures taken to relieve symptoms.

Prevention and Control

Only in training centers for military recruits are measures taken to prevent adenovirus infections. A live **attenuated vaccine** against types 4, 7, and 21 when given by the oral route to military

Attenuated vaccine
a vaccine made from living microorganisms which have been selected for their lack of virulence.

recruits, has successfully controlled the epidemics of acute respiratory disease syndrome caused by these viruses. Eye clinics should use proper methods of sterilization and asepsis to prevent the spread of adenoviruses.

POXVIRUSES

Poxviruses are large (250 x 300 nm), brick-shaped, DNA-containing viruses. Many animal species have their own specific poxvirus infections, usually in the form of lesions (pocks) on the skin. The major poxvirus of humans is the variola virus that causes the disease of smallpox (Figure 34-2).

Smallpox

Smallpox has been one of the most devasting diseases of humans. History is replete with reports of epidemics in which more than 50% of the inhabitants of a city or country developed smallpox, with as many as half the infected dying of the disease.

A new milestone in medical science was achieved with the eradication of smallpox from the world. It marked the first time that medical science had been able to eradicate a major infectious disease. Because future workers in medicine will not encounter smallpox, the pathogenesis, transmission, diagnosis, and control of this disease will not be discussed. Instead a historical synopsis of the control of smallpox is presented with emphasis on those concepts that may be helpful in understanding the control of infectious disease in general.

Figure 34-2 Lesions (pox) on the hand of a patient with smallpox. (Armed Forces Institute of Pathology, AFIP MIS #CA 44271-3)

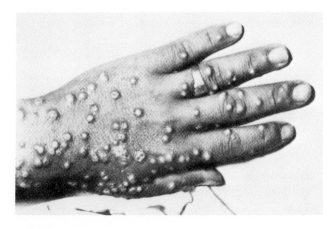

Contact Spread of Vaccinia from a National Guard Vaccinee: Wisconsin, 1985

On January 24, 1985, a 15-year-old female was referred to a dermatologist in a clinic in La Crosse, Wisconsin, for evaluation of an ulcerated lesion on her left upper lip. On examination, the patient had a 2-cm diameter ulcer on her left upper lip, five 4-mm diameter oval vesicles on the arms, and marked conjunctival injection of the left eye. She appeared mildly sick with low-grade fever, fatigue, and tender cervical lymphadenopathy. The patient was otherwise in good health, with no history of eczema, malignancy, or immunologic deficiency.

The patient has a male friend who is a member of the Wisconsin National Guard. He had received a smallpox vaccination in a U.S. Army facility in Wisconsin at the end of December 1984. In early January, the patient assisted her friend in applying compresses to ease the discomfort of a successful smallpox vaccination. As a child, the patient had received a smallpox vaccination but had never developed a reaction. She has no scar compatible with smallpox vaccination.

She was treated with trifluridine in the left eye, oral erythromycin, and topical neosporin for the ulcer on her lip. In addition, she received a total of 30 ml of vaccinia immune globulin (VIG) intramuscularly over 2 days. Vaccinia virus was cultured from the skin lesions. On follow-up visit on February 6, all lesions were healing well, and it appeared that the lesion on the left lip would heal without scarring.

An investigation conducted to determine whether the patient had transmitted disease to her contacts involved 5 immediate family members and 45 participants in a girls' gymnastics meet on January 21 in which the patient competed. By January 31, none of these 50 individuals had subsequent evidence of vesicular or pustular skin lesions (*MMWK* 34:182, 1985).

Celebration by Health Leaders to Mark a Decade Sans Smallpox: 1987

On October 26, 1977, a cook in Merka, Somalia, came down with an illness that was to make him famous—history was to record him as the last person in the world to contract naturally occurring smallpox.

The tenth anniversary of this momentous med-

The control of smallpox Before the nineteenth century, smallpox was controlled in a limited way by purposely inoculating persons who had not yet contracted it with a mild form of the disease. The severe form of smallpox was called *variola major* and the mild form *variola minor* or *alastrim*. Recovery from either form conferred immunity against both forms. Inoculation with variola minor usually caused mild symptoms with a fatality rate of "only" 1% to 2%. Many considered it an acceptable risk compared to that of conical milestone—the eradication of a disease that for centuries caused death and disfigurement—will be celebrated this week by health officials at the World Health Organization and at the national Centers for Disease Control.

The CDC, which joined the worldwide effort to eliminate smallpox in 1966, will mark 10 years of a smallpox-free world on Thursday, with an awards presentation by U.S. Surgeon General C. Everett Koop and a display of smallpox eradication memorabilia. There also will be an address by Dr. Donald A. Henderson, dean of the School of Hygiene and Public Health of Johns Hopkins University.

Henderson was the first director of CDC's smallpox eradication program. He later was assigned to WHO's headquarters in Geneva and became director of the global eradication program to which many nations, including the Soviet Union, contributed.

A smallpox case has not been diagnosed since 1977, except for a laboratory-associated case that claimed the life of a medical photographer at a Birmingham, England, hospital in 1978. The Somalia smallpox victim, Ali Maow Maalin, recovered from his illness, an isolate of the virus being quickly identified by a CDC virologist, James H. Nakano. Nakano, who joined the eradication effort at its beginning and set up the first U.S. smallpox laboratory, made the last diagnosis of a naturally occurring smallpox case.

"Towards the end (of the eradication effort) all the isolates turned out to be chickenpox," said Nakano, who is now retired. "But in this case we did see the pox virus. We were able to diagnose it fairly easily."

The International Commission on Certification of Smallpox Eradication waited for two years after the Somalia case before declaring the world free of smallpox in 1979. During that period, Nakano recalled, there were many reports of suspected smallpox but they turned out to be false alarms.

Health officials do not know when the last case of smallpox in the United States occurred but they believe it was in 1949 in the lower Rio Grande Valley of Texas.

But elsewhere in the world, millions of smallpox cases were being recorded, Nakano said. A 1966 effort by 21 countries was successful in ridding Central and West Africa of the disease and this success launched the global eradication campaign (*Desert News*, October 29, 1987).

tracting and dying of the major form of smallpox. This practice of purposely inoculating persons with variola minor, called *variolation*, was pursued in Africa and Asia from ancient times and was used to a limited extent in some areas of North America during the eighteenth century.

The most significant contribution toward the eventual control of smallpox was the development of the vaccination procedure by Edward Jenner in 1796 (see Chapter 1), using the cowpox

Freeze-dry

to process materials by freezing them and then removing the water from the frozen material without melting it.

virus. Afterward the practice of vaccination against smallpox became widespread in most developed countries and a steady decline in the total number of cases occurred over the past 190 years. The last cases of smallpox seen in the United States were in the lower Rio Grande Valley in 1949. The final struggle with smallpox began in 1966 when the World Health Organization embarked on a program of complete eradication of this disease. Much of the program's success was made possible by the development of a **freeze-dried** form of vaccine that was stable without refrigeration and was very effective; the methods of administration were easy to learn and inexpensive. These developments made it possible to carry out effective vaccination programs in remote areas of the world. As a result of this concentrated eradication program, by 1972 all countries in North and South America were free of smallpox. By 1975 only Bangladesh, Ethiopia, and surrounding areas reported cases. After a slight reversal in early 1977, this eradication program moved to its successful conclusion. The last person to have a naturally acquired case of smallpox was a hospital cook in Somalia who came down with the disease in October 1977. After a 2-year waiting period in which no new cases occurred, the world was officially declared free of smallpox in October 1979 (see clinical note). Actually, the last known cases of smallpox occurred from accidental infections in a research laboratory in England in 1978. Now only four reference laboratories possess the smallpox virus and its use is stringently controlled.

Although smallpox was a severe and highly contagious disease, it possessed features that permitted its successful eradication. First, the disease was easily recognized and few if any subclinical cases occurred. This factor was a help in detection and diagnosis. Second, the virus did not remain in the body as a latent infection after the patient recovered from the clinical disease. Third, no regular nonhuman host could act as a reservoir of the virus. Fourth, an effective, easily administered vaccine was available. And fifth, the virus did not readily mutate.

The most notable result of this eradication program in countries where smallpox was not normally found was the discontinuation of routine smallpox vaccination. The smallpox vaccination used a living virus and caused a mild infection in those vaccinated. In some persons, mostly young children with compromised host defense mechanisms, the vaccine might cause moderate to severe infections. Before smallpox vaccination was discontinued in the United States in 1971, about 500 children per year developed a serious vaccine-associated disease (**post-vaccination encephalitis**) and about a dozen deaths would occur. Thus for many years in the United States and many other countries, many more children suffered or died from the ill effects of the vaccine than from the disease itself.

Post-vaccination encephalitis

encephalitis occasionally caused in response to some viral vaccines.

CONCEPT SUMMARY

1. Over 40 types of adenoviruses have been discovered. These DNA viruses are responsible for a variety of infections in humans that may be severe but are usually self-limiting. Most common adenovirus infections occur in the respiratory tract, but conjunctivitis and intestinal infections are not infrequent.

2. Smallpox, a life-threatening infection of a DNA-containing poxvirus, has been eradicated from the ranks of human illness. Careful, thorough, and prolonged immunization efforts have apparently rid the world of this dreaded disease.

STUDY SUMMARY

1. What property of the adenoviruses make them good candidates to produce latent viral infections?

2. The fact that available adenovirus vaccine is limited to types 4, 7, and 21 suggests a number of epidemiologic considerations. List two factors that relate to this situation.

3. What features of adenovirus and adenovirus infection reduces the likelihood of the development of a general vaccine for these agents?

4. What features of the pathogenesis of smallpox made immunization such an effective means of control?

5. Not everyone in the United States has been immunized against smallpox. Why were immunizations suspended before everyone had an opportunity to be immunized?

REFERENCES FOR FURTHER STUDY

1. Human Monkeypox: Clinical Features of 282 Patients. *Journal of Infectious Diseases* 156:293, 1987.

2. *The Biologic and Clinical Basis of Infectious Diseases*, 3rd ed., G. Youmans, 1986. Saunders.

3. *Review of Medical Microbiology*, 17th ed., E. Jawietz, 1957. Appleton & Lange.

4. *Viral Infections in Humans*, A. Evans, 1982. Plenum Medical Books.

HERPESVIRUSES

Members of the family Herpesviridae are widespread in nature and infect many animal species. These viruses are usually host-specific; that is, the human herpesviruses cause natural infections only in humans and not in other animals. Likewise, the herpesviruses of lower animals do not affect humans, although on rare occasions monkey herpesviruses have caused fatal infections in humans.

The common diseases of humans caused by herpesviruses are cold sores or fever blisters, genital herpes, chickenpox, and infectious mononucleosis. Exposure to these viruses generally occurs in the first decade of life in those living in conditions of poor hygiene and the resulting infection may be apparent or subclinical. An important characteristic of these viruses is their ability to remain sequestered inside certain cells long after the primary infection is resolved. These latent infections may persist for the life of the person with no further clinical symptoms or they may cause sporadic recurrences of clinical symptoms. Such latent infections allow these viruses to remain ever present in a population, to be passed on to new susceptible individuals. Four of the human herpesviruses—herpes simplex, varicella-zoster, cytomegalo, and Epstein-Barr—are discussed in this chapter.

GENERAL PROPERTIES OF THE VIRUSES

The capsid of the herpesviruses is 100 nm in diameter, has cubical symmetry with 162 capsomers, and is surrounded by an envelope (Figure 35-1). The herpesviruses are fairly unstable and, after being shed from the body, become inactivated within hours at room temperature. The nucleic acid is double-stranded DNA and the viruses multiply in the nucleus of the host cell. This association of foreign DNA with the nucleus of host cells has provided theoret-

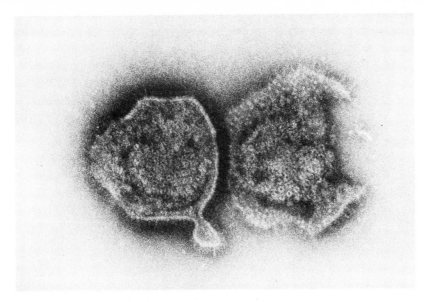

Figure 35-1   Transmission electron micrograph of herpesviruses showing icosahedral capsids (partially disrupted) surrounded by envelopes (magnified 160,000 ×). (Courtesy Robley C. Williams, University of California, Berkeley)

ical evidence that herpesviruses may induce cancer. Some forms of cancer in lower animals are associated with these viruses and several lines of evidence associate herpesviruses, particularly the Epstein-Barr virus, with certain forms of cancer in humans. Women who have cervical herpes infection have a significantly greater incidence of cervical cancer than uninfected women.

Because cancer may be induced by the double-stranded DNA of the herpesviruses, there has been a reluctance to develop vaccines produced from the whole viruses, for the use of such vaccines would result in the introduction of relatively large amounts of this DNA into the tissues of humans. It has not been economically feasible in the past to produce herpes vaccines containing only the viral protein antigens. Yet theoretical and experimental evidence strongly suggests that antibodies against these protein antigens will offer protection against primary herpes infections. Using advances in genetic engineering, several approaches are being used to develop vaccines against herpesvirus infections. The gene for the protective antigens has been cloned into microorganisms and mammalian cells where large amounts of these antigens can be produced. These purified antigens have been effective in stimulating production of protective antibodies. In addition, these genes have been cloned into vaccinia viruses, which have in turn been used to effectively immunize experimental animals. Using this technology, effective vaccines against the major herpesvirus diseases should soon be available for use in humans.

HERPES SIMPLEX VIRUSES (HSVs)

Two serotypes of herpes simplex viruses have been identified. Type 1 is generally associated with infections of the upper half of the body and type 2 with infection of the genitourinary tract and surrounding tissues. Both types may cause generalized infections in infants and compromised patients.

Pathogenesis and Clinical Diseases

Cold sores or *fever blisters* (herpes labialis) are among the most common of all human infections and are usually caused by the type 1 HSV (Figure 35-2). The recurring lesions on the lips are the clinical manifestation of a complex chronic interaction between the virus and the host. Most newborn infants are not readily infected, possibly as a result of passive immunity that offers some protection against primary infection. Once the passive immunity is gone, the infant is highly susceptible to primary infection. Susceptibility tends to decrease somewhat as the child gets older. However, in conditions of poor sanitation as many as 80% of the population has been infected before adulthood. Persons living under conditions of improved sanitation experience about a 40% infectivity rate. The primary infection is often asymptomatic or is not diagnosed as herpes. Symptoms are seen in 10% to 15% of the cases from 2 to 12 days after being exposed to the virus. The primary lesions may appear as small **vesicles** in the throat, mouth, or nose and go relatively unnoticed. The most noticeable form of primary infection involves the lips, mouth, and gums (gingivostomatitis), in which the vesicles rupture and develop into ulcerative lesions.

Vesicle
a blisterlike structure that contains a clear serous fluid.

Figure 35-2   Herpes simplex fever blister on lower lip two days after onset (Courtesy Centers for Disease Control, Atlanta)

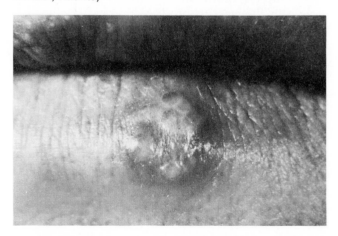

Fever, pain, and irritability usually persist for about 1 week, followed by gradual healing during the second week.

Recovery is associated with a rise in antibodies against the virus. During the primary infection, however, the virus passes along nerve fibers to regional **ganglia**. In the case of gingivostomatitis, the trigeminal ganglion is commonly involved and the virus becomes sequestered in a latent form in this tissue. While in this latent form, the virus cannot be detected by ordinary means during life. It causes no symptoms and is not affected by antibodies. Periodically, in from 20% to 30% of the general population, these latent viruses become activated and move down the nerve fiber to cause recurring skin lesions at the site of the original infection (Figure 35-3). The frequency of these recurring lesions varies from person to person, ranging from once every few years to about once a month. Various stressful stimuli, such as excessive sunlight, fever, cold winds, emotional stress, and hormonal changes, apparently trigger the reactivation of the virus. As the virus moves down the nerve fibers, it passes directly into the skin cells without becoming exposed to the host's antibodies. The antibodies usually prevent the virus from spreading systemically to other tissues of the body but are unable to prevent the recurring lesions. Primary and recurring infections may also occur in the eyes, causing a disease known as *herpetic keratoconjunctivitis*. Le-

Ganglia
a mass of nervous tissue that is not part of the CNS; major nerve trunks connecting the peripheral nerves to the CNS.

Figure 35-3   Aspects of the pathogenesis of primary and recurring herpes infections of the lips.

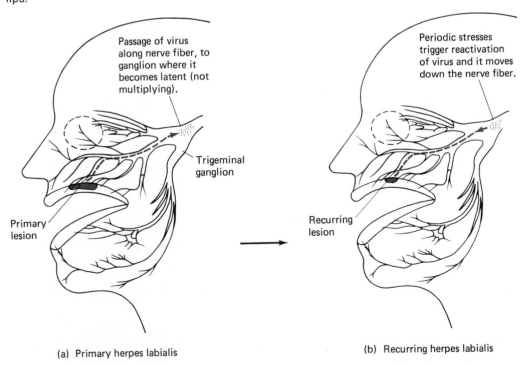

Passage of virus along nerve fiber, to ganglion where it becomes latent (not multiplying).

Trigeminal ganglion

Primary lesion

(a) Primary herpes labialis

Periodic stresses trigger reactivation of virus and it moves down the nerve fiber.

Recurring lesion

(b) Recurring herpes labialis

Eczema
inflammation of the skin, often associated with scaling, papules, crusting, and serous discharge.

sions on the cornea are most serious, for the accumulating scar tissue may lead to vision impairment.

Occasionally almost any tissue of the body may become infected with these viruses. Primary and recurring infections may occur on any cutaneous area of the body. Traumatic injury may provide a portal of entry for primary infections that may develop in both children and adults. Such infections have been seen in wrestlers (herpes gladiatorum) due to skin abrasions, or in persons following burns, or on the thumb of a thumb-sucking child or the finger of a dentist (herpetic whitlow). Children with **eczema** may acquire a serious herpes infection over large areas of the body (eczema herpeticum).Herpes simplex viruses may also infect the central nervous system, causing a severe, and often fatal, infection (herpetic encephalitis).

Genital herpes is recognized as a very common sexually transmitted disease. Over 80% of these infections are caused by HSV type 2. In females the vesicles usually occur in the mucosal tissue of the vulva, vagina, or cervix, but any of the genital or surrounding tissues may be involved. These vesicles ulcerate, producing shallow lesions. The symptoms may include malaise, urinary retention, local pain, fever, vaginal discharge, and tender, swollen inguinal lymph nodes. In males the vesicles and subsequent ulcerations develop on the penis and surrounding tissues. These infections heal spontaneously in 1 to 2 weeks. Recurrent infections are common but are generally milder than the primary infection. All ages seem susceptible to genital herpes, but most infections are seen in young adults. A disseminated form of herpes occasionally occurs in newborns, particularly premature infants, and here the virus spreads throughout the body. These infections are usually fatal. Infections are acquired most often during birth as the infant passes through an infected birth canal. Disseminated herpes may also occur in patients of any age when they become immunosuppressed.

Transmission

HSV type 1 is transmitted by direct contact or by indirect contact with such objects as eating utensils. A typical mode of transmission is for an adult with an active recurring lesion to kiss or cuddle a young child. Large numbers of viruses are present in the vesicular fluid and exudate from the ulcerative lesions. Transmission within family units is difficult to prevent. Some persons may be intermittent subclinical shedders of HSV, which further complicates attempts to prevent transmission of this agent. In general, transmission is much more efficient among persons living in crowded, unsanitary conditions.

HSV type 2 is spread primarily by sexual contact and in the current sexually permissive societies the number of cases have increased alarmingly. HSV type 2 can be isolated from 10% to 15% of the patients who visit clinics for sexually transmitted diseases. Infected females may transmit this virus to infants during delivery. Such neonatally acquired HSV type 2 infections are generally serious and may result in death of the infant.

Diagnosis

Most diagnoses are based on the clinical appearance. Disseminated infections and atypical complicated cases often require a laboratory diagnosis. This diagnosis involves isolating HSV from the lesion early in the illness. HSV multiples well in some commonly used cell cultures. HSV can be detected in cell cultures after about 24 hours by the use of specific monoclonal antibodies tagged with fluorescent dyes or enzymes that can differentiate HSV-1 from HSV-2. A correlation of **antibody titers** (showing a significant rise) is often needed to confirm a diagnosis, for these viruses may be found in normal-appearing tissues. HSV produces a characteristic inclusion body in the nucleus of infected cells; such intranuclear inclusions may be seen on microscopic examination of stained cells that are scraped from a suspected lesion. Direct fluorescent antibody tests on biopsied tissues may also give a rapid diagnosis of a HSV infection.

Antibody titer
the concentration of antibody available in the blood serum; usually measured in 2-fold dilutions.

Treatment

The herpetic infection of the cornea was the first viral infection to be routinely treated by chemotherapy. The chemical *iododeoxyuridine*, used in corneal infections, interferes with the replication of herpesviruses by inhibiting DNA synthesis. When applied to the surface of the cornea every hour or two, it greatly reduced the severity of infection. This agent has been successfully used since the mid-1960s to prevent the scarring that leads to impaired vision. Questionable success has been obtained by treating herpes infections of other tissues with this chemical.

In the 1970s, a compound called *trifluridine* became available to treat HSV keratitis. A third antiviral compound called *adenine arabinoside* is now licensed for use in the United States. This compound is also effective in treating eye infections when applied to the surface of the cornea; when given systemically (injected into the blood) early in the illness, it reduces the mortality from herpes encephalitis. A fourth compound called *acyclovir* is also available now and has advantages over the agents developed earlier. Acyclovir is less toxic to humans than the other agents, and is currently the drug of choice. An ointment of acyclovir effectively treats HSV keratitis. When given intravenously it helps treat serious disseminated herpes infections. In cream form it is able to shorten the duration of recurrent fever blisters and has some in-

Genital Herpes Infection: United States, 1966–84

Genital herpes infection remains a major public health problem in the United States. Data collected by the National Disease and Therapeutic Index (NDTI) from 1966 to 1981 showed marked increases in the numbers of patient consultations for genital herpes. Current analysis shows continued upward trends in symptomatic genital herpes infections among private patients in the United States.

The NDTI survey is a national stratified random sample of data from private practitioners' office-based practices in the contiguous United States. This survey is a continuing compilation of statistical information about patterns and treatments of various diseases and represents a sample of patient-physician interactions. Included in the data coded are "consultations" about genital herpes between patients and physicians, including office visits, house calls, telephone calls, and hospital visits; "office visits," referring to initial or repeat visits for genital herpes; and "first office visits," coded if the patient presents to a physician participating in the survey for the first time with genital herpes. No laboratory confirmation of the physicians' diagnoses is included in the survey.

The estimated number of physician-patient consultations for genital herpes increased 15-fold between 1966 and 1984, from 29,560 to 450,570. Office visits accounted for 79% of these consultations. Also, first office visits—a more likely indicator of newly acquired infection—increased nearly ninefold, from 17,810 in 1966 to 156,720 in 1984. Although a decline in consultations, office visits, and first office visits was evident from 1978 to 1980, the upward trends remain statistically significant for all three types of physician-patient interaction ($p < .004$).

The number of first office visits for genital herpes was approximately the same for both men and women. However, over the 19-year span, women made more total office visits for genital herpes than did men. In each of three time periods—1966–1972, 1973–1978, and 1979–1984—the number of consultations increased for men and women in each age group, except for men 40–44 years of age. Adults 20–29 years of age continued to account for the largest proportion of consultations in all age groups in each period (*MMWR* 35:402, 1986).

hibitory effects on genital herpes when given topically, orally, or intravenously. Acyclovir is not effective in curing the latent state of HSV.

Prevention and Control

Whenever possible, persons with active herpetic lesions should avoid contact with young children. Children with primary lesions should be isolated from other children until the lesions have healed. Pregnant females with genital herpetic infections may need to have a Caesarean delivery to help avoid infecting the newborn. Dentists and other medical personnel who come in contact with oral secretions of patients should wear gloves.

Current evidence suggests that antibodies are able to prevent the primary infection but not the recurring lesions. This finding has stimulated research on a possible vaccine that could be given to young children before they lose their passive immunity. If the primary infection were prevented in children, then it would follow that the recurring lesions later in life would also be prevented.

VARICELLA-ZOSTER (V-Z) VIRUS

The V-Z herpesvirus is the causative agent of both chickenpox (varicella) and shingles (zoster), hence the double name. For many years it was thought that these two diseases were unrelated. Now it is known that chickenpox is the acute primary form of the disease complex whereas shingles is a delayed recurrent form of the same infection (Figure 35-4). Only a single serotype of the V-Z virus exists.

Pathogenesis and Clinical Diseases

Chickenpox   The V-Z virus enters the respiratory tract by the airborne route. The virus then apparently passes through the lymphatic system and is disseminated throughout the body via the bloodstream. The extent of viral multiplication and the tissues involved during the early stages of the incubation period have not been well documented. After an incubation period of 10 to 20 days, the virus is found to be multiplying in numerous foci of the deep skin and in the throat. General discomfort, together with a sore throat, may occur a day or so before the appearance of a macular (flat) rash on the skin. Within 24 hours the rash develops into vesicles. The vesicles form into **pustules** within the next 24 hours. The lesions next form scabs that fall off after a few days. Successive crops of vesicles develop and all stages of the lesions may be seen simultaneously (Figure 35-5). After about 5 days the lesions begin to disappear. Scarring usually does not result without secondary bacterial infection. The intense itching often causes scratching that, in turn, may lead to secondary bacterial infection with accompanying inflammation and scarring.

Chickenpox rarely has serious complications in otherwise healthy children. Occasionally a serious condition called **Reye's syndrome** develops during the recovery period and consists of diffuse metabolic and neurologic malfunctions. Chickenpox, however, can be severe or fatal in newborn infants, children with leukemia, or in other immunosuppressed patients. Infections in

Pustule
a small blister that is filled with pus.

Reye's syndrome
a syndrome of organ changes that may occur following a viral infection. Most noticeable changes occur in mental status, nausea, and liver enlargement.

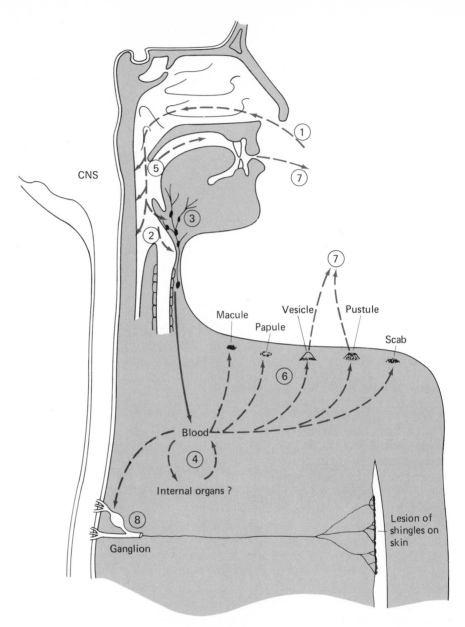

Figure 35-4 Pathogenesis of Varicella-Zoster. (1) Virus enters by airborne route. (2) Early viral multiplication in upper respiratory tract; no symptoms and patient not infectious. (3) Passage of virus into regional lymph nodes. (4) Passage of virus to blood and spread to various internal organs. (5) Several days before pock formation virus may be found in respiratory tract; patient may be infectious. (6) Virus deposited in the epithelial tissues with resultant pock formation; this occurs 14 to 21 days after exposure. (7) Virus shed from the respiratory tract and from the pocks. (8) Virus becomes sequestered in neural ganglia and remains latent. At a later time the virus may become active and moves along the sensory nerves to cause the localized lesions of shingles.

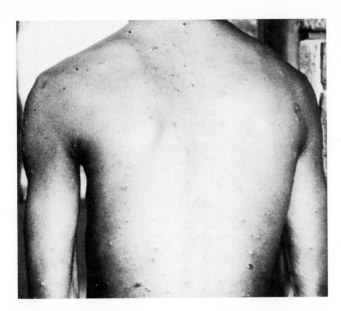

Figure 35-5   Chickenpox three days after onset of rash. Lesion in different stages of development can be seen. (Courtesy Centers for Disease Control, Atlanta)

adults are more severe than those in children, with varicella pneumonia being a much more frequent complication. Recovery confers lifelong immunity to reinfection. Nevertheless, the antibodies do not remove the viruses that become sequestered in the ganglia.

Shingles   Shingles is a recurrent clinical manifestation of a latent-dormant infection with the V-Z virus. Analogous to the latent infections with the herpes simplex virus, the V-Z virus is apparently able to become sequestered in neuroganglia following a typical acute chickenpox infection. The V-Z virus may lie dormant for many years before it becomes reactivated. More than 65% of the cases occur in persons over 45 years of age; however, reactivation may occur at any age. Usually a person has only a single attack of shingles, but second episodes occasionally develop. The mechanisms of reactivation are not understood. One theory is that it may be associated with a waning of the acquired immunity. Shingles is much more common in persons who are immunosuppressed or who have irradiation or injuries to the spine. After the virus becomes activated, it moves down the sensory nerve leading from the infected ganglion. This step is accompanied by an abnormal sensation and/or pain over the area served by the involved nerve (dermatome). Several days later the eruption occurs (Figure 35-6) and is confined to the involved dermatome. The distribution is often in a band (zoster-girdle) on one side of the body with an abrupt margin at midline (Figure 35-7). The skin involvement pro-

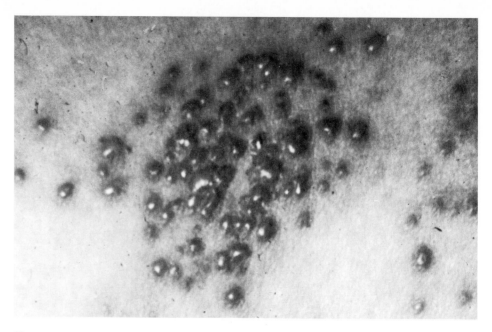

Figure 35-6   Vesicular lesions of shingles. (Courtesy Centers for Disease Control, Atlanta)

Figure 35-7   Shingles with extensive scab formation in a college-age student about 12 days after onset. Classical midline distribution is seen.

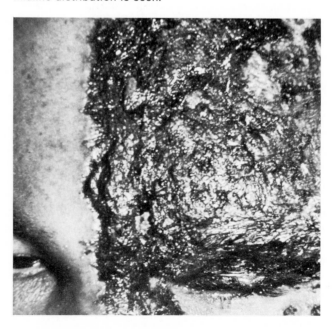

gresses through the rash, vesicular, pustular, and crusting stages, often fusing together into large lesions. Pain associated with the neurologic involvement may be severe for 1 to 4 weeks. Recovery occurs in 2 to 5 weeks with pain persisting (postzoster neuralgia) in some elderly patients for an additional period of time. The skin of the trunk and face are the areas most often affected.

Transmission

Chickenpox is one of the most communicable of all childhood diseases and most children become infected before the age of 10. The airborne route is the major means of transmission. Viruses are present in respiratory secretions, possibly a day or more before the appearance of a rash. Children are generally isolated after the rash appears; however, the V-Z virus may have already been spread by respiratory droplets to schoolmates and friends during the prodromal (onset) period. Viruses are also found in the vesicular fluid and pustular exudate during the first week of illness. Viruses are readily spread from this source by both direct and indirect contact and outbreaks are much more prevalent in the winter and spring (Figure 35-8).

Shingles is not transmitted from person to person; however, viruses are shed from the zoster lesions and susceptible children are able to contract chickenpox from this source. Thus the reactivation of the V-Z virus in zoster patients serves as a source that reintroduces the virus into a given population year after year.

Figure 35-8   Reported cases of chickenpox per month in the United States, 1982-1986. Seasonal variations are consistently seen with peak incidence rates in March, April, and May. A total of 183,243 cases were reported in 1986 (CDC Summary 1986).

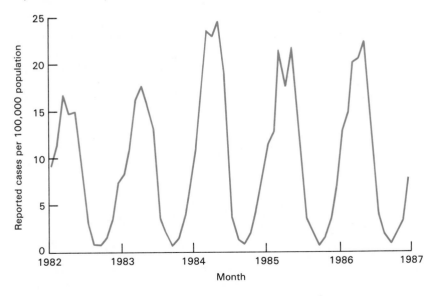

Chickenpox: Texas, 1979

A total of 7009 cases of chickenpox were reported in 1979 in Texas, a 14% increase over the 1978 figure. Eighty-five percent of the 4799 cases for which age data were available were in the 1- to 9-year age group. However, there was a 35% increase in the number of cases reported in the 10- to 14-year age group. The majority (76%) of reported cases occurred during the months of February through June, with the highest incidence in March.

In 1980, chickenpox cases continued to increase in this state. In the first 8 weeks of this year, 1452 cases were reported, a 38% increase over the total number for the same period in 1979. About 25% of the 362 cases reported during the single week ending February 23 occurred in a 5- to 9-year old group of children residing in one small town.

Editorial note: The data reported here are in general agreement with those previously published. Chickenpox is primarily a disease of school-age children that occurs in the winter and spring. The infectious agent, varicella-zoster virus, infects about 95% of the population in urban areas by early adulthood; secondary attack rates vary from 78% to 96% in susceptible household contacts. Four percent of infections are subclinical. Infection usually confers lifelong immunity, although rare cases of second attacks have been reported. Children who are not immunosuppressed may transmit the virus from as early as 1–2 days before to as late as 6 days following eruption of the first skin lesions. The incubation period is 10–23 days.

Persons at risk of severe disseminated disease include newborns whose mothers developed chickenpox less than 5 days before or within 2 days following delivery, and patients who are immunocompromised or have hematologic malignancies. These high-risk persons should be considered for attempted postexposure prophylaxis with varicella-zoster immune globulin (VZIG).

Adults who are otherwise healthy are at greater risk than children of developing complications of chickenpox, including pneumonia, encephalitis, and death. Fortunately, most adults are immune because of previous infection. Truly susceptable healthy adults who are exposed to chickenpox may be considered for prophylaxis with regular gamma globulin, which has been shown, at least in children, to reduce the severity of the incubating disease. True susceptibility may be determined by serologic tests such as the fluorescent-antibody-to-membrane-antigen (FAMA) test. The complement-fixation test is not sensitive enough for screening purposes. If serologic tests are unavailable, a high index of suspicion for true susceptibility should be maintained for those adults denying a history of chickenpox who either (1) grew up in the tropics (where the disease is less common) or (2) had relatively limited contact with children while growing up (e.g., lived in rural areas, had no siblings, or were the youngest in their sibships) (*MMWR*, 1980).

Diagnosis

Chickenpox is usually diagnosed on clinical appearance. Occasionally an atypical case may require laboratory diagnosis. Clinically chickenpox resembles smallpox; therefore when both diseases were present, it was important to make a rapid differential diagnosis. Since the eradication of smallpox, however, this is no longer a concern. Serologic tests are sometimes done on immunocompromised patients and on pregnant females near term who have no history of prior infection but have recently been exposed to chickenpox. This helps determine if they should receive passive immunization with zoster immune globulin (ZIG).

Diagnosis of zoster may be difficult in the early stages. Even in the later stages it may occasionally be confused with other skin infections. In such cases, it may be necessary to isolate and identify the virus by laboratory procedures.

Treatment

No specific antiviral treatments are normally used but acyclovir may be effective in treating disseminated infection in immunosuppressed patients. Symptomatic relief to relieve itching may be obtained with ointments. Secondary bacterial infections should be treated with antibiotic ointments.

Prevention and Control

A living attenuated vaccine is currently available and has limited use in patients who are at increased risk of developing severe, life-threatening disease. Passive immunization with ZIG, obtained from persons who have recently recovered from shingles, is sometimes used to treat near-term pregnant women who are seronegative to V-Z virus antibodies but have been exposed to chickenpox. ZIG is also administered to newborn infants of mothers who contract chickenpox just before or just after delivery and to immunosuppressed patients who become exposed, but have no prior immunity to the V-Z virus. Persons with chickenpox or zoster should be isolated for the first 5 to 7 days of illness to prevent further spread of the virus.

CYTOMEGALOVIRUSES (CMV)

The term *cytomegalo* means a cell of great size and describes the appearance of cells infected with this herpesvirus. CMV multiplies slowly and causes the host cell to swell in size. Cells up to 40 μm in diameter with a large inclusion body in the nucleus are produced.

Prevalence of Cytomegalovirus Excretion from Children in Five Day-Care Centers: Alabama, 1984

Recent studies have been done in Birmingham, Alabama, to determine the prevalence of cytomegalovirus (CMV) infection among attendees of day-care centers. Samples of urine and saliva from children attending five day-care centers were tested for CMV by viral isolation between March and June 1984. A culture was obtained from each child on a single occasion at both sites in almost all cases. Prevalence of serum antibody to CMV among parents and day-care center workers was determined using a commercial enzyme immunoassay. Centers A, B, and C served mainly middle-income families; centers D and E served primarily low-income families. Although excretion rates varied among the centers, each center had children who were shedding virus. Centers A, B, and C had at least one age cohort with greater than 50% excretion. A small number of children under 3 years of age had CMV in saliva and not in urine. Thus, the percentage of children with excretion from either site for the respective centers was 49% (A), 40% (B), 32% (C), 9% (D), and 13% (E). Frequency of viral excretion was lower in both urine and saliva

specimens from children in the lower socioeconomic centers. Questionnaires completed by parents provided past medical histories and histories of recent illness. One 3-year-old in center B had congenital CMV infection proven by viral isolation at birth. No children had histories of mononucleosislike illness, and there was no association between any specific acute illness during the preceding 6 months and CMV excretion at the time of the study. Previous CMV studies have found infection rates for preschool-aged children in the United States to range from approximately 5% to 30%. Serologic results revealed that 50% to 100% of workers from each day-care center had antibody to CMV, as did 56% to 88% of parents. These data indicate that CMV infection is common among young children in day-care centers.

Editorial note: Public awareness that maternal primary CMV infection during pregnancy can result in damaging fetal infections has increased in recent years. Although little is known about how CMV is transmitted in the community, it does not appear to be highly contagious. Acqui-

Inapparent infection

a subclinical infection. The immune response system is triggered in most inapparent infections but disease is not evident.

Pathogenesis

Most CMV infections are **inapparent** and the virus is able to persist in the body for long periods. In much of the world, the primary infection generally occurs early in life and remains subclinical in the infected person for the remainder of his or her life. The virus is shed periodically in the saliva and urine from persons with these inapparent infections.

Several clinical diseases are caused by the cytomegaloviruses. *Congenital infections* are acquired when the developing fetus becomes infected by viruses crossing the placental tissues from a mother who acquired a primary CMV infection during the pregnancy. Some of these congenitally infected infants are born with

sition appears to require close or intimate contact with persons who are excreting CMV in their urine, saliva, or other secretions. CMV can also be transmitted via blood transfusions, breast milk, sexual intercourse, and transplanted organs.

Studies have shown that infants and children acquire CMV infection from other children or from their mothers either in utero, at birth, or during the perinatal period. Intrauterine CMV infection is the most common of all recognized intrauterine infections, occurring in an estimated 0.4% to 2.3% of all live births, and it can have a variable outcome. It may result from either primary maternal infection acquired during pregnancy or from a recurrent infection (reactivation) or reinfection in a seropositive woman. Current evidence indicates that most but not all symptomatic congenital CMV infections result from primary infection of the mother. In the United States, 35% to 90% of women (depending on race and socioeconomic status) entering their childbearing years are seropositive, and thus, they are not susceptible to primary CMV infection.

CMV infection is endemic in the community, and infection in childhood is common and usually asymptomatic. Previously published results from a longitudinal study of children in a day-care center indicate that the majority of children acquired CMV after joining the center and that the estimated cumulative infection rate may reach as high as 80% for children during their second year of life. Excretion of CMV has persisted for months to years in most of the children studied at that center, as it does in congenital CMV-infected children. Another study comparing point prevalence rates of CMV excretion in urine and saliva of children attending infant development centers for the developmentally delayed and those in day-care centers demonstrated that urinary excretion occurred in 22% of children in both types of centers (*MMWR* 34:50, 1985).

severe deformities and die shortly after birth. About 1% of neonatal deaths are due to this virus. Some infants survive with serious physical and mental defects. Other congenitally infected infants survive without any obvious tissue damage. The second clinical form of this disease is an activation of an inapparent infection. It may be seen in both children and adults and is associated with prolonged immunosuppressive therapy for such procedures as organ transplants or cancer. This form of infection is frequently seen in AIDS patients and is a severe life-threatening disease in these persons. A third form of CMV disease is posttransfusion or post–organ transplant syndrome, a mononucleosislike illness that is seen in persons who had not previously been exposed to CMV but received blood transfusions or organ transplants that contained CMV. Normal adolescents may also develop a mild mononucleosislike illness when exposed to this virus for the first time.

Transmission

About 1% of newborns have congenital CMV infections. Most infections occur early in life in children who are exposed to contaminated saliva and urine. In much of the world, 80% to 100% of the population has been exposed to CMV. Some infections are transmitted by blood transfusions. As with most diseases, transmission of CMV is more efficient in environments of poor sanitation.

Diagnosis

CMV may be cultivated from the infected tissues or secretions on cell cultures. Cells taken from the site of infection may show the characteristic cytomegalic cells, and the presence of CMV antigens can be detected using immunofluorescent procedures with monoclonal antibodies.

Treatment

Chemotherapeutic agents that show some effects on other herpesvirus infections have shown little if any effect on CMV infections. Interferon treatments have possibly helped reduce the incidence and severity of reactivation of CMV infections in recipients of kidney transplants.

Prevention and Control

Because of the large number of inapparent cases of CMV infection in the general population, no specific control measures are available. No vaccine currently exists, but developmental work on a vaccine is now underway.

EPSTEIN-BARR VIRUS (EBV)

Epstein-Barr virus is a widespread herpesvirus that has been incriminated as the possible cause of several forms of cancer, and is also the cause of *infectious mononucleosis*.

Pathogenesis and Clinical Disease

Parotid glands
salivary glands located at the back of the jaw.

Infection with EBV is acquired by the oral route. Viral multiplication possibly occurs in the throat and **parotid glands**. The virus also apparently passes through the lymphatic system and into the blood where the principle target is the B cells. Most of the interactions between the viruses and B cells do not destroy the B cells but transform them into plasma cells. These plasma cells secrete a variety of immunoglobulins unrelated to the EBV. Some of these immunoglobulins are the **heterophile antibodies** that are useful in the diagnosis of infectious mononucleosis. T cells in large numbers are mobilized against the B cells that have EBV antigens on their membranes. The transformed B cells and T cells account for the increased number of **atypical lymphocytes** that are seen in infectious mononucleosis patients. The accumulation of these cells also accounts for the tonsillitis, swollen spleen, and enlarged lymph nodes associated with infectious mononucleosis. Immunity against reinfection occurs, yet, multiple copies of the EBV DNA persist in a few B cells. The immune system is not able to rid the body of these infected cells and a few of these cells shed virus. Some evidence suggests that virus may also continue to multiply intermittently in the parotid glands and be shed in the saliva, which is a principal means of spread.

Infectious mononucleosis is very mild or even subclinical in young children. From adolescence on, clinical disease occurs in about 50% of those who are infected for the first time with the EBV. And most typical clinical diseases are seen in persons between 15 and 35 years of age. The incubation period may range from 3 to 7 weeks. The onset is gradual, lasting up to 1 week, and may consist of such general symptoms as malaise, headache, fatigue, and low-grade fever. The acute phase may last 1 to 3 weeks, but it is longer in some and is characterized by intermittent high fever, generalized weakness, severe sore throat, malaise, swollen lymph nodes, enlarged spleen, occasionally a rash, and a greatly increased number of abnormally appearing lymphocytes (mononuclear cells) in the blood. The last characteristic is the basis for the name infectious mononucleosis. The convalescent phase, with accompanying malaise and weakness, may be prolonged. Death or serious complications are rare in otherwise normal patients. However, in persons on immunosuppressive treatment for organ transplants, on anticancer chemotherapy, or with some genetic defects, infectious mononucleosis may progress unchecked by the immune system, and death may result.

A condition sometimes referred to as *chronic EBV disease*, has been described in recent years. These patients have persistent or relapsing unexplained fatigue lasting for months. Sometimes this is associated with slight fever, sore throat, muscle and bone pains, and headaches. Some evidence suggests this condition is a result of a chronic EBV infection.

Transmission and Epidemiology

It now appears that most people, particularly in areas where crowding and poor sanitation exist, contract mononucleosis early in life and experience subclinical infections. The typical clinical

Heterophile antibody

an antibody that reacts with antigens other than those responsible for induction. Human heterophile antibodies will hemagglutinate sheep red blood cells.

Atypical lymphocyte

lymphocytes which are abnormal, usually enlarged with a foamy nucleus. These cells typically appear in response to certain viral infections.

disease usually occurs in adolescents and young adults who escaped infection earlier in life. About 90% of adults have been infected and the virus is found in the oral secretions of an estimated 20% of the general population.

The infection is widespread in young persons in tropical and subtropical areas as well as lower socioeconomic groups in temperate climates. People in such groups are frequently infected before school age and develop a subclinical or generalized infection that is not recognized as infectious mononucleosis. These persons may become lifelong carriers of the virus. The typical clinical disease is seen most often in adolescents and young adults; the highest incidence occurs in young persons who have had a more sheltered early life. When these individuals experience greater exposure during high school or college, they are prime candidates for the clinically recognizable form of infectious mononucleosis. Because the exchange of saliva by intimate oral contact is a most efficient means of transmitting this disease, the synonym "kissing disease" is appropriate; however, transmission may occur by other less direct routes. It is estimated that 100,000 college undergraduates contract infectious mononucleosis each year in the United States.

Diagnosis

The enlarged lymph nodes and increased number of mononuclear cells, along with the compatible generalized symptoms in persons of the appropriate age, strongly suggest infectious mononucleosis. The diagnosis is confirmed by showing a rise in antibodies. Tests are now becoming available to measure antibodies specifically against the EB virus. A nonspecific antibody test, called the *heterophile antibody test*, has been helpful in diagnosing this disease for many years. This test used sheep or horse red blood cells as the antigen. By the third week of illness 80% of the infectious mononucleosis patients develop antibodies that will agglutinate these red blood cells.

Treatment

There is no treatment for mononucleosis other than supportive therapy. Bedrest is recommended during the acute phase and is usually spontaneous as a result of the generalized weakness of the patient. Contact-type physical activities should be avoided, for the swollen spleen could rupture if bumped.

Prevention and Control

No vaccine against EBV infections is available, but some are being developed. Isolation of patients is of little value. Persons who have recently recovered from mononucleosis should not donate blood. Due to the widespread distribution of this virus in asymptomatic carriers, only a recluse could purposely avoid being infected—a price most young people are not willing to pay to prevent this nonfatal disease.

CONCEPT SUMMARY

1. Infection due to the DNA herpesvirus group is the object of considerable attention and concern today. These viruses are responsible for a wide variety of disease conditions in both humans and animals. They cause benign, latent infections, such as cold sores, and extensive life-threatening infections, such as generalized herpes.

2. Herpesviruses are widely known because of current interest in their role as agents of a sexually transmitted disease caused by herpes simplex virus type 2 and because of infectious mononucleosis due to the Epstein-Barr virus.

3. Herpesviruses are among the few viruses for which a specific antiviral therapy has been developed.

4. Although not generally well known, cytomegalovirus infection is extremely common. This agent is responsible for serious, often fatal, disease in immunocompromised patients.

STUDY SUMMARY

1. Briefly describe the host-parasite relationship commonly associated with herpesvirus infections.

2. Why isn't antibody to herpesvirus type 1 and type 2 protective against reoccurrence of the disease?

3. What is the most common site of infection for type 2 herpes?

4. Why would a viral-component vaccine be particularly useful against herpesviruses?

5. What is the likely source of an outbreak of chickenpox in a community that is apparently free of the virus?

6. What is the biggest risk factor associated with cytomegalovirus infection?

REFERENCES FOR FURTHER STUDY

1. Increased Frequency of Cytomegalovirus Infection in Children in Group Day Care. *Pediatrics* 74:121, 1984

2. *The Herpes Viruses* vols. 1–4, B. Roizman, 1982–1983. Plenum.

3. Herpes Simplex Viral Hepatitis in Adults: Review of the Literature. *Reviews of Infectious Diseases* 9:329, 1987.

4. Antiviral Chemotherapy. *Infectious Disease Clinics of North America* 1:2, 1987.

5. Serologic Markers for Epstein-Barr Virus Infection in Chronic Carriers of Hepatitis B Surface Antigen Who Live in Northern Canada. *Journal of Infectious Diseases* 156:202, 1987.

6. Herpes Simplex Virus Glycoprotein Treatment of Recurrent Genital Herpes. *Journal of Infectious Diseases* 157:156, 1988.

chapter 36

HEPATITIS VIRUSES

A lthough the clinical disease of **hepatitis** was recognized in ancient times, it was not until the early 1940s that sufficient evidence existed to distinguish at least two distinct types and to suspect that the etiologic agents were viral. One form of hepatitis was called *infectious*, for evidence indicated that it was passed from person to person by usual means, particularly the fecal-oral route. The other form was called *serum hepatitis* and was thought to be transmitted only by the injection of body fluids, such as blood, serum, and plasma, or the use of contaminated needles or syringes. Up until the late 1960s little progress was made in isolating and characterizing the viruses causing hepatitis by standard methods; since then, however, new methods have yielded significant information on the nature of hepatitis. This new information is markedly changing our understanding of these diseases; at present, our knowledge is expanding rapidly but is still incomplete. The disease previously referred to as infectious hepatitis is now called *hepatitis A* and serum hepatitis is called *hepatitis B*. When it became possible to specifically diagnose both hepatitis A and B by serologic tests, it was discovered that some cases of hepatitis were not caused by either hepatitis A or hepatitis B viruses but were apparently caused by other, as yet unidentified viruses. These cases are being referred to as *non-A non-B* (NANB) hepatitis. This chapter summarizes our current knowledge of hepatitis A and B, and other possible types of viral hepatitis.

HEPATITIS A

Virus

For many years all attempts to grow the hepatitis A virus in cell cultures failed, but such propagation is now possible. Marmosets, monkeys, and chimpanzees can be experimentally infected, but,

Hepatitis
inflammation of the liver. This condition may be due to infectious disease agents or organic causes.

in general, early experimental work involved human volunteers. In 1973 virus-sized particles were observed via the electron microscope in the feces of patients with hepatitis A. These particles were 27 nm in diameter, possessed cubical symmetry, and specifically reacted with antibodies in the serum of patients who had recently recovered from hepatitis A. This virus closely resembles the enteroviruses (Chapter 39) and has been classified as enterovirus type 72. The hepatitis A virus has single-stand RNA, is very stable, and only one serotype has been found.

Pathogenesis and Clinical Disease

The hepatitis A virus enters the body orally. Most evidence indicates that the virus first multiplies along the intestinal epithelium and may result in anorexia (loss of appetite), malaise, intermittent fever, followed by nausea, vomiting, and diarrhea. In an undetermined percentage of infected persons the virus passes to the blood and spreads to the liver. Inflammation of the liver produces the classical signs of hepatitis, such as **jaundice** (yellowness of skin due to presence of bile pigments), dark urine, and pale, offensive feces. The signs of hepatitis appear about 1 week after the initial intestinal symptoms, recovery takes 4 to 6 weeks or longer, and the general weakness continues even longer. Death rates are less than 0.1%. The disease is mild in children and usually inapparent. It is now suspected that the hepatitis A virus might be widespread in tropical and underdeveloped areas, where most persons become infected early in life. In such environments, clinical infections are most often seen in adult "outsiders" who enter the area. The extent of virus spread in countries with improved sanitation is difficult to determine at present. Clinical cases seem to increase, however, as living conditions improve, thus suggesting a condition similar to that seen with polio (see Chapter 39); that is, the lack of exposure early in life allows a greater number of susceptible persons to accumulate in the adult population. An inexpensive serological test (ELISA) is now available to measure antibodies against the hepatitis A virus. Using this test, it is possible to study and gain a greater insight into the epidemiology of this disease.

Transmission and Epidemiology

The fecal-oral route appears to be the major means of transmission. Outbreaks have been traced to contaminated water supplies and to food vendors who are carriers. Outbreaks are common in mental institutions where sanitary practices are difficult to maintain. Over 20,000 cases of hepatitis A are reported each year in the United States (Figure 36-1).

Jaundice
a symptom showing an increase in bilirubin in the blood. Jaundiced patients often develop yellow-brown skin color.

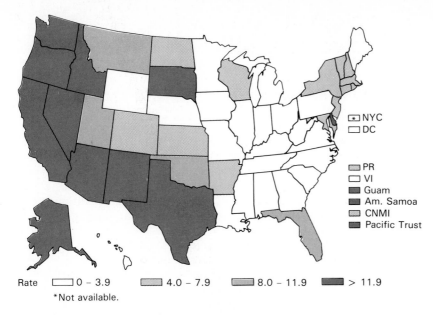

Rate ☐ 0 – 3.9   ▨ 4.0 – 7.9   ▨ 8.0 – 11.9   ■ > 11.9
      *Not available.

Figure 36-1   National distribution and occurrence of Hepatitis A.
(Courtesy Centers for Disease Control, Atlanta)

Diagnosis

Routine serological tests are available to detect the virus and measure antibodies. Diagnosis is based on both serology and clinical signs associated with inflammation of the liver. Liver enzymes called **transaminases**, which are released into the blood during liver inflammation, can be measured as an indirect sign of viral hepatitis.

Treatment

Treatment of hepatitis is symptomatic and often prolonged rest is required before complete recovery occurs.

Prevention and Control

Research programs are under way to develop vaccines for hepatitis A and a live vaccine is being tried in United States military personnel. Maintenance of good sanitary conditions is the most effective control. Passive immunization with pooled human gamma globulin may offer some protection for several months. Such passive immunizations are recommended for military or other persons going into areas where poor sanitation exists.

Transaminase
a normal tissue enzyme that can transfer an amino group from one compound to another. Increased levels of serum transaminase indicate tissue injury.

Outbreak of Food-borne Hepatitis A: New Jersey, 1981

An increase in the number of hepatitis cases in Monmouth County, New Jersey, was reported to the New Jersey Department of Health on June 15, 1981. Investigation by state and local area health departments revealed that 56 cases of hepatitis had occurred during the first 3 weeks of June in an area of Monmouth County where the usual average is 3 to 4 cases per month. Patients for whom appropriate laboratory tests had been done were confirmed to have hepatitis A.

Detailed food histories revealed that, within the appropriate incubation period for hepatitis A, 55 of the 56 patients had eaten at a Mexican-style restaurant. Interviews of a control group matched for age, sex, and neighborhood of residence, showed that 10% of the controls ate food from this restaurant over a time period comparable with that for 90% of the patients. The restaurant agreed to close voluntarily pending further investigation.

Of the patients whose illness was related to the Mexican restaurant, 71% were male, 68% were between the ages of 15 and 29 years, and 4 were children under 15 years. A case-control study using 46 non-ill patrons revealed that patients were more likely to have eaten nachos, beans, and jalapeno peppers. Both beans and jalapeno peppers were used in preparing nachos.

Ten individuals including the two owners worked in the restaurant; all handled food at one time or another. Interviews on June 18 revealed that one employee who frequently ate food from the restaurant was ill with hepatitis at the time of the interview. Another employee had symptoms compatible with hepatitis on May 9. He had worked all day May 9, but felt too ill to work thereafter; the diagnosis of hepatitis A was confirmed for him on May 16. This employee prepared food—including grating cheese, shredding lettuce, and occasionally cutting meat; measured portions of meat, beans, jalapeno peppers, onions, cheeses, and lettuce into shells; and served the customers.

Because a food handler was recently ill with hepatitis and because the restaurant was implicated in the spread of hepatitis, immune globulin was offered to all individuals who ate in the restaurant from June 5 until it closed. A total of 1430 people were immunized at a 2-day clinic held June 19 and 20.

Editorial note: Hepatitis A virus (HAV) can be transmitted by food contaminated with feces from an infected food handler. If acute hepatitis A has been confirmed in a food handler by testing for IgM-specific HAV antibody, immunoglobulin prophylaxis (IG, gamma globulin) may be considered by patrons, depending on the probability of transmission of infectious virus and the probability of successful intervention in transmission by using IG. However, few food handlers actually appear to transmit disease via food, and IG prophylaxis of patrons is seldom warranted. Although for the past few years approximately 1000 food handlers with non-B hepatitis have been reported annually to CDC, an average of four outbreaks of food-borne hepatitis A have been reported each year (*MMWR* 31:150, 1982).

HEPATITIS B

Virus

The hepatitis B virus (HBV) differs from other known viruses and has been classified into a separate family called Hepadnaviradae. It cannot be grown in cell cultures and higher primates are the only susceptible experimental hosts. In spite of the inability to readily grow this virus in the laboratory, a significant amount of information has been obtained by studying concentrations of viruses obtained from blood of infected humans. The complete **virion** is 42 nm in diameter and is sometimes called a *Dane particle* (named after D. S. Dane who first characterized it). The virion has two concentric protein capsids. The inner capsid or core is 27 nm in diameter and surrounds the nucleic acid and is made of a different type of protein than the outer capsid. The proteins comprising the outer capsid are called the *hepatitis B surface antigens* (HBsAg) and the core protein is called the *hepatitis B core antigen* (HBcAg). The HBV contains a unique circular DNA molecule that is part double-stranded and part single-stranded. The DNA and HBcAg appear to be produced and assembled in the nucleus of infected cells and then passed into the cytoplasm. The HBsAg is produced in the cytoplasm and then added over the core protein. In chronic infections, great excesses of HBsAg are produced and form into 22-nm diameter spherical and filamentous particles. These particles contain only protein and are released in large numbers into the blood. The presence of this HBsAg in the blood is a valuable diagnostic aid in the detection of persons who may be carriers of HBV. The structure of HBV is shown in Figure 36-2.

Virion
the complete, infective virus.

Figure 36-2   The various particles associated with HBV. (a) 42 nm complete virion (Dane particle); (b) 22 nm diameter spheres composed only of surface antigen; (c) 22 nm diameter filaments composed only of surface antigen.

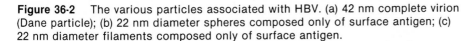

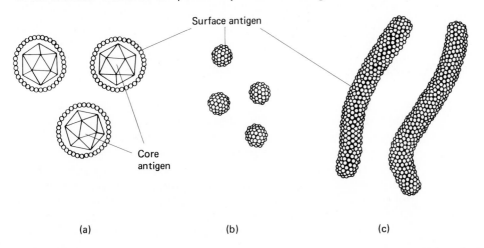

(a)   (b)   (c)

Pathogenesis and Clinical Disease

The clinical picture of hepatitis B is somewhat similar to that of hepatitis A except the incubation period is longer—6 weeks to 6 months—and the disease is more severe, with an overall death rate of about 1%. When adults become infected, most recover completely after several months. Some, 5% to 10% develop chronic forms of hepatitis that in a few cases progress to either **cirrhosis** or cancer of the liver. Some patients become asymptomatic carriers of the infection and contain large amounts of HBsAg in their serum; this condition may last from 6 months to a lifetime. In developing countries where HBV is widespread, most adults have been infected. These infections usually occur in early childhood and many (10% to 50%) become carriers of the virus. About one-third of these will eventually develop chronic forms of hepatitis.

Cirrhosis

a progressive disease of the liver characterized by granuloma/modular development and ultimate liver failure.

Transmission and Epidemiology

The most readily detected outbreaks of hepatitis B are usually transmitted by contaminated blood or blood products that are used in the treatment or immunization of patients. These cases are generally quite severe. The death rates may be from 10% to 20% in persons acquiring hepatitis B through blood transfusions, partly because of the large doses of virus received and partly because of the weakened or compromised conditions of the persons needing the transfusion. Contaminated needles, syringes, and similar items may readily transmit this virus and infectivity rates, as measured by the presence of HBsAg in the serum, may exceed 50% among drug addicts who use and share unsterilized needles and syringes. The infection is also transmitted between sexual contacts and is a particular problem for homosexual males. About 26,000 cases of hepatitis B are reported in the United States each year.

With the development of serologic methods to detect the presence of HBsAg in blood in the late 1960s and early 1970s, a better study of the epidemiology of hepatitis B was possible. The picture that is emerging indicates that this infection is widespread in certain cultures with most cases being subclinical. The infection is most widespread among population in Asia, in primitive areas, in mental institutions, and in areas where sanitation practices are inadequate. The infectivity rates run from close to 100% in some groups, less (20% to 30%) in others with improving conditions, compared to about 0.1% in the United States. HBsAg was originally discovered during a study of blood proteins of the Australian aborigines when it was thought that this protein was a common but unique component of their blood; so at first it was called the Australia antigen.

Diagnosis

Diagnosis of hepatitis, in general, is made as described for hepatitis A. When the disease occurs in a patient who has received blood transfusions or other blood products, hepatitis B is suspected. Various serologic tests to detect the presence of hepatitis B antigens and antibodies in the serum are now available and are being used as specific tools in the diagnosis of this disease.

Treatment

Hyperimmune gamma globulin may offer some passive protection to individuals who have been exposed to HBV-contaminated materials. Personnel working with hepatitis patients or blood products in the laboratory should be extra careful so as to reduce the chances of contracting hepatitis B. Treatment is symptomatic.

Prevention and Control

The major efforts to prevent hepatitis B in developed countries involve the avoidance of contaminated instruments when cutting tissues or injecting medication and transfusing blood that may contain HBV. Up until the discovery of HBsAg in the late 1960s no reliable method was available to detect the presence of HBV in the blood of donors. Once the HBsAg was isolated, it was possible to induce high levels of antibodies against this antigen in animals. These antibodies then became available for use in serologic tests to determine whether a given sample of blood contained the HBsAg. Such sensitive serologic tests as radioimmunoassays or ELISA tests have made it possible to detect and eliminate most HBV-contaminated blood products. Federal regulations now require that all blood samples used for transfusion, as well as blood products given by injection, must be tested for HBV. Such serologic tests help to reduce the cases of post-transfusion hepatitis but are irrelevant to the control of HBV infections that are widespread in areas with low standards of hygiene or where transmission is primarily by sexual contact or parenteral drug abuse.

Even though the HBV cannot be grown under experimental conditions, the HBsAg can be obtained in relatively large amounts from the serum of chronic human carriers of the infection. This formed the basis of the first vaccine developed for hepatitis B in the early 1980s. The HBsAg was extracted from the blood of known carriers (primarily from infected male homosexuals), purified, and treated with formalin to kill any active virus particles; this was then used as a killed vaccine. Such a vaccine was relatively expensive and in short supply, but was useful in protecting some high-risk individuals, such as babies born of HBsAg-positive mothers, those who require frequent blood transfusions, and ho-

Hepatitis B Associated with Jet Gun Injection: California, 1985

In March 1985, during routine investigation of hepatitis B (HB) case reports, an epidemiologist at the Long Beach (California) Department of Public Health noted that three HB patients had each received injections at the same weight-reduction clinic (clinic A) before disease onset. When review of previous case records and questioning of newly reported HB patients identified five additional HB cases among clinic attendees, the California Department of Health Services joined in the investigation of the clinic on July 1, 1985.

Clinic A belonged to a chain of 29 weight-reduction clinics located throughout southern California. Attendees at the clinic typically received a series of daily parenteral injections of human chorionic gonadotropin (HCG). Injections were usually given by jet injectors (Med-E-Jet Corp., Cleveland, Ohio), although some attendees received injections with single-use disposable needles and syringes. A standard regimen consisted of 30 injections; however, individuals varied considerably in duration of treatment and number of injections received.

The investigation focused on a cohort of 341 persons who attended clinic A during the first 6 months of 1985. Clinical history, review of risk factors for acquiring hepatitis B virus (HBV) infection, serologic testing for HBV markers (hepatitis B surface antigen [HBsAg], antibody to HB core antigen [anti-HBc], and IgM anti-HBc) and quantification of parenteral exposures at the clinic were obtained on 287 (84%) of cohort members. For comparison, 93 new attendees (after July 1, 1985) at clinic A and random samples of 100 prior attendees and 70 new attendees at the other Long Beach clinic (clinic B) were tested for markers of HBV infection.

Ultimately, 31 cases of clinical HB were identified among attendees of Clinic A. Onset dates ranged from January 1984 to November 1985, with the majority of cases occurring between February and November 1985. Only 2 (6%) of the patients with clinical HB had other identified risk factors for acquiring HBV infection in the 6 months before their illnesses.

On initial analysis of the cohort members, exposure to the jet injectors and HCG were both significantly associated with the development of acute HBV infection. However, two lots of HCG used at the clinic during the outbreak (from February 1985 onward) were negative when tested for HBsAg. Furthermore, stratification of cohort members who received HCG by type of parenteral inoculation (jet injector only, compared with syringe only) showed that 24% of those receiving injections by jet injector had developed acute HBV infection compared with none of those receiving injections by syringe only ($p <$ .01). These two groups had similar numbers of HCG exposures, with the syringe-only group averaging 31, while the jet injector–only group averaged 27 (*MMWR* 35:373, 1986).

mosexual males. With the discovery that AIDS was caused by the HIV virus, there was great alarm that persons who were both HBV carriers and infected with HIV may have provided blood for HBV vaccine. Subsequent studies have shown that while some blood may have initially contained both viruses, the process of inactivating the HBV also inactivates the HIV. Therefore HBV vaccine prepared from the blood of AIDS patients poses no threat of transmission of HIV. In 1987, HBsAg produced through genetic engineering of HBV DNA into bacteria, yeast, or mammalian cell cultures became available as a vaccine. This should make a hepatitis B vaccine readily available to population groups at risk. Work is also progressing on cloning the gene for HBsAg into vaccinia viruses for the production of a live vaccine that could be economically feasible for use in developing countries where hepatitis B is so widespread; an estimated 200 million people are infected in those countries. The concern for infection with the HIV virus has led to alteration of some male homosexual practices that were associated with transmission of HBV. The occurrence of both of these diseases has decreased in this population as a result of these changes.

OTHER TYPES OF HEPATITIS

One of the distressing discoveries in recent years has been the failure to eliminate post-transfusion hepatitis by eliminating blood that contains HBsAg. It now appears that other hepatitis viruses may be present. Such hepatitis has been referred to as *non-A non-B hepatitis* (NANB). Because of the HBV serologic screening tests used on all blood donated for transfusion, most of the posttransfusion hepatitis that does occur in the United States now is NANB (Figure 36-3). A virus particle with cubical symmetry and a diame-

Figure 36-3   Report of cases of hepatitis in the United States 1950–1987. (Courtesy Centers for Disease Control, Atlanta)

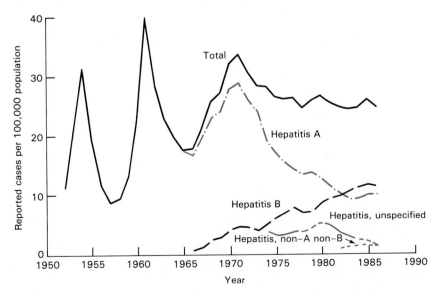

Delta Hepatitis: Massachusetts, 1984

An outbreak of hepatitis B (HB) that began in September 1983 is continuing in Worcester, Massachusetts, primarily involving parenteral drug abusers (PDAs) and their sexual contacts. As of August 1, 1984, 75 cases of acute HB have been identified, 50 of which are considered outbreak-related. Fulminant hepatitis has been a prominent feature of this outbreak. Six deaths have occurred, for an outbreak-related case fatality ratio of 12%.

Patients meeting all the following criteria were considered outbreak-related HB cases: (1) an acute clinical illness compatible with HB; (2) elevated serum glutamic-oxaloacetic transaminase (SGOT) or serum glutamic-pyruvic transaminase (SGPT) two or more times greater than the upper limit of normal (when such results were available); (3) positive serology for hepatitis B surface antigen (HBsAg); (4) residence and/or primary diagnosis and treatment within the city of Worcester; and (5) a PDA or a direct contact of a PDA.

Patients with acute HB who could be located were interviewed regarding their drug and alcohol use, as well as risk factors for HB. Serum samples were obtained to test for markers of hepatitis B virus (HBV) infection and delta virus infection.

Of the 50 outbreak-related case patients, 35 were male. Twenty-nine were white, non-Hispanic; 17 were Hispanic; 2 were black; and 2 were of unknown race. Ages ranged from 15 years to 43 years (median 25 years). Forty-three patients used needles; 6 were sexual contacts of PDAs; and 1 had direct contact with open wounds of a person with hepatitis. Of the 6 patient who died, 3 were male; 5 were white, non-Hispanic; and 1 was Hispanic. Ages ranged from 19 years to 34 years of age (median 27 years). Five were PDAs, and 1 was a sexual contact of a known PDA.

Drugs that were self-injected were primarily heroin and cocaine. No 3,4-methylene diamphetamine (MDA), a drug implicated in fulminant HB/PDA deaths in North Carolina in 1979, was used. The only potential hepatotoxin identified was alcohol.

Testing for HB markers confirmed HB in all cases. Serum specimens were available from 4 patients who died; 3 had immunoglobulin M (IgM) anti–delta virus antibodies. IgM anti–delta virus antibodies were also present in 4 of 22 PDAs with nonfulminant acute HB, 1 of 7 PDA contacts with nonfulminant acute HB, and none of 11 non-outbreak-related patients with acute HB. In addition, 2 of 13 nonill HBsAg-positive PDAs had serologic markers of delta virus infection (1 with IgG antibodies and 1 with IgM) (*MMWR* 33:494, 1984).

ter of 27 nm has been associated with NANB hepatitis and may represent a newly discovered hepatitis virus.

Another form of viral hepatitis that is being characterized is called hepatitis D. The causative agent is a 36-nm spherical virus with a single-stranded RNA genome and has a protein coat composed of HBsAg. It is called the *delta virus*. The delta virus is a defective virus, which means it is only able to replicate in association with another virus that acts as a helper virus and supplies essential components needed by the defective virus. The HBV acts as a helper virus by supplying its surface antigen (HBsAg) as a protein coat for the delta virus. This means that only persons who have infections with HBV can be superinfected with the delta virus. The person may be a chronic carrier of HBV with no clinical signs of hepatitis before the infection with the delta virus, but after the superinfection with the delta virus the hepatitis becomes clinically active and even **fulminating**. The epidemiology of hepatitis D is not clearly understood; however, preliminary evidence suggests it could be a major problem in intravenous drug users and in some primitive cultures. When these two viruses (HBV and delta) occur together the disease tends to be particularly severe with a significant increase in mortality.

Fulminating
running a rapid course with continued worsening of patient condition.

CONCEPT SUMMARY

1. Hepatitis has long been one of the most common human diseases. Today the more widely known hepatitis A form has given way in interest to hepatitis B, which is transmitted through body excretions and is associated with increased health risks to hospitalized patients and personnel. A third hepatitis virus, non-A non-B, appears to cause a disease similar to that of hepatitis B.

2. These viruses are not yet cultured effectively in in vitro systems. Some protection, however, is afforded to hepatitis A by passive immunization procedures, and a recently developed hepatitis B vaccine has been effective in reducing the incidence of this disease.

3. Diagnosis of both hepatitis A and B, as well an non-A non-B, is effectively accomplished by recently developed serologic procedures. Use of these tests has greatly reduced the risk of transfusion-associated hepatitis B.

STUDY SUMMARY

1. What characteristic of the hepatitis viruses significantly delayed the development of diagnostic serological tests?

2. Describe the essential differences between transmission of hepatitis A and hepatitis B viruses.

3. What reasons can you suggest for the extremely high rate of HBV infections in Asian populations?

4. List the primary risk factors associated with HBV transmission, and suggest a mechanism which may be useful to interrupt each.

REFERENCES FOR FURTHER STUDY

1. Detection of Hepatitis A Virus by Extraction of Viral RNA and Molecular Hybridization. *J. Clinical Microbiology* 25:1822, 1988.

2. Comparative Evaluation of Commercial Enzyme Immunoassay Kits for Detection of Hepatitis B Seromarkers. *J. Clinical Micro.* 25:432, 1988.

3. Demonstration of Hepatitis D Virus in Patients with Chronic Hepatitis. *J. Infectious Disease* 157:191, 1988.

4. Studies of Prototype Live Hepatitis A Virus Vaccines in Primate Models. *J. Infectious Disease* 157:338, 1988.

5. Delta Hepatitis: A New Scourge? *N. England Journal of Medicine* 312:1515, 1985.

6. *Viral Hepatitis and Liver Disease.* G. N. Vyas. 1984, Grune & Stratton.

7. Immunization Practices Advisory Committee: Recommendations for Protection Against Viral Hepatitis. *Morbidity and Mortality Weekly Report* 34:313, 1985.

chapter 37

ORTHOMYXOVIRUSES

T
he family Orthomyxoviradae contains the influenza viruses. Various animal species become infected with their own specific strains of influenza and, in some cases, the animal strains may produce mild infections in humans. The human strains of influenza viruses cause some of the more explosive and severe viral respiratory infections. The term "flu" is used in daily speech to refer to a wide variety of infections, ranging from mild respiratory infections, such as the common cold, to various forms of enteritis ("intestinal flu"). Yet when used correctly, the terms flu or influenza should describe a very characteristic disease that is discussed in this chapter.

INFLUENZA

Characteristics of the Viruses

Three general types of influenza viruses have been identified and are designated types A, B, and C. Type A causes the major influenzal epidemics of humans, type B causes moderate outbreaks, and type C is relatively insignificant. The following discussion is limited primarily to type A influenza.

The influenza virus has several features that need to be understood when studying the unique epidemiologic patterns of influenza. Features of the influenza virus are shown in Figure 37-1. The inner core of the virion contains a helical capsid that surrounds a ss-RNA molecule. The RNA molecule is somewhat unique in that it is made up of eight loosely connected segments and each segment contains the genetic information for the formation of a specific viral component. Of importance to the following discussion are the two protein components (peplomers) that are embedded in the lipid envelope and project out from the virus. These protein peplomers are effective antigens and the antibodies that form against them provide immunity to the host. One

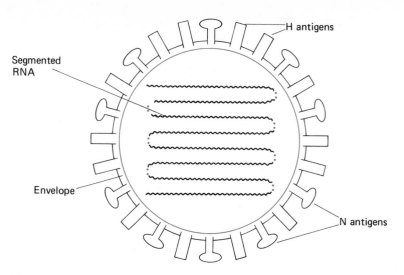

Figure 37-1 Schematic outline of an influenza virion. The H and N antigens are peplomers that protrude from the envelope. The RNA is in eight segments and is located inside a helical capsid.

Hemagglutination

a process by which an antibody or virus particle forms a bridge between two red blood cells such that they appear to be stuck together.

peplomer serves as the attachment site between the virus and the host cells and also causes **hemagglutination** (the clumping or agglutination of RBCs); thus it is called the *hemagglutinin* or simply the *H antigen*. The other peplomer is an enzyme that dissolves a component of mucus called *neuraminic acid*. This protein is thus called *neuraminidase* or the *N antigen*.

Among the influenza viruses that infect humans, three distinct antigenic subtypes exist and are designated H1, H2, and H3. Thirteen distinct H antigens are found in influenza viruses that infect animals and include H1, H2, H3 and on to H13. A total of nine N antigen subtypes (N1–N9) have been found, but only N1 and N2 are routinely found in viral isolates from humans. Antibodies formed against the H and the N antigens are the important protective antibodies.

Minor mutations occasionally occur in the RNA segments that control the configurations of the antigenic determinants of the H and N antigens. These minor changes are called *antigenic drift*. When the minor antigenic drifts occur, the antibodies in the general population are less effective in providing immunity and limited outbreaks of influenza may develop. When a new subtype of the H or the N antigen appears in a strain of influenza virus, it is called an *antigenic shift*. The origin of the antigenic shifts have been theoretically attributed to either major mutations in the viral RNA or to reassortment of RNA segment between two different influenzal subtypes that are simultaneously infecting the same host. When a major shift occurs, the protective antibodies that are already in the population are of no further value, the virus is able to spread without restrictions, and a pandemic of influenza may result. Subtypes of type A influenza viruses are given a designation that tells where and when it was first isolated, and the antigenic composition. For example, A/Hong Kong/68(H3N2) would be the influenza subtype isolated in Hong Kong in 1968 with the H3 and N2 antigens.

Pathogenesis and Clinical Disease

Humans are infected with influenza viruses primarily by the airborne route. The viruses specifically attach to the ciliated epithelial cells of the respiratory tract for the initiation of the infection. As viruses are released from the few cells that are initially infected, many adjacent cells become infected and the infection spreads along the epithelium of the respiratory tract. Widespread inflammation results. Usually the infection is limited to the upper respiratory tract, but in severe cases the lower respiratory tract may also be involved. The influenza virus rarely spreads to the blood or deeper body tissues; however, toxic products from the virus are absorbed into the blood and are responsible for the generalized symptoms of influenza. Influenza has a distinct clinical picture with an onset of 1 to 3 days after exposure. A sore throat, cough, possible hoarseness, and nasal discharge are the localized signs. The systemic manifestations caused by the toxic materials include headache, fever, chills, generalized muscular aches, and, in severe cases, prostration. Gastrointestinal symptoms may also be present. Recovery is usually spontaneous after 4 to 7 days. Deaths are rare in otherwise healthy individuals, but increased death rates are noted among the very young, elderly, and chronically ill when an epidemic of influenza is in an area. Because influenza weakens the natural defense mechanisms of the respiratory tract, secondary bacterial pneumonia is a common complication during influenzal outbreaks and is responsible for many of the resulting deaths. Reye's syndrome (Chapter 34) occurs in a very small portion of children during the late recovery phase of influenza.

Epidemiology

There are few if any parallels today to the epidemiology of influenza. When major antigenic shifts occur in virulent strains, a worldwide pandemic occurs and may involve hundreds of millions of persons. Such pandemics are accompanied by significant increases in the overall death rate. They often force the closing of schools and factories and generally disrupt the normal flow of human activities. Fortunately, these major outbreaks only occur every 10 to 15 years; less extensive outbreaks occur every 2 to 4 years as a result of antigenic drift.

Figure 37-2 shows the general epidemiological patterns of in-

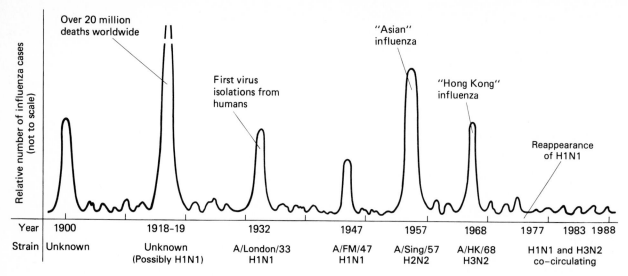

Figure 37-2 Time line showing when some of the major outbreaks and antigenic shifts occurred associated with type A influenza during the 1900s. Minor outbreaks occurred between the major outbreaks.

fluenza during the past century. The most devastating pandemic occurred in 1918–19. This strain of influenza virus was highly virulent, particularly in young adults, for some yet unexplained reason and approximately 20 million deaths occurred throughout the world. As the world population developed antibody immunity to this virus, the rate of disease decreased. The technology of 1918 was not able to isolate the virus responsible for this great pandemic but indirect evidence suggests it may have had H1N1 antigenic composition. In 1931 the first influenza virus was isolated from swine. It was noted, however, that serum taken from persons who had recovered from the 1918 influenza pandemic did contain antibodies that specifically reacted, to a limited extent, with the swine influenza virus. Whether any further relationship existed between these viruses could not be determined.

In 1932–33 epidemics occurred around the world and at that time the first influenza virus from humans was isolated. The isolates from this period had the antigenic makeup of H1N1 and over the next 20 years antigenic drifting occurred in these viruses with limited epidemics resulting every 3 to 4 years; rather extensive epidemics occurred in 1947. Originally, the 1932 and 1947 isolates were considered to be different antigenic subtypes, but more detailed studies have now shown them to be similar enough to be both classed as H1N1 subtypes. The H1N1 subtype generally disappeared from the world population in the early 1950s. Major antigenic shifts occurred in 1957 in both the H and N antigens and resulted in a new subtype with H2N2 antigens. A prototype of this subtype is A/Japan/57 (H2N2) and is commonly known as the "Asian" influenza virus. Because no antibody immunity was present in the world population against either the H2 or N2 antigen, this subtype of influenza spread very rapidly and within a year was causing major pandemics in most parts of the world. Epidemics of H2N2 subtype occurred every 3 years or so for the next 10 years. In 1968, a major shift occurred in the H antigen, creating subtype A/Hong Kong/68 (H3N2), also known as the "Hong Kong" influenza virus. Like its predecessor, the Asian flu, the Hong Kong flu spread rapidly from Asia to most parts of the world causing major pandemics. No new major antigenic shifts have occurred from 1968 to 1988. The subtype H1N1, however, made a reappearance in 1977 and has caused some epidemics through the 1980s in persons who were born since 1950 and were thus not previously exposed to this subtype. The H3N2 and H1N1 subtypes have continued to co-circulate in human populations in the 1980s.

A subtype designated A/New Jersey/76 (H1N1) that was isolated in 1976 deserves special mention. This subtype was apparently the same as or closely related to the swine influenza virus. This virus was isolated from recruits at a military camp in New Jersey in January of 1976. Because it was first detected in young adults and was related to "swine flu," there was a great deal of concern that it might be a return of the same strain that caused the great pandemic of 1918. In order to prevent a possible recurrence of such a devastating pandemic, with the possibility of millions of deaths, a massive immunization program was undertaken. By late summer and early fall of 1976 large segments of the population of the United States were being vaccinated. Fortunately, the A/New Jersey/76 subtype was not the deadly strain of 1918; it was probably a random transmission of the flu from infected swine to humans.

Diagnosis

Preliminary diagnosis is made on the basis of clinical and epidemiological observations. The diagnosis is confirmed by demonstrating the presence of the virus in throat washings. The virus can be grown in cell cultures or in embryonated eggs. Changes in antibody levels can be readily demonstrated by hemagglutination inhibition tests.

Treatment

Unlike most viral diseases, early therapy of type A influenza can be accomplished with *amantadine hydrochloride*. This compound prevents the uncoating of the virus in host cells and so restricts its replication. Unfortunately, the compound is not effective against either type B or C and is therefore not commonly used as an antiviral agent. In all cases of influenza, supportive treatment of the symptoms may be helpful in comforting the patient and antibacterial chemotherapy may be needed to treat secondary bacterial infections.

Prevention and Control

Because of the increased mobility of today's world population, the influenza virus is apparently able to spread most effectively from country to country. Quarantine measures seem of little value. The major means of controlling outbreaks is through a killed vaccine. This type of vaccine is moderately effective in that it confers protection to about 70% of those who receive it; this protection lasts from 6 months to a year. The vaccine contains the toxic products of the virus and often induces mild systemic symptoms of influenza, such as headache, fever, and muscle aches. Purified vaccines having only the H and N antigens are currently being used to a limited extent and do not contain the toxic by-products. The most important aspect of influenzal immunization is to use the proper subtype of virus for the production of the vaccine. When an antigenic shift occurs, the vaccines then in stock may be of no value. Continual worldwide surveillance programs monitor for the appearance of new subtypes. When a new subtype is found and is determined to be of significant virulence, a race begins between humans and virus with the goal being to produce large amounts of vaccine and vaccinate a significant proportion of the population before the viral pandemic arrives. The first time this race was run was with the advent of the Hong Kong flu of 1968. Unfortunately, delays occurred in the production of the vaccine, and the pandemic had circled the earth before the vaccine had become available. The next attempt was during the "swine flu" episode of 1976. In this case, the vaccine was prepared in time, but this subtype of virus was of low virulence and no significant outbreak occurred. Whether this stratagem will work in aborting a major pandemic in the future due to an antigenic shift of a virulent subtype remains to be determined. Various projects are now underway, using genetic engineering technology, to develop an influenza vaccine that contains combinations of the commonly encountered H and N antigens. It is important that individuals with increased risk of serious outcome from influenza infection receive adequate immunization. This would include elderly persons and anyone who has heart or respiratory health problems.

In the United States information is collected each week from about 120 selected cities on the deaths due to pneumonia and influenza (Figure 17-4). When deaths exceed the expected range in a given area, an investigation is undertaken to determine if an influenza epidemic is occurring and what subtype might be present. Frequent updates are reported in the *Morbidity and Mortality Weekly Reports*; an example is given in the following clinical note.

Update: Influenza Activity:
United States, Worldwide, April 15, 1983

United States: Morbidity reports collected weekly by each state indicate a continuing decline in influenza outbreaks. For the week ending April 9, 1983, two states (Kentucky and New Mexico) reported regional activity, and no state reported widespread activity. In recent weeks, reports of influenza virus isolations from collaborating laboratories have also indicated a decline in influenza activity. Most isolates (89%) continue to be type A (H3N2) virus, despite increases in influenza B and type A (H1N1). For the week ending April 9, 1983, an excess in the ratio of pneumonia and influenza deaths to total deaths were reported from 121 cities for the thirteenth consecutive week. The observed ratio was 5.2 and the expected ratio was 4.1.

Worldwide: Influenza activity during the 1982–83 season has generally been moderate and largely associated with influenza type A (H3N2) viruses, which have been reported from all five continents since October 1982. A (H3N2) has been the type most frequently isolated in all areas of the world and has been associated with sporadic cases and with outbreaks among schoolchildren. Influenza type B isolates, generally associated with sporadic cases, have been identified in several European countries. During late March and early April, influenza activity appeared to be declining in most European countries (*MMWR* 32:191, 1983).

CONCEPT SUMMARY

Influenza is the most common disease due to orthomyxoviruses. This disease while common in occurrence may prove serious in its consequences. An unusual genetic arrangement in the genome of this virus facilitates the repeated development of viruses with altered antigenic structures. These "new" viruses are the basis of periodic pandemics of the influenza. Vaccines are available against the influenza virus and consist of the most recent and common antigenic variations of the virus.

STUDY SUMMARY

1. What is the chemical composition and the physical structure of the influenza H and N antigens?
2. Discuss the epidemiologic significance of antigenic drift and antigenic shift in the influenza virus.

3. If a patient had recovered from influenza caused by an H2N3 virus, to which of the following viruses would he/she be most susceptible: H2N1, H1N3, or H1N1?

4. If type A influenza is treatable with amantadine hydrochloride, why isn't this compound commonly used in the early stages of an influenza epidemic?

REFERENCES FOR FURTHER STUDY

1. Intranasally Administered Interferon as Prophylaxis against Experimentally Induced Influenza A Infection in Humans. *Journal of Infectious Diseases* 156:379, 1987.

2. Lessons for Human Influenza from Pathogenicity Studies with Ferrets. *Reviews of Infectious Diseases* 10:56, 1988.

3. Role of Respiratory Tract Proteases in Infectivity of Influenza A Virus. *Journal of Infectious Diseases* 155:667, 1987.

4. *The Biologic and Clinical Basis of Infectious Diseases*, 3rd ed., G. Youmans, 1985. Saunders.

5. Acute Respiratory Disease Associated with Influenza Epidemics in Houston, 1981–1983. *Journal of Infectious Diseases* 155:1119, 1987.

chapter 38

PARAMYXOVIRUSES

The family Paramyxoviridae consists of related viruses that cause some common diseases of humankind. These viruses are structured somewhat like the orthomyxoviruses, but, compared to the influenza virus, they are genetically stable so that new mutant serotypes do not periodically develop. Many common viral respiratory diseases, as well as such distinct clinical diseases as mumps and measles, are caused by paramyxoviruses. The parainfluenza, respiratory syncytial, mumps, and measles paramyxoviruses are discussed in this chapter. Rubella, which is caused by a togavirus, is also described here because its clinical manifestations are much like measles.

CHARACTERISTICS OF PARAMYXOVIRUSES

The paramyxoviruses contain ss-RNA and have helical symmetry. The helical capsid is wound in a loose sphere that is somewhat irregular in shape and ranges from 100 to 300 nm in diameter. They possess an envelope and N- and H-type peplomers. Paramyxoviruses are unstable and do not survive long outside the host.

INFECTIONS DUE TO PARAINFLUENZA VIRUSES

Four serotypes of parainfluenza viruses infect humans. The infections are seen primarily in infants and young children. Illnesses range from subclinical to mild upper respiratory infections to croup or pneumonia. The viruses do not spread to the blood. Most cases are seen during the "respiratory disease season" from late fall to early spring. Many children are infected during the first

Nosocomial Respiratory Syncytial Virus Infections in an Intensive Care Nursery: California, 1978

An outbreak of upper respiratory infection and pneumonia involving nine infants and caused by respiratory syncytial virus (RSV) occurred in a 16-bed intensive care nursery (ICN) of a hospital and medical center in San Francisco, California, from February 25 through March 19, 1978.

On February 25 an 18-week-old premature infant with hyaline membrane disease and bronchopulmonary dysplasia developed fever with respiratory distress and had a convulsion. A nasopharyngeal viral culture taken then was subsequently positive for RSV. Two days later two other premature infants (aged 13 and 35 weeks) developed sneezing, cough, and rales. The 13-week-old was in isolation for a previously documented cytomegalovirus infection. Nasopharyngeal viral cultures from both infants were reported positive for RSV on March 2.

At that time the following procedures were instituted:

1. RSV fluorescent antibody (FA) screening and viral cultures were performed on nasopharyngeal swabs from all ICN patients.
2. All positive patients were isolated in a separate room.
3. Strict handwashing, gowning, and gloving procedures were required before contact with all ICN patients (masking was not required).
4. Certain nursing staff were assigned exclusively to infected infants.
5. All nursing staff with upper respiratory symptoms were considered infected with RSV. If well enough to work, they were allowed to care only for already-infected infants.

On the basis of direct FA screening, two additional infants were found positive for RSV on March 2 and were isolated. One had a collapsed right upper lobe; a culture was positive for RSV. The other patient had no respiratory symptoms; two of three FA studies were borderline positive for RSV, and none of eight viral cultures was positive.

FA screening was repeated March 6 on the remaining 11 patients in the unit, but no new cases were identified. The following day 2 patients, both aged 6 weeks, developed mild upper respiratory symptoms. Repeat FA testing was positive on both; cultures taken at this time subsequently grew RSV.

On March 19 a 6-day-old infant who had been in the ICN since birth developed nasal congestion. FA studies were negative and he was discharged from the hospital 2 days later. Viral cultures taken before discharge were later positive for RSV.

One additional infant developed RSV infection in association with this outbreak. The child, born on February 28, remained in the newborn nursery, a room adjoining the ICN, for 6 days because of neonatal hyperbilirubinemia. She was discharged on March 7 but was readmitted to another hospital ward on March 15 because of rhinorrhea and cough of 5 days' duration. FA studies and viral culture were both positive for RSV at the time of readmission. The child had had no direct contact with ICN babies during her first hospitalization. The nursing staffs of the intensive care and newborn nurseries are separate, but patients in both units are cared for by the same house staff members.

Routine viral screening of nursing and house staff members was not performed. However, from March 7 to March 21 FA studies and viral cultures were performed on 2 pediatric house officers, 11 ICN nurses, 1 nursery x-ray technician, and 1 phlebotomist, who regularly bled patients in the ICN. All 15 reported upper respiratory illnesses with onset occurring from 1 to 13 days (mean 4.9 days) before viral testing. The RSV FA test was strongly positive in 1 nurse and weakly positive in 4 additional nurses and the phlebotomist. None of the adults was positive by culture, perhaps owing to the delay in obtaining cultures after onset of symptoms (*MMWR* 27:260, 1978).

years of life so that by age 10 most children (over 80%) have antibodies against the four types of parainfluenza viruses. Reinfections may occur at all ages, but they are much milder than the primary infection and present symptoms of the "**common cold**." These viruses cause about 15% of the acute respiratory diseases seen in children under 10 years of age. Treatment is symptomatic; no vaccines are available.

Common cold
a minor upper respiratory infection caused by any one of a number of viruses. Those caused by adenovirus are often fairly severe.

INFECTIONS DUE TO RESPIRATORY SYNCYTIAL VIRUS (RSV)

The RSV is a major cause of respiratory illness in infants during the first few months of life. About 50% of **bronchiolitis** cases and about 25% of all pneumonia occurring in infants up to 2 months of age are caused by the RSV. Deaths may result from these infections. The infection is mild in older children and is limited to the upper respiratory tract (rhinitis and pharyngitis). No vaccine is available.

Bronchiolitis
inflammation of the bronchioles.

MUMPS

Mumps is one of the common communicable diseases of children and young adults. It is not as contagious as measles or chickenpox and outbreaks are generally limited to fewer cases. Along with the well-recognized swelling of the salivary glands, mumps may also involve other glands or the CNS.

Virus

The mumps virus is a typical paramyxovirus and is inactivated quite readily (within hours) once expelled from the body. Only one serotype is known and humans are the only natural host. This virus can be grown in a variety of different cell cultures and in embryonated eggs. **Primates** can be experimentally infected. Various serologic tests are available to measure antibodies against the mumps virus.

Primate
an order of upright, bipedal mammals of which humans are an example.

Pathogenesis and Clinical Diseases

Humans are infected by inhaling infected **droplet nuclei** that contain the virus. Mumps has an incubation period of 16 to 18 days and during this time the virus passes from the site of entry in the

Droplet nuclei
a small particle about which moisture and other particles may collect. Usually associated with respiratory droplets.

respiratory tract into the lymphatic system and then into the blood. The virus is deposited from the blood into the meninges and various organs, such as the salivary glands, ovaries, testes, mammary glands, and pancreas. Several days to a week before the onset of symptoms, and for about an equal length of time after the onset of symptoms, the virus may be found in the saliva, urine, stool, and blood. In about a third of these patients the infection remains subclinical or at least the infected person experiences none of the classical symptoms of mumps. In the other two-thirds the most readily recognizable sign is the swollen salivary glands (parotitis; Figure 38-1). Swelling occurs only on one side (unilateral) in 25% of the cases. Several days to a week or more following the onset of parotitis, involvement of other glands may become apparent. Inflammation of the testes (orchitis) is rare in prepubertal males (under 11 to 13 years of age) whereas 20% to 30% of males over this age may experience orchitis. Usually orchitis is unilateral and all current evidence indicates that sterility is rarely caused by this infection. Inflammation of the ovaries and mammary glands is seen in a similar percentage of infected females and permanent damage rarely, if ever, occurs. The most serious complication from mumps results from infection of the central nervous system. Mumps is one of the most common causes of aseptic (nonbacterial) meningitis and **encephalitis**. Most patients with CNS involvement recover without permanent complications.

Encephalitis
inflammation of the brain. Encephalitis is most often due to virus infection and causes a condition sometimes referred to as *"sleeping sickness."*

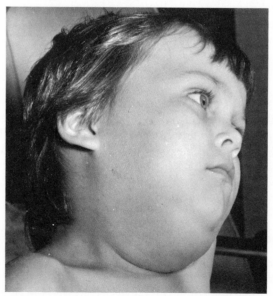

Figure 38-1 Child with diffuse swelling as a result of mumps infection. (Centers for Disease Control, Atlanta)

Deafness may result in a small percentage of cases and death occasionally occurs.

Transmission and Epidemiology

Mumps is transmitted by the airborne route and by direct contact with saliva. No documentation of transmission by virus-infected urine or mothers' milk has been observed. Those with subclinical cases, however, are able to transmit the disease. Transmission is not as effective as with diseases like measles, chickenpox, or influenza. Epidemics occur every few years in the winter or spring, but cases tend to be more sporadic and occur throughout the year. It is quite easy for a person to go through childhood without contracting this disease, and about one-fourth of the cases are seen in adolescents or young adults. About 20% of U.S. residents reach adulthood and have no antibodies against mumps. Because of this group of susceptible adults, mumps infection often occurs in recruits during the military mobilization of large numbers of persons. Since the introduction of a living vaccine in the late 1960s, the overall incidence of mumps has decreased. Recovery from mumps generally confers lifelong immunity. Reported second attacks of mumps are probably based on the assumption that any infection involving swollen salivary glands is mumps. When two attacks of mumps are reported in the same person, this assump-

Figure 38-2   Reported cases of mumps per year in the United States, 1968–1987. In 1968, the year the vaccine was licensed, 155,209 cases were reported. In 1985, 2,982 cases were reported, and in 1987, 12,299 were reported (modified from CDC annual summaries).

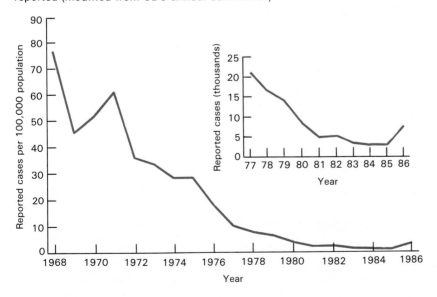

Fatal Mumps Myocarditis: England, 1979

In early 1979 in Bristol, England, a previously healthy, 8-month-old baby girl was found sweating profusely in her stroller, with mottled blue patches on her face. She was taken to a hospital by ambulance but was dead on arrival. The child was being looked after by her grandmother at the time, and no history of illness immediately preceding death was obtained. The baby had two older siblings, aged 2 and 4 years, but there was no recorded history of illness in these children during the weeks preceding the baby's death.

At autopsy the heart was enlarged due to gross dilation of all the chambers, and there was a pericardial effusion of about 5 ml of clear yellow fluid. No congenital abnormalities of the heart or main vessels were found and, apart from congestion, the other organs appeared normal. Microscopy of the heart revealed diffuse infiltration of the myocardium by lymphocytes and oc-

casional polymorphonuclear leukocytes and a mild pericarditis. The submandibular glands showed marked focal infiltration by lymphocytes and plasma cells, particularly around small ducts. The submucosa of the larynx, trachea, and nasopharynx was also infiltrated with these cells, and scattered interstitial aggregates of lymphoid cells were present in skeletal muscle.

The cause of the acute myocarditis was established when mumps virus was isolated from the myocardium and an impression smear of the myocardium, tested by indirect immunofluorescence, revealed mumps virus antigen. On retesting, mumps virus was again isolated from the heart. No virus was isolated from a nasopharyngeal aspirate, the lung or the feces, and bacteriologic and biochemical investigations revealed no other abnormalities (*MMWR* 29:425, 1980).

tion is not correct and one of the illnesses with parotitis would be assumed to be caused by an agent other than the mumps virus. The number of cases of mumps reported in the United States is shown in Figure 38-2.

Diagnosis

Typical cases of mumps with swelling of the salivary glands can be readily diagnosed on the basis of clinical appearance. Atypical cases require laboratory tests to confirm that they are mumps. The virus can be isolated from the throat, saliva, urine, or spinal fluid through cell cultures or embryonated eggs. Various serologic tests are available to measure specific mumps antibodies.

Prevention and Control

Children with mumps should be kept from school or other association with other children for about 2 weeks. A living attenuated vaccine has been available since 1968 in the United States. This vaccine is quite effective and induces immunity in over 95% of the recipients. The vaccine has few side effects. But because mumps is generally not a serious disease, vigorous campaigns to administer the vaccine have not been carried out. The vaccine should be given as part of the routine childhood vaccination series at about 1 year of age. It is usually given as part of a triple vaccine known as MMR, which stands for measles, mumps, and rubella. In training centers for military recruits mumps vaccines have been used effectively to control troublesome outbreaks. Significant decreases in mumps have been observed in areas where the vaccine has been widely used.

MEASLES (RUBEOLA)

Measles (sometimes called *rubeola*) is one of the most contagious diseases of humankind. Before the development of an effective vaccine in the mid-1960s, 98% of the U.S. population contracted measles by the age of 18. Even though measles was considered a disease that everyone had to get and ''get it over with,'' it is a serious disease and a leading cause of death in many undernourished children in developing countries where vaccination is not carried out. Cases of measles have declined significantly in the past 10 to 15 years in countries where vaccination programs are applied.

Virus

Only one serotype of measles virus exists. This virus can be adapted to grow in cell cultures and embryonated eggs. It has a short survival time outside the body but does remain viable for a long enough time in droplet nuclei to be spread effectively by the aerosol route.

Pathogenesis and Clinical Disease

The measles virus enters by the airborne route and is taken up by the draining lymph ducts of the respiratory tract. The virus passes into the blood and is deposited throughout the body. The incubation period is 9 to 12 days before the onset of prodromal signs of fever, cough, runny nose (coryza), and conjunctivitis. At this stage of the disease red macules or ulcer-type lesions, called *Koplik spots*, appear on the inside of the cheek. After about 3 days the rash appears on the skin and continues to spread and intensify over the next 1 or 2 days (Figure 38-3). General symptoms may be

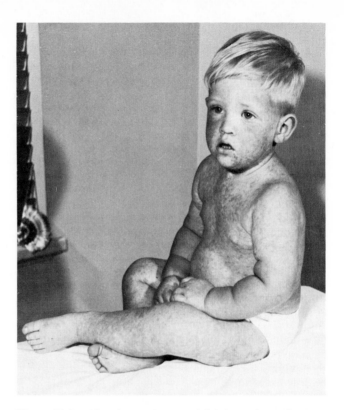

Figure 38-3 Measles rash on a child three days after onset. (Centers for Disease Control, Atlanta)

severe and such complications as secondary bacterial infections may occur. The CNS is infected and in about one out of every 1000 cases the encephalitis is severe enough to cause noticeable signs. About 15% of those with severe signs of encephalitis die; others may have permanent effects, such as epilepsy, hearing loss, and personality changes.

A rare degenerative neurological disease with the formidable name of *subacute sclerosing panencephalitis* (SSPE) develops in a few children or adolescents several years after a measles infection. All current evidence indicates that this disease is caused by measles viruses that have remained latent in the CNS.

In the mid-1970s a new dimension in the clinical picture of measles appeared. The immunity of some children who had been vaccinated waned or their vaccinations were of insufficient potency to produce full immunity; consequently, a significant number of cases of atypical measles occurred. These atypical cases resembled various other diseases and it was necessary to use serologic tests to confirm that they were measles.

Transmission and Epidemiology

Transmission is by droplet nuclei expelled from the respiratory tract, often a few days before to a few days after the onset of the rash. The disease is highly infectious. When measles is introduced into an isolated population that has not had this disease, and no acquired immunity is present, almost 100% of the inhabitants contract it. In such cases, the mortality rate is high and may reach 10% if local health care is not available and the general nutritional state of the population is poor. Such an epidemic occurred on the Hawaiian Islands during early colonization by whites.

Before the introduction of vaccination, measles epidemics would occur every 2 to 5 years in a given area, with most cases happening during the winter and early spring. This epidemiologic pattern of measles has changed significantly since the introduction of vaccines in the mid-1960s. Within a few years after initiation of vaccination programs the total number of cases in the United States decreased 90%. Through the 1970s, however, the number of cases remained about the same, at around 20,000 to 30,000 cases per year. During this time the age distribution of cases shifted, with more outbreaks occurring in teenagers and college-age persons. Such a shift was attributed to the vaccination programs that had decreased the spread of measles among young children and, in turn, allowed more susceptible to accumulate in

Figure 38-4   Reported cases of measles by year in the United States, 1950–1987. In 1958, 763,094 cases were reported compared to 1,497 in 1983; 6,282 cases were reported in 1986 and 3,588 in 1987 (modified from CDC annual summaries).

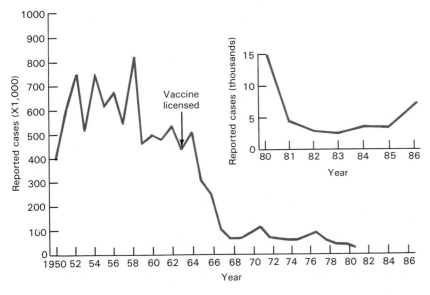

the older age groups. Increased efforts were initiated in 1979 to immunize a larger proportion of the children as they entered their first year of schooling. This program has been successful and during 1982 the number of measles cases dropped to about 1700. This was less than one-fifth the number from 1980 and less than one-tenth the number seen in any year of the 1970s (Figure 38-4). It was hoped that the number of cases of measles contracted in the United States could be reduced to close to zero by the mid-1980s. This, however, has not been attained. A low of 1495 cases was reached in 1983 and since then the numbers of cases have been increasing. Measles is still a major health problem in many developing countries and many of the cases seen in the United States are contracted outside of the country.

Diagnosis

Because of its characteristic appearance and epidemiology, measles is usually diagnosed clinically without laboratory tests. The appearance of Koplik spots is useful in diagnosing measles during early stages of the disease. But laboratory tests are needed to make a specific diagnosis in the cases of atypical measles in partially immunized children. Virus isolation can be made during the acute phase of the disease; however, most laboratory diagnoses are made by showing a significant increase in antibodies to measles virus between the acute or convalescent sera.

Treatment

No specific antiviral treatment is available. Antibiotics may be given to treat secondary bacterial infection.

Prevention and Control

The control of measles at present relies almost entirely on the use of an attenuated vaccine. This vaccine is given subcutaneously to young children after they have lost all passive immunity from their mothers, usually between 12 and 15 months of age. The measles vaccination is normally administered as part of the MMR triple vaccine. One vaccination, when given to children over 1 year of age, offers lifelong protection. For children vaccinated under 1 year of age, or for those who received inadequate protection (as determined by antibody tests) from the first immunization, it is being recommended that a second immunization be given before the child enters school at 5 or 6 years of age. All current evidence indicates that effective vaccination programs directed at preschool-age children can control measles. It is important that persons traveling outside of the United States be properly immunized.

Imported Measles with Subsequent Airborne Transmission in a Pediatrician's Office: Michigan, 1982

An outbreak of seven cases of measles was reported in Muskegon County, Michigan; rash onsets occurred from November 14 through December 10, 1982. The outbreak began with an international importation in a 7-month-old baby who arrived in the United States from Korea on October 29 for adoption. She infected four other children in a pediatrician's office, two additional measles cases occurred subsequently in family members of these four children.

The index patient (Patient A) had onset of rash on November 14 and visited a pediatrician's office on November 16. She was in the office waiting room from 11 A.M. to noon and in a single examination room from noon to 12:30 P.M. After measles was diagnosed, the pediatrician reviewed the immunization records of all children known to have been in the office at the same time and offered immune globulin (IG) to the three unimmunized children, all of whom were less than 15 months of age. Two received IG, while the third, a 6-month-old infant did not. No cases occurred among these children. However, cases did occur in patients not known to have been in the office at the same time as Patient A. One child who was subsequently infected arrived approximately 5 minutes before Patient A left the office, but did not have face-to-face contact with her; the other three arrived in the office 60 to 75 minutes after Patient A left. Only one of these four children used the same examining room as Patient A, but all four shared the same waiting room. None of the children were in contact with any other persons who had rash illnesses. No other common activities or contacts with individuals or shared objects could be identified to account for these cases. The last-known measles cases in Muskegon County had been reported in February 1981.

The patients with secondary cases ranged in age from 4 months to 2 1/2 years; none had been immunized. Two of these children transmitted measles to family members—a 14-year-old with a history of measles vaccination at 11 months and 5 years, and a 24-year-old, whose immunization status was unknown.

Of 29 children who were in the office when Patient A was present or who arrived within 90 minutes of her departure, 19 were 15 months of age or older, the recommended age for routine measles vaccination. Two of these children had not been vaccinated; both developed measles. None of the 17 vaccinated children developed measles. Of 10 children less than 15 months of age, all unvaccinated, 2 were infected, 2 received IG, and 6 remained well. Four of the 6 well patients were 6 months of age or less (*MMWR* 32:401, 1983).

RUBELLA

Rubella is a mild disease that is of little direct concern in children or adults, but it may have disastrous effects on the developing fetus should the mother become infected early in pregnancy. The terms *German measles* or *three-day measles* are also used for this disease; however, these terms often lead to confusion with regular measles and it would be better to use the name *rubella* consistently when referring to this disease.

Virus

The virus that causes rubella defied isolation by standard procedures during the 1940s and 1950s but was finally isolated in the early 1960s. The feature that made isolation difficult was the inability of this virus to cause observable changes in cell cultures (cytopathic effect) or death in embryonated eggs even though the virus will proliferate in these systems. Only a single serotype of rubella has been found. All current information indicates that the rubella virus is morphologically similar to the togaviruses (Chapter 42).

Pathogenesis and Clinical Disease

This disease has the same pathogenesis as many other diseases; that is, the virus is inhaled into the respiratory tract, followed by passage through the lymphatic system into the blood. After an incubation period of around 14 days, the signs and symptoms produced are usually trivial and include swollen lymph nodes, mild fever, and often a slight rash lasting for 2 to 3 days.

When a pregnant female is infected, the rubella virus may infect the developing fetus and cause a disease known as *congenital rubella syndrome*. This syndrome may include any of the following effects: cataracts with partial or complete blindness, loss of hearing, heart defects, mental retardation, or generalized tissue damage. The chance that the developing baby will develop serious damage due to congenital rubella is much greater if infection occurs during the first trimester of pregnancy. Severe damage results in about 50% of the fetuses infected during the first month; serious effects on the fetus are rare if the mother contracts rubella after the fourth month of pregnancy.

It is theorized that the rubella virus has such damaging effects on the fetus because of its mild nature. More virulent viruses, if they infected the fetus, would cause severe damage that would result in fetal death and lead to spontaneous abortion. On the other hand, the rubella virus, because of its mild effect, simply slows cell growth, which, in turn, leads to malformation of the tissues as they differentiate during early fetal development.

Transmission and Epidemiology

Rubella is transmitted primarily by the respiratory route with the patient being infectious several days before to about a week after the onset of the rash. Before the widespread use of the vaccine, moderate epidemics of rubella would occur every 6 to 9 years and

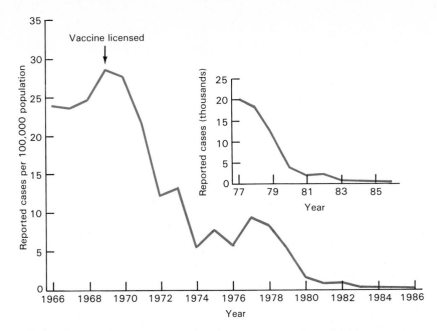

Figure 38-5 Reported cases of rubella by year in the United States, 1966–1987; 530 cases were reported in 1986 and 329 in 1987 (modified from CDC annual summaries).

major epidemics at greater intervals of up to 30 years. The last major epidemic in the United States was in 1964 when about 500,000 cases occurred. As a result of this epidemic, thousands of children were born with congenital rubella syndrome.

Rubella babies present a special problem in transmission, for they continue to shed virus in saliva, urine, and other body secretions for 1 month to 6 years after birth. The reported cases of rubella per year in the United States are seen in Figure 38-5.

Diagnosis

The major problem in diagnosing rubella centers around the concern of exposure or potential exposure of females during the early stages of pregnancy. The expense and time involved in a laboratory diagnosis are not warranted in routine nonpregnant cases. However, when a susceptible female in the first trimester of pregnancy has been exposed to a possible rubella patient, it is important to know whether the exposure was indeed to rubella. Laboratory serologic tests and viral isolation can determine if the infection is caused by the rubella virus. Routine serologic tests are available to determine whether females of childbearing age have antibodies against rubella. In some states rubella serologic tests are required when obtaining a marriage license.

Rubella Outbreak on a College Campus: Wisconsin, 1977

In the period October 12 to November 9, 1977, 45 cases of rash illness consistent with rubella were reported to the Student Health Service of Marquette University, Milwaukee, Wisconsin. Rubella virus had been isolated from the pharynx of eight students and another student had a fourfold rise in hemagglutination inhibition (HI) antibody titers to rubella.

Signs and symptoms in the reported cases were: rash (100%), adenopathy (19%), pharyngitis (76%), fever 37.4°C (99°F) (71%), headache (51%), conjunctivitis (47%), and photophobia and joint complaints (44% each). Males and females experienced the joint signs and symptoms with equal frequency. Two males noted bilateral testicular tenderness. Five of 30 students complained of itching at the onset of rash.

Of the 45 cases reported, 44 occurred in undergraduate students, an attack rate of 6 per 1000. Rates were equal in males and females and were not significantly different among the four classes. The attack rate in students living in campus dormitories, however, was twice as high as for those living off campus (8 per 1000 versus 4 per 1000).

More than 1000 students were vaccinated in a rubella immunization program prompted by these cases. Vaccine was given to all males requesting it. However, because previous testing of the university's junior and senior nursing students had revealed a 90% prevalence of antibodies to rubella, initially all women were not vaccinated. Instead, vaccine was offered only to those found to be serologically negative. When it became apparent that the outbreak was continuing and that only 70% to 85% of the women who had come to the clinic had detectable antibodies, all female students requesting it were vaccinated after appropriate counseling on the need to avoid pregnancy. Each woman's blood specimen was frozen in the event that serologic tests might later be useful.

Editorial note: Because college campuses are recognized potential sites of rubella outbreak, ideally all susceptible females should be identified and vaccinated before they enter college. Colleges and universities should consider requiring serologic screening of all incoming female students at the time of preadmission physical examinations. Susceptible, nonpregnant females should be vaccinated against rubella at a time when pregnancy will be avoided for the ensuing three months (*MMWR* 26:392, 1977).

Treatment

No direct treatment for rubella is available.

Prevention and Control

Once discoveries in the early 1960s showed that the rubella virus could be grown in cell cultures or embryonated eggs, rapid progress was made in developing a rubella vaccine. A living vaccine was first licensed in 1969 and appears to induce a high degree of immunity after a single dose. Mild infection sometimes results from the vaccine, but in nonpregnant persons it is of little consequence. There is no evidence, from 20 years of observation, that this living vaccine causes damaging infections in the developing fetus. As a precaution, however, it is still recommended that conception should be delayed until at least 3 months after a female has been vaccinated and pregnant females should not be vaccinated.

Two general approaches have been used in rubella vaccinations. One, which is used extensively in the United States, is to immunize preschool-age children, thus limiting the spread of the virus within a community and reducing the chance of exposure to expectant mothers. The other approach is to immunize girls in their early teens and older females of childbearing age who have no antibodies against rubella. Since the introduction of wide-scale vaccination, the overall incidence of rubella and congenital rubella syndrome have decreased significantly (Figure 38-5).

CONCEPT SUMMARY

1. The RNA-containing paramyxoviruses are responsible for several of the more commonly known childhood diseases. These infections include croup (epiglotitis), mumps, measles, and a not uncommon pneumonia in newborns caused by respiratory syncytial virus.

2. Disease due to these viruses has been so widespread that, although any given infection may be mild in its symptoms, the small percentage of infections with serious consequence were, in fact, quite common. This situation has spawned the development of excellent vaccines that should be used to limit the occurrence of rubella, measles, and mumps.

STUDY SUMMARY

1. What is the normal route of transmission of the paramyxoviruses?

2. In what age group is infection with the mumps virus likely to cause the most severe disease?

3. Why are so many individuals unsure as to whether or not they have had mumps, while almost everyone who has had measles is sure of this infection?

4. What procedure is available to prevent persons from developing mumps, measles, and rubella?

5. If "German measles" is such a benign disease, why has there been a major effort to ensure immunization against this disease?

6. What aspect of epidemiology has resulted in shifting the most likely age for mumps and measles from childhood to older ages?

REFERENCES FOR FURTHER STUDY

1. Time Course of Virus-Specific Macromolecular Synthesis during Rubella Virus Infection in Vero Cells. *Virology* 162:65, 1988.

2. Role of Individual Glycoproteins of Human Parainfluenza Virus Type 3 in the Induction of a Protective Immune Response. *Journal of Virology* 62:783, 1988.

3. *The Biologic and Clinical Basis of Infectious Diseases*, G. Youmans, 1985. Saunders.

4. Respiratory Syncytial Virus Epidemics: Variable Dominance of Subgroups A and B Strains among Children, 1981–1986. *Journal of Infectious Diseases* 157:143, 1988.

5. *Fundamental Virology*, B. Fields, 1986. Raven.

chapter 39

PICORNAVIRUSES

T he family Picornaviradae includes large numbers of viruses that infect humans and animals. They are among the smallest viruses and contain ss-RNA, hence the name *pico* (''small'') plus RNA (Figure 39-1). Two genera of picornaviruses are found in humans: the *rhinoviruses*, which primarily inhabit the nasal cavity, and the *enteroviruses*, which are found mainly in the alimentary tract. The rhinoviruses can proliferate only in the superficial tissues of the upper respiratory tract and are one of the frequent causes of the common cold. The enteroviruses have traditionally been subdivided into the poliovirus, coxsackievirus, and echovirus groups, but since 1970 newly discovered members have been designated simply as enteroviruses, followed by a number. Generally they produce mild or asymptomatic infections of the intestinal tract but may also cause respiratory or systemic infection. Enteroviruses are also responsible for infections of the central nervous system. The picornaviruses are stable and able to survive for long periods in sewage, water, and foods.

RHINOVIRUSES

Rhinoviruses grow best at 33°C and have thus adapted to grow in the cooler superficial tissues of the nasal cavity, thereby inducing the infections referred to as **coryza** or the ''common cold.'' These infections do not spread beyond the nasal cavity and tissue damage is usually slight to moderate. Much of the symptomatology of the common cold is due to the release of histamine from the patient's mast cells—a reaction stimulated by virus-induced tissue damage. The released histamine induces such symptoms as increased mucous secretions, watery eyes, and sneezing. Over 100 different rhinovirus serotypes have been identified.

Common colds occur year round but are most frequent dur-

Coryza
acute inflammation of the nasal mucosa accompanied by profuse nasal discharge.

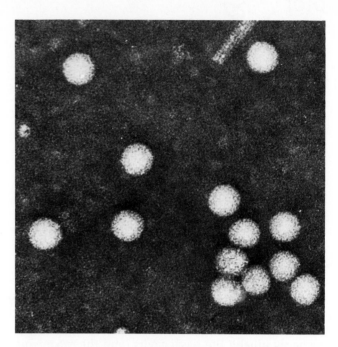

Figure 39-1 Transmission electron micrograph of polioviruses magnified 300,000×. (Courtesy Robley C. Williams, University of California, Berkeley)

ing the cooler months and it has been postulated that such factors as crowding in buildings and low relative humidity may increase the rate of infection. Attacks of the common cold occur repeatedly, partly because of the large number of serotypes of rhinoviruses. Another factor is the relatively short duration of immunity that is conferred to the superficial mucosal tissues by the IgA antibody response. Various other viruses are also able to cause common colds.

No specific treatment for the common cold is available; **antihistamines** and other medications, however, may be used to relieve symptoms. Controlled studies have failed to show any beneficial effects of vitamin C in treating and preventing colds. Vaccines are not available.

Antihistamine
drugs used to counteract allergic reaction. These compounds may be produced by the body and act to suppress histamine-induced reactions.

POLIOVIRUSES

Three serotypes of polioviruses have been identified and at present the diseases caused by these viruses constitute minor problems in developed countries. The widespread use of effective vaccines has greatly reduced the number of cases of poliomyelitis, or polio, in the United States. The conquest of polio is one of the great success stories of modern medical research. Although the disease of **paralytic polio** is no longer a threat in the developed countries, persons involved in health fields need to understand both the principles involved in the "rise and fall" of this disease during the first 65 years of the twentieth century and how these principles may still apply in underdeveloped countries. It is also important to understand why continued emphasis on immunization is needed to prevent possible future recurrences of the disease.

Paralytic polio
infection with polio virus resulting in paralysis of the patient.

Pathogenesis and Clinical Diseases

The poliovirus generally enters the body via the oral route. The virus first proliferates in the throat and small intestines and then passes through the draining lymph nodes and enters the blood, thus becoming widely disseminated (Figure 39-2). On occasion the virus passes into the CNS but infects only certain motor nerve cells of the spinal cord or brain. Varying degrees of paralysis may result, depending on the location of the destroyed nerve cells. Paralysis of lower limbs results from infection of the anterior horn cells of the spinal cord whereas infection in the brain stem, called *bulbar poliomyelitis*, may cause death due to respiratory or cardiac failure. It is now known that fewer than 1% of those infected with poliovirus show signs of CNS involvement. In over 99% of the cases the infection is limited to tissues other than the CNS and the infected persons may experience only minor nonspecific symptoms of a respiratory or intestinal tract infection. The presence of circulating antibodies is very effective in preventing the spread of the virus through the blood to the CNS.

Epidemiology

The epidemiology of paralytic polio is closely associated with the sanitary conditions of a population in a paradoxical way. That is, paralytic disease is rarely seen in populations living under conditions of poor sanitation and the paradox is explained in the following manner. Polioviruses are widespread in populations where poor sanitary conditions prevail and all persons possess specific polio antibodies. An infant born into such a culture possesses sufficient passive immunity to prevent the virus from passing through the blood to the CNS. These circulating IgG-type antibodies, however, will not prevent infections of the intestinal tract; under unsanitary conditions the infants are invariably infected with the polioviruses before they lose their passive immunity. The natural intestinal infection then stimulates lifelong natural active immunity. Only when sanitary conditions begin to improve is it possible

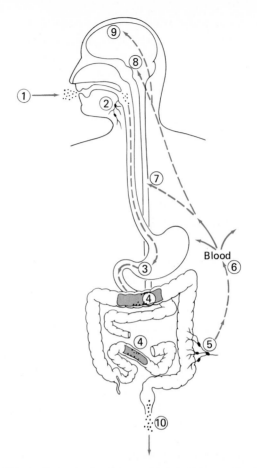

Figure 39-2 The pathogenesis of poliomyelitis. (1) Ingestion of virus. (2) Some multiplication may occur in tonsils and lymph nodes of upper respiratory tract with common cold type symptoms. (3) Virus resistant to stomach acids and digestive fluids. (4) Multiplication of virus in Peyer's patches and other lymphoid cells along the intestinal tract with clinical symptoms of enteritis. (5) Viruses drain into regional lymph nodes which stimulates antibody response. (6) Viruses may pass into blood. (7) In a small percentage of infections, the viruses may cross the blood-brain barrier into the CNS. Motor nerves (anterior horn cells) are specifically infected and result in paralysis of certain muscles. (8) Lower brain centers may be infected causing bulbar polio. (9) Motor cortex may be infected causing widespread paralysis. (10) Large amounts of virus shed in feces.

for infants to avoid the primary infection long enough for the passive immunity to disappear. Yet these infants will generally contract the natural disease fairly early in life and about 1% will develop the paralytic disease. The change from poor sanitary conditions to improved conditions began to occur during the latter part of the nineteenth century in the United States and in some European countries. At that time paralytic polio was first recognized as a specific disease; and because it occurred mainly in

Poliomyelitis: Pennsylvania and Maryland, 1979

The first paralytic poliomyelitis case in the United States with onset in 1979 was reported in a 22-year-old unvaccinated, female resident of a small Amish community in Franklin County, Pennsylvania. The patient, who had been hospitalized in Maryland, became ill on January 5 with headache, fever, and generalized myalgias. On January 6 and 7 she developed right and then left lower-extremity weakness and decreased deep tendon reflexes. She had no sensory abnormalities. On January 17 the Maryland State Department of Health and Mental Hygiene reported that type 1 poliovirus had been isolated from a stool specimen collected from the patient on January 10.

An epidemiologic investigation revealed that the patient had no known exposure to other individuals with clinical poliomyelitis or to recent recipients of the live virus vaccine. In addition, there was no history of recent travel to known polio-endemic areas. At least three Amish weddings had taken place during the period of November through January, resulting in extensive interactions among the Amish communities in Franklin and eight other Pennsylvania counties and other Amish communities in Maryland,

Ohio, Vermont, New York, and Ontario, Canada. The patient's most recent out-of-state travel had been to an Amish community in St. Marys and Charles counties, Maryland, in late November. Stool specimens were collected on January 18 and 19 from 17 asymptomatic members of this community; 12 were positive for type 1 poliovirus. In addition, stool specimens collected on January 18 through 20 from 32 individuals in the patient's own community revealed that 16 were positive for poliovirus.

Surveys by Pennsylvania and Maryland health departments revealed that few individuals had been completely immunized in the two affected Amish communities. It was strongly recommended that all members of the affected Amish communities be vaccinated with the trivalent oral poliovirus vaccine. Vaccination clinics have been set up in Pennsylvania and Maryland. Approximately 67% of the target population in Maryland was vaccinated by January 31.

Surveillance for paralytic illness and aseptic meningitis possibly due to poliovirus infection has been intensified in Pennsylvania and Maryland as well as in Amish communities in other states (*MMWR* 26:49, 1979).

young children, it was called *infantile paralysis*. As sanitary conditions continued to improve, it became possible for more and more children to avoid primary exposure for longer and longer periods and in the first decades of the 1900s more and more paralytic polio occurred in progressively older persons. The annual polio rate in the United States reached its highest level in the early 1950s and then dropped sharply after the introduction of the killed vaccine (Figure 39-3).

Prevention and Control

Polio has been controlled through the development of effective vaccines. A killed vaccine, containing all three serotypes, was first introduced in 1955 and induced adequate immunity when given

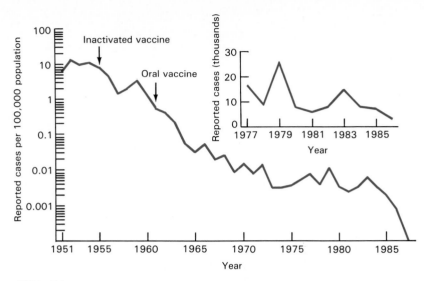

Figure 39-3   Reported cases of paralytic poliomyelitis by year in the United States, 1951–1987. The case rates since 1963 have been less than 0.06 per 100,000 population. In 1952, 57,879 cases were reported compared to 7 cases in 1974 and zero cases in 1987 (modified from CDC annual summaries).

as a series of three injections over a 3- to 6-month period, followed with booster injections every 2 or 3 years. By early 1960s a living attenuated vaccine became available and has generally replaced the use of killed vaccine in the United States and many other countries. The living vaccine provides long-lasting immunity after one administration and it can be taken orally, thus saving time and money and avoiding the discomfort of hypodermic injections.

Even though a small risk is involved with the use of the living vaccine, in that 1 out of approximately every 8 million persons receiving it may develop paralytic disease, the overall success of the polio vaccines has been phenomenal. Paralytic cases were reduced from a high of 57,879 in 1952, to 31 in 1970 and 9 in 1980. About half the cases in the 1970s in the United States resulted from infections with vaccine strains in immunosuppressed children. This prompted the remanufacture of a small supply of killed vaccine to be used for vaccinating children that may be immunosuppressed. This procedure has resulted in further reductions of paralytic polio; in 1986 three cases were reported and in 1987, for the first time, no cases were reported in the United States. Polio continues to be a problem in many developing countries, where for various reasons, effective vaccination programs have not been carried out.

ECHO 9 Outbreak: New York, 1975

During July 1975 an outbreak of illness caused by ECHO 9 virus occurred in a vacation colony in Dutchess County, New York.

All residents of the colony were surveyed and blood, stool, and throat cultures were obtained on 15 individuals with recent illness. Results of this survey revealed that from June 30 through July 23, 88 (37.6%) of the 234 colony residents became ill. Typical symptoms and signs were headache (59%), fever (53%), stiff neck (36%), and rash (36%). Other less frequent manifestations included vomiting (18%), diarrhea (16%), and sore throat (13%). Age-specific attack rates were highest in the 0 to 4 (18%) and 5 to 9 (46%) year groups. Attack rates were similar for both sexes in persons under 21 years of age, but were significantly higher for females (41%) than males (17%) in the 21 or older age groups. The dates of onset suggested person-to-person spread as the mode of transmission in this outbreak.

Analysis of the intervals between primary and secondary household cases suggested an incubation period of 2 to 4 days. ECHO 9 virus was isolated from 9 of 15 throat cultures and 11 of 13 stool specimens submitted to the New York Department of Health laboratory. Control measures taken to interrupt further transmission consisted of closure of the day camp, restriction of swimming pool use to postconvalescent persons, and temporary confinement of children to their quarters (*MMWR* 25:32, 1976).

COXSACKIEVIRUSES AND ECHOVIRUSES

The coxsackieviruses are so named because they were first isolated in 1948 from children living in the town of Coxsackie, New York. The children were thought to have mild cases of polio. The first echoviruses were discovered several years later during field trials of the killed polio vaccine. It was customary in these trials to examine many vaccinated children to determine if they were shedding the polioviruses. Besides finding some polioviruses and coxsackieviruses, a group of previously unidentified viruses was discovered. Because these new viruses were isolated from the intestinal tract, produced a cytopathic effect in cell cultures, were isolated from humans, and were not associated with any apparent diseases, they were given the name *echo*, which is an acronym for *e*nteric *c*ytopathic *h*uman *o*rphan viruses. Since that time, however, many of the echoviruses have been shown to cause a variety of disease.

About 30 different serotypes of coxsackieviruses and 33 serotypes of echoviruses are identified. Differences between these two

Enterovirus

any of a number of viruses or virus groups which have primary attachment sites on the intestinal mucosa.

groups of viruses are slight and the current procedure is not to classify new isolates into either of these groups but simply call them **enteroviruses** and give them a numerical designation—for instance, *enterovirus 70*. These viruses are transmitted by both the fecal-oral and the airborne route. Generally the enterovirus infections are subclinical or mild with generalized symptoms. Occasionally symptoms may be more severe. Such clinical diseases as common colds, fevers with skin rashes, pharyngitis, pneumonitis, meningitis, encephalitis, carditis, and diarrhea may be caused by coxsackieviruses or echoviruses. The highest rate of infection tends to occur in late summer.

CONCEPT SUMMARY

1. The picornaviruses are a large group of small RNA viruses that are responsible for both mild upper respiratory infections and severe neurological or cardiovascular disease.

2. The picornaviruses are easily transmitted by the fecal-oral route, and most of these viruses multiply in the intestine prior to further dissemination within the patient.

STUDY SUMMARY

1. Describe the picornaviruses in general taxonomic terms.

2. What rationale can you give for the present lack of a "common cold" virus vaccine?

3. To be immune to poliovirus it is necessary to receive all there serotypes in a vaccine. What does this tell you about the nature of the serogrouping antigen?

4. The name *enterovirus* refers to what characteristic of the echo and coxsackieviruses?

REFERENCES FOR FURTHER STUDY

1. The Structure of Poliovirus. *Scientific American* 256:42, 1987.

2. Rhinovirus Infection in Tecumseh, Michigan: Frequency of Illness and Number of Serotypes. *Journal of Infectious Diseases* 156:43, 1987.

3. Reemergence of an Epidemic Coxsackievirus B5 Genotype. *Journal of Infectious Diseases* 756:288, 1987.

4. Aerosol Transmission of Rhinovirus Colds. *Journal of Infectious Diseases* 156:442, 1987.

5. Case to Case Intervals of Rhinovirus and Influenza Virus Infections in Households. *Journal of Infectious Diseases* 157:180, 1988.

RHABDOVIRUSES

T his chapter discusses only one virus and one human disease caused by that virus. There are a number of viruses in the family *Rhabdovirus* and they infect various vertebrate and invertebrate hosts; however, only one, the rabies virus, causes serious widespread disease in humans. Rabies produces an invariably fatal disease of humans and is a major animal health problem throughout the world. A helical RNA virus, the rabies virus, has a unique and distinctive shape. The helix is wound in a rod shape with one end tapered which gives the virion a distinctive ''bullet'' shape (see Figure 32–2). This chapter details the epidemiology of this virus and the efforts made to prevent rabies throughout the world.

RABIES

The rabies virus appears capable of infecting and causing serious disease in most mammals. Most die, but some are able to carry and shed the virus for prolonged periods. The disease of rabies in humans was recognized and reported in ancient times as a disease transmitted by the bite of a mad (rabid) dog. Once signs of rabies begin to appear in humans, indicating infection of the central nervous system, the disease progresses in almost all cases until death results.

Pathogenesis and Clinical Disease

Generally, humans are infected by the bite of an infected animal that introduces the virus into the tissue. Infection can also occur from saliva from an infected animal that is deposited on mucous membranes or on open sores or abrasions. The virus may remain at site of entry for weeks, where some local multiplication may occur. The virus then spreads slowly from the local site of entry, moving along nerve fibers to the regional ganglia and the CNS. The incubation time—that is, the period between the time of the bite and the onset of signs of the disease in the CNS—varies greatly, depending on the site and the severity of the bite as well as other host factors. The incubation period is a reflection of the rate of spread of the virus and may range from a week to months and even a year or more (average is 1 to 2 months). The incubation period is usually longer when the bite occurs on an extremity, such as an arm or leg, and shorter when occurring about the neck and head.

The virus fails to progress from the site of entry to the CNS in approximately half or more of the persons bitten by an infected animal. Once the virus enters the CNS, however, it spreads rapidly throughout these tissues and then spreads down the peripheral nerves to other tissues. In particular, the rabies virus proliferates in the salivary glands and may be found in high concentrations in the saliva. When this stage is reached, the overt signs and symptoms of the disease begin with fever, headache, and loss of appetite. Then they progress to convulsions, excessive flow of tears and saliva, insomnia, anxiety, muscle spasms triggered by swallowing, and sometimes maniacal behavior. Ascending paralysis may be seen and death sometimes results after 2 to 6 days because of respiratory or cardiac failure. In other cases, patients lapse into a coma, followed by death. Except in a few known cases clinical rabies has invariably resulted in the death of the patient.

The pathogenesis of rabies in animals has many similarities and some differences from the disease in humans. The route of infection in animals is often by the bite of another infected animal, but disease may also result from eating a diseased animal. In many animals the virus passes to the CNS during the long incubation period. In dogs, cats, and related animals the virus appears in various excretory glands, especially the salivary glands, several days before the onset of signs of CNS involvement. Once signs of the CNS infection occur, the animal usually dies within a relatively short time. A small percentage of these animals have been found to shed rabies virus in their saliva for up to 2 years without developing the clinical disease. Bats are often infected with rabies virus and appear to tolerate the infection much better than most other animals. Some evidence indicates that bats are able to carry and shed the rabies virus for prolonged periods without showing signs of the disease.

Transmission and Epidemiology

Normally the route of transmission is by the bite of an infected animal (Figure 40-1). This route works extremely well, for the irritation of the infection in the CNS drives the animal into a frenzy

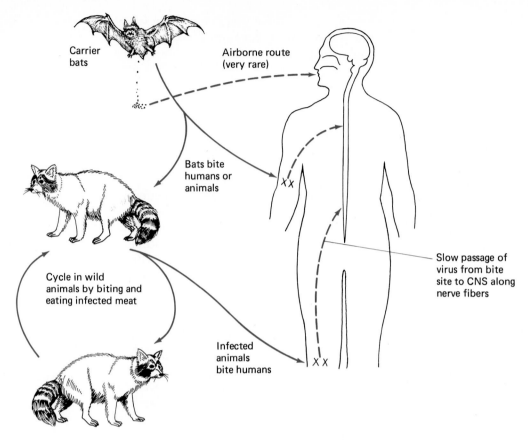

Figure 40-1   Modes of transmission of rabies viruses among animals and to humans.

that results in the biting of other animals. Such biting occurs at the time when high concentrations of virus are found in the saliva. Rabies in humans and in animals like cows or horses is usually a dead end because the infection is not conveniently transmitted to other hosts by biting. Although only a few cases of rabies are seen in humans each year in the United States (Figure 40-2), many wild animals are infected (Figure 40-3). Rabies in humans is much more frequent in many developing countries, and some studies have suggested that from 1% to 2% of all deaths in some cultures are due to rabies.

Rabies may be transmitted orally through eating infected meat and may be an important means of transmission among wild carnivores. Airborne transmission in bat caves, while rare, has occurred. Four cases have been documented in persons receiving corneal transplants from donors who had died of undiagnosed rabies. Rabies in cattle is a major economic problem in Latin America and is transmitted by the bite of infected vampire bats. Bats,

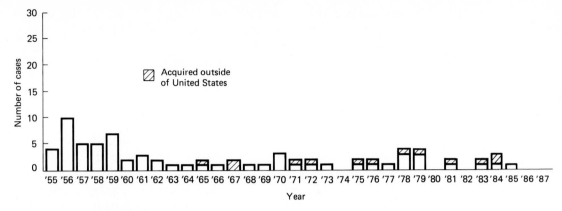

Figure 40-2 Reported rabies cases in humans by year in the United States, 1955–1987 (modified from CDC annual summaries).

in general, probably serve as the most important reservoir of the rabies virus.

Diagnosis

The most important priority is the rapid detection of rabies in an animal that has bitten a person. Whether the biting animal is infected directly determines the type of treatment that the bite victim should receive. Whenever possible, an animal that bites a person should be apprehended or killed. If domestic animals like

Figure 40-3 Reported rabies cases in wild and domestic animals by year in the United States, 1965–1986 (CDC summary 1986).

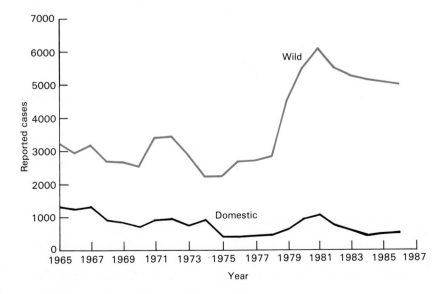

dogs or cats do not show definite signs of rabies, the animal should be placed under observation at the public health laboratory for 8 to 10 days and monitored for the appearance of clinical signs of rabies. Wild animals or domestic animals showing signs of rabies should be killed and either the intact animal or the head taken immediately to a public health laboratory. The animal should be wrapped in a plastic bag to prevent possible contamination and kept cool if possible.

The laboratory worker examines the brain cells for the appearance of clusters of viral materials (inclusion bodies) in the cytoplasm called *Negri bodies*. Negri bodies are rapidly and specifically identified by using specific fluorescent antibodies. A positive diagnosis can be made on most infected animals within a few minutes via this procedure. As a backup test, brain tissue is injected into suckling mice that will develop rabies within the next 1 to 3 weeks if the virus is present. Cell cultures may also be used to isolate the virus.

A preliminary diagnosis in humans is based on clinical signs and symptoms and on a possible history of exposure to rabies. A confirmed diagnosis may be made by showing the presence of rabies virus antigens in corneal impressions or skin biopsies (taken from the nape of the neck) using fluorescent antibodies. Diagnosis is confirmed after death by demonstrating the presence of rabies virus in the brain tissue by the fluorescent antibody method and by mouse or cell culture inoculations.

Treatment

Treatment of suspected or preclinical rabies is considered a prevention measure and will be discussed below. Treatment of clinical rabies has generally been unsuccessful. A few exceptions have occurred. The most notable was a 6-year-old boy in Ohio who was bitten by a rabid bat in 1970. He went through the Pasteur treatment (described below) but still developed clinical rabies. Through close medical supervision and such standard medical interventions as a tracheotomy to control respiration, drainage of cerebrospinal fluid to prevent excessive pressure on the brain, anticonvulsive drugs, and monitoring of heart rhythm, this patient was able to survive complications that killed most other known rabies patients. Apparently his own defense mechanisms were able to fight off the rabies virus infections and his recovery was complete.

Prevention and Control

A great deal of effort and resources go toward preventing and controlling rabies and in many countries these programs have been successful. Cases of human rabies in the United States have been reduced to only a few a year out of approximately 30,000 persons exposed to rabies each year. In developing countries, hundreds of thousands are exposed to rabies each year.

Prevention and control of rabies are carried out in the following areas:

1. Control in domestic animals by vaccination and quarantine
2. Vaccination of persons who have a high risk of being exposed
3. Postexposure immunoprophylaxis

Before the initiation of strict control measures, most human rabies were contracted by the bite of domestic cats or dogs. Leash laws, licensing of dogs, and vaccinations have reduced the cases of rabies in these animals to an insignificant number in many countries and eliminated rabies completely in such island nations as Great Britain, Australia, and Japan. Rabies is prevented from reentering these rabies-free countries by the strict quarantine of imported animals. Still, in many parts of the world rabies is widespread in wildlife and no effective methods are available to control or eliminate this reservoir of the virus. The major animal reservoirs in the United States are bats, skunks, foxes, and raccoons; yet virtually any wild animal may be infected and so any animal exhibiting abnormal behavior should be suspect. In some countries, domestic dogs and cats are still the major source of exposure for humans; for example, in 1986 in Mexico 8483 rabid dogs were reported and this made up 96% of all reported animal rabies in Mexico that year.

Several vaccine varieties are available for animals. A living attenuated vaccine is generally used to vaccinate dogs and cats. The only vaccine currently available for humans in the United States and many other countries is a killed purified human diploid cell vaccine (HDCV). This vaccine is free of most adverse reactions that were associated with the crude rabies vaccines that were used before the 1980s. Preexposure vaccination with three injections of HDCV over 4 weeks is recommended for veterinarians, animal control officers, campers, and other people who are in frequent contact with wild animals.

The prevention of rabies primarily concerns how people are handled following their exposure to rabies. Possibly because of the long incubation period, rabies is the only disease in which the initiation of active vaccination after exposure is successful. This procedure was developed by Pasteur in 1884 when he prevented the development of rabies in a boy who had been severely bitten by a rabid wolf. Pasteur infected progressively more potent preparations of rabies-infected rabbit spinal cord extracts into the boy daily over a 21-day period. The treatment worked and was referred to as the *Pasteur treatment*. Some modifications were made in the Pasteur treatment over the years, and it continued to be used up to the introduction of the HDCV in the early 1980s.

CLINICAL NOTE

Imported Human Rabies: United States, 1983

The first case of human rabies in the United States since August 1981 has been reported to CDC. The patient, a 30-year-old American architect from Waltham, Massachusetts, was exposed to rabies from a dog bite in Ososo, Nigeria, West Africa. He died on January 28, 1983, 28 days after onset of symptoms.

On October 8, the patient, who worked in Nigeria, was bitten on the right wrist by his pet Doberman pinscher while attempting to free it from a trap. The dog died later that day and was buried without laboratory examination for rabies. The patient sought medical attention at a nearby clinic and received tetanus immunization, but because the dog had recently been immunized against rabies, it was decided that postexposure prophylaxis was unnecessary.

Eleven weeks later, the patient returned to the United States and remained well until January 1, 1983, 85 days after the bite, when he developed numbness and tingling at the healed bite-site. During the next several days, the patient developed low back pain, a temperature of 38.9°C (102°F), sore throat, anorexia, and malaise. On January 5, he complained of difficulty breathing, mild chest discomfort, excessive salivation, and occasionally gagging when attempting to drink.

He was examined by a physician, who noted that he had nonspecific ST-T changes on an electrocardiogram. He was admitted to Waltham Hospital, Waltham, Massachusetts, for further evaluation.

On admission, the patient was anxious and was producing a large volume of saliva, which he refused to swallow. He suggested that a milk deficiency caused his illness, and exhibited unusual fear of some medical procedures. His pharynx was slightly erythematous, and his neck or throat structures contracted when touched with the hands or examining instruments. The remainder of the physical examination was unremarkable. Laboratory tests revealed a white blood count of 9900, with a normal differential, normal serum electrolytes and calcium, and normal chest x ray. On January 6, the patient exhibited marked hyperactivity and refused to swallow barium for a radiologic examination. On the evening of January 6, he had respiratory arrest and a generalized seizure, and an endotracheal tube was inserted. Following the respiratory arrest, his temperature rose to 41.1° C (106° F). A chest x ray showed diffuse pulmonary infiltrates. A diagnosis of rabies was considered, and the patient was placed in strict isolation. A

Hyperimmune globulin
globulin containing high levels of antibody to a specific antigen. These globulins are prepared by repeatedly immunizing animals or persons with the antigen. Blood is then donated and the globulins are obtained.

Local treatment of the wound is helpful in preventing rabies. The wound should immediately be cleansed thoroughly and flushed with soap and water. The patient should then be taken to a physician to receive antiserum treatment. A **hyperimmune globulin** known as *human rabies immune globulin* (RIG) is now available and should be instilled in the depths of the wound and infiltrated around the wound. Next, postexposure immunization with HDCV should be initiated with intramuscular injections of days 0, 3, 7, 14, and 28.

skin biopsy, taken from the back of his neck above the hairline, was sent to CDC for direct immunofluorescent antibody (FA) testing for rabies.

On January 7, the biopsy was reported positive. The patient was able to communicate rationally with hospital staff by writing notes. He demonstrated marked pharyngeal and laryngeal spasms when his face or neck was stimulated by either a wet sponge or a draught of cool air. Bacterial cultures of cerebrospinal fluid (CFS), blood, urine, and sputum were negative. Computerized tomography and electroencephalogram were normal. The patient continued to require ventilatory support and a dopamine infusion to maintain adequate blood pressure. On January 8, he was started on systemic interferon treatment. He was given human leukocyte interferon, 10 million units twice daily intramuscularly, and 5 million units once daily intraventricularly into a Rickham reservoir connected by a cannula to a lateral ventricle of his brain.

During the next 10 days, the patient became progressively less responsive and was in a deep coma by January 18. He had numerous medical complications during the course of illness, including *Pseudomonas* sepsis and keratoconjunctivitis, recurrent seizures, hypo- and hyperthermia, anemia, hypotension, abnormal blood clotting, and acute renal failure. The interferon therapy was discontinued on January 25, 17 days after the first dose was administered. The patient developed adult respiratory distress syndrome refractory to ventilation and died of cardiovascular collapse on January 28. Serum collected daily from the patient and tested at CDC for rabies antibody turned positive 1:12 on the sixteenth day of illness and remained minimally positive at 1:25 or less until his death. At postmortem, many tissues were positive for rabies virus, including specimens from brain and spinal cord, skin and nerve from the bite site, pancreas, liver, bladder, periaortic lymph node, pericardium, adrenal gland, and salivary gland.

A total of 132 persons were evaluated for potential contact with infectious secretions from the patient. Twenty-eight persons received rabies postexposure prophylaxis, including 7 physicians, 14 nurses, 3 respiratory therapists, 1 microbiologist, 2 friends and relatives of the patient, and 1 other hospital contact. In addition, 3 pathologists received preexposure prophylaxis before the patient's death (*MMWR* 32:78, 1983).

The treatment regimen should be correlated with the diagnostic program on the animal that inflicted the bite. If tests show that the animal is not infected, the immunization program should be stopped to avoid further discomfort to the patient. For this reason, it is important to apprehend the biting animal. If the animal is not apprehended, the victim usually has little choice but to go through the immunization program. About 20,000 to 30,000 postexposure immunizations are given in the United States annually.

CONCEPT SUMMARY

A bullet-shaped, helical RNA rhabdovirus is responsible for the disease rabies. This is a common disease among lower animals and in humans in foreign countries, but its occurrence is limited in people living in the United States. The disease is unusual in its mode of transmission and devastating in its consequences. Control of rabies is best accomplished by the immunization of domestic animals and individuals at high risk. Vaccines with risk of serious side effects have largely been replaced by a more useful diploid cell vaccine.

STUDY SUMMARY

1. What three preventive procedures should be taken for an individual who is bitten by a rabid animal?
2. What is the most likely source of human exposure to rabies in the United States?
3. What feature of rabies gives this disease characteristics of an occupational disease?
4. Describe the physical properties of the rabies virus.

REFERENCES FOR FURTHER STUDY

1. *The Rhabdoviruses*, R. Wagner, 1987. Plenum.
2. Is There a Risk to Contacts of Patients with Rabies? *Reviews of Infectious Diseases* 9:511, 1987.
3. *Fundamental Virology*, B. Fields, 1986. Raven.

chapter 41

AIDS

A cquired immunodeficiency syndrome, better known as AIDS, is caused by the *human immunodeficiency virus* (HIV). The appearance of this virus at the beginning of the 1980s may ultimately prove to be the most devastating medical experience in history. In terms of human life lost, AIDS may not exceed the devastation of smallpox, plague, or typhus, but in terms of economic demand, social change, and commitment of medical resources it may eclipse all previously known maladies. Even in the mass media AIDS is rapidly replacing more common and frequent disease concerns such as cancer and cardiovascular disease as the item of greatest interest. Unfortunately, such mass media reports are often contradictory, or contain only abbreviated reports on the subject. This chapter will present a review of current understanding relative to AIDS.

MICROORGANISM

Acquired immunodeficiency disease occurs in individuals infected with HIV. The virus is a single-stranded RNA virus that belongs to a group of viruses known as *retroviruses*. Retroviruses are commonly associated with animal tumors (Chapter 33). HIV, like other retroviruses depends on the presence of a *reverse transcriptase* enzyme to transcribe the virus RNA genome into DNA. With other retroviruses, when DNA is produced it readily integrates into the host cell chromosome. In such a **provirus** state, the viral DNA is able to provide genetic messages that *transform* the host cell. This type of transformed cell is characteristic of tumor cells. However, the DNA transcribed from HIV RNA does not easily integrate but proceeds as a lytic infection of the host cell. Cell lysis due to HIV may be a slow process in some cells such that the virus continues to be shed over a relatively long period of time.

Provirus
a complete viral genome that has been integrated into the host cell chromosome.

Lymphotropic
having a preference for lymphoid
cells.

HIV is a **lymphotropic** virus that preferentially infects *helper T cells* (T4 cells). These cells are killed by HIV infection, which reduces the ratio of T-helper to *T-suppressor cells* (Chapter 12). The virus can also infect other lymphoid cells such as B cells and has been found in lymphoid cells of the brain and testes. The virus will also infect monocytes, which are refractory to cytopathic change and this may provide a means whereby persons shed the virus over an extended period of time. These chronic or latent infections may be induced to develop into active disease at any time; at present, however, the type of inducing agent or agents is unknown.

In experimental in vitro studies, HIV demonstrates a high level of virulence with rapid host cell death. The virus appears to be infective for the chimpanzee but not for other animals, and the chimpanzee does not develop symptoms of AIDS. Recent reports of the isolation of *HIV-2* virus from AIDS patients in Africa and the United States raises concerns that more than a single type of virus may be involved in the epidemic.

PATHOGENESIS AND CLINICAL CONDITIONS

Lymphadenopathy
enlargement of the lymph nodes.

AIDS was first recognized in the United States in 1981. Realization that a new disease was developing was first made indirectly. A few individuals with the same, but unusual, clinical conditions raised questions as to the etiology of their disease. Each of these patients developed a rather rare form of cancer known as *Kaposi's sarcoma* (Figure 41-1), suffered from unexplained weight loss, fever, **lymphadenopathy**, and an unusual type of pneumonia caused by a parasite *Pneumocystis carinii* (Chapter 31). The other feature these patients had in common was that all were homosexual males. The clinical characteristics of these early patients set the diagnostic pattern presently associated with AIDS. Most patients suffer from malaise, diarrhea, shortness of breath, lymphadenopathy, and infection by one or more low-grade pathogens.

The normal ratio of T-helper to T-suppressor (T4 to T8) cells is somewhat greater than 1. The end result of destruction of T4 cells by HIV is to lower this ratio to values as low as 0.2. Individuals with such a small number of T4 cells are unable to maintain a proper immunologic response to their environment and they become highly susceptible to a variety of infectious agents characteristic of strongly immunosuppressed T cell functions (Chapter 12). Humoral immune response may also be diminished in these patients. The complications associated with immunodeficiency (Chapter 14, 19, 22, 30, 31, 35), include infection by microorganisms uncommonly found in other patients. Serious life-threaten-

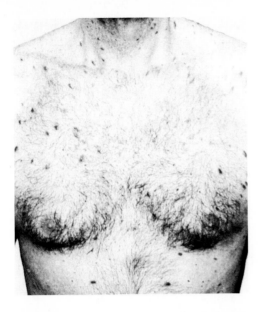

Figure 41-1 Patient with Kaposi's sarcoma. Note dark pigmented areas of skin characteristic of this disease. (Courtesy Burroughs Wellcome Co., Research Triangle Park, NC)

ing disease due to viruses such as cytomegalovirus and herpes simplex virus, bacteria such as *Mycobacterium avium* and *Salmonella*, fungi such as *Candida albicans* and *Cryptococcus neoformans*, and parasites such as *Pneumocystis carinii* and *Cryptosporidium* have become characteristics of AIDS patients. Kaposi's sarcoma, a **malignant neoplasm** manifested primarily by multiple vascular nodules in the skin and other organs (Figure 41-1), is a disease that is rare in young adults but afflicts as many as 36% of homosexuals with AIDS. Treatment of any of these complicating illnesses is made particularly difficult due to the lack of host response in these patients. The basic immune deficiency coupled with complicating factors of associated diseases has resulted in a condition with a mortality rate that is essentially 100% (Figure 41-2).

In addition to lymphotropism, HIV is also neurotropic. This results in the development of neuropsychiatric abnormalities in some patients. The virus also seems to *potentiate* some illnesses caused by other etiologic agents. For example, as noted in Chapter 19, tertiary syphilis normally takes years for development. In patients with AIDS, however, this phase of the disease may be expressed after only a few months.

Malignant neoplasm
cancer. A neoplastic growth is the growth of new cells; a malignant neoplasm is the growth of cancerous cells.

TRANSMISSION AND EPIDEMIOLOGY

There are presently three levels of diagnosis associated with HIV infection. The first of these appears in individuals with subclinical viral infection. These individuals are clinically well, but frequently

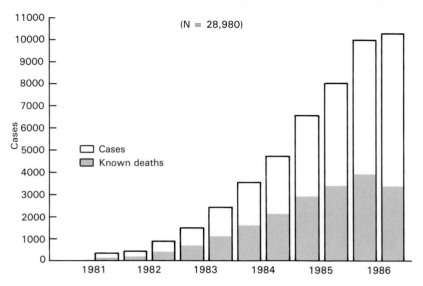

Figure 41-2   Reported cases and deaths from AIDS through 1986.
(Courtesy Centers for Disease Control, Atlanta)

have some decrease in T-helper cells and have circulating antibody to HIV. These infected individuals while well, are very important epidemiologically because of their ability to transmit the virus to others. The actual number of HIV antibody–positive persons is unknown, but is presently estimated to be as many as 2 million in the United States (Figure 41-3). The proportion of these

Figure 41-3   Distribution of AIDS cases reported in the United States. (Courtesy Centers for Disease Control, Atlanta)

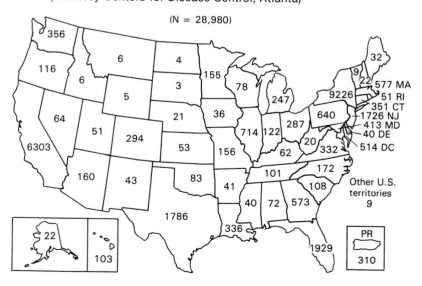

persons who will ultimately develop symptomatic disease is estimated to be in the order of 25% to 50% over a 5-year period. Whether or not all HIV-infected persons will ultimately develop AIDS is unknown.

The second level of disease is referred to a *AIDS-related complex* (ARC). Individuals in this group have persistent clinical abnormalities such as fever, diarrhea, weight loss, depressed helper T cells, fatigue, lymphadenopathy, and HIV antibody but do not meet the criteria for the diagnosis of AIDS. AIDS is the third diagnostic level. This level is associated with those conditions associated with ARC plus a rare opportunistic infection (such as *Pneumocystis* pneumonia) or the development of a rare malignancy (Kaposi's sarcoma or non-Hodgkin's lymphoma).

The incubation period for AIDS is undefined, but it may be as long as several years. Thus, the normal disease progression is for an infected individual to first become seropositive to the HIV, progress to the development of ARC, and at some interval (as short as a few months to as long a several years) enter the third (AIDS) diagnostic level.

AIDS was first described in the United States and has subsequently been found in 129 countries throughout the world (Table 41-1). It now appears that HIV infection first occurred in Africa and was transmitted to the western world by a homosexual airline steward. In the United States there were more than 54,000 cases (70% of all cases reported worldwide) with 30,000 (56%) deaths reported during the 1981–87 period (Figure 41-3). Most (67%) of the cases in the U.S. have occurred in males. This is because HIV is readily transmitted by male homosexual practices and originated in the U.S. by this means. However, as the virus can be found in the blood and semen of infected persons, transfer to the heterosexual community, to recipients of blood or blood products, and to intravenous drug users soon followed. Presently, of the cases reported in the U.S., 65% have been homosexual or bisexual males, 17% have been intravenous drug users, and 4% are heterosexuals (Figure 41-4). It is of particular public health concern that three high-risk groups continue to present with HIV infection—intravenous drug users, male homosexuals, and female sexual partners of men with HIV infection.

The estimated number of infected pregnant women varies throughout the world, but in some areas of Central and East Africa as many as 2% to 15% of pregnant women are seropositive. Between 30% and 65% of their children will be infected either prior to, or at birth. The AIDS epidemic in this part of Africa is most alarming with estimates of infection as high as 25% of individuals between the ages of 20 and 40 years. In the United States, women generally acquire HIV from infected sexual partners or from illicit intravenous drug use. Children obtain the virus in utero or at the time of birth from infected mothers. In Central Africa, the ratio

Table 41-1   Reported Acquired Immunodeficiency Syndrome Cases and Estimated Rates per Million Population, 21 European Countries, October 1, 1984–September 30, 1985

Country	Number of Cases				Rates[a]
	Oct. 1984	March 1985	June 1985	Sept. 1985	
Austria	—	13	18	23	
Belgium	—	81	99	118	3.1
Denmark	0	0	0	0	11.9
Czechoslovakia	31	41	48	57	0
Federal Republic of Germany	110	162	220	295	11.2
					4.8
Finland	4	5	6	10	2.0
France	221	307	392	466	8.5
Greece	2	7	9	10	1.0
Hungary	—	—	—	0	0.0
Iceland	0	0	0	0	0.0
Italy	10	22	52	92	1.6
Luxembourg	—	—	1	3	7.5
Netherlands	26	52	66	83	5.7
Norway	4	8	11	14	3.3
Poland	0	0	0	0	0.0
Spain	18	29	38	63	1.6
Sweden	12	22	27	36	4.3
Switzerland	33	51	63	77	11.8
United Kingdom	88	140	176	225	4.0
Union of Soviet Socialist Republics	—	—	—	0	0.0
Yugoslavia	—	—	—	1	—
Total	559	940	1,226	1,573	—

[a]Per million population based on 1985 populations.

of men to women with AIDS is about 1:1. This reflects primarily heterosexual transmission of the disease in Africa, where frequency of occurrence is related to number of sexual partners more than to sexual practices.

Prior to the development of diagnostic antibody tests, HIV was occasionally transmitted through contaminated blood or blood products to hospitalized recipients. However, present screening of blood donors to rule out high-risk individuals, and serologic testing procedures make transmission by this mode extremely unlikely. Although much controversy has existed regarding possible spread of this virus, it is becoming increasingly clear that even though the virus has been isolated from human milk, saliva, tears, urine, cerebrospinal fluid, semen, and blood, there is almost no risk of transmission except through contact with the latter two fluids. It is also now known that casual contact will not transmit the virus, and that it can not be transmitted through food prepared by an HIV-positive person or among children who at-

AIDS CASES IN THE UNITED STATES
(as of February 15, 1988)

Total diagnosed: 53,814   Total deaths: 30,158

Adults with AIDS

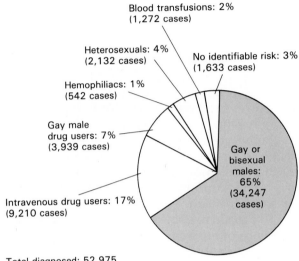

Blood transfusions: 2%
(1,272 cases)

Heterosexuals: 4%
(2,132 cases)

No identifiable risk: 3%
(1,633 cases)

Hemophiliacs: 1%
(542 cases)

Gay male
drug users: 7%
(3,939 cases)

Gay or
bisexual
males:
65%
(34,247
cases)

Intravenous drug users: 17%
(9,210 cases)

Total diagnosed: 52,975
Total deaths: 29,661

Children with AIDS

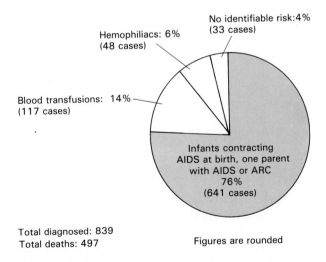

No identifiable risk: 4%
(33 cases)

Hemophiliacs: 6%
(48 cases)

Blood transfusions: 14%
(117 cases)

Infants contracting
AIDS at birth, one parent
with AIDS or ARC
76%
(641 cases)

Total diagnosed: 839
Total deaths: 497

Figures are rounded

*AIDS related complex

Figure 41-4   Case distribution of and patient demography for AIDS
in the United States as of February 1988. (Courtesy Centers for
Disease Control)

tend school or play together. With the exception of those whose lifestyles place them in the risk groups already discussed, the only individuals who are at significantly increased risk are medical and dental health professionals. Specific guidelines have been developed by the Centers for Disease Control to reduce the risk to this group of individuals. An abbreviated list of guidelines is given in Table 41-2.

DIAGNOSIS

Virus isolation from infected individuals is possible and may be undertaken in a research setting. The virus may persist for years in either symptomatic or asymptomatic persons and can be isolated from lymphocytes, bone marrow, or blood. Isolation of the virus is diagnosis for the infection. Most clinical laboratories are unprepared to do HIV isolation, and the costs of such efforts are considerable. A breakthrough in diagnostic testing came with the discovery of a procedure for producing large amounts of viral antigen in vitro. This made possible the development of tests to determine the presence of antibody in infected individuals. There are several commercially prepared antibody-detection kits now available. More recently a DNA probe that will hybridize with viral genes has become available. This probe is designed to detect the virus itself and not the host antibody response. This procedure may be able to largely eliminate the detection "window" that presently exists in HIV diagnosis.

The implications associated with test results that are *true positive* (the patient has the infection and tests positive for it), *false positive* (the patient does *not* have the infection but tests positive for it), or *false negative* (the patient has the infection but tests negative for it) are so profound that any diagnostic procedure must have a high *sensitivity* (will not produce any false negatives) and a high *specificity* (will not produce any false positives). Two tests have been developed that have both high specificity and high sensitivity. The first of these is an ELISA procedure (Chapter 13), which is commonly used by most diagnostic laboratories. This test is used to screen blood donated for transfusion and is so sensitive that some false positives (1 in 1000) result. Blood that is positive by ELISA is then sent to a reference laboratory where an antibody-detection test known as a **Western blot** is performed. This procedure has extreme specificity. Any blood specimen that is positive by both procedures is considered to be a true positive and to have come from an individual who is infected with HIV. Seropositivity rates have been determined for several groups at increased risk for AIDS; healthy homosexual men are 22% to 65% **seropositive**,

Western blot
a procedure that uses both electrophoresis and antigen-antibody reaction to identify specific antigens or antibodies.

Seropositive
having serum that tests positive for a specific antibody.

Table 41-2   Guidelines to Prevent Transmission of Aids

A. Health Care Workers
   1. General
      a. Use appropriate barrier precautions (gloves, masks, eyewear, gowns).
      b. Immediately wash any skin surfaces exposed to possibly contaminated body fluid.
      c. Use precautions to prevent personal injury from sharp objects (needles, scalpels, instruments) used in any medical procedure.
      d. Use procedures that minimize need for mouth-to-mouth resuscitation.
      e. If you have open or weeping lesions do not participate in direct patient care.
      f. Implement universal blood and body fluid precautions for all patients.
   2. Dental
      a. Consider blood, saliva, and gingival fluid from all patients as infective.
      b. Use appropriate barrier precautions (gloves, protective eyewear, etc.) for all contact with oral surfaces.
      c. Sterilize handpieces after use with each patient.
      d. Carefully clean blood and saliva from all materials that are used in the mouth. Disinfect all devices before they are placed in patient's mouth.
      e. Carefully wrap all equipment surfaces that are difficult to disinfect with impervious paper, plastic wrap, or foil and replace after each patient.
   3. Laboratory
      a. Specimens should be placed in leak-proof containers.
      b. Persons processing blood or body fluid specimens should wear gloves. Masks and eye protection should be used when appropriate.
      c. Use safety cabinet for procedures with risk of generating droplets.
      d. Use mechanical pipetting devices.
      e. Limit use of needles and syringes. Use proper discard procedures for all sharp objects.
      f. Immediately decontaminate all spills. Regularly decontaminate work surfaces.
      g. Implement universal body fluid precautions for all patients.
   4. Other
      a. Strictly follow established precautionary procedures for handling patients and patient materials in areas where there is increased risk: hemodialysis center, emergency rooms, nursing care facilities, ophthalmology and optometric centers.
B. Individual
   1. If you are HIV-positive:
      a. Use barrier (condom) protection for sexual partner.
      b. Refrain from donating blood, sperm, body tissues, or organs.
      c. Recognize that you can transmit HIV to others even if you remain asymptomatic.
      d. Properly disinfect any surface accidentally contaminated by bleeding.
      e. Notify responsible personnel of your HIV status when seeking medical or dental assistance.
   2. If you are HIV-negative:
      a. Limit sexual contacts to a monogamous relationship.
      b. If your sexual partner is HIV-positive use barrier (condom) protection.
      c. Do not share needles, toothbrushes, razors, or any item that may be contaminated with blood.
      d. Avail yourself of HIV testing if there is a possibility that you have been exposed to the virus.

Update: Human Immunodeficiency Virus Infections in Health Care Workers Exposed to Blood of Infected Persons: United States, 1986

Six persons who provided health care to patients with human immunodeficiency virus (HIV) infection and who denied other risk factors have previously been reported to have HIV infection. Four of these cases followed needle-stick exposures to blood from patients infected with HIV. The two additional cases involved persons who provided nursing care to persons with HIV infection. Although neither of these two persons sustained needle-stick injuries, both had extensive contact with blood or body fluids of the infected patient, and neither observed routinely recommended barrier precautions.

CDC has received reports of HIV infection in three additional health care workers following non-needle-stick exposures to blood from infected patients. The exposures occurred during 1986 in three different geographic areas. Although these three cases represent rare events, they reemphasize the need for health care workers to adhere rigorously to existing infection control recommendations for minimizing the risk of exposure to blood and body fluids of all patients.

Health Care Worker 1: A female health care worker assisting with an unsuccessful attempt to insert an arterial catheter in a patient suffering a cardiac arrest in an emergency room applied pressure to the insertion site to stop the bleeding. During the procedure, she may have had a small amount of blood on her index finger for about 20 minutes before washing her hands. Afterwards, she may also have assisted in cleaning the room but did not recall any other exposures to the patient's blood or body fluids. She had no open wounds, but her hands were chapped. Although she often wore gloves when anticipating exposure to blood, she was not wearing gloves during this incident.

The patient with the cardiac arrest died. A postmortem examination identified *Pneumocystis carinii* pneumonia, and a blood sample was positive for HIV antibody by enzyme immunoassay (EIA) and Western blot methods. Twenty days after the incident, the health care worker became ill with fever, myalgia, extreme fatigue, sore throat, nausea, vomiting, diarrhea, a 14-pound weight loss, and generalized lymphadenopathy which her physician diagnosed as a viral syndrome. That illness lasted 3 weeks. She felt much better 9 weeks after the incident, and, when she was examined 6 months after the incident, all signs and symptoms had resolved. She had donated blood 8 months before the incident and was negative for HIV antibody by EIA. She donated again 16 weeks after the incident and was positive for HIV by EIA and Western blot (bands p24 and gp42). Serum samples obtained 20 and 23 weeks after the incident were also positive for antibody. She stated that for over 8 years her only sexual partner had been her husband, who denied risk factors for HIV and was seronegative for HIV antibody. She denied ever receiving a blood transfusion, ever using intravenous drugs, or having any needle sticks or other significant exposures to blood or body fluids in the past 8 years. Her serologic test for syphilis was negative. Fifteen other employees who assisted in the care of the patient were seronegative at least 4 months after the exposure (*MMWR* 36:285, 1987).

persons with hemophilia A are 56% to 72% seropositive, intravenous drug abusers are 87% seropositive, and female sexual partners of men with AIDS are 35% seropositive. As is true with exposure to any antigen, individuals have some delay in antibody development following exposure to HIV. It is therefore possible for infected persons to test as seronegative if they have only recently been infected. It should be remembered that laboratory tests merely screen blood and blood products for HIV antibodies. Diagnosis of AIDS is made only when specific clinical criteria have been fulfilled.

PREVENTION AND CONTROL

There is presently no therapy that will cure HIV infection in humans. Considerable research effort is being expended to find both a chemotherapeutic treatment and a preventive vaccine. Best estimates for success in these two important areas are that such development will take at least 10 years. This presents a rather bleak outlook for those persons presently suffering from AIDS, and emphasizes the importance of using known control procedures to limit the spread of infection (Table 41-2). It is important to recognize that persons in the first diagnostic category (asymptomatic virus-positive) can transmit HIV while they themselves remain free of disease.

The economic implications associated with HIV infection are serious, with total health care costs estimated to be in the order of $20–30 billion by the end of 1991. The 1988 U.S. federal budget included $931 million for direct research into AIDS and in that year the cost of medical care for AIDS patients was greater than costs for all other infectious diseases combined.

CONCEPT SUMMARY

1. AIDS is a recently discovered, life-threatening, viral disease with worldwide distribution. The infection is readily transmitted horizontally through sexual contact and by indiscriminate use of intravenous drug paraphernalia or vertically from infected pregnant females to their offspring.

2. AIDS is caused by the human immunodeficiency virus (HIV). HIV is a RNA retrovirus that is lympho- and neurotropic. HIV reduces the T4–to–T8 lymphocyte ratio which se-

riously diminishes T cell–based immunity. These patients are highly susceptible to a broad range of pathogenic microbes.

3. AIDS can be diagnosed on the basis of clinical symptoms by isolation of the virus or by serological testing. Careful screening of blood donors, and testing for anti-HIV antibody has essentially eliminated risk of virus transmission through blood or blood products.

4. AIDS poses serious economic concerns for the health care system.

STUDY SUMMARY

1. Describe the process of HIV replication in a host cell.

2. What characteristic of the human immune response creates the "diagnostic window" in currently used laboratory diagnostic procedures for AIDS?

3. List the sociological factors presently associated with transmission of HIV.

4. List the medical factors presently associated with transmission of HIV.

5. Discuss the observation that AIDS patients suffer from "unusual" opportunistic infections.

REFERENCES FOR FURTHER STUDY

1. *Science* 239:573–622, 1988.

2. *AIDS Research*, vols. 1–4, 1985–88.

3. Salmonellosis during Infection with Human Immunodeficiency Virus. *Reviews of Infectious Diseases* 9:925, 1987.

4. Heterosexual Transmission of Acquired Immunodeficiency Syndrome: International Perspectives and National Projections. *Reviews of Infectious Disease* 9:947, 1987.

5. Opportunistic Infections in Patients with AIDS. *Reviews of Infectious Diseases* 8:21, 1986.

chapter 42

OTHER VIRUSES

T he positioning of this chapter does not reflect the relative importance of this heterogenous and interesting group of viruses. Every human on the earth has had intimate and personal experience with the reoviruses and coronaviruses which cause the "common cold." Most have also had an unpleasant association with the rotaviruses and the Norwalk group of viruses which are common agents of viral gastroenteritis. These are common viruses normally of only benign clinical significance and are contrasted in this chapter with the viral causes of fulminating and exotic diseases such as dengue, encephalitis, and Lassa fever. Although less common, this latter group of togavirus diseases make up in seriousness that which they lack in commonality. The best known, and historically most significant, of these hemorrhagic fever viruses, yellow fever, is included in this chapter along with the almost rare Argentinian and Bolivian hemorrhagic fevers caused by members of the arenavirus group.

TOGAVIRUSES

The Togaviridae family contains about 250 related viruses. They are separated into a group A, called *alphaviruses*, and a group B called *flaviviruses*. The differences between these groups are sufficient to warrant a proposed new family designation of Flaviridae for the group B viruses. The viruses in both groups contain RNA, have cubical symmetry, and possess an envelope. The presence of the envelope is the basis for the name *toga*, which means an "outer garment" or "mantle." The togaviruses constitute a major portion of a group of viruses called the *arboviruses*, which are arthropod-borne viruses. Arboviruses are able to multiply in such bloodsucking arthropods as mosquitoes, ticks, and gnats, as well as in many different vertebrate hosts including mammals, birds, and reptiles. These viruses are passed from vertebrate hosts to arthropods and vice versa during the taking of blood meals by the arthropods. Mosquitoes are the main vector involved in transmission. Most togaviruses are arthropod-borne, but also included as arboviruses are some members of the Rhabdoviridae, Reoviridae, and Bunyaviridae families. The rubella virus is morphologically similar to the togaviruses, but its pathogenesis and epidemiology are similar to that of the paramyxoviruses and so this virus was discussed with the paramyxoviruses in Chapter 38.

Pathogenesis and Clinical Diseases

Many togaviruses and other arboviruses are maintained in nature with only slight or no observable effects on their natural arthropod or vertebrate hosts. Humans are accidentally infected when bitten by an infected insect and are usually a dead end in the transmission chain. Most human infections are mild or subclinical; some togaviruses, however, are able to cause serious disease. Figure 42-1 shows an outline of the pathogenesis and general categories of togavirus diseases. The viruses first multiply in the cells lining the blood vessels (endothelial cells) and the cells of the RES. In 4 to 7 days viruses are being released into the blood. Most human infections are subclinical or relatively mild with generalized symptoms of fever, aches, and chills. Moreover, most do not progress beyond this mild or subclinical stage. A dozen or so togaviruses, however, are able to cause serious diseases that progress beyond the generalized symptoms to produce the syndromes listed next.

Fever and arthralgia The least serious of the togavirus diseases are characterized by the sudden onset of fever, headache, swollen lymph nodes, conjunctivitis, and excruciating pains in the back, muscles, and joints. A rash may or may not occur. Diseases of this category are primarily seen in subtropical and tropical areas. Deaths are rare. *Dengue fever* is the most frequently experienced disease of this type and increased numbers of cases have been seen in Mexico and the Caribbean islands in the 1970s and 1980s. Limited outbreaks that occurred in southern Texas in 1980 were the first cases reported in the United States since 1945.

Hemorrhagic fevers A few togaviruses damage the blood capillaries, resulting in subcutaneous hemorrhaging and bleeding from body openings. This type of hemorrhagic disease is found in many parts of the world but not in the United States. A second type of hemorrhagic fever causes lesions of the liver and kidney: it is the serious disease of *yellow fever*. Yellow fever was once one of the major diseases of humankind, with devastating outbreaks occurring in crews of sailing ships in tropical areas, among mili-

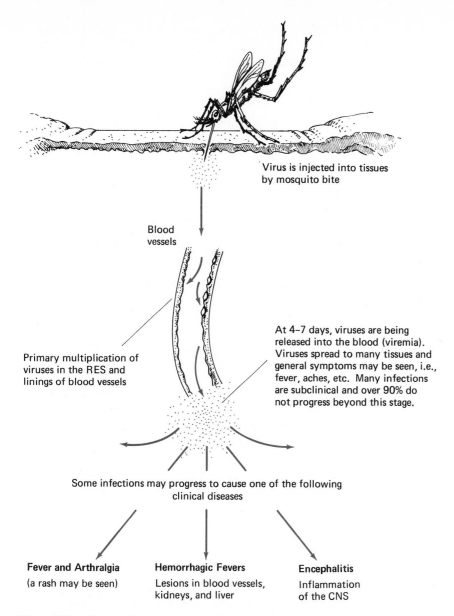

Virus is injected into tissues by mosquito bite

Blood vessels

Primary multiplication of viruses in the RES and linings of blood vessels

At 4–7 days, viruses are being released into the blood (viremia). Viruses spread to many tissues and general symptoms may be seen, i.e., fever, aches, etc. Many infections are subclinical and over 90% do not progress beyond this stage.

Some infections may progress to cause one of the following clinical diseases

Fever and Arthralgia

(a rash may be seen)

Hemorrhagic Fevers

Lesions in blood vessels, kidneys, and liver

Encephalitis

Inflammation of the CNS

Figure 42-1 The pathogeneses of togavirus infections.

tary troops, or in construction crews. Work on the Panama Canal was stopped in the late 1800s because of yellow fever. Walter Reed, a U.S. medical officer studying yellow fever in Cuba during the Spanish-American War, first demonstrated that this disease was transmitted by the *Aedes aegypti* species of mosquito. Control of the *Aedes aegypti* mosquito led to a control of yellow fever, although the disease is still prevalent in some tropical areas. An effective vaccine is available and persons traveling in endemic areas should be vaccinated. Death rates from yellow fever are about 10%.

Encephalitis Various togaviruses are able to cause encephalitis. This disease begins with generalized symptoms and then after several days develops into encephalitis. The symptoms of encephalitis include drowsiness and stiff neck; severe cases may progress to confusion, paralysis, coma, and death. The term *sleeping sickness* is sometimes applied to these diseases but they should not be confused with the protozoal disease of African sleeping sickness. Some residual effects, such as mental retardation, deafness, and blindness, may result. These infections occur in all parts of the world and several thousand sporadic cases are seen in the United States during the summer months. Rates are highest when large numbers of mosquitoes are present, as during very wet summers. Mosquito-borne encephalitis is the only type generally found in the United States. Tick-borne, as well as mosquito-borne, cases appear in other countries. The major types seen in the United States are Eastern, Western, St. Louis, and Venezuelan equine encephalitis. Eastern equine encephalitis is the most severe and causes frequent deaths. The others are less severe in humans, death rates being around 1%. The term *equine* is attached to the name of these diseases because they were first recognized in horses. Horses are often infected and the disease may be quite severe with relatively high death rates. Equine encephalitis can be a major problem to the equine industry because it forces the cancellation of races, rodeos, and horse shows and results in the death of valuable animals.

Transmission and Epidemiology

Togaviruses, as well as the other arboviruses, are transmitted in a complex ecosystem that involves the bloodsucking arthropod vectors and animal reservoirs. The viruses are usually passed in these natural hosts with few consequences. Problems result when these infections "spill over" from these natural hosts into humans and horses. This spillover occurs when environmental conditions permit a large buildup in the numbers of insect vectors and natural animal hosts and when the viruses are introduced into this environment. Such conditions frequently occur in swampy areas and in other areas that have extra wet summers. The reported cases of encephalitis from California serogroup viruses are shown in Figure 42-2; the marked increases during the summer are due to togavirus infections.

Western Equine Encephalitis: Minnesota and North Dakota, 1975

In the early summer of 1975 the Red River flooded into the valley area of eastern North Dakota and northwestern Minnesota. Subsequently health officials initiated a mosquito surveillance program that indicated an unusually high mosquito-population density in the area. Of 96 mosquito pools collected in three North Dakota counties in mid-July, 9 yielded isolation of Western equine encephalitis (WEE) virus. Because of the predominance of the mosquito vector and the resultant increased risk of virus transmission, officials intensified disease surveillance in horses and humans.

Horse surveillance. Cases of equine encephalitis were first observed in early June and a total of 192 cases of clinical encephalitis were reported through August 9, 1975. Of the 192 ill horses, 24 unvaccinated ones had sera collected, and 17 of these horses had high hemagglutination inhibition (HI) and serum neutralization (SN) antibody titers to WEE and no titers to Eastern equine encephalitis. Paired sera from 2 of the 192 ill horses showed a fourfold rise in HI antibody titer to WEE. Of 165 ill horses, 3 (1.8%) were known to have been vaccinated more than 2 weeks before the onset of clinical encephalitis.

Human surveillance. Surveillance in North Dakota and Minnesota uncovered 27 cases of acute, febrile central nervous system (CNS) disease, with onset dates from July 10 to August 6, 1975. All cases were associated with an increased number of cells in the cerebrospinal fluid and most were reported from hospitals in the Red River Valley. Of the 27 cases, 15 were diagnosed as aseptic meningitis and 12 as clinical encephalitis. Four deaths from suspected encephalitis have occurred, all in North Dakota. In 3 cases, including 2 of the deaths, the diagnosis of WEE infection was serologically confirmed by fourfold or greater HI antibody titer rises.

In addition to intensive local and state mosquito control measures that began in Minnesota on July 26, aerial spraying of ultra-low-volume malathion over population centers was begun August 1. Twelve counties in eastern North Dakota received two applications of insecticide; spraying of 11 Minnesota counties began August 12. The gradual natural reduction of breeding sites in the postflood period, combined with spraying, resulted in a substantially decreased mosquito population, but levels remained greater than normal.

Other states reporting seropositive cases of WEE in horses are: Colorado (20), Kansas (18), South Dakota (16), Oklahoma (13), Nebraska (11), Oregon (2), Montana (1), and Iowa (1). To date, no cases of WEE in humans have been reported from these states (*MMWR* 24:270, 1975).

Diagnosis

The generalized nonspecific togavirus infections usually go undiagnosed. The severe infections are tentatively diagnosed on clinical and epidemiological findings. Confirmed diagnoses are made by viral isolation and/or showing specific increases in serum antibody levels.

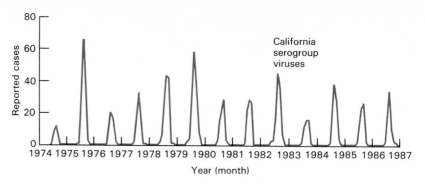

Figure 42-2   Reported cases of viral encephalitis due to arbovirus. Seasonal occurrence is distinctly demonstrated. (Courtesy Centers for Disease Control, Atlanta)

Treatment

No specific treatment for togavirus infections is available.

Prevention and Control

The major control methods are to prevent exposure to mosquitoes or ticks. Eradication or reduction in the number of mosquitoes is routinely carried out in many areas during the summer. Immunization is required for persons traveling to areas where yellow fever is present. Vaccines against other togavirus encephalitides have been developed but are not licensed for human use in the United States. Such vaccines, however, are widely used for the immunization of horses.

ARENAVIRUSES

In the late 1960s accumulated evidence demonstrated that some previously unclassified viruses shared a common morphology. These viruses are pleomorphic with diameters ranging between 50 and 300 nm. They contain dense, ribosome-sized (20 nm) particles that give the appearance of sand particles when viewed by the electron microscope (Figure 42-3). This is the basis for the name Arenaviridae (*arenosus* = sandy), for this family of viruses.

These viruses are normally found in various wild rodents where they cause persistent, lifelong infections, usually without acute clinical signs. The viruses are shed in the feces and urine of the rodent and contaminate food or water. Humans coming in major contact with the contaminated materials may contract an acute

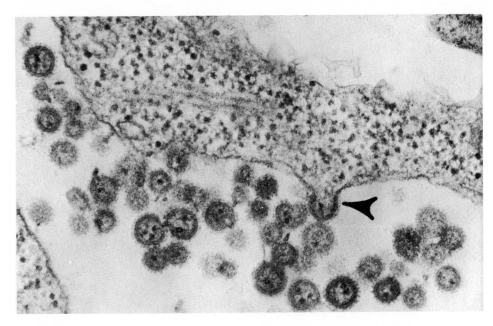

Figure 42-3   Transmission electron micrograph of granule-containing arenaviruses. Arrow points to a virus budding from the infected cell. (Centers for Disease Control, Atlanta)

viral infection. No vaccines are available against any of the arenavirus infections. Proper sanitation and antirodent measures are the most effective means of prevention.

The major arenavirus infections of humans are discussed next.

Lymphocytic Choriomeningitis

Lymphocytic choriomeningitis virus is widespread in domestic house mice throughout the world. In rural areas about 1% of the human inhabitants show serologic evidence of having been infected. The illness is usually nondescript or asymptomatic and rarely is a specific diagnosis made.

Argentinean and Bolivian Hemorrhagic Fevers

Argentinean and Bolivian hemorrhagic fevers occur in limited geographic areas of the respective countries and are caused by closely related arenaviruses. Most outbreaks occur in farm workers during the harvesting of crops when they apparently come in contact with contaminated urine and feces of infected rodents. These disease are quite severe in humans, causing widespread damage to the linings of blood vessels and capillaries. The result is internal hemorrhaging and death rates between 15% and 20%.

Lassa Fever

Index case

first known case of an infectious disease.

Lassa fever was first characterized in 1969 when this disease was dramatically brought to the attention of the world through extensive press coverage of an outbreak among American missionaries in Nigeria, Africa. The first case was reported in a missionary nurse and the disease was transmitted to two attending nurses. The **index case** and one of the attending nurses died. Clinical specimens were flown to the United States, where two laboratory personnel working with these specimens contracted the disease. One died and the other was saved by receiving passive immunization from serum taken from the original attending nurse, who had recovered from Lassa fever. Lassa fever rapidly developed the label of a severe new West African killer virus disease. In the intervening years this disease was studied in greater detail, using stringent safety precautions, and was found to be present in a variety of wild rodents in Nigeria, Liberia, and Sierra Leone. Both mild and severe cases occur among humans. The mild cases usually go undetected whereas those severe enough to require hospitalization have a death rate of 30% to 66%.

CORONAVIRUSES

The human coronaviruses were first discovered in the mid-1960s and were shown to be a frequent cause of common cold–type infections. The structure of these viruses resembles that of the paramyxoviruses except that the projections (peplomers) are more prominent with knoblike structures on the ends. When viewed by the electron microscope, these projections give the appearance reminiscent of the solar corona—hence the name Coronaviridae for this family of viruses.

Usually the human viruses cannot be isolated on regular cell cultures but require a more difficult procedure that uses organ cultures of tracheal ciliated epithelium. Consequently, the amount of research that can be carried out on these viruses is limited. All current evidence indicates that the coronaviruses cause about 15% of the mild upper respiratory tract infections, such as the common cold. All ages are infected and immunity seems to be short-lived; a person can be reinfected with the same serotype periodically throughout life. Two different serotypes have been identified.

REOVIRUSES

Reoviridae (Figure 42-4) is a family of viruses that contain a ds-RNA molecule as the genome. These viruses also possess a double-layered protein coat. The first reoviruses of humans to be discovered were found in both the respiratory and intestinal tracts but were not associated with a specific disease and the name *reo* is an acronym of *r*espiratory *e*nteric *o*rphan viruses. A second type of reovirus, now called *oribivirus*, is widespread in insects and may be transmitted to humans or animal by the bite of the virus-carrying tick. Colorado tick fever virus is the only known oribivirus to cause disease in humans. The symptoms are much like those of dengue fever except that no rash is produced.

Rotaviruses, a third type of reovirus, were discovered in 1973. The double-layered protein coat of these viruses gives a characteristic appearance of a wheel (Latin *rota*) when viewed with an electron microscope. Five serotypes have been identified. Initially rotaviruses were detected only by electron microscope examination of tissues and feces. It is now possible to grow these viruses in cell cultures. Rotaviruses are now recognized as causing about 50% of the cases of diarrhea in infants and young children in all countries. To put this figure in perspective, it is estimated that in

Figure 42-4 Transmission electron micrograph of reoviruses magnified 110,000×. (Courtesy Robley C. Williams, University of California, Berkeley)

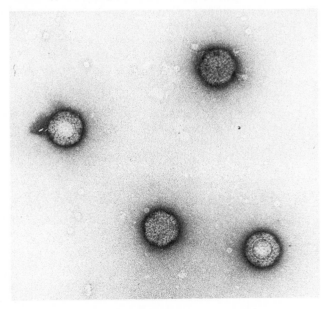

Gastroenteritis Outbreaks on Two Caribbean Cruise Ships: 1986

Three outbreaks of gastroenteritis occurred on two Caribbean cruise ships between April 26, and May 10, 1986. More than 1200 persons developed gastrointestinal illness; no deaths were reported. At least one of the outbreaks appears to be associated with Norwalk virus.

Two outbreaks occurred on two consecutive 1-week cruises of the *Holiday*, a Carnival Cruise Line ship. Between April 26 and May 3, a total of 392 (25%) of 1550 passengers and 30 (4%) of 679 crew who completed questionnaires developed gastroenteritis. Eighty-six percent had diarrhea; 62%, vomiting; 36%, headache; and 26%, subjective symptoms of fever. The outbreak peaked on the fifth and sixth days of the cruise. On the next voyage, from May 3 to May 10, a second outbreak occurred on the *Holiday* in which 321 (22%) of 1470 passengers and 48 (7%) of 658 crew developed gastroenteritis. A sanitation inspection initiated by CDC on May 3 revealed deficiencies related to water chlorination record-keeping, food preparation and holding, and potential contamination of food. A detailed account of these deficiencies was provided to the ship's management at the end of the investigation on May 3, and recommendations were made to prohibit food-service personnel from working while ill and to correct the sanitation deficiencies. A week later, when the inspection was completed, several deficiencies similar to those of the previous week were noted. The final vessel sanitation inspection score on May 10 was 18 out of a possible 100 points (passing = 85).

An outbreak of gastroenteritis also occurred on Holland America Cruises' *Rotterdam*. Between May 3 and May 10, 405 (37%) of 1108 passengers and 35 (6%) of 554 crew who completed questionnaires had a gastrointestinal illness. Eighty percent of ill passengers had diarrhea; 78%, vomiting; 41%, headache; and 32%, subjective symptoms of fever. Mean duration of illness was 2.4 days, and 76% of ill passengers were confined to their cabins during the illness. A sanitation inspection by CDC on May 9 and May 10 revealed numerous deficiencies related to food and water sanitation; the sanitation inspection score was 16 out of a possible 100 points. A detailed account of the deficiencies was presented to the ship's management on May 10 following the inspection, and recommendations were made to prohibit food-service personnel from working while ill and to correct the sanitation deficiencies.

Bacterial cultures of stool specimens from the first *Holiday* outbreak did not yield any recognized pathogens. However, an eightfold or greater rise in antibodies to Norwalk virus was demonstrated by biotin-avidin immunoassay in paired sera obtained from three ill *Holiday* crew members who had suffered gastroenteritis during the April 26–May 3 voyage; Norwalk antigen was detected by biotin-avidin immunoassay in two of six ill passengers from the same voyage. Laboratory studies of specimens and epidemiologic analysis of questionnaires from ill passengers and crew from all three outbreaks are continuing (*MMWR* 35:383, 1986).

Asia, Africa, and Latin America alone over 400 million episodes of diarrhea from all causes occur each year in children under 5 years of age and result in 10 to 15 million deaths. Although diarrhea is also a frequent disease in children in developed countries, death rates are much lower because of a greater number of children who are better nourished and who receive proper medical treatment and supportive therapy. Rotavirus illness is characterized by vomiting, diarrhea, and dehydration. Treatment is directed primarily at replacing body fluids and electrolytes that are lost from vomiting and diarrhea. Often hospitalization is required. Diagnosis can be made by serologic tests that are able either to detect the presence of the rotavirus antigen in feces or measure an increase in antibody levels between acute and convalescent sera. Diagnosis can also be made by demonstrating the presence of the characteristic wheel-shaped virus particles in fecal samples examined with an electron microscope. No vaccine is available; the best control measure involves good sanitation to reduce transmission by the fecal-oral route.

NORWALK GROUP OF VIRUSES

The Norwalk group of viruses has not been well characterized but appears similar to the Caliciviridae (Table 33-1) in size, shape, and other physical characteristics. Some studies have suggested that these viruses may be associated with about one-third of all outbreaks of viral gastroenteritis in some population groups. Infections are associated more with gastroenteritis in older persons and less with infections in infants and young children. These viruses cannot be cultivated in cell cultures. Diagnosis is made by demonstrating the viral antigens in feces with serologic tests or by detecting antibody in serum.

FILOVIRUSES

The filoviruses are filamentous viruses that are tentatively classified in a new family called Filoviridae. Two filoviruses have been identified. The first, called the *Marburg virus*, was isolated from persons in Marburg, Germany, who contracted an unrecognized disease while working with tissues from African monkeys. Seven of the 25 patients who contracted this disease died. The disease is characterized by fever, hemorrhages, diarrhea, vomiting, myalgia, pharyngitis, and conjunctivitis. Mortality is about 25%. Some sporadic cases have been seen in Africa. The natural reservoir for this infection has not been identified.

The second filovirus is called the *Ebola virus* and was discovered in 1976 when a hemorrhagic fever broke out in hospitals in Zaire and the Sudan. Over 500 people were infected, with death rates from 53% to 88%. Serologic studies have shown the Ebola virus infections may be mild or subclinical in some African villages.

CONCEPT SUMMARY

1. Togaviruses are widespread in nature and some cause important diseases of humans and animals.
2. An arenavirus causes Lassa fever, a killer disease found in Africa.
3. Coronaviruses cause about 15% of the common colds.
4. Rotaviruses are a frequent cause of severe infantile diarrhea.
5. Norwalk viruses are associated with gastroenteritis in older persons.

STUDY SUMMARY

1. What characteristic of the togaviruses is responsible for their unusual name?
2. Many of the viruses presented in this chapter are capable of producing serious, life-threatening illness. What feature of these viruses limits their discussion to only a few paragraphs?
3. What are the major encephalitis viruses in the United States?
4. What epidemiologic feature is shared by the togaviruses?
5. How are the coronaviruses, rotavirus, and Norwalk viruses transmitted?
6. What features are similar among the Ebola, Lassa fever, Marburg, and Bolivian hemorrhagic fever virus diseases?

REFERENCES FOR FURTHER STUDY

1. *The Togaviruses: Biology, Structure, Replication*, W. Schlesinger, 1980. Academic Press.

2. Epidemiology of Rotaviral Infection in Adults. *Reviews of Infectious Diseases* 9:461, 1967.

3. *Principles and Practice of Infectious Diseases*, 2nd. ed., G. Mandell, 1985. Wiley Medical.

4. *The Biologic and Clinical Basis of Infectious Diseases*, 3rd ed., G. Youmans, 1985. Saunders.

5. *Fundamental Virology*, B. Fields, 1986. Raven Press.

chapter 43

INFECTION CONTROL IN HOSPITALS

The hospital constitutes a special environment with relationship to microbial infections. Within this single complex environment are many patients who have compromised host defense mechanisms against infections, patients who are subjected to procedures that could introduce microbes into the deep body tissues, and still other patients admitted to the hospital suffering from an infectious disease who may be shedding large numbers of pathogenic microbes. This chapter describes some problems associated with the spread of microorganisms within the hospital environment and the role of hospital personnel in preventing or minimizing such spread.

COMPROMISED PATIENTS

Many patients admitted to hospitals have an illness or other medical problem that may impair one or more of their basic defense mechanisms. These patients are much more susceptible to diseases than healthy persons and special precautions must be taken to protect them from harmful microorganisms. Often, microbes of low virulence (those that are usually unable to cause diseases) can cause serious infections in these compromised patients. These low-virulence microbes may be from either exogenous or endogenous sources.

Some of the more common causes of compromise in patients are diabetes, kidney diseases, chronic heart or lung diseases, cancer, and extensive burns or other wounds. Generally, recipients of organ transplants are given immunosuppressive drugs to prevent rejection of the organ and such drugs usually render the patient highly susceptible to infectious agents. Corticosteriods and radiation used in treating various diseases are also immunosuppressive. Therefore the possible benefits given through these procedures must be weighed against the increased risk that the patient will develop a serious infection, such as pneumonia. Some tumors and most anticancer treatments increase the susceptibility of these patients to infection. Most elderly patients also have reduced resistance to infections; at the other age extreme, because of the immaturity of their immune system, neonates and premature infants are highly susceptible to infections, too. Such patients should receive special attention to protect them from infecting microbes. All hospital patients should be considered compromised in one way or another, and continual efforts should be made to protect them from disease-producing microbes.

MEDICAL PROCEDURES

Many modern medical procedures increase the chance that infections will occur. Such procedures as total hip-replacement operations, open-heart surgery, and brain surgery may expose susceptible deep tissues to the external environment for prolonged periods. Various forms of catheterization, biopsies, and bone marrow aspirations are additional procedures that may introduce microbes into deeper body tissues. Blood transfusions and hemodialysis treatments with artificial kidney machines may introduce microorganisms directly into the blood. All medical procedures, particularly those that penetrate the epithelial barriers, must be carried out in such a way as to minimize or completely prevent the introduction of microbes into the body.

INFECTIOUS PATIENTS

The relative number of patients admitted to hospitals for treatment of infectious diseases is much lower today than in the period before chemotherapy. Yet many patients with infectious diseases are still admitted. Patients with pneumonia constitute 10% of all current hospital admissions and infectious diseases are the fourth leading cause of deaths in the United States, ranking just behind cancer, cardiovascular diseases, and accidents. Over 300 million cases of infectious disease that are serious enough for medical attention occur per year in the United States. Most, however, are handled in outpatient clinics.

Hospital personnel and visitors may also carry infectious agents into hospitals. A constant responsibility of hospital personnel is to develop and follow procedures that will minimize cross infections among patients who come together in the common hospital environment.

HOSPITAL-ACQUIRED INFECTIONS

Hospital-acquired infections are, of course, those contracted by patients after they enter a hospital. The term *nosocomial* (from Latin *nosocomium* = hospital) is frequently used when referring to hospital-acquired infections. Various studies have shown that about 5% of the patients who enter a hospital in the United States contract a nosocomial infection (Table 43-1). This percentage amounts to about 1.5 million infections per year and results in or is a contributing factor in about 30,000 deaths. The added costs in treating these patients were estimated at $1 billion in 1988. Postoperative wound infections, the most common nosocomial infections, develop in from 3% to 8% of surgical patients.

PROCEDURES TO REDUCE THE SPREAD OF INFECTION

Although it may not be possible to eliminate all nosocomial infections, they can be significantly reduced if medical personnel conscientiously follow procedures that are designed to prevent the spread of infectious agents. Some of these procedures are discussed next.

Direct Contact

Contact between patients is a potential source of nosocomial infection. The most hazardous contact would be between highly compromised patients and any infected patient who is shedding large

Table 43-1 Commonly Isolated Nosocomial Pathogens

| Pathogen | Percent of Isolates from Nosocomial Infection | | | | | |
	Urinary Tract	Surgical Wound	Lower Respiratory	Cutaneous Tissue	Blood (bacteremia)	All
E. coli	31.7	11.4	7.1	7.7	9.5	18.6
S. aureus	1.6	19.0	12.8	33.3	12.8	10.8
Enterococcus	14.9	11.4	1.6	9.5	7.3	10.7
P. aeruginosa	12.5	8.1	15.1	7.2	6.1	10.6
Klebsiella	7.6	4.8	12.8	4.4	9.1	7.4
S. epidermidis	3.7	8.4	1.1	9.5	14.2	6.1
Enterobacter	4.4	6.9	10.0	4.1	6.9	5.8
Proteus	7.3	5.0	4.4	3.5	1.7	5.4
Candida	5.1	1.4	4.2	4.5	5.6	5.1
Serratia	1.2	2.0	5.6	1.8	2.8	2.2
Others	10.0	21.6	25.3	14.5	24.0	17.1
Total	100.0	100.0	100.0	100.0	100.0	100.0

numbers of virulent microorganisms. Hospital personnel may serve as symptomatic or asymptomatic carriers of pathogens that may be transmitted to patients. Conversely, patients with infectious diseases may transmit an infection to attending medical personnel. Moreover, housekeeping personnel or visitors may be involved in an exchange of potentially dangerous microbes with patients.

Various means are used to reduce person-to-person transmission of infections in hospitals. First, patients who are compromised and those who have infectious diseases should be isolated from each other and from other patients. This requires a rapid diagnosis of the patient's illness. Whenever possible, particularly when dealing with a patient who might have a communicable disease, the patient should be isolated at least until a specific diagnosis is made. Once it is determined which patients are infectious and which are compromised, appropriate methods of separation are applied. The infectious patient should be placed in a room that is designed to prevent any microorganisms from escaping—a situation called *regular* or *forward* isolation. Various levels of isolation may be used. Strict isolation is necessary for patients who have highly contagous diseases. The conditions of isolation are modified, depending on the type of infection; that is, a respiratory infection would be handled differently from an enteric infection. Isolation rooms should be posted with a sign giving instructions on the procedures to follow when entering or leaving the room (Figure 43-1 and Table 43-2). For strict isolation, gowns, masks, and shoe covers must be worn by all persons entering the room. Gloves must be worn when examining the patient. All articles used in the room, such as thermometers and stethoscopes, must be left in the room or placed in a container to be sterilized before being reused. When personnel leave the room, items like gown, mask, and gloves must be placed in a receptacle that will later be sterilized. Disinfectant-impregnated mats may be placed in the entrance to remove contaminants from the bottom of shoes. Hands should be washed with a disinfectant soap before leaving the room. The isolation room should have negative air pressure relative to the corridor so that no air flows out. Exhaust air should be passed through absolute filters that remove all airborne particles.

Compromised patients should be placed in *protective* isolation, also called *reverse* isolation, to protect them from microbes that might be transmitted from other patients or hospital personnel. These rooms should be under positive air pressure so that no air from the corridor can flow into the room. The same gowning, masking, and other procedures used for strict isolation should be applied. For severely compromised patients, such as those with extensive burns, completely enclosed canopies may be placed around the patient to isolate them more effectively from microbial

Table 43-2   A Listing of the Information Given on the Front and Back of the Warning Signs Posted by Isolation Rooms in Hospitals

Enteric Precautions	Protective Isolation	Respiratory Isolation	Strict Isolation	Wound & Skin Precautions
Visitors—Report to Nurses' Station Before Entering Room	Visitors—Report to Nurses' Station Before Entering Room	Visitors—Report to Nurses' Station Before Entering Room	Visitors—Report to Nurses' Station Before Entering Room	Visitors—Report to Nurses' Station Before Entering Room
1. **Private Room**—*necessary for children only.*	1. **Private Room**—*necessary; door must be kept closed.*	1. **Private Room**—*necessary; door must be kept closed.*	1. **Private Room**—*necessary; door must be kept closed.*	1. **Private Room**—desirable.
2. **Gowns**—must be worn by all persons having direct contact with patient.	2. **Gowns**—must be worn by all persons entering room.	2. **Gowns**—not necessary.	2. **Gowns**—must be worn by all persons entering room.	2. **Gowns**—must be worn by all persons having direct contact with patient.
3. **Masks**—not necessary.	3. **Masks**—must be worn by all persons entering room.	3. **Masks**—must be worn by all persons entering room if susceptible to disease.	3. **Masks**—must be worn by all persons entering room.	3. **Masks**—not necessary except during dressing changes.
4. **Hands**—must be washed on entering and leaving room.	4. **Hands**—must be washed on entering and leaving room.	4. **Hands**—must be washed on entering and leaving room.	4. **Hands**—must be washed on entering and leaving room.	4. **Hands**—must be washed on entering and leaving room.
5. **Gloves**—must be worn by all persons having direct contact with patient or with articles contaminated with fecal material.	5. **Gloves**—must be worn by all persons having direct contact with patient.	5. **Gloves**—not necessary.	5. **Gloves**—must be worn by all persons entering room.	5. **Gloves**—must be worn by all persons having direct contact with infected area.
6. **Articles**—special precautions necessary for articles contaminated with	6. **Articles**—*see manual text.*	6. **Articles**—those contaminated with secretions must be disinfected.	6. **Articles**—must be discarded, or wrapped before being sent to Central Supply for disinfection or sterilization.	6. **Articles**—special precautions necessary for instruments, dressings, and linen.
	Conditions Requiring Protective Isolation	7. **Caution**—all persons susceptible to the specific disease should be excluded	Diseases Requiring Strict Isolation	
	1. Agranulocytosis.			
	2. Severe and			

674

urine and feces. Articles must be disinfected or discarded.

Diseases Requiring Enteric Precautions

1. Cholera.
2. Enteropathogenic *E. coli* gastroenteritis.
3. Hepatitis, viral (infectious or serum).
4. Salmonellosis (including typhoid fever).
5. Shigellosis.

extensive, noninfected vesicular, bullous, or eczematous dermatitis.
3. Certain patients receiving immunosuppressive therapy.
4. Certain patients with lymphomas and leukemia.

from patient area; if contact is necessary, susceptibles must wear masks.

Diseases Requiring Respiratory Isolation

1. Chickenpox.
2. Herpes zoster.
3. Measles (rubeola).
4. Meningococcal meningitis.
5. Meningococcemia.
6. Mumps.
7. Pertussis (whooping cough).
8. Rubella (German measles).
9. Tuberculosis, pulmonary—sputum-positive (or suspect).
10. Venezuelan equine encephalomyelitis.

1. Anthrax, inhalation.
2. Burns, extensive, infected with *Staphylococcus aureus* or Group A streptococcus.
3. Diphtheria.
4. Eczema vaccinatum.
5. Melioidosis, pulmonary, or extrapulmonary with draining sinus(es).
6. Neonatal vesicular disease (Herpes simplex).
7. Plague.
8. Rabies.
9. Rubella (German measles) and Congenital rubella syndrome.
10. Smallpox.
11. Staphylococcal enterocolitis.
12. Staphylococcal pneumonia.
13. Streptococcal pneumonia.
14. Vaccinia, generalized and progressive.

Note: *See manual for Special Dressing Techniques to be used when changing dressings.*

Diseases Requiring Wound & Skin Precautions

1. Burns, extensive, not infected with *Staphylococcus aureus* or Group A streptococcus.
2. Gas gangrene.
3. Impetigo.
4. Staphylococcal skin and wound infections.
5. Streptococcal skin infection.
6. Wound infection, extensive.

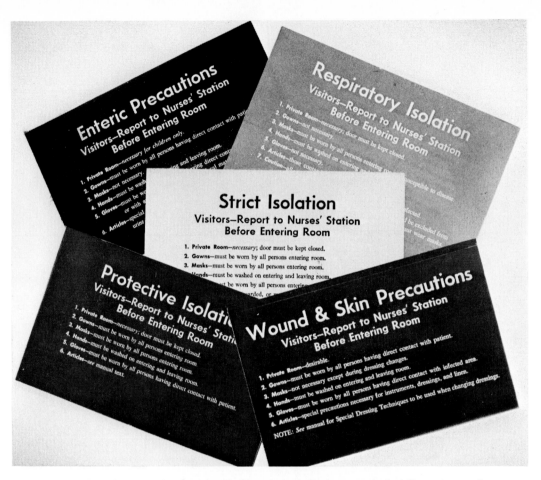

Figure 43-1 Standard warning and instructional signs that are posted at the entrance to different types of isolation rooms in hospitals.

contaminants. Visitors should preferably be restricted from isolation rooms; if admitted, they should follow the same gowning procedures as medical personnel. Housekeeping personnel, as well as all others who enter these rooms, must also follow the same procedures.

Medical personnel with infections, including respiratory disease or skin lesions as cellulitis, should be excluded from duty until their infections are resolved. Persons working in surgery or with highly compromised patients may periodically have their nares cultured to determine if they are carriers of antibiotic-resistant *Staphylococcus aureus*. If found to be positive, they should be relieved from duty with these patients until their carrier state is resolved. Similarly, visitors with infections should not be permitted to visit patients. Many hospitals do not allow children under 14 years of age to visit because, among other reasons, they are frequently carriers of a variety of infectious agents and are themselves more susceptible to infection.

Contaminated Objects

Any object that comes in contact with an infected patient or that patient's surroundings may become contaminated with pathogenic microbes. If the same object later comes in contact with another patient, some microbes may be successfully transmitted. Such items as bedding, books, and toys may indirectly transmit infections. Medical paraphernalia, such as stethoscopes, bronchoscopes, and thermometers, as well as equipment used for administering anesthesia or inhalation therapy, have been incriminated as transmitters of some nosocomial infections. Almost any items used in patient care have the potential to transmit infectious agents.

Much has been done in the past few years to prevent the transmission of infectious agents by inanimate objects. Individualized personal-care kits containing a water pitcher, thermometer, and other items for use of only one patient have reduced the need for repeated disinfection of these items, and eliminated any chance that they will become a means of transmitting infections to other patients. Many other disposable items, such as gloves, syringes, hypodermic needles, catheters, and tubes, have further reduced the chance of patient-to-patient transmission of microbes (Figure 43-2). Special care must be taken with items like bronchoscopes that are not disposable and that connot be sterilized by autoclaving or ethylene oxide. Such items must be throughly cleaned and sterilized or disinfected with a liquid disinfectant, usually by soaking in 2% glutaraldehyde for 12 hours.

Persons working directly with patients or who prepare materials to be used around patients must have a basic understanding of the possible modes of transmission of microbes and then be continually aware of how each procedure may either contribute to or prevent the spread of infection. Well-managed hospitals have outlined procedures designed to prevent the spread of microbes during routine activities involving patients. It is important that all medical personnel understand and follow these procedures. Yet not every procedure used to prevent transmission of microbes can be easily outlined and each person involved in patient care must use his or her own knowledge or microbiology to eliminate the possible spread of microbes while carrying out daily activities.

Endogenous Spread

The various routes of endogenous spread of microbes were discussed in Chapter 10. Special care must be taken when working with patients with wounds or burns to reduce or prevent cross

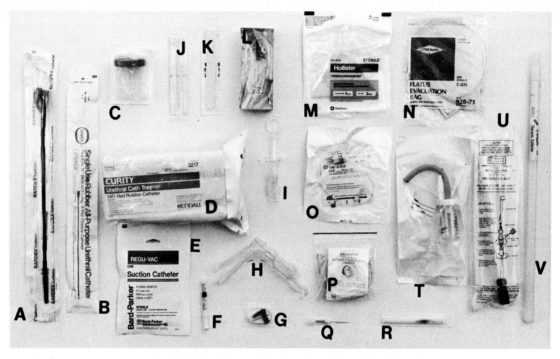

Figure 43-2   Some of the disposable items used in patient care that help reduce the chance for transmission of infections. A & B, urethral catheters; C, specimen cup; D, urethral catheter tray; E, suction catheter; F, hypodermic syringe; G, intravenous infusion needle; H, speculum; I, rectal speculum; J, cotton-tipped applicators; K, tongue depressor; L, intravenous kit; M, wound drainage set; N, evacuation bag; O, intravenous tubes; P, nasal cannula; Q, intravenous needle; R, hypodermic needle; T, specimen trap; U, sigmoidoscopy kit; V, thoracic catheter.

contamination from one part of the body to another. Bandaging of open lesions is an effective method of preventing some endogenous spread. Education of the patient as to the modes of endogenous spread and how to reduce this spread is helpful.

Airborne Transmission

Droplet nuclei from coughing or sneezing and microbe-containing dust or fine particles may be carried in air currents from person to person or from one part of the hospital to another. Changing contaminated bandages or shaking contaminated bedding may send massive numbers of microbes into the air. Sweeping floors, walking, and various types of movements result in large numbers of microbe-containing dust particles being disseminated into the air.

Airborn contaminants can be greatly reduced by handling contaminated materials carefully. Such items as bandages should be carefully removed with forceps and placed in a plastic bag. All soiled bedding, linens, and trash should be placed in airtight plastic bags for transport to laundry or disposal areas. Care must be used in sorting soiled laundry to avoid creating clouds of pathogens that might cause infection in workers. Contaminated materials should be autoclaved before being sent to the laundry. Floor should be cleaned with wet vacumms or mops that prevent the generation of dust.

All properly designed hospitals should have air systems that prevent the recirculation of contaminated air from one area to another. The use of positive or negative air pressure in isolation rooms has been discussed. Air entering critical areas like surgeries (Figure 43-3), nurseries, and intensive care areas should be filtered or irradiated with ultraviolet light to remove or destroy the airborne microbes and the airflow should carry airborne particles away from patients (Figure 43-4).

INFECTION CONTROL PROGRAMS

Each hospital must have an effective infection control program. This program is under the direction of an *infection control committee*, which should include the following members:

Figure 43-3 An operating room equipped with an aseptic air system. The ceiling is made of perforated panels through which filtered and ultraviolet light irradiated air passes. Air return ducts are located all around the base of the room. The air moves downward and out of the room at sufficient velocity to prevent airborne particles from drifting over and onto the surgical wound. (Courtesy Joseph R. Luciano)

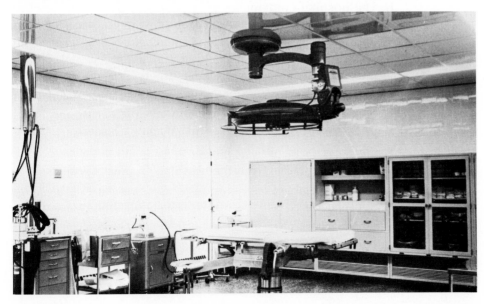

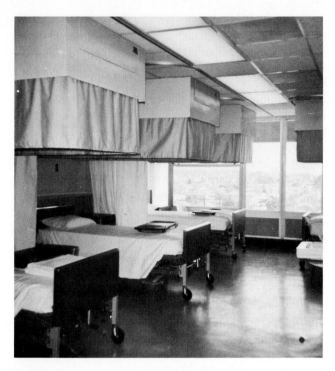

Figure 43-4 A hospital ward equipped with aseptic air canopies over each bed. A mass of microbial-free air moves down over each patient and is drawn out of the room through return ducts at the head of the beds. Such downward air movement prevents lateral movement of airborne microorganisms between patients. (Courtesy Joseph R. Luciano)

1. The hospital epidemiologist, who is a physician or another person with knowledge of and interest in epidemiology and infectious disease

2. A representative from each of the major clinical departments—for example, medicine, surgery, and pediatrics

3. A member of the pathology/microbiology laboratory

4. The infection control nurse, who is an R.N. trained in the principles of epidemiology and infectious disease

5. The director of nursing and/or nursing supervisor

6. A respresentative from the hospital administration

7. Liaison members from various services, such as pharmacy, housekeeping, central supply, inhalation therapy, and local health departments

The functions of this committee are as follows:

1. Determine the methods to be used for effective surveillance of nosocomial infections.

2. Determine what control measures need to be taken when dealing with isolation procedures or other special procedures where highly susceptible patients are involved.

3. Make proper use of the microbiology laboratory for environmental surveillance and identification of isolated pathogens.

4. Delegate authority to the hospital epidemiologist and the infection control nurse.

5. Convey the infection control policies to those who must carry them out and assess the completeness and effectiveness of the implementation of these policies.

6. Meet once a month or more often to review infection control procedures and policies and so on.

The infection control nurse and hospital epidemiologist should be primarily responsible for directing the day-to-day implementation of the environmental surveillance, infection control procedures, and inservice training of other hospital personnel relative to infection control procedures.

CONCEPT SUMMARY

1. The control of infection in the hospital environment centers around two main factors: (a) the introduction of highly virulent, easily transmissable infectious agents into the hospital environment by patients, visitors, or hospital personnel and (b) the transmission of relatively avirulent normal flora-type organisms to compromised patients either through self-inoculation or routine hospital procedures.

2. Stringent control procedures have been adopted by most hospitals in order to reduce the occurrence of nosocomial infections.

STUDY SUMMARY

1. Make a list of factors present in modern hospital care that can directly increase the frequency or seriousness of nosocomial infections.

2. What procedures can be used to reduce the possibility of airborne transmission of infectious agents in a hospital?

3. What are the principles behind the use of (a) protective isolation and (b) isolation?

4. Explain why endogenous organisms are not subject to isolation procedures used to prevent nosocomial infections.

REFERENCES FOR FURTHER STUDY

1. Microbiology—1985, L. Leive, 1985. American Society for Microbiology.

2. Manual of Clinical Microbiology, 4th ed., E. Lennette, 1985. American Society for Microbiology.

3. Significance of Microbiology in the Care of Patients, V. Lorian, 1977. Williams & Wilkins.

BIOCHEMICAL PATHWAYS

This appendix is included to give further details of some biochemical reactions outlined in Chapter 5.

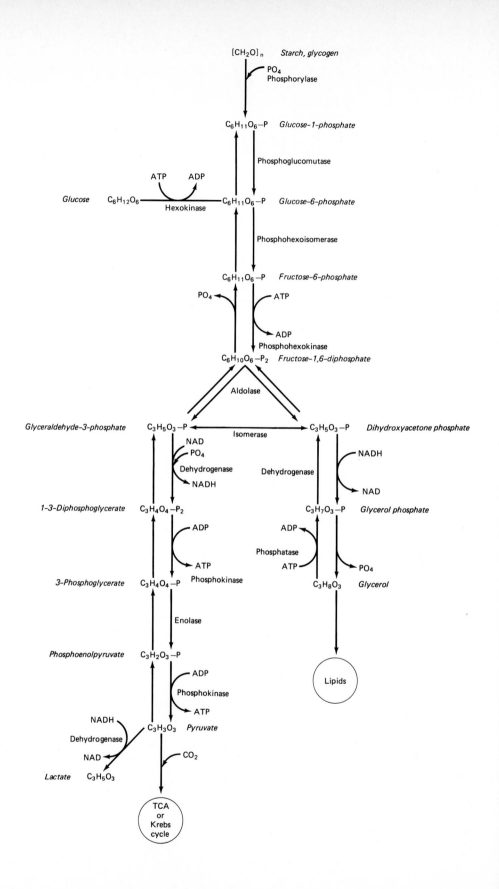

Figure A-1 This diagram indicates the most common pathway for carbohydrate metabolism. This glycolytic pathway is shown in some detail, including the names of the various metabolic intermediates and common enzymes involved in the reactions. Arrows indicate direction of reactions. This sequence is known as the Embden-Myerhoff pathway, and usually terminates in the citric acid cycle for aerobic organisms and lactate or other end products for anaerobic organisms.

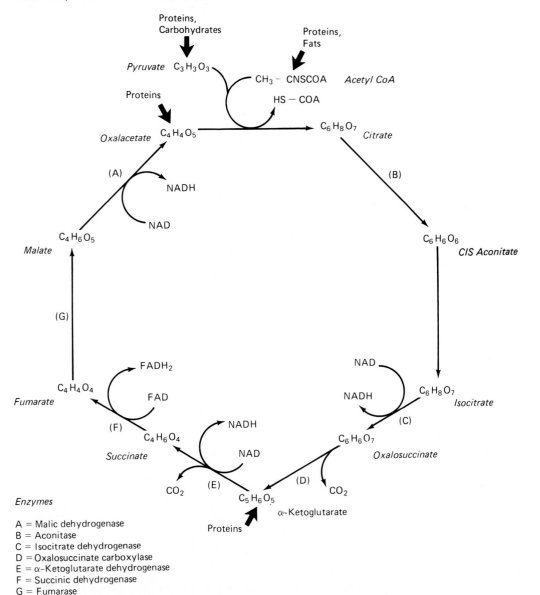

Enzymes

A = Malic dehydrogenase
B = Aconitase
C = Isocitrate dehydrogenase
D = Oxalosuccinate carboxylase
E = α-Ketoglutarate dehydrogenase
F = Succinic dehydrogenase
G = Fumarase

Figure A-2 The biochemical reactions associated with the citric acid cycle. This metabolic sequence is frequently called the Krebs cycle. A single passage through the cycle results in the loss of three carbon atoms from pyruvate. Therefore, two complete turns of the cycle will remove all the carbon from a glucose molecule entering into glycolysis. Enzymes associated with the cycle are shown.

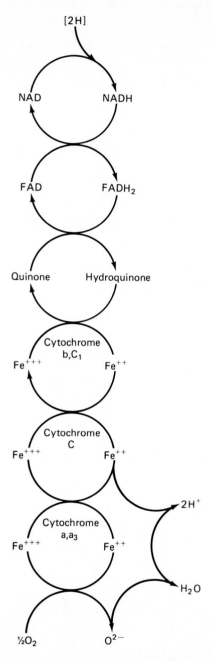

Figure A-3 Electron transport system or pathway of oxidative phosphorylation. The energy associated with the reduced carrier molecules NAD and FAD are brought to this sequence of reactions. Here, by removing the energy in a series of oxidation-reduction reactions, it is captured into ATP molecules. Most of the ATPs derived from the oxidation of glucose to CO_2 and H_2O are produced in this system.

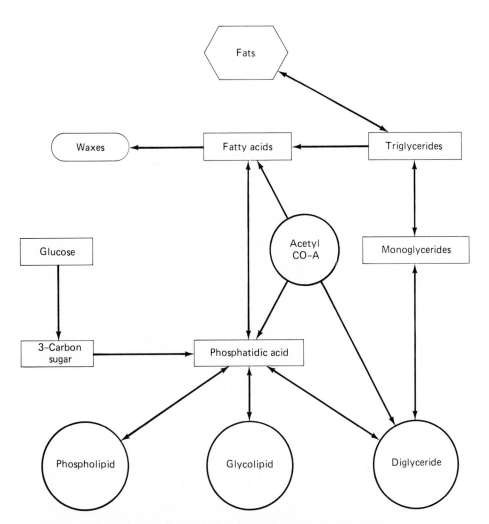

Figure A-4   This is a schematic diagram indicating the direction of catabolism and anabolism of lipids. While the details are not given, this system interlocks with most of the energy-storing systems in the cell. Note that acetyl CO-A and the 3 carbon sugar can be found in the diagram of the citric acid cycle—Figure A-2.

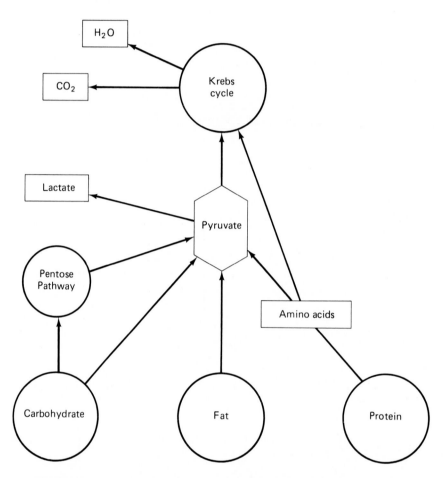

Figure A-5 A schematic diagram indicating the interactions among the major metabolic pathways and classes of macromolecules. This interrelationship allows the cell to convert a plentiful supply of a metabolite into a needed metabolite which may be limited in its availability.

HUMAN PARASITES

Here is a list of the most common parasitologic organisms found in humans. The list includes scientific and common names of the parasite or disease as well as the source from which infection is most commonly derived.

Protozoa

Type	Species	Relationship	Common Name	Source
Amebae	*Entamoeba histolytica*	Intestinal pathogen	Amebiasis	Human feces
	E. hartmanni	Intestinal commensal		Human feces
	E. coli	Intestinal commensal		Human feces
	E. polecki	Intestinal commensal		Human feces
	Endolimax nana	Intestinal commensal		Human feces
	Iodamoeba butschlii	Intestinal commensal		Human feces
	Naegleria fowleri	CNS pathogen	Encephalitis	Freshwater swimming
	Pneumocystis carinii	Tissue pathogen		Unknown
Ciliate	*Balantidium coli*	Intestinal pathogen		Pig feces
Coccidia	*Isospora belli*	Intestinal pathogen		Human feces
	Sarcocystis bovicanis	Tissue pathogen		Poorly cooked meat
	Toxoplasma gondii	Tissue pathogen		Cat feces
	Cryptosporidium species	Intestinal pathogen		Animal feces
Flagellates	*Dientamoeba fragilis*	Intestinal pathogen		Human feces
	Trichomonas hominis	Tissue commensal		Human
	T. vaginalis	Tissue pathogen		Human
	Chilomastix mesnili	Intestinal commensal		Human feces
	Giardia lamblia	Intestinal pathogen	Giardiasis	Mammalian feces
	Leishmania donovani	Tissue pathogen	Leishmaniasis	Sandfly bite
	L. tropica	Tissue pathogen		Sandfly bite
	L. braziliensis	Tissue pathogen		Sandfly bite
	Trypanosoma gambiense	Tissue pathogen	Sleeping sickness	Fly bite
	T. rhodesiense	Tissue pathogen	Sleeping sickness	Fly bite
	T. cruzi	Tissue pathogen	Chagas disease	Bug bite
Sporozoa	*Plasmodium falciparum*	Tissue pathogen	Malaria	Mosquito
	Plasmodium malariae	Tissue pathogen	Malaria	Mosquito
	Plasmodium ovale	Tissue pathogen	Malaria	Mosquito
	Plasmodium vivax	Tissue pathogen	Malaria	Mosquito

Metazoa

Type	Species	Relationship	Common Name	Source
Cestodes	*Diphillobothrium latum*	Intestinal pathogen	Tapeworm	Uncooked fish
	Dipylidium caninum	Intestinal pathogen	Tapeworm	Dog feces
	Echinococcus granulosis	Tissue pathogen	Tapeworm	Dog feces
	Hyminolepsis nana	Intestinal pathogen	Tapeworm	Human feces
	Taenia saginata	Intestinal pathogen	Tapeworm	Uncooked beef
	Taenia solium	Intestinal pathogen	Tapeworm	Uncooked pork
Nematode	*Angiostrongylus cantonensis*	Tissue pathogen		Mollusks
	Ancylostoma duodenale	Intestinal pathogen	Hookworm	Human feces
	Ascaris lumbricoides	Intestinal pathogen		Human feces
	Brugia malayi	Tissue pathogen	Elephantiasis	Mosquito
	Capillaria hepatica	Tissue pathogen		Rodent feces
	C. philippinensis	Intestinal pathogen		Raw fish
	Dipetalonema perstans	Intestinal pathogen		Midge bite
	Enterobius vermicularis	Intestinal pathogen	Pinworm	Human feces
	Loa Loa	Tissue pathogen	Eyeworm	Fly bite
	Mansonella ozzardi	Tissue pathogen		Fly bite
	Necator americanis	Intestinal pathogen	Hookworm	Human feces
	Onchocerca volvulus	Tissue pathogen	River blindness	Fly bite
	Strongeloides stercoralis	Intestinal pathogen		Human feces
	Toxocara canis	Tissue pathogen	Larva migrans	Dog feces
	Trichinella spiralis	Tissue pathogen	Trichinosis	Uncooked pork
	Trichuris trichiura	Intestinal pathogen	Whipworm	Human feces
	Wuchereria bancrofti	Tissue pathogen	Elephantiasis	Mosquito
Trematode	*Clonorchis sinensis*	Tissue pathogen	Liver fluke	Raw fish
	Fasciola hepatica	Tissue pathogen	Sheep liver flukes	Freshwater plants
	Fasciolopsis buski	Intestinal pathogen	Intestinal fluke	Human feces
	Metagonimus yokagawi	Intestinal pathogen		Raw fish
	Paragonimos westermani	Tissue pathogen	Lung fluke	Uncooked shellfish
	S. japonicum	Tissue pathogen		Water
	Schistosoma mansoni	Tissue pathogen	Bilharziasis	Water

GLOSSARY

Abscess Pus accumulated in a localized area, often associated with inflammation

Acid fast A property by which some bacterial cells fail to decolorize when washed with an acid alcohol solution

Acute A disease of short duration or exhibiting sharp clinical signs

Adenosine triphosphate A nucleotide containing two high energy chemical bonds

Adjuvant A compound (often lipid) added to an antigen to increase the antibody response

Aerosol The creation of an airborne suspension of particles

Agar A polysaccharide extracted from algae that is used as a solidifying agent in bacteriological culture media

Agglutination Clumping or bunching of particulate antigens resulting from the presence of a specific antibody

Albumin A water-soluble protein commonly found in animal sera

Allergy An altered (often damaging) reaction, the result of an antigen-antibody interaction in hypersensitive animals

Alveolus A small air sac located in the lung

Amino acid An organic compound with both amino and carboxyl groups as part of the same molecule. The monomeric components of protein

Anaerobe A bacterium that does not use oxygen as a metabolic hydrogen acceptor. Often unable to grow in the presence of atmospheric oxygen concentrations

Anamnestic A secondary or booster phenomenon observed following a primary immunologic response

Anaphylaxis A severe, systemic hypersensitivity response to an antigenic challenge

Anorexia Loss of appetite

Anti- A prefix suggesting opposition or against. The use of this prefix in medicine relates to curative processes

Antibacterial A compound or process detrimental to bacterial growth or survival

Antibiotic A substance produced by a living organism or cell system which is useful for therapy of infectious diseases

Antibody A serum protein made by an individual in response to an antigenic stimulus

Anticodon A triplet nucleotide base sequence associated with transfer RNA that is complementary to the codon triplet of messenger RNA

Antigen A substance capable of eliciting an antibody from an immunocompetent animal

Antigenic determinant The portion of an antigen molecule that determines the specificity of antibody synthesis

Antimicrobial A compound or process detrimental to microbial growth or survival

Antiseptic Literally, against sepsis (infection). A compound that can be applied to animal tissues in order to reduce the likelihood of infection

Antitoxin Antibody produced in response to a toxin or toxoid

Arbovirus RNA virus, transmissible by insect vector, frequently associated with encephalitis

Arthralgia Severe joint pain

Arthropod An invertebrate having jointed legs, commonly acting as infectious disease vectors

Aseptic Free from microorganisms

Aspirate Material removed from a patient by suction

ATP (Adenosine triphosphate) A molecule containing two high-energy phosphate bonds that act as an energy transport and exchange molecule in metabolic reactions

Attachment site Position at which an organism attaches itself to host tissues

Attenuation Reduction in virulence. Microorganisms that have lost virulence but have retained antigenicity are attenuated

Autotroph An organism which can obtain energy from sunlight or simple, nonorganic compounds

Avirulent Not virulent. Refers to microorganisms that are not capable of producing an infectious process

Bacilli Bacteria which are elongated or rod shaped

Bacteremia A condition in which living bacteria are found to be present in the bloodstream

Bactericidal A condition or compound that results in the killing of bacteria

Bacteriophage Virus that infects bacteria

Bacteriostatic A condition that prevents the growth of bacteria but does not directly kill these microorganisms

Bactiuria A condition in which bacteria are found in urine

Balanced growth Growth during which the number and composition of cells remain constant

BCG (Bacille Calmette-Guerin) An attenuated mycobacterium used as a vaccine against tuberculosis

Beta lactamase An enzyme that hydrolyzes the beta lactam ring structure essential to the antibacterial activity of penicillins and cephalosporins

Binary fission The form of cellular division associated with bacteria, resulting in equal distribution of cellular content between the daughter cells

Bipolar stain Bacteria which stain more intensely at the poles (ends) of the cell than in the center. This often gives cells a ''safety pin'' shaped appearance

Bloom The occurrence of a major outgrowth of algae

Botulism Food poisoning; specifically that due to the toxin produced by *Clostridium botulinum*

Broad spectrum Antimicrobial agents that are effective against a large number of different types of bacteria, usually including both gram-positive and gram-negative genera

Bronchi Major air passageways that branch from the trachea

Broth A liquid culture medium

B-cell A group of bone-marrow-derived lymphocytes that produce immunoglobulins

Capnophile A microorganism requiring carbon dioxide for growth

Capsid A viral protein coat

Capsomere The subunit of a capsid. Capsomeres occur in repetitive sequence in order to form the capsid

Capsule A polysaccharide or rarely a polypeptide layer surrounding bacterial cells peripheral to the cell wall

Carbohydrate A sugar molecule

Carrier Generally an individual who has recovered from an infection but who continues to shed the etiologic agent into the environment

Carrier rate The number of individual carriers in a specific population who are infected by a microorganism

Caseous Having a cheeselike consistency. Associated with tuberculous lesions termed caseation necrosis

Catabolism Metabolic breakdown of organic compounds

Catalyst A molecule that lowers the energy of activation of a chemical reaction

Catheter A tube, usually of rubber or plastic, which can be placed into a body cavity or a blood vessel to allow easy drainage of body fluids or the placement of medications into the body

Cellulitis Inflammation or infection of connective tissue. Usually resulting in a typical inflammatory lesion

Cerebral spinal fluid (CSF) A watery fluid which is produced in the brain and forms a cushion surrounding the central nervous system

Chancre A superficial ulcer generally occurring at the site of primary syphilis infection

Chemotaxis The movement of cells toward or away from a chemical stimulus

Chemotherapy The use of chemical compounds in the treatment of disease. Usually associated with cancer therapy

Chronic Lasting for a long time. Such as the disease tuberculosis

Ciliated epithelium Epithelial tissues containing numerous ciliated cells, such as the tracheal surface

Cistron A structural gene. A unit of DNA that codes for a single function

Clone A population of cells derived from a single progenitor cell. A bacterial colony

CNS (Central Nervous System) The brain and spinal cord

Code Genetic information associated with the triplet base sequence of DNA

Codon A base triplet found in messenger RNA that codes for a single amino acid

Coenzyme A molecule involved in the transfer of small molecules between enzymic reactions

Cold agglutinins Proteins produced in response to some infectious diseases which are able to agglutinate red blood cells at low (refrigerator) temperatures

Colitis Inflammation of the colon

Colon The large intestine

Colony A visible accumulation of bacterial cells that are the progeny of one cell on solid culture media

Commensal An organism that exists without rendering either harm or benefit to its environment

Communicable An infectious disease that can be transmitted between susceptible individuals

Competitive inhibition An enzymic reaction that can be stopped by the reversible interaction of an inhibitor with the free enzyme

Complement A system of serum proteins, activated in sequence, which produce a variety of biological effects

Complement fixation A serological reaction which depends on the binding of complement in an antigen-antibody complex

Compromised host An individual with decreased resistance to infection

Conjugation The process whereby bacterial DNA is transferred between individual cells through a pilus

Conjunctivitis Inflammation of the conjunctiva (tissue surrounding the eyeball)

Contagious See communicable

Cortex The outer portion of an organ such as the brain

Croup An upper respiratory obstruction, usually produced by swelling of the epiglottis or pharynx. Characterized by a hoarse cough

Cyst A dominant life stage of some parasites. Cysts have increased resistance to environmental changes or antibiotic processes

Cystitis An infection of the bladder

Cytopathic effect Observable changes in in vitro cells resulting from viral infection

Dark field A form of microscopy where light is reflected from an object such that it appears as a light against a black background

Daughter cell A cell which is produced by binary fission or budding directly from another cell

Delirium A state of disordered mentality, often associated with high fever

Denaturation To change from a natural to unnatural state. This term is often used to describe the process of alteration of the tertiary or secondary configuration of a protein

Deoxyribose The five-carbon sugar present in DNA

Desensitize Reduction in the hypersensitivity state resulting from exposure to small repeated doses of antigen

Detergent A compound used as a cleaning agent but not made from fats

Determinant group The portion of an antigen that determines antibody specificity

Diffusion The movement of molecules from an area of high to low concentration

Dimorphic Having two structural or anatomical forms

Disease An abnormal state of health

Disease reservoir A natural source of a disease agent

Disinfect The removal of some or all microorganisms from an environment

Dissemination The development of a generalized from a localized infection. The involvement of additional organ systems secondary to a primary focus of infection

DNA (Deoxyribose nucleic acid) A polynucleotide consisting of four nucleotide bases in a random sequence. The informational molecule of chromosome

DNA ligase An enzyme which can join to pieces of homologous (complimentary) DNA together

Dye A colored compound from which a stain can be made

Electrolyte A substance that readily conducts an electric current when dissolved. In medicine these substances are ions like K^+ and Na^+ in serum

Electron microscope A microscope that uses an electron beam to illuminate the object under study

Electrophoresis The separation in an electrical field of molecules having differences in electrical charge

Empirical Not founded in experimental data

Encephalitis An inflammation of the brain resulting in neurological changes

Endocarditis Inflammation of the endocardial lining of the heart

Endogenous From an internal source. Associated with self

Endonuclease An enzyme that will hydrolyse DNA

Endoplasmic reticulum A reticular membrane formation found in cellular cytoplasm, often associated with protein synthesis

Endospore A bacterial spore, associated with resistance to environmental inactivation

Endothelial cell A cell lining a cavity or tube

Endotoxin A lipopolysaccharide associated with Gram-negative cell wall

Enterotoxin A bacterial toxin that is absorbed by and acts primarily on the intestinal tract

Envelope A lipid covering found peripheral to the viral capsid on some virions

Enzyme A protein catalyst that facilitates biochemical reactions

Epidemic The occurrence of a specific disease in greater than normal or expected numbers

Epidemiology The study of disease, its occurrence, control, and effects on the environment

Epiglotitis Inflammation of the epiglotis, frequently producing a severe croup

Epithelium The nonvascular (no blood vessels) cellular layer covering internal and external body surfaces

Erysipelas A severe streptococcal infection of the skin

Erythema Redness of the skin resulting from dilation of capillaries

Eschar A deep dark crust or scab that develops at the site of an injury, such as a burn

Etiologic agent The cause of a specific infection

Eucaryotic Refers to a true nucleus that is bounded by a nucleus membrane

Exotoxin A powerful, proteinaceous toxin produced by any of several different genera and species of bacteria

Exudate A fluid (cellular or acellular) that passes through blood vessels into surrounding tissues

Fastidious Selective, usually refers to those bacteria requiring special nutrients for growth

Febrile To have a fever

Fermentation The anaerobic breakdown of carbohydrates

Fibrinous A structureless, insoluble protein exudate, such as a blood clot, resulting from cellular injury

Fimbriae A slender hairlike structure found on the surface of some bacteria that are used for attachment

Fission To divide or split into two or more parts. An asexual reproduction process

Flagella A relatively long proteinaceous projection extending from some bacteria that provides a mechanism for propelling the organism through its environment

Fomite An inanimate object involved in the transmission of disease agents

Food poisoning Illness resulting from consuming food that has been contaminated by a disease-producing microorganism

Gamma globulin Serum proteins with antibody activity

Ganglion A group of nerve cells located outside the central nervous system

Gangrene The process whereby tissues die because of a lack of blood supply

Gastroenteritis Infection of the intestinal tract, often accompanied by diarrhea

Generation time The time required for an organism to produce one new generation of progeny

Gene sequence The linear arrangement of functional genetic units along the chromosome

Genetic code The genetic information contained in the nucleotide sequence of DNA. The code is based on triplet sets of nucleotide bases

Genetic engineering The intentional alteration of genetic structure through addition or subtraction of nucleotides

Genome The nuclear content of a virion

Genotype The genetic makeup or structure of a cell

Germ A term used to refer to microorganisms capable of producing infection

Germacide A chemical compound that kills microorganisms

Germination The process whereby a bacterial endospore forms a vegetative bacterium

Globulins A group of proteins found in human serum

Glycolysis The metabolism of glucose to pyruvic acid

Granulocyte One of a series of white blood cells that contains granules in the cytoplasm. A polymorphonuclear leukocyte

Granuloma A nodule of fibrous tissue, resulting from an inflammatory reaction

Growth rate The number of generations produced in 60 minutes

Halophile A microorganism which prefers high concentrations of salt in its growth medium

Hapten A compound that can stimulate an antibody response and act as a determinant group when combined with a large molecular carrier molecule

Heat sensitive Material which will be damaged or destroyed by heat

Heavy metal Any of a group of elements found in periods 4, 5, or 6 of the periodic table constituting groups 1 to 8

HeLa cell Tumor cells taken in 1953 from Helen Lane and maintained in in vitro cell culture

Helix A spiral structure

Hemagglutination A serologic procedure that uses the agglutination of red blood cells as an indicator for a positive test

Hemolysis Breaking of red blood cells

Hemorrhagic Lesions or conditions associated with bleeding. Hemorrhagic lesions are usually dark and may be internal or external

Herbivore A plant-eating organism

Heterotroph A system of nutrition that requires preformed organic molecules as a source of energy

Histamine A small molecule found in some tissue cells that, when released, acts to produce a number of immunologic phenomena. A substance that will promote shock

Host An individual serving as a source of food for a parasite

Host range The kinds of hosts which can be infected by a specific microorganism

Humoral Pertaining to body fluids

Hybridoma A clone of cells arising from an artificial combination of two cells into a single unit

Hydrophobic A compound that repels water

Hyperimmune sera Serum with a high antibody titer prepared by the repeated immunization of an animal

Hypersensitivity Being abnormally sensitive to antigens. Usually associated with allergic reactions to environmental antigens

Hypha A single filament of a fungal colony

Immune Possessing specific resistance to disease

Immunize To make immune, usually through the injection of antigen

Immunodiffusion A serologic procedure that determines the presence of either antigen or antibody by diffusing both materials through an agar or semisolid medium

Immunoglobulin Antibodies. Globulin proteins produced in response to an antigenic stimulus

Immunosuppressed A condition in which the normal immune response has been reduced or eliminated

Impetigo An infection of the skin characterized by a vesicular lesion that often breaks and crusts

Inanimate Objects which are not capable of self movement; usually, but not always, non-living

Inclusion body Bodies or structures of high density, often stainable, and microscopically visible that occur in the cytoplasm or nucleus of cells infected by an intracellular parasite

Infectious   A living agent capable of producing disease in a host

Inflammation   A localized tissue response to injury or infection, characterized by redness, swelling, and an accumulation of phagocytic cells (pus)

Initiation complex   An arrangement of the 30s ribosome and mRNA in a configuration such that the 50s ribosome can attach and make the synthesis of protein possible

Innate   Naturally occurring

Inoculation   Injection, often by needle, of material into a host. The process of placing bacteria on a culture medium

Interferon   Protein produced by virus-infected or polynucleotide-stimulated cells that can inhibit viral development in other cells

Intravenous   Located inside a blood vessel (vein)

In vitro   Outside the host, without life

In vivo   In life; specifically, inside a living host

Iodophore   A carrier molecule complexed with iodine and used as an antiseptic

Ionizing radiation   Radiation of sufficient energy to produce ionization of atoms when they are struck

Latent   A hidden infection. One that is not manifest

Ligature   A cord used to tie a vessel or tube

Lipid   A fat. A water-insoluble compound generally soluble in chloroform, ether, or alcohol

Lipopolysaccharide   A complex molecule containing both lipid and polysaccharide

Lipoprotein   A complex molecule composed of both lipid and protein

Lymph   A colorless, acellular fluid found in the vessels of the lymphatic system

Lymphatic   A vessel that carries lymph

Lymphocyte   A leukocyte with a large nucleus and small amount of cytoplasm, having a primary immunologic function

Lymphokine   Any of a number of peptides that are produced by T cells and affect the behavior of target cells, such as B cells or other T cells

Lysogenic   A bacterial cell which has the DNA of a bacteriophage integrated into its chromosome

Lysosome   A membrane-bound intracellular vacuole that is primarily filled with digestive and hydrolytic enzymes

Lysozyme   An enzyme found in tears and other body fluids that can hydrolyze bacterial cell walls

Macromolecule   A very large and often complex molecule. Usually associated with cell function and includes proteins, lipids, nucleic acids, and polysaccharides

Macrophage   A large mononuclear phagocytic cell associated primarily with the reticuloendothelial system

Malaise   The feeling of illness

Mantoux test   The intradermal injection of antigen used to measure hypersensitivity to the tubercle bacillus

Mating bridge   A bridge formed between the walls of two adjacent bacteria through which a chromosome may be transferred

Meningitis   An infection of the meninges surrounding the brain

Mesophile   A microorganism that grows best between 20 and 40°C

Mesosome   An invaginated and convoluted area of bacterial cell membrane that carries out functions similar to the mitochondria of higher cells

Metabolism   Chemical processes occurring within a cell

Metabolite   A product of intermediary metabolism

Microaerophilic   A microorganism that grows best at reduced oxygen concentrations

Monoclonal antibody   Antibody produced in vitro by a clone of antigen-stimulated B cells. Having a single determinant specificity

Monolayer   An in vitro cell culture forming a single cell layer on the surface of a container

Monomer   A small molecule that forms the basic subunit of a polymer

Mucosa   A mucous membrane

Mucus   A thick, viscous liquid secreted by cells of the mucosa

Mutagen   Any environmental influence which will increase the rate of mutation

Mutation   A random alteration in the genetic structure of a cell

Mycelium   The hyphal mat produced by growing mold (a mold colony)

Mycoses   A fungal infection

NAD (Nicotinamide adenine dinadeotide)   A coenzyme that acts to transfer hydrogen atoms

Necrosis   The death of cells due to injury or disease

Neutralization   A serological procedure used to detect the presence of antibody by inhibiting (neutralizing) growth of a pathogen

Neutrophile   A granulocyte that is heavily involved in the inflammatory response and a major component of pus

Nonsense codon   Codons which do not correlate with any amino acid. A nonsense codon occurs whenever a termination sequence occurs

Nosocomial   An illness that is acquired incident to hospitalization

Nucleotide   Compounds which contain one of several possible organic nitrogen atoms. The most common Nucleotide molecules include adenine, thymine, cytosine, guanine and uridine

Objective lens   The lens of a compound microscope that makes the first magnification of an object under observation

Ocular   The lens of a compound microscope nearest the eye of the viewer

Oncogenic   A tumor-inducing material

Opportunist   An organism of low virulence that depends on a reduction in normal host defenses in order to produce disease. Frequently an organism of normal flora

Organelle   A functional macromolecular structure that is subcellular but associated with a primary singular cellular activity

Organic   A molecule composed of one or more carbon atoms and one or more hydrogen atoms

Osmotic pressure   The pressure created across a semipermeable membrane by solvents containing differing concentrations of solute

Osteomyelitis   An infection of bone

Otitis   An infection of the ear. *O. media,* an infection of the inner ear

Oxidation   An increase in oxygen. The loss of a hydrogen atom (electron) from a molecule

Pandemic   An outbreak of infection involving more than one nation

Parasite   An organism that depends on some other organism to supply an essential nutrient. This relationship is gained at no expense to the parasite and no benefit to the host

Parenteral   The body spaces outside the intestine

Paroxysm   A spasmodic or sudden attack of symptoms

Pasteurize   A process of decontaminating liquids that uses heat at less than boiling temperatures. Most often used for milk

Pathogen   An organism that can cause a disease in its host

Pelvic inflammatory disease   A serious infection of the female involving the internal reproductive organs as well as peritoneal spaces

Penicillinase   An enzyme that will destroy the effectiveness of penicillin by breaking the beta lactam ring

Peptidoglycan   The rigid structural molecule of bacterial cell walls

Peptide bond   A covalent bond joining adjacent amino acids in a polypeptide

Peritoneal   Pertaining to the abdomen

Petri plate   A small circular dish with a close fitting lid used to cultivate microorganisms

Phage   Bacterial virus

Phage transformed cells   Cells which produce proteins such as diphtheria toxin under the direction of an integrated bacteriophage genome

Phagocyte   A cell that has the primary function of ingesting and destroying foreign matter found in the body

Phagosome   A membrane-bound vesicle containing material ingested by phagocytosis

Pharyngitis   An infection of the throat

Phenetic   A system of classification of organisms based on their visible features and their apparent ability to modify their environment

Phenol   A chemical material used as the basis of a number of disinfectants (C_6H_5OH)

Phenol coefficient   The ratio of effectiveness of a disinfectant when compared to that of phenol

Phenotype   The actual expression of the information present in the genome

Phosphorylation   The addition of phosphorus to a molecule. This process is usually accompanied by a transfer of a relatively large amount of energy

Photosynthetic   Organisms which are capable of using light to provide their requirement for energy

Pili   The same as fimbrae but also involved in bacterial conjugation with the exchange of DNA

Plasma   The liquid (noncellular) portion of the blood, primarily composed of water, proteins, and salts

Plasma cell   Lymphocytic cells that function to produce immunoglobulins

Plasmid   A dense, circular extrachromosomal DNA not essential to cell function, often found in those bacteria having antibiotic resistance

PMN   Polymorphonuclear leukocyte, a neutrophilic phagocyte

Pneumonia   An inflammation of the lungs resulting in an accumulation of exudate in the alveolar spaces

Polymer   A large molecule primarily composed of a number of similar subunit molecules

Popypeptide   A chain of amino acids, not as large as a protein

Polyribosome   (Polysome) A complex of ribosomes found on a single messenger RNA

Polysaccharide   A large, complex carbohydrate consisting of numerous smaller sugar monomers

Precipitin test   A serological reaction in which a soluble antigen combines with an antibody to produce a visible precipitation

Procaryotic   An organism with a rudimentary nucleus that lacks a membrane

Prophylaxis   Use of an antimicrobial to prevent infection from occurring

Prosthetic device   A man-made substitute for a failed body structure

Prostration   A loss of strength, exhaustion

Protein   A large polymer composed of amino acids

Protozoa   Microscopic, single-celled animals. Most are free living, but some are responsible for human disease

Pruritis   Itching due to irritation of sensory nerve endings

Psychrophile   An organism that grows best at temperatures less than 20°C

Pure culture   A culture containing only a single species of microorganism

Purulent   Pus forming or pus containing

Putrefaction   The decomposition (usually bacterial) of organic matter with an attendant foul aroma

Pyelonephritis An infection of the kidney

Pyoderma Infection of the skin by a pus producing (pyogenic) bacterium

Quellung The apparent increase in size of a bacterium caused by the interaction of the capsule with its specific antiserum

Radioactive A compound that emits subatomic particles in the very short wavelength regions of the electromagnetic spectrum

Receptor A chemical complex on the cell surface that is recognized by a corresponding chemical group, resulting in specific adherence between the two

Recombination The process by which DNA from one chromosome is integrated into the DNA of another chromosome

Refractive index A numerical value used to indicate the ability of a substance to transmit light

Replication The process of viral multiplication within a cell. The duplication of the DNA molecule

RES (Reticulo endothelial system) A system composed of phagocytic macrophages present in sinuses and reticulum of various organs and tissues, such as the lung, spleen, and bone marrow. Important in prevention of and recovery from infectious diseases

Resistant An organism that is not inhibited by an antimicrobial agent is said to be resistant

Respiration The process of obtaining nutrient energy by breaking down sugar compounds

Restriction endonuclease An endonuclease that hydrolyzes DNA at points of specific nucleotide sequences

Rheumatic fever A disease characterized by chorea, arthritis, and carditis resulting as a sequelae to streptococcal pharyngitis

Ribosome An RNA-protein particlelike structure that serves as the site for mRNA-tRNA interaction and protein synthesis

RODAC An acronym for replicate organism detection and counting (RODAC) plate—a petri dish with a raised agar surface for impression sampling of environmental surfaces or wounds

Salpingitis Infection of the fallopian tube

Sanitation The establishment of conditions that are favorable to health

Saphrophyte An organism that does not produce infectious disease

Secondary infection Infections which occur as a consequence of other disease processes in the host

Sensitize To develop specific antibody as the result of an antigenic stimulus

Sepsis A toxic, febrile condition associated with bacterial infection and characterized by bacteremia

Septum The divided membrane structure between two cellular or body cavities

Serology The study of serum. Usually associated with approaches to the diagnosis of present or past disease based on measurement of antibody content

Serotype A strain of bacteria with a unique antigen such that it induces antibody specific for that organism

Serum The liquid portion of blood remaining after the clotting proteins have been removed from plasma

Sexually transmitted disease (STD) Diseases normally transmitted by sexual intercourse

Shingles A severe vesicular eruption resulting from latent viral infection of dorsal root ganglia by the virus that causes chicken pox

Shock A condition manifested by a decreased blood pressure, circulatory insufficiency, and a weak pulse

Single-cell protein Protein used as a nutritional source derived from microorganisms

Sinus An anatomical space or cavity

Sinusoid Small open cavities through which body fluids travel

Slide A thin, rectangular piece of glass used to support material for microscopic examination

Spectrum The range of organisms inhibited by an antimicrobial agent

Spinal fluid A clear, waterlike fluid that bathes the brain and spinal cord

Spirillus Any of a number of bacteria that have a curved or spiral shape

Spontaneous generation The development of life from nonliving materials without the assistance of living life forms

Sporadic An infrequent or irregular occurrence of an event

Spore The asexual reproductive cells produced by fungi

Sporulation The process of spore formation

Sputum A collection of mucus, host and parasite cells coughed up from the lung in cases of pneumonia or bronchitis

Stain A solution of dye which can be used to color objects to improve their visibility

Stationary phase A culture in which the number of new cells is equal to the number which die

Sterile Without life or free from life

Streaking The process of inoculation of solid media by sweeping a wire loop through the inoculum and across the agar

Subclinical The occurrence of an infection wherein the symptoms of the disease are not manifest

Substrate The compound acted on by an enzyme, resulting in a product

Subtype A designation used to distinguish among members of a species which have one or more differentiating characteristics

Sulfonamide A sulfa drug. Antimicrobials containing the sulfanilamide group

Superinfection A second infection which develops in addition to a previous infection

Suppuration Pertaining to the production of pus

Svedberg A unit of sedimentation coefficient, equivalent to 10^{-13} seconds

Syndrome A number of symptoms occurring together that characterize a specific disease

Synergistic A condition where two organisms may be able to produce a host response greater than the added effects of both organisms if they were to act alone

Synovial fluid A thick, transparent fluid found in association with synovial membranes and often occupying bone joint spaces

Systemic Relating to the entire organism and not its separate parts

T-cell A thymus-derived lymphocyte primarily involved in cellular-type immunity

Taxonomy The organization or classification of objects into logical relationships

Temperate phage A bacterial virus that can become integrated into host cell DNA or replicate as a virulent virus

Termination sequence A sequence of three bases that does not code for an amino acid, but terminates the length of the mRNA molecule as it is formed on the DNA template

Thymus An endocrine gland located behind the breastbone near the throat

Tincture A mixture containing alcohol as a solvent

Titer The concentration of a substance in a solution as determined by measuring its presence in a series of increasing dilutions. The highest dilution containing the substance is the titer

Toxic Poisonous

Toxin A biologically produced poison

Toxoid A toxin that has been modified in order to reduce toxicity without altering antigenicity. Used as a vaccine

Trachea Windpipe

Transcription The transfer of genetic information from DNA to messenger RNA

Transduction The transfer of bacterial genetic information between bacteria by means of a bacterial virus

Transformation The nonmediated transfer of bacterial DNA between bacterial cells

Translation The transfer of genetic information from messenger RNA into a protein molecule

Translocation Movement of a ribosome along the mRNA such that the tRNA attached to the newly formed peptide chain is moved one codon away from its anti-codon

Transovarian passage The transmission of infectious agents to offspring through the ovary by infection of the egg cell

Trichous Hairlike

Triplet code A set of three nucleotide bases that code for one amino acid

Trophozoite An active, vegetative, form of a parasite as opposed to its cyst

Tubercle A firm granulomatous lesion resulting from an infection with *Mycobacterium tuberculosis*

Turbid Cloudy, a solution that is not clear

Ulcer An area of inflammation where the epithelial layer has been lost

Ultracentrifugation Centrifugation at very high speeds

Ultraviolet Area of the electromagnetic spectrum whose wavelength is between 4 and 400 nm

Urethritis Infection of the urethra

Vaccination The process of using a vaccine to immunize against disease

Vaccine An antigen used in the process of vaccination

Vector An insect, often an arthropod, that can transmit disease producing agents

Vehicle An object that can serve to transmit an infectious agent

Venereal Relating to or resulting from sexual intercourse

Viable Living or capable of being alive

Virion The complete viral particle, including both capsid and genome as well as envelope if present

Virulence Relating to the capacity of an organism to overcome host resistance factors

Vitamin An organic compound that is essential for health but that cannot be synthesized by the cells of the individual

Volutin A polyphosphate complex found in some bacterial cells that stains with analine dyes

Zoonosis Diseases of lower animals that can be transmitted to humans

INDEX

Rabies, 636
radioim munoassay, 236
recombinant DNA, 137
recombination, 129
Redi, Francesco, 10
reduction, 91
refractive index, 29
relapsing fever, 339
replication, 112
resolving power, 24
respiration, 97
respiratory syncytial virus, 613
restriction endonuclease, 137
reticuloendothelial system, 230
Retrovirus, 645
reverse transcriptase, 645
Reye's syndrome, 577
Rhabdovirus, 636
Rhinovirus, 627
ribonucleic acid (RNA):
    codon, 115
    messenger, 115
    ribosomal, 78, 85, 115
    terminator, 117
    transcription, 115
    transfer, 119
Rickettsia, 465
    prowazekii, 474
    rickettsii, 478
    typhi, 476
Rifampicin, 193
Rocky Mountain spotted fever, 473
RODAC, 40
Rous sarcoma, 553
rubella, 621

Salmonella, 412
    cholerae-suis, 417
    enteritidis, 471
    gastroenteritis, 417
    typhi, 415
saprophyte, 206
scalded skin syndrome, 283
scarlet fever, 295, 300
secondary immune response, 240
sedimentation constant, 79
selective toxicity, 181
Semmelweis, Ignas, 5
sensitivity, 338
septic arthritis, 284
serologic tests for syphilis, 337
serology, 257
Serratia marcescens, 430
sex pilus, 133
Shigella, 112

dysenteriae, 421
dysentery, 420
neurotoxin, 420
shigellosis, 422
shingles, 579
smallpox, 6, 565
Snow, John, 6
Spallanzani, Lazzaro, 10
specificity, 338
spheroplast, 72
spirilla, 66
spirochete, 329
spore, 82
Sporothrix schenckii, 505
sporozoa, 524
sporulation, 81
sputum, 308
Staphylococcus:
    aureus, 280, 288
    epidermidis, 281
    methicillin resistant, 287
    saprophyticus, 81
stem cell, 238
sterile, 145
sterilization, 164
Streptococcal disease:
    erysipelas, 296
    glomerulonephritis, 297
    impetigo, 296
    pneumonia, 304
    puerperal sepsis, 296
    pyoderma, 297
    rheumatic fever, 297
    scarlet fever, 295
streptococci:
    group A, 293
    group B, 301
    group D, 302
    viridans, 302
Streptococcus:
    M-protein, 293
    pneumoniae, 110, 293, 304
    pyogenes, 293
Streptomyces somaliensis, 400
sulfonamide, 182
sulfur granules, 399
superoxide, 161
superinfection, 200
suppuration, 282
synergy, 208
syphilis:
    congenital, 334
    latent, 334
    primary, 331
    secondary, 332
    tertiary, 334
systemic disease, 283

T-cell, 235, 646
taxonomy, 46
termination sequence, 118
tetanus, 345
thermophil, 160
thumine, 112
thymus, 226
tincture, 175
tinea, 502
titer, 257
Togavirus, 657
toxic shock syndrome, 276, 284
toxin, 52, 273
toxoid, 252
Toxoplasma gondii, 529
toxoplasmosis, 531
trachoma, 467
transduction, 129
transformation, 128
translation, 118
translocation, 121
transmission, 210
transovarian passage, 478
Treponema pallidum, 329
Trichomonas vaginalis, 521
triplet code, 117
trophozoite, 517
Trypanosoma, 523
tuberculosis:
    AIDS and, 390
    latent, 382
    miliary, 382
    PPD, 386
    reactivation, 383
    secondary, 383
    skin test, 386
    vaccine, 390
tularemia, 492
turbidity, 38
typhoid fever, 415
typhus:
    endemic, 476
    epidemic, 474

ultracentrifuge, 80
undulant fever, 486
Ureaplasma, 455

vaccination, 7
vaccine, 251
vancomycin, 195
varicella-zoster, 577
variola, 566
vector, 138
vehicle, 211